DATE DUE

DEMCO 38-297

D1293849

The
OMAHA SYSTEM

Applications for
Community Health Nursing

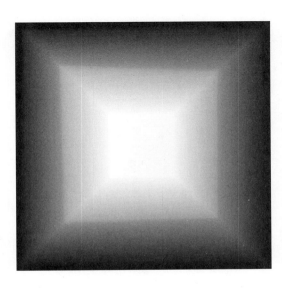

The
OMAHA SYSTEM
Applications for Community Health Nursing

KAREN S. MARTIN, RN, MSN, FAAN
Director of Research

NANCY J. SCHEET, RN, MSN
Director of Hospice and Special Programs

THE VISITING NURSE ASSOCIATION OF OMAHA

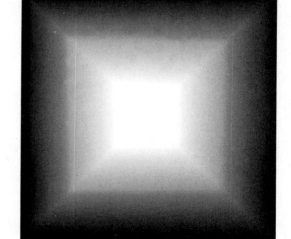

W.B. SAUNDERS COMPANY
A Division of Harcourt Brace & Company
Philadelphia London Toronto Montreal Sydney Tokyo

W.B. SAUNDERS COMPANY
A Division of
Harcourt Brace & Company

The Curtis Center
Independence Square West
Philadelphia, Pennsylvania 19106

Library of Congress Cataloging-in-Publication Data

Martin, Karen S.
    The Omaha system : applications for community health nursing
/ Karen S. Martin, Nancy J. Scheet.
        p. cm.
    ISBN 0-7216-6126-2
    1. Community health nursing.   I. Scheet, Nancy J.   II. Title.
    [DNLM: 1. Community Health Nursing—methods.   2. In-
formation Systems—organization & administration.   WY 106
M381o]
RT98.M276   1992
610.73′43—dc20
DNLM/DLC   91–18590

Editor: Ilze Rader

Developmental Editor: Miriam McCauley

Cover Designer: Ellen Bodner-Zanolle

Production Manager: Linda R. Garber

Manuscript Editors: Karen Okie and Tom Stringer

Illustration Coordinator: Peg Shaw

Indexer: Anne Cope

The Omaha System:
Applications for Community Health Nursing   ISBN 0-7216-6126-2

Printed in the United States of America.

Last digit is the print number: 9   8   7   6   5   4   3   2

To community health nurses everywhere:

May the tradition of strength, courage, and convictions established by community health nurses of the past guide us all today and in the future as we grow in numbers and power.

CONTRIBUTORS

Cathy Aden, RN, MSN
(Formerly) School Nurse, Visiting Nurse Association of Omaha, Omaha, Nebraska
Contributed to Chapter 11

Virginia Aita, RN, MSN
Instructor, Bishop Clarkson College of Nursing, Omaha, Nebraska
Contributed to Chapter 13

Shirley Alcoe, BA, RN, BEd, MA, MEd, EdD
Professor, Faculty of Nursing, University of New Brunswick, Fredericton, New Brunswick, Canada
Contributed to Chapter 13

Pamela Bataillon, RN, MSN
Director of Clinical Services, Visiting Nurse Association of Omaha, Omaha, Nebraska
Contributed to Chapter 12

Anne Becker, RN, BSN
Coordinator of Quality Assurance and Allied Health, Visiting Nurse Association, Inc., Trenton, New Jersey
Contributed to Chapter 2

Kay Bennett, RN, BSN
Student Learning Center Coordinator, Visiting Nurse Association of Omaha, Omaha, Nebraska
Contributed to Chapter 13

Kathleen Blomquist, RN, PhD
Assistant Professor and Contract Researcher/Evaluator, University of Kentucky College of Nursing, Lexington, Kentucky
Contributed to Chapter 12

Paula Cell, RN, MPH
Administrator, Visiting Nurse Association, Inc., Trenton, New Jersey
Contributed to Chapter 2

Elizabeth Cernech, RN, BA
Supervisor of School Health Program, Visiting Nurse Association of Omaha, Omaha, Nebraska
Contributed to Chapter 11

Suzanne Clarke, RN, BSN
Assistant Director, The Block Nurse Program, Inc., St. Paul, Minnesota
Contributed to Chapter 12

Jean Denton, RN, MA
Director of Health Ministries, St. Paul's Episcopal Church, Indianapolis, Indiana
Contributed to Chapter 12

Mary Dooling, RN, MSN
Instructor, University of Missouri–St. Louis School of Nursing, St. Louis, Missouri
Contributed to Chapter 13

Theresa DuPuis, RN, MPH, MBA
Director, Bureau of Nursing, State of Delaware, Department of Health and Social Services, Dover, Delaware
Contributed to Chapter 9

Esther Dworak, RN, MSN
Director of School Health Program, Visiting Nurse Association of Omaha, Omaha, Nebraska
Contributed to Chapter 11

Barbara Friedbacher, RN, MS
Nursing Center Program Manager, University of Wisconsin–Milwaukee Nursing Center, Milwaukee, Wisconsin
Contributed to Chapter 15

Valerie Gilbey, BN, RN, BEd, MSc
Associate Professor, Faculty of Nursing, University of New Brunswick, Fredericton, New Brunswick, Canada
Contributed to Chapter 13

Joan Goldsberry, RN

Director, Home Health, Spaulding Rehabilitation Hospital, Boston, Massachusetts
Contributed to Chapter 10

Marjorie Jamieson, RN, MS

Executive Director, The Block Nurse Program, Inc., St. Paul, Minnesota
Contributed to Chapter 12

Carolyn Jorgensen, RN, BSN

Intake Supervisor, Visiting Nurse Association of Omaha, Omaha, Nebraska
Contributed to Chapter 14

Margie Knappenberger, RN, MSN

Clinical Nurse Specialist, Corrections, Visiting Nurse Association of Omaha, Omaha, Nebraska
Contributed to Chapter 12

Prudence Kobasa, RN, MSN

(Formerly) Assistant Director, Bureau of Nursing, State of Delaware, Department of Health and Social Services, Dover, Delaware
Contributed to Chapter 9

Nancy Kreuser, RN, MS

Nursing Center Program Manager, University of Wisconsin–Milwaukee Nursing Center, Milwaukee, Wisconsin
Contributed to Chapter 15

Mary Jule Kulka, RN, MS

Clinical Services Director, Nursing Assessment Referral Network, Illinois Migrant Council, Aurora, Illinois
Contributed to Chapter 12

Norma Lang, RN, PhD, FAAN

Dean and Professor, University of Wisconsin–Milwaukee, School of Nursing, Milwaukee, Wisconsin
Contributed to Chapter 14

Beverly Larson, RN, MPH

Director, Polk County Public Health Nursing Service, Balsam Lake, Wisconsin
Contributed to Chapter 9

Sally Lundeen, RN, PhD

Nursing Center Director, University of Wisconsin–Milwaukee Nursing Center, Milwaukee, Wisconsin
Contributed to Chapter 15

Karen Marek, RN, MSN

Project Assistant/Doctoral Candidate, University of Wisconsin–Milwaukee, School of Nursing, Milwaukee, Wisconsin
Contributed to Chapter 14

Adrienne Massel, RN, MSN

Public Health Nurse, Beloit Health Department, Beloit, Wisconsin
Contributed to Chapter 12

Marilyn Maud, BSN, MHEd

Community Health Nursing Consultant, State Health Office, Florida Department of Health and Rehabilitative Services, Tallahassee, Florida
Contributed to Chapter 8

Kathleen McLaughlin, RN, MPH, CDE

Consultant, Health Education, Sparta, New Jersey
Contributed to Chapter 10

Christine Merritt, RN, MS, MPH

(Formerly) Assistant Professor, University of Nebraska Medical Center College of Nursing, Omaha, Nebraska
Contributed to Chapter 13

Helen North, RN, BSN

Public Health Nurse Consultant, Wisconsin Division of Health, Department of Health and Social Services, Milwaukee, Wisconsin
Contributed to Chapter 2

Sharon Rolph, RN, BSN, MPA

Director of Public Health Nursing, Yolo County Public Health Department, Woodland, California
Contributed to Chapter 9

Mary Jane Running, BSN, MPH, CNAA

Senior Executive Community Health Nursing Director, State Health Office, Florida Department of Health and Rehabilitative Services, Tallahassee, Florida
Contributed to Chapter 8

Gail Scoates, RN, MS

Director of Professional Practice, Visiting Nurse Association of Omaha, Omaha, Nebraska
Contributed to Chapter 14

Rose Marie Serra, RN, BSN

Assistant Director/Director of Clinical Services, Visiting Nurse Services, Des Moines, Iowa
Contributed to Chapter 10

Marcia Stanhope, RN, DSN, FAAN

Professor and Principal Investigator, University of Kentucky College of Nursing, Lexington, Kentucky
Contributed to Chapter 12

Sandra Warner, RN, PhD

Associate Professor, University of Texas Health Science Center at San Antonio, San Antonio, Texas
Contributed to Chapter 12

JoAnn Weidmann, RN, BSN

Director of Public Health Nurses, Waukesha County Health Department, Waukesha, Wisconsin
Contributed to Chapter 2

Bridget Young, RN, BSN

Client Service Manager, Visiting Nurse Association of Omaha, Omaha, Nebraska
Contributed to Chapter 14

Rita Zielstorff, RN, MS

Assistant Director, Laboratory of Computer Science, Massachusetts General Hospital, Boston, Massachusetts
Contributed to Chapters 8, 12

FOREWORD

I am convinced that contributions to community health nursing that are of any substance emanate from, are developed, and then are nurtured by those individuals who practice that fine art. So it has been and continues to be with "The Omaha System." In 1972, the Record Committee of the Council of Home Health Agencies and Community Health Services of the National League for Nursing began one of the first intensive studies of the documentation processes for community health nursing. Input from staff throughout all National League for Nursing member agencies called for a systematic and universal approach for patient records. Concomitantly, nursing seized upon the Weed approach to the problem-oriented system as a means to utilize the nursing process. Such efforts resulted in the first research contract the VNA secured to develop the classification system. This book is the culmination of 15 years of research, development, testing, refinement, and utilization. More importantly, it reflects the commitment and efforts of thousands of practitioners — all seeking the best methodology to ensure exemplary practice. To those practitioners who care so deeply, this book is dedicated.

DeLanne A. Simmons, RN, MPH
President/CEO, The Visiting Nurse
Association of Omaha

PREFACE

This book was written to celebrate the past, present, and future of community health nursing. Although our specialty faces many challenges, we are optimistic for both clients and practitioners. Community health practitioners may be direct delivery staff, supervisors, administrators, students, and faculty members. Regardless of the practitioners' roles and responsibilities, the use of effective tools increases their contributions to health services at the local, state, and national levels. This book was written to share the Omaha System, a systematic clinical- and research-based tool that can be used to meet the increasing complexities and growth opportunities within community health nursing. Use of the System can increase accountability of nurses and improve the quality of community health nursing practice, documentation, and data management in diverse settings. As use of the Omaha System increases continuity and consistency of communication and service, we anticipate that enhanced client outcomes will follow.

The chapters of this book are organized to be user-friendly. Readers may choose to read the book in its entirety or may select only those chapters specific to their interests and needs. Readers may duplicate materials and forms from the VNA of Omaha and other sources for immediate use or adapt materials to meet their own, client, staff, and program requirements.

Chapters 1, 2, 3, and 4 highlight historical, conceptual, and research linkages to the Omaha System. Chapters 5, 6, and 7 include a systematic description of the organization, terms, and definitions of the three components of the Omaha System. These components are the Problem Classification Scheme, Intervention Scheme, and Problem Rating Scale for Outcomes. Chapter 8 consists of practical, specific suggestions for implementing the Omaha System successfully. Chapters 9 through 12 are designed to illustrate direct application of the Omaha System by community health nurses and members of other disciplines who practice in diverse settings. Chapter 13 is intended for use by students, faculty members, and agency personnel involved in nursing education. The focus of Chapter 14 is quality assurance activities related to the Omaha System. Chapter 15 includes a synthesis of current and future issues related to community health nursing practice, documentation, and research and a summary of potential benefits of the Omaha System use. All chapters of this book were designed to provide comprehensive information and materials specific to community health practice, documentation, and data management. Additional materials such as blank record forms and instructions for completing documentation are located in the Appendix. Because the forms in the chapters and Appendix were developed for diverse purposes, the language and style are not always consistent. Glossaries of general and Omaha System–specific terms follow the Appendix. Readers are encouraged to familiarize themselves with the glossaries before beginning the book.

Some readers and users of the Omaha System will find a different version of this book beneficial, especially those who are primarily concerned about how to use the System. They may have less interest in the benefits of using the Omaha System, the steps of the implementation process, case studies with diverse forms amenable to the Omaha System, or the possibilities for computerization. Therefore, a companion, small handbook has been developed. *The Omaha System: A Pocket Guide for Community Health Nursing* includes a brief description of the Problem Classification Scheme, Problem Rating Scale for Outcomes, and Intervention Scheme. Examples, adapted from actual client data, are organized in an outline format for each of the three components of the Omaha System. These examples and care planning guidelines are the primary focus of the pocketbook.

The production of this book was truly a team effort. The number of individuals and groups who reviewed the manuscript and who gave materials, expertise, and support to the effort was astounding. Included were staff members, supervisors, and administrators from the VNA of Omaha and many other agencies/institutions and colleges of nursing. Some are identified by name in the book; others remain anonymous. We are indebted to all, including reviewers Kathy Kelly and Mary Hardy from the University of Iowa, Nancy Kuzmich from Naperville Good Samaritan Medical Center (IL), Patricia Mahovich from the Visiting Nurse Service of Akron (OH), and Valerie Swigart Courchene from the University of Pittsburgh (PA). We are especially indebted to Delanne Simmons, visionary leader, and Ruth Pieken, secretary extraordinaire.

KAREN MARTIN
NANCY SCHEET

CONTENTS

SECTION III
USING THE OMAHA SYSTEM

SECTION IV
LOOKING AHEAD

APPENDIX

LOCATION OF FORMS

PROBLEMS/RATINGS/PLANS FORMS

VISIT REPORTS

Skilled Visit Report

Long Term Care Visit Report

Family Visit Report

Public Health Nurse Record of Service

Student Health Record

Health Maintenance Center Record
Problems/Plans/Ratings/Progress

Home Health Aide Progress Note

Health Ministries Project Clinical Record

Law Enforcement Center Progress Notes

Migrant Health Project Individual Health Care Plan

Interim Notes

DISCHARGE SUMMARIES

Discharge Summary

Dismissal/Transfer Summary

The authors and the publisher gratefully acknowledge the following organizations for allowing them to adapt agency forms for use in the Appendix:

Polk County (WI) Public Health Nursing Service,
        Forms 15 and 16
Midland County (MI) Health Department, Form 20

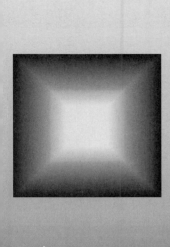

SECTION I

LINKING HISTORY, THEORY, RESEARCH, AND THE OMAHA SYSTEM

CHAPTER ONE

*P*ublic health nursing in the latter 20th century must adapt itself to a different world — to automatization, to rapid cultural change, to the stresses of cold war, to family mobility and suburbanization. It must take advantage of the benefits of fabulously rapid scientific discovery in the midst of a new appreciation of the practical as well as ethical values of the old-fashioned virtues of love and family solidarity and self-determination. (Freeman, 1957, p. 3)

A single word — explosive — describes the changes in today's community health industry and its agencies (Martin, 1988). Community health nurses face challenges and opportunities unlike any other period in history. The number of clients and complexity of needs are increasing, as are the number and types of community health staff members, agency programs, and methods of operation. Concomitantly, consumer demands for comprehensive, economical services are increasing as the availability of prepared staff and reimbursement is decreasing. These trends are expected to continue, or even escalate, with the advent of the twenty-first century.

More than 11%, or 188,000, of US nurses are currently employed in community health settings. Such settings include home care agencies, school systems, industry and alternative delivery systems, and official public health agencies. Table 1 – 1 shows the estimated numbers of nurses employed in each setting and their educational preparation.

The explosive, changing nature of community health care provided the stimulus for the development of the Omaha System. Nursing supervisor Joyce Sandin, Visiting Nurse Association (VNA) of Omaha, is credited with initiating action concerning the agency's client record and the manner in which staff nurses used that record early in the 1970s. As she communicated with others throughout the agency, it became apparent that her concerns about documentation were related to other complex emerging issues. These included the changing clinical practice of community health nurses, the value of automated management information systems, and alterations in the entire health care delivery system. Medicare and Medicaid, enacted through federal legislation in 1965, were affecting community health agency referral, service, dismissal, and reimbursement processes more than any other previous legislation.

The VNA narrative-type client record was not desirable in 1970 and was expected to become less desirable.

Agency staff, supervisors, and administrators recognized that:

- Nurses were spending too much time documenting care in a lengthy, even rambling, manner
- Primary nurses and supervisors were not able to evaluate client progress by reviewing records
- Health care professionals were not reading extensive entries written by their peers and had difficulty interpreting narrative recording
- Supervisors and administrators could not obtain aggregate clinical data to produce meaningful information about services or future trends

The impetus provided by Sandin and agency director DeLanne Simmons enabled VNA of Omaha personnel to embark on a long-term project. The purposes of the project were to improve the clinical practice and documentation of community health staff and to initiate plans for an automated management information system.

This book delineates 20 years of effort, four research projects, and 10 years of federal funding that have resulted in national recognition for VNA of Omaha staff, supervisors, and administrators. The evolution of the Omaha System, the System components, varied examples of application, and reactions of diverse users are described throughout these chapters. This book is designed to convey three additional themes: first, the autonomy of community health nursing practice; second, the merits of a holistic, nurse-client focused documentation and data management system; third, the linkages between the Omaha System and the entire health care industry.

HISTORICAL PERSPECTIVES

The Omaha System emerged because of events in society, health care, and nursing that occurred through-

Community Health Nursing and the Omaha System:
Past and Present

out the centuries. The development of the Omaha System was possible because of:

- Accomplishments of nursing and public health pioneers
- Traditions established within community health nursing
- Evolution of the scientific method, research projects, and quality assurance concepts
- Interest in the diagnostic process, nomenclature, and classification systems
- Advent of automated community health management information systems

A review of history in health care literature offers a bridge for today's administrator, nurse, and student as they acquire an understanding of and perspective about current health care issues. A historic bridge is useful not only to avoid repeating mistakes of the past, but also to enhance professionalism and convey inspiration and pride in the accomplishments of other nurses. A study of history provides insight into the development of nursing in general as it evolved from an avocation to a vocation to an occupation to an emerging profession.

Nursing Heritage

Nursing is the oldest of arts and the youngest of professions. It is compassion personified. Nursing has a long and rich international heritage, filled with colorful events and people. Nurses, with their unique, divergent opinions and talents, have made many valuable individual and collective contributions to society. Not infrequently, nurses have faced opposition and criticism. Thus, the heritage of nursing includes successes, advances, and unity as well as failures, regression, and conflicts. Most contemporary practice and professional concerns are not unique to the current era. Whereas the influence of Florence Nightingale should

not be understated, the art and science of nursing began long before her birth. Likewise, nurses practiced community health nursing for centuries before the advent of Medicare and diagnosis related groups (DRGs).

Nursing has not always progressed with steady, forward motion. Often crises such as wars, natural disasters, and personal circumstances forced nurses to take actions that accelerated general advances and reforms. Many courageous, dynamic nursing leaders have emerged during times of crisis. Strangely, some of the profession's most notable achievements were associated with the violence of war because of the increase in nurses' visibility and value. During other periods, changes in society led to regression in nursing practice. A review of historic nursing literature reveals significant linkages between societal events, the development of nursing, and the status of nurses. The cycles of political, economic, environmental, religious, and technologic constraints and advances throughout the world have profoundly affected nursing practice, education, and research.

Origins of Nursing

Evidence of nursing care precedes recorded history. The first human nurse was probably a mother caring for her children. In most ancient cultures, the wise women of the tribes served as nurses. The social status of females, and therefore nurses, was usually below that of males.

It is not known when formal home visitation to the sick began. By 1300 BC, ancient Hebrew nurses were part of carefully planned, family-centered programs that were based on principles of prevention and treatment. In accordance with the health code of Moses, Hebrew nurses provided physical and spiritual care to the sick and their families. Deborah is the first nurse recorded in history, as noted in Genesis, Chapter 24.

Phoebe of Cenchrea (60 AD) is the first visiting nurse identified by name. Like the Roman matrons who fol-

TABLE 1-1 ■ Employment Sites and Education Levels of Community Health Nurses: 1988

EMPLOYER	NUMBER OF COMMUNITY HEALTH NURSES	PERCENT PREPARED AT OR ABOVE BSN LEVEL
Home care agencies	54,000	44
School systems	48,000	
Industry/emerging systems	46,000	41
Official public health agencies	40,000	55
Total	188,000	

Data from Moses (1990).

lowed her, she was from a wealthy, powerful family. Flaccilla (352–385 AD), daughter of the King of Spain, was the first volunteer visiting nurse. She devoted her life to the poor, making daily visits to the sick and continuing her royal responsibilities. During this era, the earliest hospitals began when bishops and powerful Roman noble matrons opened their homes to the sick. One of these matrons, Fabiola, is credited with making nursing a vocation.

As monasteries, convents, and military nursing orders thrived during the first century, so did nursing. Nursing developed roots, purpose, direction, and leadership (Dolan, Fitzpatrick, & Herrmann, 1983). Periodically, women's religious privileges, education, and responsibilities were curtailed by male priests who preferred to limit the rights of women and the freedoms of the early church. Freedom to visit homes and provide care outside the convents also varied over time. Three hospitals constructed as almshouses in France and Italy still stand today. Wayward women and widows were often recruited as nurses.

Reformation and Renaissance

Protestant groups began to flourish during the Reformation of the 1500s. In countries where Protestant leaders established control, Catholic monasteries were suppressed and health care deteriorated markedly. The quality of medical care was better within some societies, particularly among those of the Moslems and southern Europeans.

A significant societal change occurred at the beginning of the 1600s. There emerged a new social consciousness and feeling of responsibility for the welfare of the sick and the poor for their own sake, distinct from the personal benefit of providing service. The first Poor Law, enacted in England in 1601, imposed a compulsory tax on all citizens.

The change in societal values also stimulated community health nursing, especially in France. About 1610, Madame de Chantal and Francis de Sâles organized the Order of the Virgin Mary, a group of women free to visit the homes of the sick without restriction. The Order existed for only 4 years; the Catholic church opposed the unconventional idea of freedom outside the walls of a monastery. This group, more like a modern visiting nurse association than any previous organization, became a model for others to follow.

St. Vincent de Paul has been credited with introducing the modern principles of visiting nursing and social service. In 1617, he founded an order that later became the Sisters of Charity. Like Madame de Chantal and Francis de Sâles, he was determined that his visiting nurses not take solemn vows, remain within the confines of a monastery, devote extensive hours to religious exercises, or be completely subordinate to the clergy. As the nurses made visits, he wanted them to encourage families to help themselves.

French explorers and priests traveled to North America in 1605, establishing their first settlement in Nova Scotia. Three sisters from the Order of St. Augustine established the Hôtel Dieu in Quebec in 1639. Jeanne Mance, a lay nurse, provided nursing care at a Montreal fort and founded the Hôtel Dieu in Montreal in 1644.

Eighteenth and Nineteenth Centuries

Innovation and change were particularly difficult during this era because of social revolts and economic crises. Some leaders emerged, however, to make important contributions to the advancement of medical classification, contributions that made contemporary taxonomies possible. The first known attempt, the London Bills of Mortality, was mandated by the king of England. Using quantitative methods, John Graunt analyzed the mortality rate for children under 6 years and, in 1700, published a listing of causes of death. He is credited with founding the science of biostatistics and epidemiology. Between 1735 and 1763, Carl von Linné (Linnaeus) originated binomial nomenclature for scientific classification as he wrote concise descriptions for plants, animals, and minerals (Garrison, 1929). Jacques Bertillon of Paris classified causes of death and is credited with originating the International Classification of Diseases, Adapted (ICDA). This standard nomenclature was first adopted for statistical use in 1893 and 1900.

The home continued to be the usual setting for the provision of health care. Few advances occurred in hospitals. Reformers used terms such as "squalid," "inhuman," and "appalling" to describe hospital conditions. Few women resembling the Roman matrons were interested in nursing. Among the leaders who made significant contributions to nursing were Elizabeth Gurney Fry and the Fliedners. Fry initiated prison reforms, persuading others to provide health care to prisoners and their families. Theodor Fliedner, a Lutheran minister in Kaiserwerth, Germany, and his parishioners revived the ancient order of deaconesses. In 1836, Theodor and Frederike Fliedner founded the Kaiserwerth Institute for the Training of Deaconesses. Students, especially those assigned to district nursing, were encouraged to use a problem-solving approach during classroom instruction and when providing care. Despite the leadership of Elizabeth Fry in England and the Fliedners in Germany, medical and nursing practice continued to deteriorate.

Florence Nightingale

Florence Nightingale has been called a genius and the founder of secular, modern nursing. During the Crimean War of 1854, she became the Superintendent of the Female Nursing Establishment of the English General Hospitals in Turkey. Upon arrival at Scutari, she and her staff of 39 nurses faced the nearly insurmountable tasks of setting up a hospital, overcoming opposition of male army officers including physicians, and contending with the political turmoil in England. Nightingale described the situation as calamity unparalleled (Dolan, Fitzpatrick, & Herrmann, 1983). Within 2 months, she had used her administrative skills and demands for complete authority to transform the hospital into an efficient institution.

The remarkable, radical achievements of Florence Nightingale only continued after Scutari. These achievements were even more noteworthy because Nightingale and her nurses "violated the gender norms of the day and threatened male power" (Bullough, 1990, p. 6). Nightingale wrote clearly and extensively, establishing principles and standards of sound nursing care as well as instruction, supervision, and control of nursing by nurses. She described important concepts such as primary prevention, health maintenance, sick-nursing, and health-nursing; she repeatedly noted nurses' professional responsibility and the resulting economic benefits of depauperizing the poor. Florence Nightingale influenced nursing education markedly beginning the Nightingale system with the Training School at London's St. Thomas' Hospital in 1860. Similar to the Fliedners' program, nursing education there included classroom instruction, hospital experience, and home visits for sickness care and health education.

Nightingale consistently used the scientific method; she originated interest in the nursing process. Her own practice, administration, and writing consistently reflected assessment, intervention, and evaluation. Because of her background in science and mathematics, she had the tools to gather data systematically and document evidence graphically for herself and others. She used and advanced theory, research, and the sciences of statistics and epidemiology.

William Rathbone

William Rathbone founded the first public health nursing association in 1859. Under his direction, nursing services were provided to the rich in their homes only after the poor and those who came to the Royal Liverpool Infirmary (England) were treated. By 1863, 18 nurses were employed in Rathbone's Community Nursing Association. He required that nurses be trained as social reformers as well as attendants for the sick; they could not dispense material relief or interfere with religious views of their patients. This philosophy was radical for the era.

Colonial America

Nursing developed more slowly in the US than it did in Europe. Because educated nurses were members of religious and nursing orders, they were not included among the early Protestant colonists. Families were expected to care for their own members; their religious beliefs did not encourage social welfare concerns. Clergymen, often the most highly educated members of the community, became self-taught physicians.

The first US hospitals, founded in the 1730s, were established as poorhouses and insane asylums with care and conditions that matched or exceeded the neglect, cruelty, and filth that existed in any of England's almshouses. Hospital nurses were described as far superior to their counterparts in the poorhouses. However, nursing services at most hospitals were disorganized, and no systematic nursing education program existed in this country until a training school was established at the New England Hospital for Women and Children of Boston in 1872. Prior to that program and the beginning of medical schools, nurses and physicians were educated in Europe or received training by apprenticeship. Often, patients who received no medical care or the care of community health nurses were more likely to recover than those who were treated by physicians or admitted to hospitals.

Organizing Community Health Nursing

North American community health nursing services were first organized in Canada. In 1738, Madame d'Youville founded the Grey Nuns, a group of Quebec women who provided home nursing services. Early dispensary services in the US colonies were initiated by the Quakers of Philadelphia in 1786. Dispensaries based on the Philadelphia model were opened in New York in 1791 and in Boston in 1796. The dispensaries flourished until hospital care improved and became more accessible.

Several small home visit programs were organized in this country at the beginning of the nineteenth century. In 1797, Elizabeth Seton and other society matrons established the Widow's Society in New York. Because these matrons raised money for poor widows and made home visits, the Society was described as the Protestant equivalent of St. Vincent de Paul's Ladies of Charity. When Catherine Spalding established the Sisters of Charity of Nazareth, Kentucky, in 1812, nurses rode on horseback to visit the sick in their homes. In addition to providing sickness care, members of other religious nursing orders cared for unwed mothers, the mentally ill, victims of epidemics, and the sick in hospitals.

Post-Revolutionary and Civil War Era

The status of women diminished during the years that followed the Revolutionary War. Men were becoming midwives or obstetricians, a role previously held only by women. Male physicians were primarily responsible for excluding females from medical education and practice. In the mid-nineteenth century, Susan B. Anthony and others began to oppose the values of the Victorian society and to fight for women's rights, including the right for entry into colleges and the professions such as medicine. Although Elizabeth Blackwell established a milestone when she was admitted to medical school in 1847, she faced much criticism and opposition while in school, which continued as she attempted to establish a practice (Bullough, 1990).

Nursing care for injured and sick soldiers at the beginning of the Civil War was provided by the few existing religious orders. Because nurses were needed desperately for both Confederate and Union soldiers, many wealthy or politically active women volunteered. They became powerful, visible nursing leaders during and after the war and advanced the profession.

Environmental Health

Throughout the centuries, environmental health issues have received little public attention. The Romans are remembered for their exceptional concern about public health and their engineering skills during the first 5 centuries AD. They built drains, aqueducts, central heating systems, and proper cemeteries; they drained marshes in order to advance sanitation and decrease infection. Societies that followed the Romans did not continue their practices. Major epidemics and high mortality were frequent, especially in heavily populated areas.

Concern about environmental health issues increased in England and the US in the nineteenth century. Chadwick, the pioneer of modern public health, wrote an influential 1842 publication about the deplorable sanitary conditions of the English laboring classes. The first US health department, the Massachusetts State Board of Health, was established in 1869. Environmental concerns resulted in the organization of the American Public Health Association in 1872 and the beginning of the modern public health era.

Problems developed early in New York City because of the size and population density of the urban area. In 1796, ordinances were finally established regarding garbage disposal. The ordinances did little, however, to decrease extensive public health problems, especially among the poor. Finally, in 1866 a Board of Health was established. It enforced actions that were credited with reducing epidemics. Although Board physicians went to the tenements to care for sick children and to provide infant care instruction, no nurses were involved. After 2 months, the urgent need for nurses was recognized and they were permitted to make visits.

Early Nursing Education

Various individuals and groups attempted to develop nursing education programs soon after the first medical programs were established. Valentine Seaman, a New York physician, developed a nursing program in 1798 for 24 students.

By the time of the Civil War, about 68 hospitals existed, which were staffed by one or more nurses. The serious medical and nursing needs of soldiers and their families during that war aroused public interest and resulted in expanded nursing education and improved medical education.

Members of the American Medical Association (AMA) discussed the value and independence of nursing in 1869; they resolved to encourage the establishment of nursing education programs and associations. By 1872, the number of hospitals rose to 178, increasing the demand for nurses. That year, two physicians, Marie Zakrzewska and Susan Dimock, established a training school for nurses at the New England Hospital for Women and Children in Boston. Linda Richards graduated in 1873, received a certificate, and became the first American trained nurse.

All of the early nursing schools had problems and opponents. Directors had difficulty convincing applicants who were 25 to 35 years of age that they needed to devote 1 year to an educational program, often followed by 6 months to 2 years of service to a hospital. Many students left, exhausted due to the long hours and hard work; others were dismissed for anything less than total obedience. Power struggles between nursing and medicine were frequent; the tradition of medical control over nursing education and practice was well established. The question of priorities, whether students were to provide nursing service or to receive education, frequently arose. Even the term "trained nurse" was controversial. As the number of graduates increased, more were employed as private duty nurses in homes where conditions, including independence in nursing practice, were usually better. Although problems and opposition continued, schools of nursing increased; more than 200 existed at the end of the century.

The New Century and Community Health Nursing

Spectacular advances in community nursing occurred late in the nineteenth century and early in the twentieth. During this era, the specialty became one of three recognized divisions of nursing; hospital nursing and private duty were the other two. The emergence of community health nursing as a specialty was linked to a population explosion, social and environmental crises, and a renewal of humanitarianism. A sense of community responsibility grew with the proliferation of volunteers and voluntary agencies.

The role of nurses in the community became firmly established when the Women's Board of the New York City Mission and Tract Society organized home visiting by Bellevue graduates in 1877. The first nurse employed was Francis Root. Another employee was Lavinia Dock, who previously worked as a visiting nurse in Connecticut; more of her extensive contributions to nursing will be described later. Root, Dock, and other nurses visited the sick poor while providing nursing care and religious instruction.

Autonomous nursing associations that offered similar home visit programs were organized, especially during the late 1800s. Historians disagree about the names and founding dates of early agencies because few records were kept and definitions varied markedly. The staff of early organizations, now known as visiting nurse associations, were frequently referred to as district or instructive nurses, based on Rathbone's model, which emphasized client education (Gardner, 1917). In Canada, the English influence resulted in the formation of the Victorian Order of Nurses and a national organization of voluntary agencies.

Lillian Wald

Lillian Wald brought vision, skill, and determination to the evolving specialty of community health nursing, just as Florence Nightingale had done for nursing in general. She described the poverty, illness, and filthy living conditions as a baptism of fire that provided the stimulus for Lillian and her classmate Mary Brewster to live in a tenement. In 1893, they established the Henry Street Settlement as an experiment in public health nursing.

Collaboration between the Henry Street staff and the New York City Mission home visit staff followed, and it resulted in formation of the New York Visiting Nurse Service. Staff were concerned about acute and chronic health problems of all ages, nutrition, prostitution, public parks, public education for children, school nursing, unemployment, and unfair labor practices, especially for women and children.

The practice of Wald and her staff represented a major advance in nursing autonomy and authority. Sound nursing judgment was essential as staff offered comprehensive preventive, curative, and social services. Families were referred to physicians as appropriate, and staff accepted referrals from physicians. Services were available to all, regardless of ability to pay. Lillian Wald sought and received financial support for the agency from wealthy persons in the community. To ensure adequate educational preparation of community health nurses, Wald and the faculty of Teacher's College, Columbia University, offered public health classes beginning in 1902.

Lillian Wald's commitment to a community-based reform was equivalent to a crusade. During her 40-year tenure at Henry Street, Wald convinced physicians, politicians, and community leaders to support her efforts. Her vision of public health nursing services was not limited to the poor; she viewed the entire community as the client. She established the first school nursing program in 1902, initiated school lunches in 1905, and contracted with Metropolitan Life Insurance Company for nursing services in 1909. Wald encouraged enactment of labor codes and founded the Rural Nursing Service of the American Red Cross in 1912. She proposed the idea of a federal Childrens' Bureau that was established within the US Department of Commerce and Labor in 1912.

Early Community Health Nursing Leaders

Mary Adelaide Nutting and Lavinia Dock made many important contributions to nursing in general and community health nursing in particular. They coauthored the first history of nursing. Dock is remembered as a radical feminist who picketed, paraded, and protested, and as a community health nursing leader who worked with Lillian Wald at the Henry Street Settlement (Christy, 1969). Nutting is credited with initiating the transition from apprenticeship training to education of nurses as she followed the philosophy of her mentor, Isabel Hampton Robb.

In the community health tradition established by Lillian Wald and Lavinia Dock, Margaret Higgins Sanger became a nurse, developed a profound concern for the poor, and became a social activist. She began her career as a public health nurse in New York City and observed that unplanned pregnancy was a major problem associated with poverty. Reliable contraceptive information and skilled practitioners were available only to affluent and literate women; poor women resorted to dangerous or lethal methods to terminate pregnancy. Sanger went to France, studying and preparing to open the first birth control clinic in Brooklyn. One hundred fifty women came to the clinic on the first day in 1916. After 1 week, she was arrested and sentenced to 30 days in the workhouse.

Margaret Sanger continued her crusade for women's rights and free dissemination of contraceptive information. She founded several organizations, one of which eventually became the Planned Parenthood Federation. On behalf of women, Margaret Sanger initiated change that challenged the political and social institutions and led to new interpretations of existing laws. She was jailed seven more times. Her work was opposed by conservatives and various religious groups. Nursing historians rarely mention her or her contributions even though her promotion of contraception was directly related to a 38% decline in the birth rate between 1910 and 1930 (Kalisch & Kalisch, 1986).

Another community health pioneer of the era was Mary Breckinridge. In 1925, she established the Frontier Nursing Service in Kentucky as a demonstration project. She instructed staff nurses to provide care to women during pregnancy, labor, and delivery and to infants and children. Nurses rode horses to make visits in remote areas until years later when horses were replaced by jeeps.

Visiting Nurse Movement

The success of community health nurses stimulated rapid expansion of the specialty throughout the US. In 1895, Ada Mayo Stewart was hired as a district nurse by the owner of the Vermont Marble Company, becoming the first industrial nurse. Nursing settlement houses similar to the Henry Street facility were established between 1900 and 1903 in Richmond, VA, San Francisco, CA, and Orange, NJ. Those receiving care included many immigrants with diverse health values and beliefs. In 1907, Alabama was the first state to recognize the public health nurse as a legitimate employee of an official agency. By 1910, milk stations were initiated in at least 30 cities, offering germ-free milk to everyone. The first fulltime county health departments were established in the states of North Carolina and Washington in 1911.

The visiting nurse association movement expanded rapidly, resulting in the formation of 71 agencies prior to 1900. Nurses offered home care to the sick poor, whereas middle and upper class families were expected to hire their own private duty nurses. Yssabella Waters (1909), the first nursing statistician, carefully compiled details about the number of agencies, locations, names, and founding dates.

The proliferation of agencies early in the twentieth century was phenomenal. By 1912, 2,500 nurses were employed by 900 independent agencies; often a sole nurse was the only employee (Kalisch & Kalisch, 1986). By 1916, almost 2,000 organizations existed and the number of nurses reached 5,000 — a 50% increase in 3 years (Gardner, 1917). To prevent conflicts between the agency and special interest groups, leaders encouraged broad, nonsectarian community support. Fundraising projects such as lawn parties, band concerts, teas, and annual tag or donation days were used as means to generate income. As other projects were eliminated and annual tag campaigns became more successful, they were called Community Chest drives and, eventually, United Way campaigns.

The nurses from most agencies used a standard client record form. Documentation included sex, ethnicity, age, medical diagnosis, occupation, marital status, place of birth, number of nursing visits made, and condition on dismissal. No attempt was made to describe nursing services or document the effectiveness of care.

Agency staff were expected to complete 8 to 12 visits per day, providing comprehensive, therapeutic care to the sick and teaching family members about sickness care, environmental sanitation, and protection of milk and water supplies. In addition to home visits, nurses distributed milk at stations, established summertime open-air baby camps for infant care and teaching, and weighed and measured infants at baby stations or clinics (Lyons-Barrett, 1989). Nursing salaries ranged from $45 to $60 per month for an 8- to 10-hour workday. Overtime compensation was not expected by or given to staff. Traditionally, nurses carried a black bag containing an apron, bandages, thermometer, and catheter for those who were ill, as well as broth and jellies for the malnourished.

Community Health Organizations and Publications

Many community health nurses were concerned about formidable issues such as consistent practice standards, the client record, collection of statistics, minimum employment qualifications, financial stability of agencies, and extension of services throughout the country. Nurses argued about specialization versus generalization and the use of graduates versus students as agency staff. In 1911, national leaders and members of various nursing school alumni organizations who were concerned about these issues established the American Nurses' Associations (ANA). In 1912, prominent community health nursing leaders began to organize a separate national association. The founders selected the title National Organization for Public Health Nurses (NOPHN), noting that it was the most inclusive choice. Membership was open to public health nurses, agencies, and interested citizens. These are nine of the influential founders:

- Lillian Wald, first president of NOPHN
- Ella Phillips Crandall, first NOPHN executive secretary; supervised Henry Street Settlement and directed the first public health nursing program at Teachers College (NY) and Simmons College (MA)
- Mary Lent, superintendent of the Baltimore Instructive District Nursing Association; organized public health nursing services for World War I soldiers
- Edna Foley, superintendent of the Chicago Visiting Nurse Association and, later, president of NOPHN
- Mary Gardner, founder and superintendent of the Providence (RI) District Nursing Association, a prolific writer, and the second president of NOPHN
- Katharine Tucker, superintendent of the Philadelphia VNA and, later, president and general director of NOPHN
- Lystra Gretter, director of the nursing school at Harper Hospital in Detroit; established the 8-hour day for students
- Mary Beard, director of the Boston VNA, the health division of the Rockefeller Foundation, and the Red Cross Nursing Service; wrote *The Nurse in Public Health* in 1929
- Elizabeth Fox, administrator of the Red Cross Nursing Service and, later, president of NOPHN

Publications offered an important method of communication and education for community health nurses. The first journal specific to the specialty was established by the staff of the Cleveland Visiting Nurse Association at the beginning of the century. Gardner's standard community health nursing textbook of 1917 included an extensive overview of public health nursing history, principles, organization, and staffing, as well as responsibilities of the nurse in homes, schools, and industry. While Gardner did not use the terms "nursing process" or "scientific method," she referred to the concepts. She made a strong plea that staff members record client care in a reasonable and thoughtful manner, generating data that could lead to valuable conclusions. NOPHN staff wrote the first edition of

Manual of Public Health Nursing in 1926 as a comprehensive guide. Therapeutic and educational nursing responsibilities during a home visit, recording, and administration were emphasized.

The Great War

World War I served as a force both to interrupt and briefly accelerate nursing progress. The Victorian era ended, a 1920 constitutional amendment gave women the right to vote, and the general public expected women to join the labor force, especially in factories. The public image of nursing deteriorated, however, particularly when the war ended. The public viewed nursing as a female occupation with limited prestige. Many nurses wanted to marry and stop working; few wives or mothers were employed as nurses.

Some influential people, especially physicians, suggested methods to solve the nursing shortage such as suspending all admission standards to schools of nursing. Others urged the introduction of nurses' aides. Nursing leaders united in opposition and developed alternative plans including the first doctoral program for nurses. Columbia University Teachers' College, which had established the first collegiate postgraduate public health course 10 years before, introduced the doctoral program.

Before the end of the war, community health nursing became a visible specialty. Mary Lent organized 200 community health nurses to serve in military camps throughout the US. Nurses inspected sanitary conditions and water supplies and provided care to soldiers who had developed communicable diseases such as malaria, venereal disease, and tuberculosis. In Europe, Mary Breckinridge and Red Cross nurses helped introduce public health practices, in addition to providing care to sick and wounded American soldiers.

Post World War I

After World War I, another milestone in college-based nursing education occurred when Yale University opened a School of Nursing, the first autonomous nursing school within a university. Annie Goodrich, Dean, and Bertha Harmer, an early nursing theorist, were among the progressive faculty members. Harmer emphasized Nightingale's and Wald's concepts as she defined nursing in her books about the principles and practices of nursing, first published in 1922. In relation to public health nursing practice, she emphasized the need for an educational approach. By 1926, more than 2,000 nursing schools were operating, compared to 15 programs in 1880 (Dolan, et al., 1983). Whereas some programs were excellent, most nursing education of the era was inadequate. Furthermore, not all nurses and physicians supported advances and independence in nursing education or interest in scientific solutions; many opponents viewed nurses as manual laborers who should remain under the benevolent dictatorship of physicians.

Nursing and medical education was intensively evaluated before and after World War I. The Flexner Report indicated the need for reforming medical schools. In 1923, the Rockefeller Foundation funded and published one of the best known nursing studies, the Goldmark Report. Findings included the need for less apprenticeship, for better prepared instructors, and for grading of schools. While the Goldmark Report and most nursing leaders favored general community health nursing practice, controversy increased and a proposal emerged to separate the role of the public health nurse from that of the visiting nurse. Those who favored specialization indicated that a public health nurse should focus on health education, whereas the visiting or home health care nurse should provide therapeutic bedside care to the sick. Some leaders suggested that public health nursing was the responsibility of government and the voluntary or private sector should support visiting nurse services.

A survey conducted by staff and members of NOPHN in 1924 was designed to elicit census data regarding community health nursing practice. The census indicated that there were more than 11,000 full-time graduate nurses employed by over 3,000 agencies. Just over 50% of the agencies were public or official; the others were private or voluntary agencies, branches of the Red Cross, and tuberculosis associations. The increase of official agencies indicated a significant organizational change. The problems related to immigration and infectious diseases that had stimulated the development of visiting nurse associations were decreasing; public and professional interest in maternal-child health was thriving. The definition of public health nursing varied markedly among the agencies responding to the NOPHN survey, a conclusion also noted in the Goldmark Report.

Depression Years

At the end of the 1920s and during the 1930s, the Depression caused a disastrous degree of unemployment and hardship throughout the country. Nurses did not escape the effects of the Depression; many accepted decreases in salary or were unable to find work. The demand for private duty nurses in homes decreased in direct relationship to increasing public confidence in hospitals and inability of families to pay for private services. For the first time, graduate nurses began to work in hospitals, often over the objections of student nurses. In exchange for room and board, the graduates provided personal care to patients and cleaned the equipment and the building itself. Nurses performed few skilled procedures.

The relationship between the health of the individual and economic security of the community became generally recognized. As a result, private and governmental public works programs were developed to provide incentives for employing health professionals and re-establishing health care services. In 1934, Pearl McIver became the first public health nurse employed by the US Public Health Service to provide consultation services to state health departments. One of her important contributions was to help plan and conduct a research project comparing recorded data generated by groups of staff (Derryberry, 1939). Although previous evaluation of community health service was based on volume and intensity, this study focused on client progress and quality of service. McIver also directed the development of categorical public health nursing services mandated by the Social Security Act of 1935.

A second survey of community health nursing agencies was completed by NOPHN staff in 1934. The findings indicated that 20,000 community health nurses were employed by 5,000 voluntary and official agencies (Tucker & Hilbert, 1934). At the beginning of the century, most community health nurses provided comprehensive curative and preventive services, were employed by visiting nurse agencies, and enjoyed autonomy in practice. The trend shifted as official public health agencies became prominent during this era. Health officers, often physicians or sanitarians, administered official agencies and public health nursing activities.

Just as advances in nursing practice were hindered by the impact of the Depression, so too were those in medicine. An exception was public health medicine, which expanded beyond the initial issues of sanitation and communicable disease and into the areas of maternal and infant health. Contributing to expansion was the development of diphtheria, pertussis, and tetanus immunizations as well as the availability of federal funds.

Other advances in medicine during the Depression era involved nomenclature and classification. In 1928, members of the League of Nations examined and expanded the causes-of-death listing. This expansion of the International Classification of Diseases (ICD) represented the first effort to use the terminology for morbidity statistics and causal association studies, an effort that was conceptually related to the nursing process. In an attempt to make the ICD more applicable to clinicians and to hospital record rooms in this country, the Standard Nomenclature of Diseases and Operations (SNODO) was developed through efforts of AMA members. It was designed to systematically link a specific disease to an area of the body, differentiate disease from symptoms, and facilitate retrieval of case histories related to specific variables. Formulated between 1928 and 1932, SNODO and the revisions that followed were widely used until the late 1960s.

Modern Advances in Nursing Education and Practice

The end of the Depression at the beginning of the 1940s marked a time of significant transition in the US. Individual independence, voluntary support, and local control were established traditions. Social reforms originating in the 1900s and intensifying during the Depression precipitated changes. By the time of World War II, federal intervention, regulation, and support were accepted as desirable and necessary. These trends affected the entire health care delivery system and caused the programs, organization, and funding of community health nursing agencies to change.

Educational and practice opportunities for nurses improved in direct relationship to public and federal support of two wars. During World War II, the US Cadet Nurse Corps was designed and administered by Lucile Petry Leone, one of the most influential nurses of the era. The Corps represented the first use of federal funds to subsidize nursing education. The status of nursing also improved during the Korean conflict in the 1950s. Nurses were assigned to duty everywhere, from hospitals in the continental US to the battle zone, and they emerged as an integral part of the war effort. Many educational and practice opportunities became available to black nurses because of the nursing shortage created by the wars.

Esther Lucile Brown, an anthropologist, completed *Nursing for the Future* in 1948. Financed by the Carnegie Foundation, this controversial study included recommendations for differentiating professional nursing from vocational nursing. Brown's report and the establishment of the National Nursing Accreditation Services led to improved nursing education programs as well as to the introduction of associate degree programs and specialized preparation at the master's degree level. Brown's report added to the impetus necessary to create two distinct national nursing organizations in 1952. The organizations, the American Nurses' Association (ANA) and National League for Nursing (NLN), were established through merger and restructuring of four national organizations, including the NOPHN.

Pioneers in Nursing Research and Theory

Interest in research, statistics, and theory increased during this era, interest that would precipitate developments during the 1960s involving quality assurance and evaluation. In 1944, the Division of Public Health Nursing was created within the US Public Health Service. Nurses employed by the Division began to conduct research studies, a process that increased the national visibility of health care issues. In 1956, an extramural nursing research grant program was established. Helen Bunge and other leaders initiated the first research journal for nurses, *Nursing Research*, in 1952. A nursing research pioneer, Harriet Werley, established the Walter Reed Army Institute of Research and served as a member of federal review panels and a mentor to nursing colleagues. Doris Schwartz was among community health nursing leaders who became interested in evaluation and research. Schwartz in 1958 conducted a nationally recognized study with a sample of 50 nonconforming patients who obtained medical and nursing services at an outpatient clinic. The study was intended to reveal the characteristics of patients who staff judged "nonconforming" to care. Myrtle Aydelotte and Marie Tener (1960) conducted a landmark study at the University of Iowa that was designed to establish criteria for evaluating nursing services in relationship to client outcomes.

During the same era, pioneers struggled to identify a unique body of knowledge relevant to nursing practice. Hildegard Peplau in 1952 described four phases of nurse-client relationships. Virginia Henderson and her colleague, Bertha Harmer, revised Harmer's book. Henderson's 1966 definition of nursing has become an international classic: "The unique function of the nurse is to assist the individual (sick or well), in the performance of those activities contributing to health or its recovery (or to peaceful death) that he would perform unaided if he had the necessary strength, will, or knowledge. And to do this in such a way as to help him gain independence as rapidly as possible" (p. 15).

Vera Fry and Faye Abdellah were two of the first nurses to focus on the concept of nursing diagnosis as a means of articulating nurses' special contributions to client care. Fry in 1953 described the concept as a creative and necessary approach to understanding a client as an individual. Abdellah investigated nursing problems and in 1957 concluded that nursing faculty needed to de-emphasize procedure instruction and, instead, emphasize identification of significant overt and covert client behaviors and conditions. Abdellah's efforts paralleled those of the physicians who began to classify medical diagnoses as early as 1893.

Community Health Nursing Leaders

Community health nursing education continued to advance, primarily in conjunction with early schools of public health. Ruth Freeman had a profound influence as a renowned educator, national leader, and prolific writer. She helped to establish community health nursing agencies throughout the country while she was the nursing service administrator of the American Red Cross. During her tenure at Johns Hopkins University, Freeman served as the principal investigator of a 1961 study designed to measure the effectiveness of public health nursing service (Freeman, 1961; Mickey, 1958). Incorporating concepts of the nursing process, she defined effectiveness as the relationship between goals and achievement.

Ruth Freeman's first book is a classic that included comprehensive guidelines for agency supervisors. Seven more of Freeman's books, published between 1950 and 1981 as basic and graduate nursing texts, were used by most college-based students because baccalaureate programs included public health in the curriculum. The book titles reflect the change in generally accepted terminology from "public health" nursing to "community health" nursing.

Maria Phaneuf, another community health nurse, contributed to the development of quality assurance and evaluation of care. She conducted a demonstration project for Associated Hospital Service of New York (Blue Cross) and originated the Phaneuf Nursing Audit Format and Pattern (Wandelt & Phaneuf, 1972). As a result of Phaneuf's efforts, the New York State insurance law was revised in 1959 to permit insurance plans to pay for home care. By late 1964, more than half of the Blue Cross Plans in the US provided payment for visiting nurse care; some plans contain parts of Phaneuf's instrument today. Several of her recommendations were incorporated into 1965 Medicare legislation. In addition to her individual contributions, Phaneuf collaborated with Mabel Wandelt to develop tools to measure effectiveness and quality of care.

Community Health Nursing Trends

Trends associated with World War II, the Korean conflict, and national priorities precipitated change in both voluntary and official community health nursing agencies. With increasing frequency, adequate health care was viewed as a basic human right. The total number of voluntary nursing agencies and staff remained constant. In contrast, the number of tax-supported, official agencies and staff escalated; this trend, begun during the previous decade, continued into the 1970s. Fewer than 10,000 registered nurses were employed by local health departments before the Depression; by the 1970s almost 20,000 were employed (Roberts & Heinrich, 1985). The staff of local and state health departments usually consisted of a sanitarian, a nurse, and a physician with the physician functioning as a clinician, and an administrator.

1960s

The 1960s were an era of national turmoil. The health care industry did not escape the effects of this turmoil. Community health nurses and administrators developed a sense of urgency about documentation and accountability.

Simultaneously, physicians were struggling to more precisely describe and measure medical care. Avedis Donabedian in 1966 described the structure, process, and outcome framework for evaluating the quality of medical care that has become known internationally. Because of Lawrence Weed's (1968) concerns about the continuity and effectiveness of medical care, he developed a problem-oriented medical record system (PROMIS) that was adaptable to computerization. Almost immediately, nurses, including those at the VNA of Omaha, recognized the potential applicability of Donabedian's and Weed's systems to the practice of community health nursing and the issues of documentation and accountability.

Changes in Nomenclature and Classification

Many other physicians advanced systems for nomenclature and classification. The Standard Nomenclature of Diseases and Operations (SNODO), developed during the 1930s, was replaced by the 1965 Systematized Nomenclature of Pathology (SNOP). SNOP was designed to define disease in relation to the four categories topography, morphology, etiology, and function. Because SNOP was developed by pathologists, the system required expansion for other physicians and hospitals; two fields, procedure and disease, were added to revise SNOP into Systematized Nomenclature of Medicine (SNOMED).

Development of the International Classification of Diseases (ICD), begun in 1893, continued through the eighth revision in 1964. Classification was based upon three-digit codes; specific conditions were identified by etiology or manifestation. The ICD is intended to facilitate collection and distribution of statistical morbidity and mortality information throughout the world. It has provided the basis for specialized classification systems such as the Diagnostic and Statistical Manual of Mental Disorders, third edition (DSM-III), which has been sponsored by the American Psychiatric Association. The ICD has been accepted as the official United States index for coding death records.

Federal Initiatives

The staff of the Division of Nursing, US Department of Health, Education, and Welfare (DHEW), investigated ways to document client progress and community health nursing services beyond the traditional tally of number of visits and number and types of individuals served. Beginning in 1959, Doris Roberts and Helen Hudson (1964) developed a method of reporting that incorporated family, client, nursing service, and client progress data. By 1964, the tool was tested, refined, and used in 33 agencies that included the VNA of Omaha. The agencies were located in nine states and served 5,000 clients. In addition, the study was replicated in Canada.

A new health care era began when the Social Security Amendments were initiated in 1966. Increased federal funds became available for programs involving mothers and infants, children and youth, handicapped children, and low-income preschoolers. Medicare benefits provided financial assistance to people 65 years and older who needed hospitalization, nursing home, home health, medical equipment, and physician services or outpatient services.

The advent of Medicare and Medicaid programs had a revolutionary effect on community health nursing. Local agency directors quickly recognized the need for increased communication and mutual support as they were asked to justify services and expenditures. Often they did not have the necessary data to respond. At the state level, the Illinois Council of Home Health Services was established in 1960, uniting providers and agencies who were concerned about the effects of Medicare. At the national level, restructuring of the NLN resulted in formation of councils. Community health nurses and agencies became members of the Council of Home Health Associations and Community Health Services (CHHA/CHS). Many agencies began to participate in the new NLN-American Public Health Association agency accreditation program as another way to increase their credibility.

Controversies

Controversy was associated with nursing practice and education issues during the mid-1960s. Nurses participated in collective bargaining and organized strikes even though nonprofit hospitals were exempted until 1974 under the Taft-Hartley Act. Also controversial was the 1965 ANA Position Paper proposing that nursing education by provided at established educational institutions. Nursing specialization developed as nursing roles expanded. Advanced educational programs were developed to increase the expertise of clinical nurse specialists or nurse clinicians. In 1964, the ANA defined the public health nurse as a graduate of a baccalaureate program in nursing. Specialized public health baccalaureate programs were eliminated when public health theory and practice were required as part of all NLN-accredited baccalaureate nursing programs. To circumvent the issues of educational preparation for practicing nurses, the term "community health nurse" was used increasingly within many agencies.

Nursing Theory and Process

Nursing educators began to recognize the need for a more coherent, integrated, and comprehensive theoretical structure of nursing knowledge that was relevant to nursing practice. Leaders such as Ida Orlando, Imogene King, Myra Levine, Dorothea Orem, and Martha Rogers explored, developed, and tested nursing theories to enhance nursing science. Nursing theory and research were integrated into college programs, signifying an extensive campaign to achieve full professional status independent of medicine. Simultaneously, the number of master's degree programs escalated and doctoral nursing programs were introduced.

The significance of the nursing process and its components to theory and practice was clearly recognized by certain nursing leaders. Helen Yura and Mary Walsh (1967) used a human needs theoretical approach to write their text, which was one of the first comprehensive presentations of the nursing process. Delores Little and Doris Carnevali (1969) described their ideas about systematic planning of nursing care, as did members of the Western Council on Higher Education for Nursing (WCHEN). WCHEN member Lucile Lewis (1968) described the nursing process as a key to the kind of care that characterizes professional nursing; she noted that it included assessment, intervention, and evaluation. However, whereas exploration of nursing process was acceptable to most nurses, nursing diagnosis continued to be very controversial. Unlike some other evolving theories, the nursing process offered relevance for service delivery nurses because it explained the realities of nursing practice. Concurrently, the nursing process offered a method of decreasing the gap between theory and practice. Documenting the steps of the nursing process in clients' records was an innovative commitment to evaluating the effectiveness of service.

1970s

The national turmoil of the 1960s changed to the resolution and tranquility of the 1970s. Nurses entered their third and current phase of evolution. Nursing salaries continued to rise in comparison to nonprofessional wages although inequities persisted, especially in relation to comparable but male-dominated professions. Nurses were attempting to identify nursing diagnoses, resolve quality assurance issues, and develop nursing as a science. Faculty was strengthened within nursing education programs; 874 of 1,492 programs were accredited by 1974. The development of nursing involved a continuing struggle by practitioners for respect, credibility, recognition, and power. Many, including some nurses, viewed nursing as a practice discipline only, a threat to the medical hierarchy, and a group lacking a body of scientific knowledge.

Racial Integration and Professional Autonomy

Black nurses were integrated into nursing schools and employment settings during the decade. With integration, all nurses shared professional opportunities, as they had prior to the 1870s. The need for a professional organization for black nurses continued, however. In 1971, the National Black Nurses' Association was established with a structure complementary to ANA. As black nurses and specialty groups developed independent associations, debate increased regarding the fragmentation of power and advantages of one large inclusive organization versus many small specialized organizations.

Nurses gained autonomy and independence when, in 1971, Idaho became the first state to broaden the Nurse-Practice Act by including nursing diagnosis and treatment of problems under certain circumstances. Today, most states have nursing practice acts that incorporate diagnosis and treatment of human responses to actual and potential problems, case-finding, health teaching and counseling, and provision of care. Although many states authorized the expanded role for nurses, only a few included independent prescriptive authority.

Community Health and the NLN

Community health agencies proliferated, especially those that were hospital-based and private. Many new agencies, proprietary or for-profit, were established by entrepreneurial groups with no previous interest or experience in health care. Nurse administrators of nonprofit community health agencies continued to develop networks. A group of 10 agencies was organized in 1973 through the NLN Council, CHHA/CHS. During the next 10 years, the participating executives exerted significant influence on community health nursing as they perpetuated the traditional values of the specialty. They provided mutual support, offered leadership expertise to other agency directors, and discussed ways to control costs. Because these executives tended to share their expertise informally, their names appear infrequently in the nursing literature. In 1979, the members included:

Margaret M. Ahern, Visiting Nurse Association of Chicago

Alice M. Dempsey, Visiting Nurse Association of Boston

Jean D. Galkin, Visiting Nurse Association of Baltimore

Elsie I. Griffith, Visiting Nurse Association of Dallas

Margaret C. Kauffman, Community Nursing Services of Philadelphia

Jane D. Keeler, Visiting Nurse Association of New Haven

Lillian H. O'Brien, Visiting Nurse Association of Los Angeles

Sylvia R. Peabody, Visiting Nurse Association of Metro Detroit

Eva M. Reese, Visiting Nurse Service of New York

DeLanne A. Simmons, Visiting Nurse Association of Omaha

Members of the 10-agency group and NLN staff addressed topics of mutual concern such as client records, use of client statistics, computerized management information systems, performance evaluation, and quality assurance. They reviewed classification and evaluation models as well as nursing applications of the problem-oriented system and computer technology. The activities of the group stimulated DeLanne Simmons and her staff to initiate research investigations which, at the VNA of Omaha, integrated the nursing process, documentation, and data management. These studies, funded by the Division of Nursing, US Department of Health and Human Services (DHHS), are the basis of the Omaha System and this book.

Developments in Diagnosis and Theory

Related issues, including the concepts of nursing assessment and nursing problem or nursing diagnosis, were examined by nurses during the 1970s. Nursing diagnosis remained controversial, although it was no longer a new idea. Because of their interest in the concept, faculty at St. Louis University organized the First National Conference on Classification of Nursing Diagnoses in 1973. Through small group sessions and consensual validation, the 100 conference participants approved 30 diagnostic labels with defining characteristics and etiology. The movement grew to the extent that the North American Nursing Diagnosis Association was formed before the sixth conference was held in 1984. The history of the Association, the text of biennial conference presentations, and transcripts of Association discussion are documented in seven volumes of Conference Proceedings.

Medical diagnosis and classification, initiated long before comparable efforts by nurses, continued to require refinement. Physicians explored their diagnostic art and science, noting potential therapeutic and educational benefits. Alvan Feinstein in 1970 described the goals of clinical medicine, which included reducing observer variability, developing new systems of taxonomy, establishing criteria for clinical judgments, and improving quantification.

Advances related to nursing process and quality assurance occurred because of individual and group efforts, often related to efforts begun during the 1960s. Norma Lang (1980) helped to use and disseminate a quality assurance and nursing process model with her 1974 doctoral dissertation, her many publications, and her efforts on behalf of ANA. Many nurses conducted studies during the 1970s because they recognized that the generation of research-based knowledge was critical to the progress of the profession. The staff at Medicus and VNA of Omaha were among those who conducted ongoing research related to community health nursing practice and nursing process. The Omaha research is described in Chapter 4. A Medicus team began an extensive research project and developed a method to monitor quality of nursing care in acute care settings. Their method has been widely adopted by nursing staff in many hospitals.

Just as theory-building must occur to increase the scope and depth of nursing science, so must replication, extension, and sharing of research. In 1978, Harriet Werley became the founding editor of *Research in Nursing and Health* and in 1983, the *Annual Review of Nursing*. These publications provided nurses with more opportunities to share research-based knowledge.

1980s

Nursing literature of the 1980s included frequent references to complex issues. These included continuing economic recession, spiraling health care costs, decreasing insurance benefits, increasing denials of Medicare claims, disputes over direct payment for nurses, increasing competition among providers, fragmentation of services, and quality of life concerns. Consumers recognized the economic benefits of healthful living and illness-preventive behaviors. Reimbursement for nursing and medical care, however, rewarded secondary and tertiary prevention. Nurses became aware that health services throughout this country were interrelated to complex international economic, political, religious, and technologic concerns. An urgent need became apparent for individual and collective involvement of nurses in broad health care matters such as acquired immune deficiency syndrome (AIDS) and homelessness.

Effects of Legislation and Regulations

Reports, legislation, and regulations increasingly affected nurses in both positive and negative ways. When the US DHHS was created, health issues received more national funding and visibility. The 1981 National Commission on Nursing report included recommendations for baccalaureate education as entry-level nursing preparation, inclusion of nurse administrators in top management, and collaboration between nurses and physicians. The 1988 Commission report emphasized nursing's responsibility for promoting a positive image of the profession as well as the need for increasing nursing autonomy, support systems, and salaries to

ensure adequate levels of staffing. A 1983 Institute of Medicine report suggested that nursing research be in the mainstream of scientific investigation; further, the report stated that the nursing shortage was over. Almost as soon as the report was issued, however, another serious shortage began.

Nurses experienced almost immediate effects of regulation when Congress passed the Tax Equity and Fiscal Responsibility Act (TEFRA) in an attempt to control escalating Medicare costs. This 1982 Act initiated a prospective payment system for hospital-based care. With the advent of diagnosis related groups (DRGs) hospitals were paid based on 470 diagnosis categories rather than on actual costs. The categories were based on the language of the ICD-9-CM.

The management and staff of community health nursing agencies felt the effects of DRGs as referrals from hospitals increased. Existing agencies added staff, and new agencies proliferated. For the first time, the number of employed community health nurses exceeded 100,000. As the number of agencies peaked in 1986, staff in more than 6,000 Medicare-certified home health agencies were providing millions of home visits. Blurring of program distinctions increased, especially among those agencies that were Medicare-certified. This led to a confusing assortment of fragmented, duplicated, and competitive services within most communities.

The entire Medicare system became financially troubled at the time when the number of community health nursing agency referrals as well as the cost of services increased dramatically. Since 1965, agency costs have increased, particularly in relation to the extensive, complex reimbursement procedures required by Medicare regulations. The national average cost for a community health nursing visit was $8 in 1968, $26 in 1979, and $62 in 1989 (Hoyer, 1990; *Survey of Community Health Nursing 1979*, 1982).

Coalitions and joint ventures were developed during the 1980s among community health agencies and other health care institutions to control and increase referrals. Agencies also diversified services, initiating new community health programs for age-specific groups and social needs. Services were offered at more convenient locations, including shopping centers. Many agencies increased their hours of service to 24-hour days, 7 days a week. In order to provide continuous service, nurses, home health aides, and companions were employed, often on a contractual arrangement resembling the nursing registries popular earlier in the century.

Community Health Organizations

The need for communication among community health nursing agency directors increased during the 1980s. An organization that became the Visiting Nurse Associations of America (VNAA) originated in 1982. The VNAA was the first formal organization of VNAs and was established to foster communication, promote a national image, and pool resources. By 1987, VNAA had evolved into a national association designed as an affiliation model. It had 107 member agencies. Also in 1982, the National Association for Home Care (NAHC) was created by the merger of the National Association of Home Health Agencies and the NLN Council, CHHA/CHS. Between 1982 and 1987, member agencies increased from 500 to more than 5,000; membership was open to all community health agencies. NAHC was designed to be a trade rather than a professional organization. Staff and members lobbied in Congress, developed public relations campaigns, established a journal, communicated with state associations, and conducted annual conventions and legislative conferences.

Nursing Research

In the 1980s, trends emerged that were associated with community health nursing research studies and theory development. Various authors identified quality assurance as an area for continuing attention. During the decade, the number, diversity, and sophistication of research studies increased and included new areas of inquiry such as home infusion, the client-caregiver dyad, and agency referrals and reimbursement (Martin, 1988). Phillips, Fisher, MacMillan-Scattergood, and associates (1987) examined the differences between referrals and services in a public and a private agency, concluding that the public agency's decreasing financial base had negative implications for future consumers and professionals.

In general, nursing research became more diverse, interdisciplinary, and rigorous during the decade. Researchers and theorists increased exploration in practice-related areas such as problem-oriented recording, nursing process, nursing minimum data set, and diagnostic reasoning; summaries of their conclusions are included in Chapters 3 and 4. After years of effort, a National Center for Nursing Research was established in 1986 as part of the National Institutes of Health (NIH) with Ada Sue Hinshaw as the first director. Members of Sigma Theta Tau and other nursing organizations increased their efforts to facilitate wider dissemination and use of research-based knowledge by practitioners as well as educators and researchers.

The dilemmas related to reimbursement and productivity provided the impetus for research in acute care settings. Nurses recognized the urgency to separate or unbundle nursing service costs from total hospital charges. Classifying clients and identifying discrete nursing costs were considered initial steps toward establishing direct charges for nursing care and predicting nursing costs, independent of a medical model such as DRGs. Giovannetti and Mayer (1984) and Horn (1985) were among nurses who refined patient classification systems to address allocation of nursing personnel, acuity, and intensity. Sovie, Tarcinale, Vanputee, and associates (1985) conducted an extensive correlation study to examine the relationships among nursing patient classification, DRGs, and other significant patient variables, and total costs of care. Findings suggested that DRGs were useful for measuring nursing costs. Romano, McCormick, and McNeely (1982) described the value of developing a management information system that could integrate client data with other cost and management data. Although the age of informatics had arrived, continuing problems and expense with software development limited direct benefits to nurses.

SUMMARY

Ever changing demands, trends, and cycles have occurred in community health nursing since the time of Phoebe. Nurses have differed markedly in relation to age, marital status, socioeconomic status, and educational preparation as well as professional commitment, autonomy, and unity. The orientation of community health nursing practice has varied from the individual to the family to the community. Because of technologic advances, the orientation is now extending to the world or even the universe. Throughout the history of community health nursing, and nursing in general, the status and strength of the specialty was directly related to the vision, strength, and caring of the leaders. Leaders who were nurses, and some who were not, were influential in shaping advances in service, education, and research. A smaller but very significant group of leaders concentrated on fundraising, politics, organizations, and writing. The influence of articulate, provocative journal editors on the profession has been especially notable.

Slowly, progress is being made toward the international goal of holistic health care services for all. Progress will be affected by the quality of leadership provided by nurses and by political, economic, environmental, religious, and technologic changes. All nurses, including community health nurses, need practice, documentation, and data management tools such as the Omaha System. These tools enable community health professionals to meet changing public and professional requirements, to articulate professional contributions to the general public, and to increase the visibility of the profession. The resources of community health nurses rarely exceed those needed for the number of clients, the intensity of those clients' health-related problems, and the severity of service delivery constraints. Community health nurses must become excellent promoters for the specialty to thrive. Such promotion must occur at all levels, from the locations where care is provided, to boardrooms, and to newspapers and television.

REFERENCES

Abdellah, F. (1957, June). Methods of identifying covert aspects of nursing problems. *Nurs. Res.,* 6:4–23.
Aydelotte, M., & Tener, M. (1960). *An Investigation of the Relation*

Between Nursing Activity and Patient Welfare. Iowa City, IA, University of Iowa.

Bullough, V. (1990, Spring). Nightingale, nursing and harassment. *Image, 22:*4–7.

Christy, T. (1969, June). Portrait of a leader: Lavinia Lloyd Dock. *Nurs. Outlook, 17:*72–75.

Derryberry, M. (1939). Nursing accomplishments as revealed by case records. *Public Health Rep., 54:*2035–2043.

Dolan, J., Fitzpatrick, M., & Herrmann, E. (1983). *Nursing in Society: A Historical Perspective* (15th ed.). Philadelphia, W. B. Saunders.

Donabedian, A. (1966, July). Evaluating the quality of medical care. *Milbank Memorial Fund Q., 44*(2):166–206.

Feinstein, A. (1970). What kind of basic science for clinical medicine? *N. Engl. J. Med., 283:*847–852.

Freeman, R. (1957). *Public Health Nursing Practice* (2nd ed.). Philadelphia, W. B. Saunders.

Freeman, R. (1961, October). Measuring the effectiveness of public health nursing service. *Nurs. Outlook, 9:*605–607.

Fry, V. (1953, March). The creative approach to nursing. *Am. J. Nurs., 53:*301–302.

Gardner, M. (1917). *Public Health Nursing.* New York, Macmillan.

Garrison, F. (1929). *An Introduction to the History of Medicine* (4th ed.). Philadelphia, W. B. Saunders.

Giovannetti, P., & Mayer, G. (1984, August). Building confidence in patient classification systems. *Nurs. Manag., 15:*31–34.

Henderson, V. (1966). *The Nature of Nursing.* New York, Macmillan.

Horn, S. (1985). Severity of illness: Case mix beyond DRGs. In Schaffer, F. (Ed.), *Costing Out Nursing: Pricing Our Product* (pp. 225–235). New York, National League for Nursing.

Hoyer, R. (1990, May). [1989 home health agency cost per visit.] Personal communication regarding unpublished data.

Kalisch, P., & Kalisch, B. (1986). *The Advance of American Nursing* (2nd ed.). Boston, Little, Brown.

Lang, N. (1980). *Quality assurance in nursing: A selected bibliography.* Hyattsville, MD, DHEW, Bureau of Health Manpower, Division of Nursing.

Lewis, L. (1968). This I believe . . . about the nursing process. *Nurs. Outlook, 16:*26–29.

Little, D., & Carnevali, D. (1969). *Nursing Care Planning.* Philadelphia, J. B. Lippincott.

Lyons-Barrett, M. (1989, Winter). The Omaha Visiting Nurses Association during the 1920s and 1930s. *Nebraska Hist., 70:*283–296.

Martin, K. (1988, June). Research in home care. *Nurs. Clin. North Am., 23:*373–385.

Mickey, J. (1958, July). Studying extra-hospital nursing needs: A preliminary report. *Am. J. Public Health, 48:*880–887.

Moses, E. (1990, March). [Survey of RNs in U.S.] Personal communication regarding unpublished data.

Peplau, H. (1952). *Interpersonal Relations in Nursing.* New York, G. P. Putnam's Sons.

Phillips, E., Fisher, M., MacMillan-Scattergood, D., et al. (1987, June). Home health care: Who's where? *Am. J. Public Health, 77:*733–734.

Roberts, D., & Heinrich, J. (1985, October). Public health nursing comes of age. *Am. J. Public Health, 75:*1162–1172.

Roberts, D., & Hudson, H. (1964). *How to Study Patient Progress.* US DHEW Publication No. 1169. Bethesda, MD, PHS–National Institutes of Health, Division of Nursing.

Romano, C., McCormick, K., & McNeely, L. (1982, January). Nursing documentation: A model for a computerized data base. *Adv. Nurs. Sci., 4:*43–56.

Schwartz, D. (1958, January). Uncooperative patients? *Am. J. Nurs., 58:*75–77.

Sovie, M., Tarcinale, M., Vanputee, A. et al. (1985, March). Amalgam of nursing acuity, DRGs, and costs. *Nurs. Manag., 16:*22–42.

Survey of Community Health Nursing 1979. (1982). Hyattsville, MD: DHHS, Bureau of Health Professions, Division of Nursing.

Tucker, K., & Hilbert, H. (1934). *Survey of Public Health Nursing.* New York, The Commonwealth Fund.

Wandelt, M., & Phaneuf, M. (1972, August). Three instruments for measuring quality of nursing care. *Hosp. Topics, 50:*20–29.

Waters, Y. (1909). *Visiting Nursing in the United States.* New York, Charities Publication Committee.

Weed, L.. (1968, March 14–21). Special article: Medical records that guide and teach. *New Engl J. Med., 278:*593–600, 652–657.

Yura, H., & Walsh, M. (1967). *The Nursing Process: Assessing, Planning, Implementing, Evaluating.* New York, Appleton-Century-Crofts.

BIBLIOGRAPHY

American Nurses' Association. (1990, February). *The American Nurse.*

Brainard, A. (1922). *The Evolution of Public Health Nursing.* New York, Garland.

Brown, E. (1948). *Nursing for the Future.* New York, Russell Sage Foundation.

Buhler-Wilkerson, K. (1985, October). Public health nursing: In sickness or in health? *Am. J. Public Health, 75:*1155–1161.

Buhler-Wilkerson, K. (1987, January/February). Left carrying the bag: Experiments in visiting nursing, 1877–1909. *Nurs. Res., 36:*42–47.

Buka, M. (1976). A survey of nomenclatures and classifications systems. In Gebbie, K. (Ed.), *Summary of the Second National Conference: Classification of Nursing Diagnoses.* St. Louis, National Group for Classification of Nursing Diagnoses.

Bullough, B. (1976, March). The law and the expanding nursing role. *Am. J. Public Health, 66:*249–253.

Carroll-Johnson, R. (Ed.). (1989). *Classification of Nursing Diagnoses: Proceedings of the Eighth Conference.* Philadelphia, J. B. Lippincott.

Chambers, W. (1962, November). Nursing diagnosis. *Am. J. Nurs., 62:*102–104.

Chaska, N. (Ed.). (1978). *The Nursing Profession: Views Through the Mist.* New York, McGraw-Hill.

Christy, T. (1970, August). Portrait of a leader: Annie Warburton Goodrich. *Nurs. Outlook, 18:*46–50.

Clark, M. (1984). *Community Nursing Health Care for Today and Tomorrow.* Reston, VA, Reston.

Codman, E. (1918). *A Study in Hospital Efficiency: The First Five Years.* Boston, Thomas Todd.

Daubert, E. (1979, July). Patient classification system and outcome criteria. *Nurs. Outlook, 27:*450–454.

Diers, D. (1988, Fall). On money. . . . *Image, 20:*122.

Dock, L. (1912a). *A History of Nursing* (Vol. 3). New York, G. P. Putnam's Sons.

Dock, L. (1912b). *A History of Nursing* (Vol. 4). New York, G. P. Putnam's Sons.

Dock, L., & Stewart, I. (1938). *A Short History of Nursing* (4th ed.). New York, G. P. Putnam's Sons.

Donahue, M. (1985). *Nursing the Finest Art: An Illustrated History.* St. Louis, C. V. Mosby.

Douglas, E. (1970). *Margaret Sanger: Pioneer of the Future.* New York, Holt, Rinehart & Winston.

Durand, M. & Prince, R. (1966, April). Nursing diagnosis: Process and decision. *Nurs. Forum, 5:*50–64.

Fitzpatrick, M. (1975). *The National Organization for Public Health Nursing, 1912–1952: Development of a Practice Field.* New York, National League for Nursing.

Freeman, R. (1944). *Techniques of Supervision in Public Health Nursing.* Philadelphia, W. B. Saunders.

Fulmer, H. (1902, March). History of visiting nurse work in America. *Am. J. Nurs., 2:*411–425.

Gebbie, K. (Ed.). (1976). *Summary of the Second National Conference: Classification of Nursing Diagnoses.* St. Louis, National Group for Classification of Nursing Diagnoses.

Gebbie, K., & Lavin, M. (Eds.). (1975). *Classification of Nursing Diagnoses.* St. Louis, C. V. Mosby.

Goodnow, M. (1938). *Nursing History in Brief.* Philadelphia, W. B. Saunders.

Gough, H. (1971). Some reflections on the meaning of psychodiagnosis. *Am. Psychol., 26:*160–167.

Griffith, E. (1986, August). The home health agency: Past, present, and future. *Caring, 5:*12–15.

Hamilton, D. (1988, Fall). Faith and finance. *Image, 20:*124–127.

Hanlon, J., & Pickett, G. (1984). *Public Health Administration and Practice*. St. Louis, Times Mirror/Mosby.

Harris, M. (1988). *Home Health Administration*. Owings Mills, MD, Rynd Communications.

Haupt, A. (1953, January). Forty years of teamwork in public health nursing. *Am. J. Nurs., 53*:81–84.

Hegyvary, S., & Haussmann, R. (1969, November/December). Nursing characteristics and patient progress. *Nurs. Res., 18*:484–501.

Huffman, E. (1972). Disease and operation nomenclature. In Price, E. (Ed.), *Medical Record Management* (6th ed.) (pp. 247–284). Berwyn, IL, Physicians Record Company.

Hurley, M. (Ed.) (1986). *Classification of Nursing Diagnoses: Proceedings of the Sixth National Conference*. St. Louis, C. V. Mosby.

Kim, M., McFarland, G., & McLane, A. (Eds.). (1984) *Classification of Nursing Diagnoses: Proceedings of the Fifth National Conference*. St. Louis, C. V. Mosby.

Kim, M., & Moritz, D. (Eds.) (1982). *Classification of Nursing Diagnoses: Proceedings of the Third and Fourth National Conferences*. New York, McGraw-Hill.

Komorita, N. (1963, December). Nursing diagnosis. *Am. J. Nurs., 63*:83–86.

Marriner, A. (1989). *Nursing Theorists and Their Work* (2nd ed.). St. Louis, C. V. Mosby.

McLane, A. (Ed.) (1987). *Classification of Nursing Diagnoses: Proceedings of the Seventh National Conference*. St. Louis, C. V. Mosby.

Melosh, B. (1982). *The Physician's Hand*. Philadelphia, Temple University Press.

Mundinger, M., & Jauron, G. (1975, February). Developing a nursing diagnosis. *Nurs. Outlook, 23*:94–98.

National League for Nursing (NLN). (1976). *State of the Art in Management Information Systems for Public Health/Community Health Agencies*. New York, National League for Nursing.

National League of Nursing Education. (1922). *Early Leaders of American Nursing*. Syracuse, NY, Gaylord Brothers.

The National Organization for Public Health Nursing (NOPHN). (1926). *Manual of Public Health Nursing*. New York, Macmillan.

Nightingale, F. (1859a). *Notes on Hospitals: Being Two Papers Read Before the National Association for the Promotion of Social Science*. London, John Parker and Son.

Nightingale, F. (1859b). *Notes on Nursing: What It Is and What It Is Not*. London, Harrison.

Nightingale, F. (1860). *Notes on Nursing*. New York, D. Appleton & Company.

The Nursing Development Conference Group (1973). *Concept Formalization in Nursing: Process and Product*. Boston, Little, Brown.

Nutting, M., & Dock, L. (1907a). *A History of Nursing* (Vol. 1). New York, G. P. Putnam's Sons.

Nutting, M., & Dock, L. (1907b). *A History of Nursing* (Vol. 2). New York, G. P. Putnam's Sons.

Rathbone, W. (1890). *Sketch of the History and Progress of District Nursing from its Commencement in the Year 1859 to the Present Date*. New York, Macmillan Company.

Reverby, S. (1987). *Ordered to Care*. Cambridge, Cambridge University Press.

Rosen, G. (1958). *A History of Public Health*. New York, MD Publications.

Sanger, M. (1922a). *The New Motherhood*. London, Jonathan Cape.

Sanger, M. (1922b). *The Pivot of Civilization*. Elmsford, NY, Maxwell Reprint Company.

Secretary's Commission on Nursing (1988a, December). *Secretary's Commission on Nursing:* Final Report (Vol. I). Washington, DC, DHHS.

Secretary's Commission on Nursing (1988b, December). *Secretary's Commission on Nursing: Support Studies & Background Information* (Vol. II). Washington, DC, DHHS.

Shapiro, S. (1967, April). End result measurements of quality of medical care. *Milbank Memorial Fund Q., 45*(1):7–30.

Simmons, D. (1975). Quality assurance in a home health agency. *Quality Assurance—a Joint Venture* (pp. 7–11). New York, National League for Nursing.

Simmons, D. (1980). *A Classification Scheme for Client Problems in Community Health Nursing*. Hyattsville, MD, DHHS, Bureau of Health Professions, Division of Nursing.

Stanhope, M., & Lancaster, J. (1988). *Community Health Nursing: Process and Practice for Promoting Health* (2nd ed.). St. Louis, C. V. Mosby.

Stewart, M., Innes, J., Searls, et al. (Eds.). (1985). *Community Health Nursing in Canada*. Toronto, Ontario, Gage.

They Caught the Torch. (1939). Milwaukee, WI, Will Ross.

Tucker, K., & Hilbert, H. (1934). *Survey of Public Health Nursing*. New York, The Commonwealth Fund.

Wald, L. (1915). *The House on Henry Street*. New York, Henry Holt.

Wald, L. (1934). *Windows on Henry Street*. Boston, Little, Brown.

Welsh, M. (1936, May). What is public health nursing? *Am. J. Nurs., 36*:452–456.

Wilner, D., Walkley, R., & Goerke, L. (1978). *Introduction to Public Health* (7th ed.). New York, Macmillan.

Winslow, C. (1920). The untilled fields of public health. *Science, 51*:23–33.

CHAPTER TWO

*T*he keeping of accurate records will characterize the competent public health nursing agency. Records bear a definite relationship to both cost and quality of nursing service. "The maintenance of accurate records of nursing activities and results is an application of good business methods. The directors of a successful business concern recognize that careful records of their operations are essential in evaluating results and in guiding the course of their organization along sound lines. Fully as necessary are adequate and accurate records for the wise direction of an organization engaged in the care and prevention of sickness and the promotion of public health" (Hiscock, 1927; NOPHN, 1932, p. 61).

The practice of community health nursing has been dynamic and complex since the specialty was established by spirited leaders such as Phoebe and Lillian Wald. The scope of community health nursing practice has been more diverse, independent, and comprehensive than that of any other nursing specialty. Community health nursing practice focuses on clients as individuals and aggregates. Although aggregates can be defined as families and groups, the entire community is also a client of a community health nurse. A practice setting includes the home, clinic, school, worksite, and community. Community health clients range in age from the newborn to the elderly and cover the entire health-illness continuum. Clients include (1) pregnant females, infants, school children, and people of all ages who are healthy, at risk, or may have a disease in an asymptomatic stage; (2) those acutely ill; (3) those chronically ill; and (4) those terminally ill.

CHANGE AND CRISIS

The rate and type of change in the entire community health care system have escalated during the past three decades. Recruitment and retention of well qualified nurses, capable of functioning in staff, supervisory, and administrative positions, have become more difficult. Intelligent, motivated women and men have many career options, often with attractive job responsibilities and benefits.

Rising health care costs are affecting community health agencies as well as other health care providers. Shorter hospital stays associated with diagnosis related groups (DRGs) and other reimbursement constraints are directly influencing the number and acuity of refer-

rals to community health nursing agencies. Throughout the nation, increasing client referrals to these agencies have resulted in a proliferation of the number of agencies and nurses, especially in proportion to the number of nurses employed in acute care settings. As agency referrals, costs, and technology issues are increasing, reimbursement for services is decreasing. Individuals and groups are beginning to address the ethical dilemmas associated with the provision, rationing, and denial of health services. Whereas political trends are influencing the knowledge, practice, and productivity requirements of the individual community health nurse, these trends are affecting administrators and entire agencies even more. Agency instability, and even agency closures, have followed significant, rapid changes in community alliances, competition, governmental regulation, and reimbursement requirements.

How can motivated community health agency managers and staff deal with change and crisis? No single nursing strategy, management style, or system can ensure individual or collective community health nursing excellence and success, a fact recognized by leaders of the past and present. Early in the 1970s, however, Visiting Nurse Association (VNA) of Omaha staff and administrators began to anticipate the critical need for practice, documentation, and data management systems. They channeled their energy into efforts that resulted in the Omaha System.

Various facts and philosophies guided the Omaha System efforts. To make work satisfying, VNA of Omaha and other community health administrators need to reduce uncertainty in the workplace by (1) stabilizing schedules and work groups, (2) providing clear expectations regarding responsibility and performance requirements, (3) articulating expectations, (4) orga-

The Omaha System:
Bridging a Gap in Community Health Nursing

nizing work, (5) developing a delivery system that empowers staff and provides maximum opportunities for job satisfaction, (6) teaching staff to care for themselves and each other, (7) building a strong team, and (8) making it a safe environment for risk-taking (Manthey, 1989).

Professional independence and autonomy are essential (Stewart, Innes, Searl, et al., 1985). Certain characteristics have been associated with high performance individuals, programs, and agencies that are intensely committed to the concept of quality. The following four characteristics are essential for success in a community health environment.

- Vision — must be based on knowledge and clinical expertise. As professionals, individual providers and the entire staff of agencies are responsible for identifying what is truly in the best long-term community health interests of the public and the profession.
- Inspiration — loyalty, communication skills, and the commitment to work well with others within and outside the organization will assist an individual or agency to eliminate barriers that impede continuation and growth.
- Flexibility — an individual and agency must be willing to take risks, reconsider, and change as needed.
- Mobilization — agency survival depends on the ability to implement innovative and creative strategies involving staff, skills, materials, and programs.

NEEDS MET BY THE OMAHA SYSTEM

The growth of the community health industry and predictions of even greater crises in community health nursing prompted the VNA of Omaha staff and management to consider changes within the agency. Beginning in 1970, VNA personnel explored alternative methods and tools related to practice and documentation. Before the decade was over, it was apparent that any new methods and tools must be computer-compatible yet consistent with the community health tradition of a nursing-driven system (Crews, Connolly, Whitted et al., 1986). During the 1980s, the burden of paperwork intensified. Concerns about legal and reimbursement implications of documenting client data and health care services escalated. Furthermore, community health professionals acknowledged the benefits of considering epidemiologic principles in relation to client data and for examining pattern recognition. According to Gruber and Benner, "Pattern recognition is an essential component of nursing expertise" (Gruber & Benner, 1989, p. 503). Increasingly, nurses must make these patterns more legitimate and visible elements of their practice.

Nursing must be able to name itself and to describe what it does in order to function effectively in a world where computerized information is used to establish everything from diagnosis related groups (DRGs) to cardiac output. Until nurses can name what they do and assign a computer code to that name, we may be neither reimbursed nor recognized as a profession with unique skills and knowledge. (American Nurses' Association, 1989, p. 3)

The Omaha System evolved because of 15 years of effort, 7 years of federally funded research, and the combined labors of many health care and data processing professionals. It was developed to consist of the *Problem Classification Scheme, Intervention Scheme,* and *Problem Rating Scale for Outcomes.* The Problem

Classification Scheme is a taxonomy of nursing diagnoses that provides consistent language for collecting, sorting, classifying, documenting, and analyzing data about client concerns. The Intervention Scheme is a taxonomy of community health nursing actions or activities that offers a method of describing services provided to clients. The Problem Rating Scale for Outcomes is an evaluation tool designed to measure client progress in relation to specific problems or nursing diagnoses. The three components of the Omaha System represent a structured, comprehensive approach to community health practice, documentation, and data management. Therefore, the System offers the following six capabilities and characteristics for community health nursing:

- Advances the scientific practice of nursing
- Offers capabilities to quantify community health nursing
- Is practical for general community health application
- Is congruent with the nursing process
- Minimizes redundancy in the client record
- Limits documentation time

The Omaha System offers interrelated benefits to the staff and administrators of community health agencies and to nursing students and faculty members who affiliate with agencies. The Omaha System provides a tool that administrators can use to obtain standardized data. These data can be aggregated and integrated into manual and automated information management systems or systems that combine manual and automated elements. System reports provide a critical source of information to administrators, especially as the requirements for costing data increase.

The Omaha System can and has been used extensively by various professionals. Examples of application involving nurses, physical therapists, social workers, nutritionists, physicians, geriatrician consultants, houseparents, and police officers will be given in this and later chapters. For simplicity, and because nurses continue to represent the largest category of community health agency employees, benefits and application in relation to nursing will be emphasized. The primary benefits that will be described in this chapter include:

- Framework for an integrated practice and documentation system
- A method of organizing and inputting client data into a manual or computerized management information system

A PRACTICE AND DOCUMENTATION SYSTEM

The Omaha System serves as a tool for novice as well as expert community health nurses, other health care professionals, and administrators. As a system of effective feedback loops, the tool provides a structure or framework for those professionals to provide client care and document that care. Such tools are relevant to current professional practice, quality assurance, and legal, productivity, and reimbursement issues.

The need for a precise, uniform, and professionally acceptable method of communication and documentation has become increasingly important. King states, "One of the functions of the registered nurse, according to law, is to observe, record, and report information about patients or clients, including any change in their status. . . . The function involves analysis and integration of data, to making decisions with and for patients through interactions and transactions" (King, 1989, p. 43). As noted by Morrissey-Ross (1988), the primary purpose of the record is to ensure continuity of quality care to the client. Based on that primary purpose and the needs of community health professionals who provide services in the community setting, the record must reflect a holistic model. Medical diagnoses, physicians' orders, and physician communication are important in community health documentation systems. Physicians, however, infrequently document their work in these records. Instead, client records in a community health setting are traditionally designed by and for community health nurses as well as members of other disciplines. Therefore, the client record model typically used in the community health setting is in sharp contrast to the medical model or medical record that is traditionally used in the acute care setting.

Documentation is becoming a key to financial success for all community health services—home visits, school-based care, and clinic services. In relation to productivity, community health personnel must document their actions consistently in a detailed, yet brief, manner. In relation to reimbursement, staff and supervisors must be cognizant of ever changing third-party regulations. Regulations involving home health services and Medicare reimbursement are of special concern. Many reimbursement denials occur after reviewers deem documentation to be inadequate or inappropriate. Medicare reviewers are looking for documented evidence of (1) frequency and type of services provided in relation to referral data and medical diagnoses, (2) homebound status, (3) justification for every visit, (4) skilled services, (5) negative findings, and (6) client responses (Boesch, 1989). The staff can and must record client status and services in a professional manner that is also acceptable to reviewers.

Benefits for New Staff

New community health agency employees or nursing students beginning a community health course often function at the level of novice or advanced beginner (Benner, 1984). These people need to be introduced to the world of community health practice using a nonthreatening, yet comprehensive, approach. Sometimes, new staff nurses have made shared or independent home visits a part of a previous student experience. Often, a new employee has had no exposure to community health practice. A supervisor, staff development coordinator, and peers need to structure the orientation process using a tool such as the Omaha System to provide immediate help to the new employee. A less experienced practitioner must develop or enhance insights, knowledge, and skills rapidly in order to function independently in the community health setting.

Newly employed community health nurses experience some degree of "culture shock." The extent varies in relation to previous personal and professional experiences, especially to the extent that these experiences have involved autonomy and independent decision-making opportunities. Gaining confidence and a feeling of comfort is a time-consuming and even threatening experience for a new employee. Most new practitioners who are functioning as neophytes expect to go through such a process during their early months of employment. Nurses who have developed professional competence and have been functioning at advanced, even expert, levels in settings such as intensive care units may experience culture shock equal to or greater than a novice. Developing basic skills such as locating addresses and gaining entrance into homes and providing service to clients with diverse personal values and lifestyles may be frustrating to the newly employed nurse. The process may be more perplexing or traumatic to an accomplished nurse, causing that nurse to consider resignation or to actually terminate community health employment.

Movement along the proficiency continuum is enhanced through practice and documentation tools such as the Omaha System, tools that new staff find coherent and comprehensible. In all settings, tools are needed to help new staff direct or focus their energy. Furthermore, tools allow new nurses to see the linkages between the nursing process and the realities of the practice setting. The Problem Classification Scheme helps introduce the student, new graduate, and new employee to the world of community health nursing. The Scheme is composed of *Environmental, Psychosocial, Physiological,* and *Health Related Behaviors* Domains; 40 problems, modifiers, and signs/symptoms (see Chapter 5). The Scheme provides a system for streamlining or sorting out essential information, sparing the novice the sensation of drowning in client data. The *categories, targets,* and *client-specific information* of the Intervention Scheme allow the new employee to clearly articulate proposed and completed actions (see Chapter 6). The *Knowledge, Behavior,* and *Status* ratings of the Problem Rating Scale for Outcomes help the new community health nurse focus on client/nurse goals as well as significant, observable, and measurable client changes (see Chapter 7).

Benefits for Experienced Staff and Administrators

Experienced community health agency staff can derive benefits from the practice and documentation framework of the Omaha System. Agency staff include (1) competent, proficient, and expert nurses (Benner, 1984); (2) members of other disciplines; and (3) administrators (see Chapters 5, 6, & 7). Although community health practice has changed dramatically during this century, some aspects have remained constant. "Agony" related to documentation has been described as one such constant (Morrissey-Ross, 1988). As noted by Gardner in 1917:

The subject of record-keeping has probably never been discussed at a convention without some agitated nurse arising to ask if she is expected to neglect her patients in order to write down information about them. . . . Records are kept for two purposes; first as a form of indispensable bookkeeping which will enable those managing the work to know whether or not it is being run on good business principles, and secondly, as a means of gathering data which will give accurate information concerning the various aspect of illness and health. (p. 342)

Specific benefits can be achieved through the Omaha System and other tools. Of concern to both experienced and new employees, these benefits relate to practice, documentation, and management information systems. Furthermore, these benefits reflect the practice-based origins of the Omaha System and the continuation of that philosophy. Agency staff, supervisors, and management have similar, yet different, data needs. Moreover, their data needs are not totally compatible. If agency personnel are willing to work collaboratively, the following benefits can be achieved:

1. Allow staff nurses to track client care over time in a simple, efficient manner.
2. Allow supervisors to monitor care provided by one nurse to one client as well as multiple nurses to multiple clients.
3. Allow agency management and external personnel to evaluate delivery of care as a basis for diverse decisions.

The Omaha System is a comprehensive, yet simple, documentation framework. It meets the generally accepted professional and legal standards for a recording system. According to Stanhope and Lancaster (1988):

Records provide complete information about the client, indicate the extent and quality of services being rendered, resolve legal issues in malpractice suits, and provide information for education and research. (p. 245)

The Omaha System can help narrow the discrepancy between the quality of care that is delivered and care that is documented (Schmele, 1986). When implemented in an agency whose personnel are willing to make the commitment to quality documentation, use of the Omaha System will produce a client record that is:

- Comprehensive
- Brief
- Precise
- Timely
- Essential, but secondary to service

The Omaha System offers standard language to enhance community health practice and improve the quality of documentation. Uniformity of client records was of great concern to community health nurses in 1934 (Tucker & Hilbert, 1934). More recently, community health nurses, especially supervisors and administrators, are recognizing the importance of language and communication skills. Because the staff members of most agencies are functioning in a multidisciplinary environment, effective communication with others regarding client services is crucial. The Omaha System provides common language that has meaning to all disciplines and enhances collaboration.

Improving the clarity, precision, and conciseness of the client record increases that record's potential to serve as a professional and legal documentation trail for others to follow. Those who analyze the documentation trail can identify meaningful relationships among the data, especially when those data are uniform and quantified. Analysis is part of the evaluation process and involves decision-making and critical thinking.

The admission and dismissal decisions made by home health and public health staff on a daily basis provide another example of essential, complex, critical thinking. These decisions are increasingly regulated by reimbursement systems. Too often clients can be served for only short periods of time even though their health problems involve a high degree of acuity, are severe, and have developed over many years. Concurrently, the use of the Omaha System and other tools is becoming critical as visionary agency managers and administrators address issues such as economy, efficiency, and productivity to ensure their agency's continued operation. Faculty are beginning to recognize that nursing students in all programs must be exposed to these issues in order to cope with the practice realities that they will encounter after graduation. Use of the Omaha System offers benefits that include:

- A practice framework
- A standard terminology
- Precise recording
- An evaluation method
- Efficiency
- Improved reimbursement

Benefits for Agencies

This book is based on Omaha System experiences involving VNA of Omaha clients, staff, supervisors, and administrators. In order to offer a wide variety of perspectives and experiences, many chapters include brief contributions written by people not employed at the VNA of Omaha. The following paragraphs are such contributions, illustrating the similarities and differences experienced by people who implemented the Omaha System in Wisconsin and in New Jersey. JoAnn Weidmann and Helen North describe the value of the Problem Classification Scheme in an agency where staff provide public health and home health services; Paula Cell and Anne Becker delineate their experiences in an agency that offers home health services.

A FRAMEWORK FOR PRACTICE: WISCONSIN EXPERIENCES*

by JOANN WEIDMANN, RN, BSN, Director of Public Health Nurses, Waukesha County Health Department, Waukesha, WI; and HELEN NORTH, RN, BSN, Public Health Nurse Consultant, Wisconsin Division of Health, Department of Health and Social Services, Milwaukee, WI

. . . Until the mid 1970s, the nurses in the Waukesha County Health Department, Waukesha, Wisconsin, recorded observations, findings, and nursing care in their own individual ways. A format was recommended but compliance was low. As a result the nursing records were lengthy, dissimilar, and unstructured. In the hope of finding ways to improve these unwieldy records, late in 1974 two agency nursing supervisors attended workshop on nursing diagnosis and record audit.

There they learned that other nurses were beginning to study more systematized recording methods. Following the workshop, an audit committee was formed to study the agency's current recording practices and to devise a better system. Input from the staff nurses was solicited throughout the change process. Committee members studied the work of many nursing theorists . . . and familiarized themselves with the concept of nursing diagnosis. They then explored ways to introduce the concept to the staff of 21 public health nurses.

. . . The nursing director looked for a format to more uniformly record nursing diagnoses. The early nursing diagnoses from the National Conferences, which were to become known as North American Nursing Diagnosis Association, or NANDA, labels, were then incorporated with agency gener-

---

*The following contribution is taken from Weidmann, J., and North, H. (1987). Implementing the Omaha classification system in a public health agency. *Nursing Clinics of North America*, 22 (4), 971–979.

ated labels. However, this combination led the nurses to an even more time-consuming, diverse, and variously structured recording mixture. The NANDA list proved inadequate for public health nursing because it was too "acute care" oriented.

In 1981, the Omaha Classification Scheme was presented at a meeting of midwestern nursing directors, which the Waukesha public health nursing director attended. The system had been developed and tested in four community health nursing agencies. It appeared to have the potential to standardize and systematize nursing diagnosis in community health, replacing the NANDA labels in that setting.

However, since the NANDA list appeared to be the "officially" evolving taxonomy, there was concern about implementing a different system that would divert interest or focus from the NANDA effort. Those fears were set aside when several nursing leaders, recognized for their work with nursing diagnosis, were consulted. It was their opinion that nursing diagnosis was in such an early evolutionary phase that use and testing of the Omaha labels would be very appropriate.

. . .The advantages of this coded, problem-oriented nursing diagnosis recording system versus the free-lance method it replaced are that the Omaha Classification System:

1. Standardizes terminology, facilitating understanding for all record users
2. Saves time in recording nursing observations and client problems
3. Enables nurses to plan appropriate interventions based on observed, documented data

4. Provides dates for expected client progress
5. Identifies client progress for both client and nurse
6. Validates case closure
7. Enables audit of care for quality assurance
8. Provides clear and understandable problem identification to assist in program planning.

An appealing aspect of the Omaha Classification System is that it provides an open system. . . . Nurses can develop a diagnostic label for observations when the system does not provide one specific to the signs and symptoms encountered.

Another very positive feature of the Omaha Classification System is that it can be used with existing agency records. A major shortcoming of the Omaha Classification System is that there are not, as yet, any standard nursing interventions or standard care plans.

. . . During the implementation period there were frequent opportunities for agency personnel to have dialogue with nurses from other agencies about Omaha Classification System and NANDA labels. Similarities and dissimilarities were identified. To explain and clarify the dynamics of the Omaha Classification System versus the NANDA taxonomy, in 1985 Helen North correlated the Omaha Classification System list of labels with the 1984 National Conference list. . . .

Even though there is much congruence between the separately evolving systems, the correlation findings emphasize the need for continued development and refinement efforts on both systems.

A FRAMEWORK FOR PRACTICE: NEW JERSEY EXPERIENCES

by PAULA CELL, RN, MPH, Administrator, Visiting Nurse Association, Inc., Trenton, NJ;
and ANNE BECKER, RN, BSN, Coordinator of Quality Assurance and Allied Health, Visiting Nurse Association, Inc., Trenton, NJ

The 53-year-old Visiting Nurse Association of Trenton (NJ) is a diversified, progressive community agency with a tradition of commitment to excellence. Agency programs include (1) traditional reimbursable skilled and paraprofessional services, (2) grant-supported programs such as case management, (3) nurse-managed treatment of incontinence, (4) meals-at-home, and (5) nonreimbursable private pay care. In 1973, the Trenton VNA was one of the first agencies in the country to be accredited by the National League of Nursing. In 1983, when the Home Health Agency Assembly of New Jersey initiated implementation of the Problem Classification Scheme (PCS) in home health agencies throughout the state, the VNA was the second agency to participate. Since that initial exposure, agency staff have viewed the PCS as an ideal structure for focusing nursing care. The PCS has provided a "framework for practice."

The agency data base was refined by 1987, providing a good structure for standard and consistent identification of client problems. Tools used by the staff to monitor quality were outdated because they were designed for structure and process evaluation with no emphasis on outcomes. There-

fore, VNA staff focused attention on the development of a broad-based Quality Assurance Program that used the PCS as the base for establishing professional practice standards against which client outcomes could be measured. The newly hired Quality Assurance Coordinator worked closely with the Director of Nursing and a graduate student to develop, study, and design a tool that would ultimately produce practice standards. Although these three nurses considered developing a totally research-based tool, constraints dictated that the opinions of experienced staff would be used to supplement empirical data.

A clinical record audit was conducted to determine the type of care delivered, nursing interventions performed, and client problems most frequently identified. A tool was developed to sort the data according to medical diagnoses. From this assessment of 48 records, it was evident that most VNA clients had medical conditions that fell into six major categories: acute cardiac, chronic cardiac, respiratory, gastrointestinal, orthopedic, and cancer. Although some client problems identified were specific to medical diagnoses, other problems and interventions were common to all clients in the sample. Thus, these client problems were used to develop minimum care standards that formed the basis of the generic care plan and the client record audit materials. The care plan was tested by a small group of experienced community health nursing staff during a 6-month period.

The final standard care plan generally reflects the agency's client population, its particular standards of client care, and its commitment to achieving a consistent level of documentation. The plan may be used independently or in conjunction with supplemental care plans based on other nursing diagnoses from the Problem Classification Scheme. Recently, the care plan was revised to incorporate Knowl-edge, Behavior, and Status ratings from the Problem Rating Scale for Outcomes. The agency now has a tool to collect outcome data. These data, when combined with structure and process data, complete the framework for practice.

The development of standard nursing care plans using the PCS has enabled the VNA staff to accurately describe the true domain of nursing practice in home care. Implementation has resulted in greater accountability for professional practice and has reduced the burden of documentation. This achievement is significant for the VNA of Trenton and could be of value to other home care agencies.

A MANAGEMENT INFORMATION SYSTEM

The Omaha System offers a method of organizing and entering client data into a manual or automated community health agency management information system. This benefit is comparable in importance to a framework for an integrated practice and documentation system. During the last several decades, the requirements for comprehensive, accurate, and timely health-related data have increased dramatically. Romano (1987) noted that these data are "prerequisite for quality and continuity of care, for the documentation and collection of fees, for the effective management of health institutions, for the protection of public health, and for the conduct of biomedical, epidemiological, and evaluative research" (p. 99).

Increasingly, administrators of public and nonprofit community health agencies realize that technologic support systems are essential to manage and control operations (Knollmueller, 1985), especially when many nurses in clinical settings spend 40% of their time managing and communicating information (Zielstorff, McHugh, & Clinton, 1988). For many community health agencies, 40% may be a conservative estimate. ". . . the modern nursing role is to take the explosion of new information and find new and better ways to deliver care. Nursing has a role of innovator in the 1990s" (Romano, 1990, p. 99).

Changing Data Needs

Most community health agency administrators are recognizing the need for more sophisticated management information systems as one or more of the following four conditions emerges: First, the relationship between the agency and the Medicare fiscal intermediary grows more burdensome. More claims are being denied or procedural demands are straining agency personnel resources. If intermediary mandates require new forms, electronic billing, or a radically revised reporting structure, the agency must comply. Perhaps more than any other single factor, governmental insistence on more detailed accountability has stimulated community health agency directors to upgrade their management information systems to the point that computerization is a necessity. The requirements of other third parties such as insurance companies, health maintenance organizations, or preferred provider organizations have also influenced the trend toward more sophisticated client management information systems.

Second, agency accounting practices may be inadequate in relation to current requirements. Cash flow may be restricted and the budgetary process may be requiring inordinate amounts of time. For most agencies, standard accounting practices require some degree of automation. The number and comprehensiveness of the required internal and external audits have grown considerably in recent years. Tightened budgets, stringent Internal Revenue Service (IRS) rulings, and demands for more precision and detail in accounting procedures are all serving to make the exacting nature of computers more of a necessity than a luxury.

Third, the effectiveness and productivity of agency primary care delivery staff may have eroded because of the growing demands for documentation required by a growing bureaucracy. The practice of nursing has changed substantially over the years, but one thing has remained constant: few in the profession have much respect for the time spent on paperwork, a disparaging term often denoting anything other than the direct delivery of care. Any method that can decrease this load would pay substantial dividends in morale as well as money (Morrissey-Ross, 1988).

Finally, marketing decisions and strategic plans made by agency personnel may have gone awry. Plans may have been aborted. Rapid changes in regulations, legislation, and political coalitions make past decisions obsolete. For agency growth, and even survival, managers must have current, accurate, and complete information. The manager's need to know, while not insatiable, grows with each added challenge in the areas of marketing and competition as well as regulation and cost.

A management information system, whether computer-based or manual, is only a tool. A system can impair the data management process or it can improve it. A well designed management information system offers the following benefits to community health agency administrators and staff:

1. It facilitates organization and tracking of client care data

2. It provides the statistical and predictive data base that can enable managers to make informed decisions
3. It supplies a foundation for administrators to build a more powerful structure that can support growth in clients, personnel, and programs
4. It expedites the agency billing process and reduces the number of errors
5. It smooths and speeds agency reporting to third-party payors and accelerates payment.

Automation

Advances in technology have contributed to the advent of the information revolution permeating industrialized societies. Such advances in technology may be the most important trend influencing nurses and other health care providers today. The advent of the informatics era has resulted in altered patterns of (1) direct client care, (2) communication, (3) data availability and retrieval, (4) quality assurance programs, and (5) health care costs. These altered patterns suggest the need for improving practice, documentation, and data management by using tools such as the Omaha System.

Most nurses recognize the lasting significance of computer applications and are attempting, although with some hesitation, to become familiar with the field. Some nurses are willing to accept the "role of innovator" suggested by Romano. This interest represents a recent change.

The importance of rational, systematic, and economical use of information has not always been recognized in nursing. Laudable as nursing concern has been for the care of patients and families, nurses have tended to be myopic when it came to influencing the system of which they are critical components. Because of the economic benefits to be realized, it was hospital administration that introduced computer technology into the health care system; medicine and nursing were slower to realize the benefits that could accrue to practice through the use of computerized information systems. But recognition of the value of these tools has been dawning, and more and more nurses are developing interest and expertise in this specialized field. (Werley & Grier, 1981, p. ix)

The trend to automate is so significant that computerization will soon be essential for delivery and management of client care regardless of setting (Zielstorff et al., 1988). A 1962 American Hospital Association study found that 39 hospitals were using digital computers (Veazie & Dankmyer, 1977). By 1976, the number of hospitals that rented, leased, or owned data processing equipment had increased to almost 4,000. During the 1980s, automation escalated in both acute care and community health settings. The greatest proliferation of hardware, however, was in personal computers, while interest in mainframe and minicomputers declined. Increasingly, personal computers were integrated into the primary data bases of many institutions (Packer, 1987). A 1990 review included a description of the specific applications that facilitate nursing practice and documentation in six large hospital-based systems (Hendrickson & Kovner, 1990).

The intensified effects of computerization on nursing are evident in nursing literature. As early as 1972, Wesseling described an experimental attempt to automate nursing history and care plans, a concept that was innovative and unique in nursing literature. Zielstorff (1980) identified three reasons for nurses to be interested in computers: (1) computers are indeed a valuable resource for nursing in terms of improved patient care, (2) computers can serve as a catalyst in bringing about positive changes in the practice and profession of nursing, and (3) computer systems will be developed for nurses by non-nurses if nurses are not involved. The number of articles and degree of sophistication in those articles are escalating; most nursing journals include one or more computer-related articles in each issue. When *Computers in Nursing* was initiated in 1982, it was a newsletter-type publication. It is now a standard-sized journal, published six times a year. The contrast between Zielstorff's 1975 and 1985 publications emphasizes the rapid growth of the field.

Many community health administrators have computerized at least a portion of their operations due to the effects of the information revolution and the increasingly pressing need to organize records and analyze data. Zielstorff (1985) made a strong case for computerization and stated, "the increasingly complex financial environment, reporting requirements of outside agencies, communication needs of an expanded health care team, and explosion of knowledge related to all facets of patient care have overpowered our antiquated information management systems" (p. 22).

Computers and computer experts must have concrete, concise, and objective data. The three components of the Omaha System were designed to assist in producing such client and provider data. Computers offer limitless potential to programmers for collating and linking related data, enabling programmers to produce significant statistical and graphic outputs. Nurses must realize that "until voice recognition technology and natural language processing are perfected, there will always have to be compromises in how much data can be structured to take most advantage of computer capabilities while imposing the least burden on the clinician" (Zielstorff et al., 1988, p. 33). Relating care to cost and to staffing are significant current concerns noted frequently in publications. Thus, computers offer users the potential to analyze data in diverse ways, including the application of an epidemiologic approach to client data.

Costs of Automation

Cost is a crucial factor that community health agency administrators must consider in relation to automation. The major expenses incurred when changing any operating procedures, whether or not the changes relate to computerization, involve personnel, time, training, and job disruption. Although computer hardware and software do represent a major expense for an agency, the cost of computer power is on a steep, downward spiral, a spiral that is expected to continue. "As costs go down, capital expense will become less of an issue and buyers will concentrate on acquiring the most flexible, well-tested, and powerful system available for the money" (Zielstorff, 1985, p. 25).

The costs of a totally or partially automated versus a manual system must be weighed against anticipated benefits of a computerized system. Such benefits may include:

■ Greater timeliness and accessibility of data
■ The ability to combine data rapidly into multiple formats for analysis
■ Time savings for service delivery, management, and support staff
■ Improved staff morale

VNA Information System

A management information system design was delineated by VNA of Omaha staff in conjunction with the Omaha System research project (Fig. 2–1). The purpose of the system design is to enhance efficient handling of information required by community health agency personnel as they administer the care of clients and manage the business affairs of the agency. Personnel, financial, and client data are essential system inputs. Use of the system allows for integration and sorting of data elements into client, service, personnel, and financial management data sets. Unique client and employee information is sorted into the client management data set, whereas aggregate client and staffing in-

formation is sorted into the service management data set. Employee salary and benefit information is sorted into the personnel data set; total agency income and disbursement information is sorted into the fiscal management data set. Elements from the four data sets can then be reintegrated to produce timely documentation that includes client records and agency reports. Such records and reports, critical to the agency's existence, are used by staff, supervisors, and management.

System Modules

The management information system design consists of 11 modules. Unlike the structure of most community health agency management information systems, the client record comprises the pivotal module. The Omaha System enables coding of client record data from the referral through the dismissal process. Coded client data are combined with personnel and agency data, becoming an integral part of the total information system. Thus, the system is useful for management of client care as well as agency business affairs. The remaining 10 modules are part of typical management information systems and are described below.

The general ledger module consists of a chart of accounts used to record all the financial transactions of the agency. Transactions flow into the module from the billing/accounts receivable, accounts payable, and personnel/payroll modules in the form of journal entries, cash disbursements, cash receipts, and purchase orders. Information flows out via a trial balance, balance sheet, and statement of revenues and expenses.

The billing process is the initial step used to create

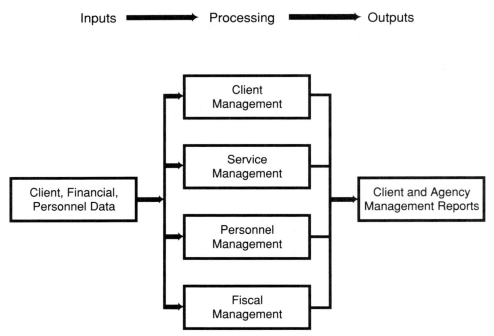

FIGURE 2–1 ■ The VNA Information System. This diagram shows the flow of information as it enters the system and is processed to produce client and agency reports.

data for the billing/accounts receivable module. Generation of client bills requires information regarding who provided the service, the date and time of service, supplies used, and the type of service provided. When the billing process is complete, the charges generated are grouped, totaled, and transferred to the general ledger. In addition, the detailed data of each client account is transferred to the appropriate accounts receivable file. (Accounts receivable files indicate the money owed to the agency by clients and third-party payors.) Information flows out via a monthly statement of each account and an aged trial balance that lists the amount owed by each client and the length of time the balance has been outstanding.

The accounts payable module is designed to handle all agency expenditures except payroll and petty cash. The module has the capability to (1) assign vendor codes, (2) produce reports of purchases by vendor, (3) produce checks to pay for agency purchases, (4) distribute costs of purchases to the appropriate accounts, (5) produce lists of invoices and scheduled payment data to assist in cash flow planning and establishing an audit trail, (6) produce a check register, (7) process adjustments, and (8) provide detailed records of all transactions.

The personnel/payroll module is used to produce payroll checks and to handle related payroll deductions. Payroll costs are distributed and recorded in the appropriate general ledger accounts. In addition to the basic function of producing reports summarizing gross salaries and deductions, a more sophisticated payroll/personnel module generates reports that analyze employee productivity and cost accounting.

The primary functions of the inventory/supply module are to (1) allow agency personnel to manage inventory of supplies, (2) assign a monetary value to the existing quantity of supplies, and (3) assign a monetary value to supplies withdrawn from inventory and used in provision of client service. The module accepts data from accounts payable and produces data for increasing inventory. In addition, it transfers disbursement of supplies to the billing system and provides a running balance of type, amount, and dollar value of inventory.

The durable medical equipment module is designed for use by agencies that rent and sell durable medical equipment. The module tracks items rented to clients and costs recoverable under various third-party pay arrangements. The module interfaces with the clinical record and the billing/accounts receivable modules to produce reports required by various third-party payors.

The system maintenance, report generator, and user help modules interface with all other modules of the management information system. The system maintenance module is used to update information utilized by the other modules. Because the report generator module interfaces with all files in the system, agency personnel can use it to create reports required on a one time only basis. The user help module provides detailed on-line operating instructions for each module within the management information system.

Reports

Data abstracted from client records are essential for many reports generated within community health agencies. The major types of reports involving client data can be classified as individual and aggregate. Such statistical reports are useful in measuring and describing services provided and in relating the services to recognized community needs and resources. While agency preferences vary, as do local, state, and federal requirements, many similarities exist. Typical purposes of community health nursing reports identified in 1977 are still pertinent today. They are:

- To describe the characteristics of the caseload at time of admission, while under care, and at time of discharge
- To learn what tasks are faced by the professional staff and what skills are used in accomplishing them
- To set various standards for administrative control
- To provide information for use by mass media
- To solicit financial support from public and private sources
- To assess the impact of proposed and new legislation on agency caseload
- To become aware of the need for new programs and to evaluate them after inception
- To assess changes in patient condition while under agency care (National League for Nursing, 1977, p. 26)

The focus of an individual report is the service provided to a specific client. The report may consist of the entire clinical record or portions of the record. Use of the Omaha System to document services in the client record produces two benefits relative to review of records by external sources: first, the clinical components assist the practitioner in differentiating and recording pertinent data that can present a clear picture of client status and care provided. Second, the clinical components use standard language that can facilitate understanding on the part of reviewers.

Individual client data are required by third-party payors, utilization review committees, peer review organizations, and licensing and accrediting bodies. Occasionally, client records are subpoenaed by attorneys as legal evidence. Examination of agency records by these external reviewers often results in important decisions that affect the agency's public image, competitive advantages, and financial strength.

Aggregate reports use data collected on groups of clients or staff as a method of providing information about agency services. Traditionally, these reports have reflected client data based on periods of time and client demographics, as well as on types and amounts of services provided. Examples of these reports include (1) clients by age and sex, (2) visits by medical diagnosis, (3) visits by discipline, (4) cost by discipline, (5) clients by care provider, and (6) clients by program.

The traditional approach to aggregate reporting does not fully describe the client's status or the health care provider's interventions. Use of the Omaha System enables coding of data regarding client problems, client status, and interventions. Data can be compiled into reports that provide a more definitive picture of clients and services. Reports can be generated to depict (1) urgency and complexity of client needs and (2) changes in client status over the course of care. Examples of these reports include client problems by age, interventions by problem, and client status related to length of stay.

Aggregate reports are required by three different groups of reviewers. First, organizations that certify, accredit, and license community health agencies require statistical reports related to client demographics, agency services, and reimbursement. Second, other individuals and groups outside the agency are interested in statistical reports, including Health Officers, Boards of Health, Boards of Directors, and professional and utilization review committees. Finally, aggregate reports serve as a vital tool for agency administrators and managers. Statistical data are used in (1) evaluating the effectiveness of services, (2) long- and short-term planning, (3) designing marketing strategies, (4) determining personnel and other resource needs, and (5) developing inservice education programs for staff.

HEALTH CARE COSTS

The costs of health care in the US have risen rapidly during the last decade, a phenomenon that also has occurred in other countries. Efforts to slow the rise in those costs led to an emphasis on cost-effectiveness, cost-containment, and productivity as well as to the proposal of new reimbursement systems. "The inability to define, compare, and contrast the use of nursing services frequently is cited as a distinct concern in managing the cost of health care" (Lant, 1988, p. 325). As early as 1975, Jelinek and Dennis developed the following definition: "The concept of productivity encompasses both the effectiveness of nursing care, which relates to its quality and appropriateness, and the efficiency of care, which is production of nursing output with minimal resource waste" (p. 3).

A prospective pay Medicare reimbursement system (PPS) was established in 1983 for hospitals. The system was designed to slow the growth rate of federally reimbursed hospital costs. The implementation of the PPS system resulted in a rapid shift from inpatient to community-based care. The success of prospective pay is slowing the growth rate of hospital costs. Hospice care providers, durable medical equipment suppliers, and some skilled nursing facilities and nursing homes are now subject to some form of prospective payment. Home health care is one of the few forms of health care that does not currently have some form of prospective pay for Medicare clients. Some experts predict that home health care will have some sort of prospective pay system within the next 5 years. Others predict that home health agencies will simply experience increasing regulation and reimbursement constraints, at least partially related to outcome effectiveness initiatives.

Most experts do not believe that a prospective pay reimbursement system based on medical diagnosis would be efficient for home health agencies. The proportion of labor costs in the budget of community health agencies exceeds that of hospitals. The amount and type of home care services required for a particular client tend to depend more on the severity of illness and the client's functional limitations and support system than on the illness itself (Staebler, 1988). The variables affecting home care costs are less subject to control than are variables affecting hospital costs (Martin & Scheet, 1985).

Public health agencies and administrators, like their counterparts in the home health industry, have experienced reimbursement constraints and financial crises in the last decade. Federal block grant funds, traditionally distributed to local and county health departments by state health departments, have not grown in proportion to population changes or escalating health care needs. Simultaneously, elected officials have increased demands upon administrators. Recently, officials from two Nebraska counties conducted a competitive bidding process before awarding the contracts for public health nursing services. Many experienced public health staff nurses, supervisors, administrators, and educators are alarmed about current and future programs; they are recognizing that they need better methods to interpret the contributions of community health nurses to the total community.

Public health professionals are told with increasing frequency to justify their existence. In 1962, Roberts asked, "How Effective is Public Health Nursing?" Many professionals and nonprofessionals are asking related questions at the present time. The extensive research conducted by Olds and associates produced findings that supported the value of the public health nurse. Both research and documentation are becoming critical to justifying current or increased levels of funding.

Use of the Omaha System enables agency administrators to accurately identify case mix based on nursing diagnoses in the domains of environment and psychosocial and health-related behaviors as well as physiologic status. Specifically, the Problem Rating Scale for Outcomes can provide data relative to the severity of clients' health-illness circumstances. Finally, use of the Intervention Scheme can provide accurate data regarding the types of services provided. When combined with data regarding cost, information gained through use of the Omaha System can be of vital importance to agency administrators in determining costs of community health care. Such interrelated data sets as the three just described can become the basis for administrators and researchers to prove the value of community health nursing services to third-party payors, politicians, and the public.

SUMMARY

Tools such as the Omaha System have been developed to generate client and provider data in ways that are timely, comprehensive, and logical. These data must meet basic professional, management, and legal standards, all increasingly critical to the continuation and growth of community health agencies. Although the specific data management needs of staff, supervisors, and administrators differ, generally they are related. The Omaha System is a tool that provides agency personnel with (1) a framework for an integrated practice and documentation system and (2) a method of organizing and entering client data into a manual or computerized management information system.

Community health nurses from Wisconsin and New Jersey described their experiences with the Omaha System and identified specific benefits to their agencies and staff members. Benefits included the ability of the staff to focus their documentation on the most pertinent data and to increase professional accountability of the staff.

REFERENCES

American Nurses' Association (1989). *Classification Systems for Describing Nursing Practice.* Kansas City, MO.

Benner, P. (1984). *From Novice to Expert.* Menlo Park, CA, Addison-Wesley.

Boesch, D. (Ed.) (1989, February). Prevent claims denials with effective documentation. *Hosp. Home Health, 6:*13–16.

Crews, C., Connolly, K., Whitted, P., et al. (1986, January/February). Computerized central intake: Streamlining community health-care admissions. *Nurs. Econom., 4:*31–36.

Gardner, M. (1917). *Public Health Nursing.* New York, Macmillan.

Gruber, M., & Benner, P. (1989, April). A dialogue with excellence: The power of certainty. *Am. J. Nurs., 89:*502–503.

Hendrickson, G., & Kovner, C. (1990, January/February). Effects of computers on nursing resource use: Do computers save nurses time? *Comput. Nurs., 8:*16–22.

Jelinek, R., & Dennis, L. (1976, November). *A Review and Evaluation of Nursing Productivity* (Vols. I, II, & III). DHEW Publication No. (HRA) 77-15. Bethesda, MD, US DHEW.

King, I. (1989). King's systems framework. In Henry, B., Arndt, C., DiVincenti, M., et al. (Eds.), *Dimensions of Nursing Administration: Theory, Research, Education, and Practice* (p. 43). Boston, Blackwell.

Knollmueller, R. (1985, January). The growth and development of homecare: From no-tech to high tech. *Caring, 4:*3–8.

Lant, T. (1988). Use of the nursing minimum data set to determine nursing care cost. In Werley, H., & Lang, N. (Eds.), *Identification of the Nursing Minimum Data Set* (pp. 325–333). New York, Springer.

Manthey, M. (1989). What satisfies nurses enough to keep them? In Glover, S. (Ed.), *Recruitment and Retention* (Vol. 1) (pp. 61–71). Baltimore, Williams & Wilkins.

Martin, K., & Scheet, N. (1985). The Omaha system: Implications for costing community health nursing. In Shaffer, F. (Ed.), *Costing Out Nursing: Pricing Our Product.* New York, National League for Nursing.

Morrissey-Ross, M. (1988, June). Documentation: If you haven't written it, you haven't done it. *Nurs. Clin. North Am., 23:*363–371.

National League for Nursing (1977). *Statistical Reporting in Home and Community Health Services.* New York.

The National Organization of Public Health Nursing (NOPHN) (1932). *Principles and Practices in Public Health Nursing Including Cost Analysis.* New York, Macmillan.

Packer, C. (1987, February 20). Information management. *Hospitals,* 98.

Roberts, D. (1962, July). How effective is public health nursing? *Am. J. Public Health, 52:*1077–1083.

Romano, C. (1987, May/June). Privacy, confidentiality, and security of computerized systems. *Comput. Nurs., 5:*99–104.

Romano, C. (1990, May/June). Innovation: The promise and the perils for nursing and information technology. *Comput. Nurs., 8:*99–104.

Schmele, J. (1986, July/August). Teaching nurses how to improve their documentation. *Home Healthcare Nurse, 4:*6–10.

Staebler, R. (1988, February). Hospital DRGs: What do they mean for home care? *Caring, 7:*29–31.

Stanhope, M., & Lancaster, J. (1988). *Community Health Nursing: Process and Practice for Promoting Health.* St. Louis, C. V. Mosby.

Stewart, M., Innes, J., Searls, S., et al. (Eds.) (1985). *Community Health Nursing in Canada.* Toronto, Ontario, Gage.

Tucker, K., & Hilbert, H. (1934). *Survey of Public Health Nursing.* New York, The Commonwealth Fund.

Veazie, S., & Dankmyer, T. (1977, October). HISs, MISs, DBMSs: Sorting out the letters. *Hospitals, 51*(16):80–84.

Weidmann, J., & North, H. (1987, December). Implementing the Omaha classification system in a public health agency. *Nurs. Clin. North Am., 22:*971–979.

Werley, H., & Grier, M. (Eds.) (1981). *Nursing Information Systems.* New York, Springer.

Zielstorff, R. (Ed.) (1980). *Computers in Nursing.* Rockville, MD, Aspen.

Zielstorff, R. (1985, February). Cost effectiveness of computerization in nursing practice and administration. *J. Nurs. Admin., 15:*22–26.

Zielstorff, R. (1988). Considerations in data capture, storage, and retrieval for the nursing minimum data set. In Werley, H., & Lang, N. (Eds.), *Identification of the Nursing Minimum Data Set* (pp. 67–76). New York, Springer.

Zielstorff, R., McHugh, M., & Clinton, J. (1988). *Computer Design Criteria for Systems That Support the Nursing Process.* Kansas City, MO, American Nurses' Association.

BIBLIOGRAPHY

Ahmadi, K. (1990). The American health-care "system": A structural nightmare. In Wold, S. (Ed.), *Community Health Nursing: Issues and Topics* (pp. 57–79). Norwalk, CT, Appleton & Lange.

Andersen, E., & McFarlane, J. (1988). *Community as Client: Application of the Nursing Process.* Philadelphia, J. B. Lippincott.

Avillion, A., & Mirgon, B. (1989). Quality assurance and home health care. In *Quality Assurance in Rehabilitation Nursing* (pp. 151–178). Rockville, MD, Aspen.

Aydelotte, M. (1987, May/June). Nursing's preferred future. *Nurs. Outlook, 35:*114–120.

Barkauskas, V. (1983, May). Effectiveness of public health nurse home visits to primiparous mothers and their infants. *Am. J. Public Health, 73:*573–580.

Berwick, D. (1989, January 5). Sounding board: Continuous improvement as an ideal in health care. *New Engl. J. Med., 320:*53–56.

Bocchino, C. (1990, March/April). An interview with Stuart H. Altman and Uwe E. Reinhardt. *Nurs. Econom., 8:*72–82.

Booth, R. (1985, January/February). Financing mechanisms for health care: Impact on nursing services. *J. Prof. Nurs., 1:*34–40.

Branch, L., Wetle, T., Scherr, P., et al. (1988, March). A prospective study of incident comprehensive medical home care use among the elderly. *Am. J. Public Health, 78:*255–259.

Brennan, P., & Romano, C. (1987, December). Computers and nursing diagnoses: Issues in implementation. *Nurs. Clin. North Am., 22:*935–941.

Brett, J. (1989). Outcome indicators of quality care. In Henry, B., Arndt, C., DiVincenti, M., et al. (Eds.), *Dimensions of Nursing Administration: Theory, Research, Education, and Practice* (pp. 353–369). Boston, Blackwell.

Buday, R. (1984, November). Making your way through that computer decision. *Home Health Age, 2:*15–22.

Burns, J., Fox, A., Shelby, I., et al. (1987, April). The survival of the community health nurse in a Medicare environment. *Caring, 6:*81–83.

Caserta, J. (1987, September/October). People, not paper. *Home Healthcare Nurse, 5:*1.

Chapman, C. (1988, June). Of mice and Merle. *Am. J. Nurs., 88:*938.

Deming, W. (1986). *Out of the Crisis*. Cambridge, MA, Massachusetts Institute of Technology.

Diers, D. (1988, Fall). On money. . . . *Image, 20*:122.

Drucker, P. (1985). *Innovation and Entrepreneurship: Practice and Principles*. New York, Harper & Row.

Edwardson, S. (1989). Productivity measurement. In Henry, B., Arndt, C., DiVincenti, M., et al. (Eds.), *Dimensions of Nursing Administration* (pp. 371–385). Boston, Blackwell.

Ervin, N. (1982, July/August). Public health nursing practice—An administrator's view. *Nurs. Outlook, 30*:390–394.

Freeman, R., & Heinrich, J. (1981). *Community Health Nursing Practice* (2nd ed.). Philadelphia, W. B. Saunders.

Gardner, J. (1961). *Excellence: Can We be Equal and Excellent, Too?* New York, Harper & Brothers.

Gebbie, K., & Lavin, M. (1974, February). Classifying nursing diagnoses. *Am. J. Nurs., 74*:250–253.

Glancey, T., Brooks, G., & Vaughan, V. (1990, March/April). Hospital information systems. *Comput. Nurs., 8*:55–59.

Glover, S. (Ed.) (1989, March). *Recruitment and Retention* (Vol. 1). Baltimore, Williams & Wilkins.

Griffith, E. (1986, August). The home health agency: Past, present, and future. *Caring, 5*:12–15.

Grobe, S. (1984a). *Computer Primer and Resource Guide for Nurses*. Philadelphia, J. B. Lippincott.

Grobe, S. (1984b). Conquering computer cowardice. *J. Nurs. Ed., 23*:232–239.

Gulino, C., & LaMonica, G. (1986, June). Public health nursing: A study of role implementation. *Public Health Nurs., 3*:80–91.

Hales, G. (1984, July/August). Paleontology. *Comput. Nurs., 2*:115–116.

Hannah, K., Gullemin, E., & Conklin, D. (Eds.) (1985). *Nursing Uses of Computers and Information Science*. New York, North-Holland.

Henderson, V. (1964, August). The nature of nursing. *Am. J. Nurs., 64*:62–68.

Henry, B., & LeClair, H. (1987, January). Language, leadership, and power. *J. Nurs. Admin., 17*:19–25.

Hoffman, F. (1988). *Nursing Productivity Assessment and Costing Out Nursing Services*. Philadelphia, J. B. Lippincott.

Jackson, S. (1989, June). Peer review—why and how to do it. In Glover, S. (Ed.), *Performance Evaluations* (Vol. 1) (pp. 60–86). Baltimore, Williams & Wilkins.

Jewell, M., & Peters, D. (1989, September/October). An assessment guide for community health nurses. *Home Healthcare Nurse, 7*:32–36.

Jones, K. (1989, November/December). Evaluation of the prospective payment system: Implications for nursing. *Nurs. Econom., 7*:299–305.

Keating, S., & Kelman, G. (1988). *Home Health Care Nursing*. Philadelphia, J. B. Lippincott.

Kohler, C. (1988). Management information systems. In Harris, M. (Ed.), *Home Health Administration* (pp. 517–551). Owings Mills, MD, Rynd Communications.

Kovner, C. (1989, March). Public health nursing cost in home care. *Public Health Nurs., 6*: 3–7.

Lampe, S. (1989, March). Nursing documentation: A new prospective. *J. Nurs. Admin., 19*:3,19.

Laxton, C. (1988, February). Editorial. *Caring, 7*:2–3.

Leahy, K., Cobb, M., & Jones, M. (1982). *Community Health Nursing* (4th ed.). New York, McGraw-Hill Book Company.

Lentz, J., & Meyer, E. (1979, September). The dirty house. *Nurs. Outlook, 27*:590–593.

Lohn, K. (Ed.) (1990). *Medicare: A Strategy for Quality Assurance* (Vol. 1). Washington, DC, National Academy Press.

Lunney, M. (1990, January–March). Accuracy of nursing diagnoses: Concept development. *Nurs. Diagnosis, 1*:12–17.

Magnan, M. (1989, February). Listening with care. *Am. J. Nurs., 89*:219–221.

Martin, K., & Scheet, N. (1989). Nursing diagnosis in home health: The Omaha system. In Martinson, I., & Widmer, A. (Eds.), *Home Health Care Nursing* (pp. 67–72). Philadelphia, W. B. Saunders.

McCloskey, J. (1989, January). Implications of costing out nursing services for reimbursement. *Nurs. Manag., 20*:44–49.

McCloskey, J., & Grace, H. (Eds.) (1990). *Current Issues in Nursing* (3rd ed.). St. Louis, C. V. Mosby.

Mehmert, P. (1987, December). A nursing information system: The outcome of implementing nursing diagnoses. *Nurs. Clin. North Am., 22*:943–953.

Meisenheimer, C. (1989). *Quality Assurance for Home Health Care*. Rockville, MD, Aspen.

Mowry, M., & Korpman, R. (1987, January/February). Evaluating automated information systems. *Nurs. Economics, 5*:7–12.

Mundinger, M. & Jauron, G. (1975, February). Developing a nursing diagnosis. *Nurs. Outlook, 23*:94–98.

Naisbitt, J. & Aburdene, P. (1985). *Re-inventing the Corporation: Transforming Your Job and Your Company for the New Information Society*. New York, Warner.

Oda, D. (1989, March/April). Home visits: Effective or obsolete nursing practice? *Nurs. Res., 38*:121–123.

Oda, D., & Boyd, P. (1987, September). Documenting the effect and cost of public health nursing field services. *Public Health Nurs., 4*:180–182.

Olds, D., Henderson, C., Jr., Tatelbaum, R. et al. (1986a, January). Improving the delivery of prenatal care and outcomes of pregnancy: A randomized trial of nurse home visitation. *Pediatrics, 77*:16–28.

Olds, D., Henderson, C., Jr., Tatelbaum, et al. (1986b, July). Preventing child abuse and neglect: A randomized trial of nurse home visitation. *Pediatrics, 78*:65–78.

Olds, D., Henderson, C., Jr., Tatelbaum, R., et al. (1988, November). Improving the life-course development of socially disadvantaged mothers: A randomized trial of nurse home visitation. *Am. J. Public Health, 78*:1436–1445.

Orem, D. (1971). *Nursing Concepts of Practice*. New York, McGraw-Hill.

Ozbolt, J., McHugh, M., Schultz, S., II, et al. (1985). Designing the CYBERNURSE system: A proposed information system to support nursing practice, administration, research, and quality assurance. In Hannah, K., Gullemin, E., Conklin, D. (Eds.), *Nursing Uses of Computers and Information Science* (pp. 285–292). New York, North-Holland.

Pasquale, D. (1987, Winter). A basis for prospective payment in home care. *Image, 19*:186–191.

Peters, T. (1987). *Thriving on Chaos: A Handbook for Management Revolution*. New York, Random House.

Peters, T., & Waterman, R. (1982). *In Search of Excellence: Lessons from America's Best Run Companies*. New York, Harper & Row.

Pettey, S. (1988, February). Defining the scope: The HHSSA/health policy alternatives discussion. *Caring, 7*:20–21.

Phillips, E., Fisher, M., MacMillan-Scattergood, D., et al. (1987, June). Home health care: Who's where? *Am. J. Nurs., 77*:733–734.

Roberts, D., & Heinrich, J. (1985, October). Public health nursing comes of age. *Am. J. Public Health, 75*:1162–1172.

Rothberg, J. (1967, May). Why nursing diagnosis. *Am. J. Nurs., 67*:1040–1042.

Roy, C. (1975). The impact of nursing diagnosis. *AORN J, 21*(6):1023–1030.

Saba, V. (1988). Overview of nursing information systems. In Werley, H., & Lang, N. (Eds.), *Identification of the Nursing Minimum Data Set* (pp. 89–102). New York, Springer.

Saba, V., & McCormick, K. (1986). *Essentials of Computers for Nurses*. Philadelphia, J. B. Lippincott.

Simmons, D. (1984). Computer implementation in ambulatory care: A community health model. In *Computer Technology and Nursing*. Bethesda, MD, US DHHS.

Simmons, D., & Hailey, R. (1988). Management information systems. In Benefield, L. (Ed.), *Home Health Care Management* (pp. 39–51). Englewood Cliffs, NJ, Prentice Hall.

Sovie, M., Tarcinale, M., Vanputee, A., et al. (1985, March). Amalgam of nursing acuity, DRGs, and costs. *Nurs. Manag., 16*: 22–42.

Stagger, N. (1988, July/August). Using computers in nursing. *Comput. Nurs., 6*:164–170.

Stephany, T. (1990, April). A death in the family. *Am. J. Nurs., 90*:54–56.

Tinkham, C., Voorhies, E., & McCarthy, N. (1984). *Community Health Nursing: Evolution and Process in the Family and Community* (3rd ed.). New York, Appleton-Century-Crofts.

von Windeguth, B., Urbano, M., Hayes, J., et al. (1988, September). Analysis of infant risk factors documented by public health nurses. *Public Health Nurs.*, 5:165–169.

Werley, H., & Lang, N. (Eds.) (1988). *Identification of the Nursing Minimum Data Set.* New York, Springer.

Wesseling, E. (1972, May/June). Automating the nursing history and care plan. *J. Nurs. Admin.*, 2:26–30.

Wold, S. (Ed.) (1990). *Community Health Nursing: Issues and Topics.* Norwalk, CT, Appleton & Lange.

Worth, C. (1989, February). Handle with care. *Am. J. Nurs.*, 89:197–198.

Zielstorff, R. (1975, July/August). The planning and evaluation of automated systems: A nurse's point of view. *J. Nurs. Admin.*, 5:22–25.

CHAPTER THREE

*I*n practice, we are concerned with making the best clinical judgements possible; we must prepare nurses to make astute clinical judgements, to make accurate and relevant observations, to draw inferences from those observations, and to determine appropriate nursing actions. . . . We have much to learn from practice and from experts in practice. (Tanner, 1988, p. 206, 214)

The nursing process is widely accepted and respected as an essential component of nursing theory and professional practice. It is the foundation of a powerful epidemiologic or deliberative puzzle-solving process. It is a relatively simple system of feedback loops. The nursing process reflects the application of the scientific method to practice. Kuhn (1970) described the application process for science in general, and nurses have advanced their profession's scientific revolution by using the nursing process to expand crucial discoveries and knowledge. The nursing process defines characteristics of practice in language that is clear and acceptable to most nurses. It serves as the organizing framework for practice, documentation, and management. The nursing process enables nurses to standardize care while providing individual service. Furthermore, it provides the basis for the American Nurses' Association (ANA) Standards of Nursing Practice.

Nurses since Florence Nightingale have described creative adaptations of the nursing process. Often nurses define the interrelated concepts as both processes and products. Theorists and researchers have identified components of the nursing process in various ways. These are shown in Table 3–1.

Recently, nurses began to question if the nursing process captures the total essence of clinical judgement and nursing practice. Writers have emphasized the art and craft as well as the science of the profession. Nurses, working independently and collaboratively, are exploring caring, intuition, clinical knowledge, diagnostic reasoning, artificial intelligence, expert systems, and other related conceptual frameworks. They are examining the complex linkages between theory and practice as the foundation of nursing. To investigate these issues, Benner and Wrubel (1989) conducted several large research projects, interviewing many practitioners. Participating nurses are explicitly depicted as using clinical judgement and skill acquisition characteristics in exemplars or vignettes. A primary purpose of the research was to delineate nurses' pattern recognition skills, their salience or ability to prioritize data.

These are essential competencies developed during the practice of nursing. Benner described nurses as practicing on a continuum from novice to expert. Schultz and Meleis (1988) differentiated among clinical, conceptual, and empirical knowledge when they examined the basis of nursing as a practice discipline. Although some of the underlying concepts in theories associated with nursing process and clinical judgement may be contradictory, most are congruent.

CONCEPTUAL FRAMEWORK

The concepts included in nursing process and clinical judgement are closely related to the art and science of community health nursing practice. Beginning in 1978 and throughout the second and third VNA of Omaha research projects, these concepts were extensively reviewed and incorporated into a model or conceptual framework (see Fig. 3–1). The model was the basis for developing the three clinical components of the Omaha System: the Problem Classification Scheme, the Problem Rating Scale for Outcomes, and the Intervention Scheme. The model provides a conceptual bridge by which the Omaha System can be integrated into community health practice, documentation, and data management. The Omaha System is useful to community health practitioners, supervisors, administrators, students, and educators. This chapter includes a description of the model and a review of the related literature; the application and value of the Omaha System are delineated in other chapters.

Many sources were examined to ensure that the conceptual framework of the Omaha System was grounded in and congruent with current practice, education, and research standards. Guiding the work was the belief that theory is born in practice, is refined in research, and must and can return to practice in a continuing cycle. Information was obtained through an ongoing, extensive literature review that emphasized the work of

Conceptual Framework
of the Omaha System

nursing theorists and researchers. Portions of the literature review are included in this chapter. Formal and informal discussions with staff and supervisory nurses at the VNA of Omaha and community health nursing educators provided valuable data.

The following assumptions were formulated as part of the research process:

1. Most community health nurses have the skills necessary to identify client problems, utilize nursing interventions, and measure client progress.
2. Mutuality of concern and effort between the community health nurse and the client is needed to identify, use, and record realistic client problems and outcomes as well as nursing interventions.
3. The health status of the client is influenced by complex forces; the community health nurse recognizes, but may not be able to control, these forces.
4. Most individuals and families are interested in increasing their competence, enhancing control over their own lives, and promoting their functioning at the highest possible level.
5. The problem-oriented system and record can be adapted to and provide for an effective approach to the delivery of community health nursing services.
6. Community health nurses understand basic principles of community health practice and recording.
7. Community health nurses have the expertise to develop a valid and reliable system of practice, documentation, and data management.
8. Community health nurses, other health care providers, supervisors, and administrators will implement the Omaha System in diverse settings regardless of agency organization, size, services, or client population; the System is beneficial to users, clients, and external personnel.

A circular model was chosen to depict the dynamic, interactive nature of the nursing process, the nurse-client relationship, and related theories of diagnostic reasoning and clinical judgement. Because the concepts of the nursing process overlap and sometimes co-

incide as the community health nurse makes decisions and provides client care, a circular rather than linear model was chosen, as shown in Figure 3–1. The significance of a caring, appropriate nurse-client relationship is indicated by the outer circle surrounding the diagram. The importance of the client is emphasized by placement at the center of the model. The client is defined as an individual, family, or group; group is not listed on the model because the VNA of Omaha research investigations were limited to individual and family. Although nurse-client progress and problem-solving often occur in a sequential pattern, the broken lines depict an open system that allows frequent, multidirectional movement. The constant motion and the changing health status of the client are influenced by many complex forces. The remaining concepts of the model reflect the nursing process:

1. Collect and assess data — to accurately and systematically gather client information in relation to a defined data base through observation and interviews with clients and other health team members and to analyze the data in relation to environment, psychosocial status, physiologic status, and health-related behaviors.
2. State problem (nursing diagnosis) — to delineate a matter of doubt or difficulty that (a) historically, presently, or potentially adversely affects any aspect of a client's well-being; and (b) is amenable to and appropriate for nursing intervention.
3. Identify admission problem rating — to designate a numeric rating for the concepts of client knowledge, behavior, and status in relation to a specific problem at the time of admission.
4. Plan and intervene — to establish priorities and select a course of action to address a specific client problem and to implement the action in order to improve, maintain, or restore health or prevent illness.
5. Identify interim/dismissal problem rating — to designate a numeric rating for the concepts of client

TABLE 3-1 ■ Three Conceptualizations of Nursing Process

I	II	III
Collection of data	Assessment	Assessing
Problem identification/ diagnosis	Problem identification/ diagnosis	
Goal-setting		
Plan of nursing care	Plan	Planning
Nursing action	Intervention	Implementing
Reassessment and revision of the plan	Evaluation	Evaluating

knowledge, behavior, and status in relation to a specific problem at periodic intervals during the course of service and at discharge.

6. Evaluate problem outcome—to measure client progress in relation to a specific problem by comparing admission, interim, and dismissal problem ratings.

APPLICATION OF THE CONCEPTUAL FRAMEWORK

A community health nurse begins service to a client following an intake or referral process. During a nurse's initial visit and all other visits, the vital importance of establishing and maintaining a positive nurse-client relationship is recognized. Freeman and Heinrich (1981) emphasized that a positive relationship is developed, not discovered. Such a relationship promotes quantity and quality of data and enhances the potential for suc-

cess and client progress in relation to all components of the nursing process.

A nurse's initial activities include data collection, assessment, and analysis. This process involves gathering, clustering, combining, summarizing, and validating diverse subjective and objective information relative to each family member, the family as an interacting unit, and the sociocultural and physical environment. A community health nurse uses principles of epidemiology to enhance systematic data collection and assessment and to identify patterns within client data. Application of epidemiologic principles assists a nurse in examining the relationships of the agents of illness, human host, and environmental factors during the course of illness (Leavell & Clark, 1965). The conclusion and logical end product of the data collection and assessment process is problem identification or diagnosis, which involves interpretation of the acquired data.

Planning and intervening are two of the most important concepts of the model to both a client and a nurse. Campbell (1984) described a broad interpretation of planning and intervention involving nurse and family collaboration to:

■ Set priorities
■ Identify client status and expected outcomes-outcome criteria or goals relative to specific nursing problems and time frames
■ Delineate alternative courses of action
■ Choose and take action

In relation to community health nursing interventions, the major categories of action have been described as: sickness care; health teaching, guidance, and counseling; coordination and collaboration with other workers; referral; and family advocacy (Corrigan, 1983). In addition, a community health nurse uses principles of epidemiology to identify appropriate plans and intervention strategies associated with primary, secondary, and tertiary prevention (Leavell & Clark, 1965).

Identification of admission, interim, and dismissal ratings quantifies the evaluation process. Each rating provides a baseline for contrast with later ratings during the period of client service. The evaluation component of the Omaha System allows a nurse to compare a client's health status at different points in time to determine the degree of nursing effectiveness. Through evaluation, a nurse has feedback that can be used to revise and modify plans and interventions with an individual, family, or group. Thus, evaluation is both ongoing and terminal.

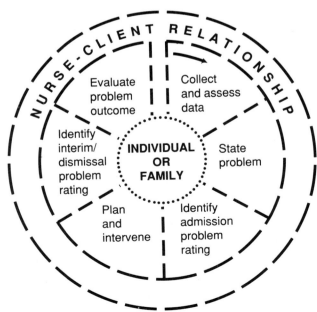

FIGURE 3-1 ■ Conceptualization of the family nursing process.

LITERATURE REVIEW

The literature review focuses on the concepts of problems, plans, interventions, and evaluation. These concepts are directly associated with the conceptual model and the Problem Classification Scheme, the Intervention Scheme, and the Problem Rating Scale for Outcomes of the Omaha System. The literature review incorporates references by clinicians, educators, and researchers.

Client Problems

The term "problem" has been used in nursing literature to mean "client problem," "nursing problem," and "nursing diagnosis." Nursing diagnosis has been defined as the end product of assessment (Gebbie & Lavin, 1975). A problem has been described as a difficulty or concern experienced by a client at a given point in time that is predictable or typically expected for a certain diagnosis or illness-wellness context (Mayers, 1983). Nursing diagnoses have been described as actual or potential health problems that nurses, by virtue of their education and experience, are capable and licensed to treat; nursing diagnoses require a problem-etiology-sign/symptom format (Gordon, 1987). Yura and Walsh (1988) noted that the assessment phase begins with a nursing history and ends with designations of potential or actual nursing diagnoses. In contrast, some writers de-emphasized illness and emphasized wellness in their descriptions of nursing diagnosis.

Abdellah (1957) and other early writers recognized the controversial nature of nursing problems and nursing diagnosis. These writers differentiated between medical and nursing diagnosis because of the unique perspective and knowledge base of each discipline. Nursing diagnosis has been described as distinct from medical diagnosis, anticipated in certain medical conditions, or identical to a medical diagnosis in emergency situations. Nurses have also emphasized the need to consider the value of both nursing and medical diagnoses during the problem identification component of the nursing process.

Client Problems and the Nursing Process

The identification of a client problem, nursing problem, or nursing diagnosis has generally been viewed as a step in the nursing process that follows data collection and precedes planning. Nursing diagnoses are derived from health status and health-related behavior data, leading to goals and subsequent planning of nursing interventions. Gough's steps (1971) in formulating a psychological diagnosis were adapted by Brown (1974) as she recommended an approach to formulating all nursing diagnoses. Brown's approach included: identifying the present problem, gathering facts about the problem, formulating a hypothesis to explain the problem, checking the implications of the hypothesis and/or making new observations, and confirming or disproving the diagnosis.

Additional consensus regarding the essence of nursing problems appears in nursing literature. Problems must be identified from a client's verbal and nonverbal communication and must be defined from a client's perspective. Problems may be classified as actual or potential as well as individual or family. Nursing problems or nursing diagnoses are means to an end, not ends in themselves; their use enhances the provision of care, increases nursing accountability, and facilitates recording.

Client Problems and Nursing Practice

The Problem Classification Scheme and related concepts of nursing diagnosis, problem-oriented recording, diagnostic reasoning, and nursing process have been implemented in multiple settings. Approximately 220 agency, college or school of nursing, and other users of the Omaha System have been identified in 41 states. Cell, Peters, and Gordon (1984), Hays (1990), Schmele (1986), Aden and Warren (1991), Weidmann and North (1987), Peters (1989), Mundt (1988), and Feldman and Richard (1988) are among those who have conducted research, implemented, and computerized the Omaha System at various locations. More details about users are included in other chapters of this book.

Writers have described widespread application of North American Nursing Diagnosis Association (NANDA)-approved diagnoses and other diagnostic systems. Most involved acute-care settings, although some authors have described use in a community health nursing agency. In addition, nurses have demonstrated use of nursing diagnoses with population groups such as chronically ill or developmentally disabled clients in long-term care settings.

Documentation of the nursing process, including client problems or nursing diagnoses, has been fostered by advances in automation and artificial intelligence. An example of a hospital information system with a significant nursing component is Technicon, a system originating in California hospitals (Mayers, 1983). At the University of Michigan, CYBERNURSE has been developed as an information system to support nursing practice, administration, research, and quality assurance (Ozbolt, McHugh, Schultz, et al., 1985). Nursing faculty assisted in designing Creighton University's On-Line Multiple Modular Expert System (COMMES), a decision-support system intended to provide consultation to nurses in acute care and educational settings (Evans, 1984). All groups are considered pioneers in the field.

Client Problems and Nursing Research

A marked increase in the research studies related to nursing problems and nursing diagnoses occurred in the US and Canada during the 1980s. A review of nursing diagnoses used when hospital nurses referred clients to community health nurses showed nurses from both settings reported more satisfaction when they used nursing diagnoses in addition to medical diagnoses (Gordon, Sweeney, & McKeehan, 1980). The generic, differentiation, and condition features of nursing diagnosis were analyzed using Delphi methodology and a

Soltis paradigm (Shoemaker, 1984). According to the findings, a nursing diagnosis has the following essential generic features: it is a statement of a client problem, refers to the health state, refers to a potential health problem, is a conclusion resulting from identification of a pattern or cluster of signs and symptoms, and is based on subjective and/or objective data that can be confirmed.

Gordon (1987) is among those who have described numerous validation studies specific to individual NANDA-approved diagnoses. In contrast, a small number of research studies have been designed to explore the entire group of diagnoses. In a comparison of medical and nursing diagnoses of clients in an acute care Chicago hospital, nursing diagnoses were found to be strong predictors of nurse-client time and length of hospital stay (Halloran, 1985). The relationship between all 65 NANDA-approved diagnoses and nursing resources was examined as one portion of a large pilot study (McKibbin, Brimmer, Clinton, et al., 1985). Since the researchers found a lack of strong or consistent relationships between nursing diagnoses and nursing resources, they identified a need for further analyses.

Werley and Lang (1988) compiled research studies involving nursing diagnoses and other concepts of the nursing process. They also initiated a series of investigations designed to produce uniformly defined and collected nursing data that could be shared and analyzed across all care settings. The concepts and other nursing care elements served as the framework for a proposed nursing minimum data set.

The applicability of nursing diagnoses to chronically ill clients has been examined. Investigators validated a list of 51 diagnoses for a large client sample, using a human needs framework (Hoskins, McFarlane, Rubenfeld, et al., 1986). Another study was conducted at a long-term care facility (Maas, Hardy, & Craft, 1990). The purposes were to identify nursing diagnoses in the client population and to examine methodologic problems and issues inherent in descriptive nursing diagnosis studies.

Consensus

The nursing diagnosis paradigm has not been developed without criticism. Writers questioned the dangers of packaged categories — diagnoses that may simplify and even obliterate the client's experience — and the implications of prefabricated lists of labels for empowering professionals and diminishing the power of clients during the course of client service (Hagey & McDonough, 1984). Others described concerns about the negative, deviant, or pathologic implications of nursing diagnosis (Gleit & Tatro, 1981; McLane & Fehring, 1984). Some writers have focused their criticism on specific nursing diagnoses as knowledge deficit (Dennison & Keeling, 1989; Jenny, 1987). Another nursing leader questioned the utility of NANDA diagnoses to practicing nurses (Roy, 1984). Shamansky and Yanni (1983) suggested that nursing diagnosis in the current form limits nursing practice, creates obstacles to clear communication, and constrains inference and intuition. Lunney (1986) offered a different view. She supported the efforts of NANDA but suggested clarifying and simplifying the diagnostic language into a more usable system.

Some nurses have strongly supported the diagnostic process but have urged peers to clearly differentiate between data that do and do not need to be collected. Others have noted that sophisticated nursing judgment and tools such as a defined data base are necessary for this differentiation. After studying the diagnostic abilities of 26 graduate nursing students, investigators concluded that nursing diagnosis was a weak link of the nursing process (Andersen & Briggs, 1988). Physicians have experienced similar needs and dilemmas in relation to the practice of medicine (Densen, 1970; Weed, 1968).

The terms "client problem," "nursing problem," and "nursing diagnosis" have been used increasingly by nursing authors since the 1960s. Many vocal proponents have been attracted to the movement since that time. According to advocates, objections to nursing diagnosis are related to errors in use rather than to the concept itself. Supporters suggest that nursing diagnosis will enjoy the same relationship to nursing that medical diagnosis does to medicine. Advocates indicate that nursing diagnosis can lead to improved management of nursing care, identification of staffing requirements, justification for third-party payments, development of quality assurance programs, establishment of standard terminology between nurses, and generation of an extensive and valid research data base.

Plans

Many books and articles have been written about the importance of nursing plans and interventions for the autonomous and collaborative functions of professional nurses. Often the terms "plan" and "intervention" have been used conjointly in these publications. Care plans have been described as essential to nursing practice. Various authors have indicated that plans are needed by the nurse to: (1) make care individual, (2) assist with priority setting, (3) facilitate systematic communication, (4) coordinate care among groups of health care personnel, (5) assist in evaluation of care, (6) contribute to staff development, and (7) increase continuity of care. Kramer (1972) contends that care plans have only two realistic purposes: to foster continuity and comprehensiveness of client care.

Planning Process

Urwick (1943), a management authority, stated that planning is fundamentally an intellectual process; it is a mental predisposition to do things in an orderly way, to think before acting, and to act in response to facts rather than by conjecture. According to Urwick, a good plan has the following characteristics: (1) is based on a clearly defined objective, (2) is simple, (3) establishes standards, (4) is flexible, (5) is balanced, and (6) uses available resources to the utmost before creating new authorities and new resources. Others have written that planning consists of setting goals, weighing alternatives, proposing intervention, and predicting outcomes (Walter, Pardee, & Malbo, 1976). According to another writer, the planning process is a method of determining what to do, when to do it, who shall do it, and what is needed to accomplish the task (Bower, 1982). A plan has also been defined as the determination by the nurse and client of those goals that must be achieved to promote adaptation (Perry, 1982). Planning involves goal-setting and establishing priorities. Planning is concerned with (1) choosing among possible courses of action, (2) selecting appropriate types of nursing intervention, (3) identifying appropriate resources for care, and (4) developing an operational set of interventions (Freeman & Heinrich, 1981). "Planning is an action word implying a problem-solving process . . . Planning . . . initiates activities designed to channel all available resources appropriately and effectively" (Braden, 1984, p. 311). Others noted that a plan provides a valuable asset as a nurse works with a client to achieve optimal wellness (Yura & Walsh, 1988).

Plans and Nursing Practice

Nurses in practice settings have addressed planning in various ways; they have written mixed reviews about their experiences with both standard and individual care plans. As early as 1972, Kramer criticized the written, individual plans required by the Joint Commission on Accreditation of Hospitals. Kramer questioned the efficiency and effectiveness of individual nurses developing individual client care plans, noting that these care plans could not be expected to meet dozens of goals and purposes. Instead, she suggested that group nursing plans for patients with common sets of limitations are preferable. Many of Kramer's concerns have been repeated by others, including researchers who developed a study to examine the use of standard care plans throughout the 27 units of University of California Hospitals, San Francisco (Nichols & Barstow, 1980). Some authors have recommended use of client-specific nursing care plans. Others, however, have suggested that these plans are practical only if problem-specific, standard interventions are developed and implemented.

Other nurses have developed comprehensive care plans in relation to nursing diagnoses approved by NANDA. Some of those were developed for use by community health nurses.

Cornell and Brush (1971) were among the first to describe a computerized recording system. The system, designed for their small rehabilitation hospital, included 56 basic care plans stored in computer memory. As staff nurses retrieved a plan, it could be changed to fit individual clients. No recent description of their system is noted in nursing literature. Additional descriptions of automated care planning are appearing in the literature with increasing frequency. Included is a system that integrated care plans into the hospital information system (Albrecht & Lieske, 1985). Another example involved the faculty and students at University of North Florida, who developed an expert system prototype to generate plans based on nursing diagnoses (Bloom, Leitner, & Solano, 1987).

Nursing literature contains many references to definitions and descriptions of planning in relation to nursing. Planning is identified as an integral part of problem-solving when applied to nursing practice or any other endeavor. Because planning, however, is essentially an intellectual process, it continues to be controversial and difficult to investigate through research studies.

Interventions

Intervention describes activity that follows a thought process or written exercise usually referred to as planning. Intervention is often used simultaneously with terms such as "approach," "order/prescription," "care/service," "strategy," and "treatment." While client-nurse negotiation and mutuality are important when problem-solving or applying the family nursing process, they are critical when implementing interventions.

Florence Nightingale (1859), writing about nursing, described specific environmental and dietary actions to decrease the spread of infectious diseases. Recently, nurses defined nursing intervention as a nursing action specific to a diagnosis and designed to improve, maintain, or restore health or prevent illness (Gebbie & Lavin, 1975). Other writers viewed intervention as the direct or indirect action taken (Walter, Pardee, & Malbo, 1976).

Interventions and the Nursing Process

Intervention has been defined as the use of nursing therapy necessary to accomplish the defined plan and to promote adaptation of the individual, the family, and the community (Perry, 1982). A nurse must be knowledgeable regarding: (1) scientific rationale for the selected intervention, (2) additional health care resources to assist the client in achieving adaptation, and (3) psychomotor skills for use in implementing the planned intervention. Another writer referred to intervention as prescribing the best solutions after considering options, constraints, and resources. She described nursing orders as those specific, itemized, nurse-initiated prescriptions for care (Mayers, 1983).

A nursing intervention has been defined as a single-action nursing measure designed to fulfill the unmet human needs that are inferred from the patient's problem (Campbell, 1984). Others supported a broader approach and defined a nursing intervention as an autonomous action based on scientific rationale that is executed to benefit the client in a predicted way related to the nursing diagnosis and stated goals (Bulechek & McCloskey, 1985). Intervention has been described as a symbolic concept, a goal-specific treatment for a nursing diagnosis. Interventions are "what nurses do with and for clients to solve a problem or prevent a possible problem" (Bulechek & McCloskey, 1985, p. 8).

Gordon (1987) stated that interventions are actions taken to help a client move from a present state to the state described in the projected outcomes. Interventions must be specific to the client and the client situation based on the following data: personal client factors, client's perception, current level of compensation, problem magnitude and urgency, extended effects, and cost-benefit factors.

Corrigan (1988), who adapted definitions from others (Gebbie & Lavin, 1975; Freeman & Heinrich, 1981), described an intervention as a nursing action specific to a diagnosis and designed to promote, maintain, or restore health or prevent illness or injury. Interventions have been categorized as supplemental, facilitative, and developmental (Freeman & Heinrich, 1981). Supplemental interventions involve services that the individual, family, group, or community cannot do for itself. Developmental interventions relate to the capacity of clients to act on their own behalf. Facilitative interventions, situated between those that are supplemental and developmental, involve the removal of barriers to care.

Intervention Models

Some nurses have considered interventions and developed models at a global level — that of an entire specialty or the entire scope of nursing practice. One model includes life-sustaining care, remedial care, personal/custodial care, restorative care, preventive care, and health-promoting care as implications for intervention (Bircher, 1982). Another model of nursing interventions lists prescriptive, structuring, mutual participation, indirect approach, and discretionary nonaction modes of therapeutic influence (Benoliel, Ellison, Kogan, et al., 1985). Participants at the Nursing Minimum Data Set Conference designated a seven-category intervention classification scheme. Included were surveillance and/or observation, supportive measure, assistive measure, treatment and/or procedure, emotional support, teaching, and coordination (Werley & Lang, 1988). Taylor's (1989) extensive review of interventions identified models developed by Bulechek and McCloskey (1985, 1990), Snyder (1985), and Pender and Pender (1986). Although the latter authors viewed nursing interventions as means of health promotion and protection from illness, the review contained few references specific to community health nursing.

Community health nurses have explored nursing interventions. In relation to public health nursing services, Roberts (1962) divided interventions into four categories: direct care, instruction and counseling, evaluation and supervision, and referral. A nursing ed-ucator noted the major community health nursing categories of action as: sickness care; health teaching, guidance, and counseling; coordination and collaboration with other workers; referral; and family advocacy (Corrigan, 1983). Other educators listed community health nursing functions as direct nursing care, health teaching, referral, health counseling, anticipatory guidance, planning, collaboration, coordination, and health advocacy (Tinkham, Voorhies, & McCarthy, 1984).

Many nursing clinicians and researchers have examined and written about interventions specific to their practice and interest areas. Sometimes these areas were discrete and isolated. Sometimes they overlapped other nursing and medical practice areas. On occasion, interventions were referred to as nursing orders (Mayers, 1983). Evidence that nurses are beginning to study interventions in greater depth appears in nursing literature. Studies are being conducted in various settings including general hospitals, critical care units, and homes or related community health settings.

Young children and their mothers have served as the focus of intervention studies conducted in home settings. Seven intervention categories were identified in conjunction with a study of mothers and infants (Barkauskas, 1983). These included: (1) assessment of mother, (2) assessment of infant, (3) assessment of family, (4) instructions, (5) followup of problems, (6) referrals, and (7) miscellaneous activities. Nursing interventions were explored in relation to parents of premature infants (Barnard, 1984). The four discrete interventions identified were: (1) monitoring, (2) information, (3) support, and (4) therapy.

Campbell (1984) has developed an extensive list of nursing diagnoses. Each diagnosis is associated with assessment (subjective, objective, and relative data), possible etiology, planning (patient needs and primary nurse-patient goals), nursing interventions (nursing treatment, nursing observations, and health teaching), and evaluation. Campbell's three categories of independently initiated nursing interventions are (1) nursing treatments, (2) nursing observations, and (3) health teaching. The interventions apply to nursing in general and medical-surgical nursing in particular. Campbell also categorized nursing interventions as assistive, hygienic, rehabilitative, supportive, preventive, observational, and educative. Other authors have developed extensive lists that are similar to Campbell's and are designed for use in acute care settings; these efforts are described in Chapter 6.

Snyder (1985) investigated the complex process of nursing intervention and practice as well as specific nursing actions or activities. Her book is divided into four sections: movement and proprioceptive interventions, cognitive interventions, sensory interventions, and other interventions that include play and humor. Twenty general interventions are categorized and described within the sections. Snyder's approach is similar to that of others as she emphasizes the value of independent nursing practice, diagnostic reasoning, and decision-making (Benner & Wrubel, 1989; Tanner, 1988).

A system called Nursing Intervention Tools has been developed; it is oriented toward community health nursing (Stanhope & Lancaster, 1988). The system is based on age groups, medical diagnoses, and nursing problems. The interventions are labeled as nursing anticipatory guidance, nursing interventions, or management.

Interventions and Current Nursing Research

Growing interest in nursing interventions is producing an increase in research and publication. Broad interventions have been categorized into stress management, lifestyle alteration, acute care management, and communication (Bulechek & McCloskey, 1985). Among the 26 interventions in the four categories are relaxation training, truth-telling, music therapy, patient contracting, preoperative teaching, and discharge planning. A team of University of Iowa faculty led by Bulechek and McCloskey is conducting research and continuing to explore interventions in an acute care setting (1989, 1990). Their research efforts resulted in identification of seven types of nursing activities. They have elected to focus their efforts on three types:

(a) Nurse-initiated treatments in response to nursing diagnoses (including those nursing treatments that result from the clients' responses to medical interventions). (b) Physician-initiated treatments in response to medical diagnoses. (c) Daily essential function activities (e.g., bedmaking, help with tray setup, watering plants) that may not relate to either medical or nursing diagnoses but are done by the nurse for the client who cannot do these things for her/himself. (Bulechek & McCloskey, 1989, p. 24)

One of the most comprehensive research studies including interventions is being conducted at the University of Texas (Grobe, 1989). The focus of the study involves the importance of language and how that language reflects the state of knowledge of the profession. During the 1988–1993 study, important nursing terms will be identified, especially in relation to chronically ill clients. In addition, interrelationships between terms and methods of analyzing language will be examined.

Literature review reveals a similarity between the current developmental stages of interventions and nursing diagnoses in the early 1970s. Five reasons have been given to explain why interest and research concerning interventions have proceeded more slowly than those related to nursing diagnoses (Snyder, 1985). The reasons were: (1) basic nursing texts focus on nursing skills needed to carry out physicians' orders; (2) faculty work to assure employers that students can carry out these skills safely; (3) independent nursing interventions are viewed as extras, not essentials; (4) clinical research is difficult; and (5) some nurses hesitate to accept autonomy. Deciding what intervention data is essential and how to organize that data will require extensive involvement of clinicians, administrators, and educators (Werley & Lang, 1988).

Consensus on the nominal level is not followed by consensus on the operational level in relation to interventions. "Three problems have been identified: lack of acceptance by other health care workers of nursing's value of prevention, lack of a research base, and lack of classification schemes" (Bulechek & McCloskey, 1989, p. 28). Some authors have advocated interventions for specific client populations, whereas others have advocated them for general populations. Measurable, documented evidence of quality, cost, or time benefits to nurses and clients is noticeably limited or absent, even though nursing literature suggests the need to identify and record interventions.

Evaluation

Evaluation is generally viewed as a process designed to ascertain value or amount or to compare accomplishments with some standards. Phaneuf noted that the purposes of the evaluation process are to:

1. Account for the level of care provided
2. Make comparisons (of different situations, settings, or times)
   a. Determine the effects of changes made in care practices
   b. Determine the extent to which objectives of a program have been attained
3. Provide bases for planning for improvement. (Phaneuf, 1976, p. 149)

Concern with evaluation and quality of care is not a new phenomenon. Health care providers have historically sought to measure the impact of health care employees or programs on individual clients or client aggregates. Individuals and groups have been challenged by the desire to evaluate the many intangibles of health care in valid, reliable, and definitive ways.

Evaluation Frameworks

Some evaluation attempts have been related to the concept of outcomes. In 1918, a surgeon suggested that end results of patient care be examined in light of (1) the physician or surgeon responsible for the treatment, (2) the organization carrying out the details of the treatment, (3) the disease or condition of the patient, and (4) the personal or social condition augmenting or preventing the cooperation of the patient (Codman, 1918). By 1939, the concept of outcomes was elaborated in relation to nursing care evaluation that focused on the changing state or behavior of the client (Derryberry, 1939). In community health nursing, two national leaders, Freeman (1961) and Roberts (1962), developed early evaluation approaches and encouraged other community health nurses of their era.

Other evaluation attempts have focused on structure and process alone or a combination of structure, process, and outcome. Donabedian's (1966) structure, process, and outcome frameworks for evaluating client care were widely published and adapted by others; this framework triad is considered classic. The focus of a structural framework is the environment, the institution with its organization and facilities; the focus of a process framework is the manner in which personnel deliver care; and the focus of an outcome framework is the client and that client's progress or measurable change.

Outcomes

Evaluation based on client outcomes has been described as both formative and summative, suggesting the need for concurrent as well as retrospective review of client progress. Evaluation is the analysis of the efficiency of the plan based on predicted outcomes (Walter, et al., 1976). The predicted behavior or nursing goal can be compared and contrasted with realized behavior at a later point in time. An evaluation framework assumes that changes in client health status and behavior result from or are consequences of care. Additional data are required as part of the evaluation framework. For example, data regarding all previous concepts of the nursing process, as well as medical diagnosis and treatments, must be considered. By nature, the behavior and relationships of nurses and clients as individuals, families, and communities are complex.

Two trends in outcome evaluation were noted after 1960. First, emphasis increased on health care evaluation in general and nursing care evaluation in particular. Donabedian's framework (1966) was incorporated into quality assurance — a construct resulting from the 1972 Social Security Amendments. Quality assurance, peer review, and audit entered the vocabulary, educational curricula, and institutions of health professionals (see Chapter 14). Second, interest in evaluation began to shift from the practitioner and process to the client and outcome. New accreditation and federal regulations, legislation, escalating health care costs, and increasingly vocal consumers intensified the emphasis on outcome. "This current wave of concern focuses not on raising or improving care, but rather on preserving quality while efforts to reduce costs are made" (Peters, 1989, p. 133). As a result of the interest within the profession, two large invitational conferences were sponsored by the ANA to address evaluation research, especially in relation to client outcomes. Nursing literature suggests that this emphasis will continue.

Consensus

The quantity of published references to client outcomes, as well as the number of projects supported by individuals, agencies, and institutions, suggests general consensus among nurses and other health professionals. Nursing or nursing-sensitive outcome has been defined as "a patient or client health status (condition, behavior, or functional ability) that is influenced by nursing treatment (action, intervention, procedure, or therapy) at specific times for an episode or encounter of care" (Werley & Lang, 1988, p. 391). When referring to a nominal definition of client outcomes, most writers

have attempted to develop a comprehensive client focus, that is, the physical, emotional, and social health/wellness status that results from or is a consequence of care.

Outcomes have been organized in various ways. One nurse used Riehl and Roy's adaption model to group outcomes into physiologic needs, self-concept, role function, and interdependence (Laros, 1977). Outcomes have been further described as those desired effects or benefits defined by specific clinical manifestations, mobility levels, client knowledge, self-care skills, recovery rates, mortality rates, and client satisfaction. Outcomes may also be described as points along a health status continuum or terminal points.

In contrast to the nominal level just described, consensus regarding outcomes decreases markedly when valid measurement of actual implementation is involved. Thus, health care publications suggest many current, complex issues and unresolved questions about the use of outcomes in evaluating nursing practice. The following represents a synthesis of questions that concern community health nurses and other health professionals:

1. Which dimensions or categories are essential in evaluating the physical, emotional, and social health state of a client?
2. Which dimensions should and/or do nurses influence?
3. How and when can nursing care be measured? Have valid and reliable instruments and methods been developed for evaluating the impact of community health nurses and/or other health professionals? Do all community health nurses affect clients similarly or differently? If not, what variables are significant?
4. How do multiple factors and persons, over which health professionals have no jurisdiction or control, influence outcomes?
5. From the standpoint of nursing practice, what commonalities do widely divergent samples of clients possess? Are clients sufficiently divergent that it is logical, sound, and practical for sets of outcome criteria to be developed for discrete subgroups of client populations?
6. What unifying framework can be applied to outcomes that considers multiple care settings and the perspective of a client as an individual, family, group, or community?

Evaluation and Nursing Research

The state of evaluation efforts has led many authorities to urge further outcome development and research. The need to develop outcome measures specific to community health nursing practice was a major recommendation included in a 1976 American Public Health Association Nursing Section study (Januska, Engle, & Wood, 1976). Contributing data to the study were 566 purposively selected community health agencies and institutions that varied as to geographic location, size, structure, and programs. Daubert (1979) described a classification system or method of measuring client outcome that was developed at the VNA of New Haven (CT). All clients were classified into one of five groups based on the client's rehabilitation potential, regardless of the client's number of medical diagnoses. The nursing staff of the Hartford (CT) Visiting Nurse and Home Care (1987) created a tool called Self Management Outcome Criteria. The tool consisted of five self-management categories: (1) level of knowledge, (2) reduction of risks to health, (3) functional ability/activities of daily living (ADL) management, (4) behavior-mentation-emotion, and (5) support from significant others. The staff of Washington home health care agencies participated in a research project to develop outcome scales (Lalonde, 1988). Their seven scales included (1) general symptom distress, (2) discharge status, (3) prescribed medications, (4) caregiver strain, (5) functional status, (6) physiologic indicators, and (7) knowledge of diagnosis/prognosis. Marek (1989) completed a literature review on community health nursing projects and expressed optimism about the future.

Outcome development and research have been conducted in acute care and community health settings. An extensive outcome study was conducted by the staff of Rush Hospital and Medicus between 1972 and 1977 (Haussmann, Hegyvary, & Newman, 1976). The focus of the study was quality of nursing care in the hospital setting as defined by a client-centered instrument. The instrument, currently implemented in many institutions, is often described as a patient classification system. The Rush Medicus Study and related systems are designed to group patients "according to their requirements for nursing care, and the express purpose of nursing resource determination and allocation" (Giovannetti, 1988, p. 103). Patient classification systems are closely related to various measures of severity of illness, patient acuity, and nursing intensity through tools that were developed for use in hospitals. In general, implementation of the classification tools is related to Joint Commission on Accreditation of Healthcare Organizations requirements and to the effects of diagnosis related groups (DRGs) (Shaffer, 1986). Of note are the investigations of Peters (1988, 1989) and Hays (1990), which address similar issues in the community health setting and are based on the VNA of Omaha's Problem Classification Scheme.

Horn and Swain (1977) developed 539 outcome criteria or health status dimension statements to measure effectiveness of care for hospitalized patients. The measurement tool includes universal demands or physical-emotional needs and health deviations. Others applied the ANA Outcome Standards to rheumatology nursing practice (Pigg & Schroeder, 1984).

Campbell (1984) developed principles of criterion-referenced measurement for an expected outcome standard framework. Each expected outcome or goal was accompanied by criteria as well as examples of objective and subjective data indicating that criteria were met. Although the principles of criterion-referenced measures were incorporated into a methodology and a lengthy text designated to enhance nursing practice, no attempt to test and validate this methodology was included. Therefore, continuing research and instrument development is needed for Campbell's work, and for the work of others, to clarify health status and behavior dimensions and suggest valid levels of client achievement.

Evaluation of client care is an evolutionary process that needs to be systematically validated by applying research findings in service settings. Concurrently, there is a need to maintain structure and, especially, process, as interrelated and necessary components of comprehensive client care evaluation. To disregard structure and process in favor of outcome would be erroneous, especially since research findings on outcome are few and sometimes contradictory. Acknowledging the complexity inherent in evaluating quality nursing care and the elusive nature of outcomes, Lang (1976) suggested that the measurement and implementation portions of evaluation frameworks are in infancy and even labor stages. Although the process is slow, continued commitment and involvement of nurses are necessary. Persistent efforts will enable nurses to develop improved, sound, and practical evaluation techniques that may establish norms or statistical performance averages for nursing.

SUMMARY

Concepts of the nursing process, in conjunction with diagnostic reasoning, were used to develop a model or framework for the Omaha System projects. For development, information was obtained from nursing theorists and researchers, community health nursing educators, and staff and supervisory nurses of the VNA of Omaha. When completed, the cyclical Conceptualization of the Family Nursing Process was congruent with generally accepted nursing theories as well as with community health nursing practice and documentation. The model provided a systematic framework for developing research-based nursing diagnosis, intervention, and evaluation components of the Omaha System. Throughout the remainder of this book, those components are referred to as the Problem Classification Scheme, the Intervention Scheme, and the Problem Rating Scale for Outcomes.

REFERENCES

Abdellah, F. (1957, June). Methods of identifying covert aspects of nursing problems. *Nurs. Res.*, 6:4–23.

Aden, C., & Warren, J. (1991). A validation study of NANDA's taxonomy I. In Carroll-Johnson, R. (Ed.), *Classification of Nursing Diagnosis: Proceedings of Ninth National Conference.* Philadelphia, J. B. Lippincott.

Albrecht, C., & Lieske, A.M. (1985, July). Automating patient care planning. *Nurs. Manag.*, 16:21–26.

Andersen, J., & Briggs, L. (1988, Fall). Nursing diagnosis: A study of quality and supportive evidence. *Image*, 20:141–144.

Barkauskas, V. (1983, May). Effectiveness of public health nurse home visits to primiparous mothers and their infants. *Am. J. Public Health,* 73:573–580.

Barnard, K. (1984). *Newborn Nursing Models: Final report of project supported by grant number RO1 NU-00719.* Division of Nursing, Bureau of Health Manpower, Health Resources Administration, DHHS. Seattle, WA, University of Washington.

Benner, P., & Wrubel, J. (1989). *The Primacy of Caring.* Menlo Park, CA, Addison-Wesley.

Benoliel, J., Ellison, E., Kogan, H., et al., (1985). Report of the clinical therapeutics task force. Seattle, University of Washington, School of Nursing.

Bircher, A. (1982). The concept of nursing diagnosis. In Kim, M., & D. Moritz, (Eds.), *Classification of Nursing Diagnoses: Proceedings of the Third and Fourth National Conferences* (pp. 30–46). New York, McGraw-Hill.

Bloom, K., Leitner, J., & Solano, J. (1987, July/August). Development of an expert system prototype to generate nursing care plans based on nursing diagnoses. *Comput. Nurs.,* 5:140–145.

Bower, F. (1982). *The Process of Planning Nursing Care* (3rd ed.). St. Louis, C. V. Mosby.

Braden, C. (1984). *The Focus and Limits of Community Health Nursing.* Norwalk, CT, Appleton-Century-Crofts.

Brown, M. (1974). The epidemiologic approach to the study of nursing diagnosis. *Nurs. Forum,* 13:346–359.

Bulechek, G., & McCloskey, J. (1985). *Nursing Interventions: Treatments for Nursing Diagnoses.* Philadelphia, W.B. Saunders.

Bulechek, G., & McCloskey, J. (1989). Nursing interventions: Treatments for potential nursing diagnoses. In Carroll-Johnson, R. (Ed.), *Classification of Nursing Diagnoses: Proceedings of Eighth National Conference* (pp. 23–30). St. Louis, C. V. Mosby.

Bulechek, G., & McCloskey, J. (1990). Nursing intervention taxonomy development. In McCloskey, J., & Grace, H. (Eds.), *Current Issues in Nursing* (3rd ed.) (pp. 23–28). St. Louis, C. V. Mosby.

Campbell, C. (1984). *Nursing Diagnosis and Intervention in Nursing Practice* (2nd ed.). New York, John Wiley & Sons.

Cell, P., Peters, D., & Gordon, J. (1984, January/February). Implementing a nursing diagnosis system through research: The New Jersey experience. *Home Healthcare Nurse,* 2:26–32.

Codman, E. (1918). *A Study in Hospital Efficiency: The First Five Years.* Boston, Thomas Todd Company.

Cornell, S., & Brush, F. (1971, July). Systems approach to nursing care plans. *Am. J. Nurs.,* 71:1376–1377.

Corrigan, M. (1983). *Conceptualization of Family Nursing Practice.* [Mimeograph]. Omaha, NE, University of Nebraska.

Corrigan, M. (1988). *Glossary of Terms.* NU 840-841, Nursing of Families in Health and Illness in the Community: Course Syllabus. [Mimeograph]. Omaha, NE, University of Nebraska.

Daubert, E. (1979, July). Patient classification system and outcome criteria. *Nurs. Outlook,* 27:450–454.

Dennison, P., & Keeling, A. (1989, Fall). Clinical support for eliminating the nursing diagnosis of knowledge deficit. *Image,* 21:142–144.

Densen, P. (1970). Some practical and conceptual problems in appraising the outcome of health care services and programs. In Hopkins, C. (Ed.), *Outcomes Conference I–II: Methodology of Identifying, Measuring, and Evaluating Outcomes of Health Service Programs, Systems, and Subsystems* (pp. 15–30). Rockville, MD, DHEW, Health Service & Mental Health Administration.

Derryberry, M. (1939, November). Nursing accomplishments as revealed by case records. *Public Health Rep.,* 54:2035–2043.

Donabedian, A. (1966, July). Evaluating the quality of medical care. *Milbank Memorial Fund Q.,* 44(2):166–206.

Evans, S. (1984). A computer-based nursing diagnosis consultant. In Cohen, G. (Ed.), *Proceedings: The Eighth Annual Symposium on Computer Applications in Medical Care.* New York, IEEE Computer Society Press.

Feldman, J., & Richard, R. (1988). The measurement of nursing outcomes for home health care. In Waltz, C., & Strickland, O. (Eds.), *Measurement of Nursing Outcomes, Vol 1, Measuring Client Outcomes* (pp. 475–495). New York, Springer.

Freeman, R. (1961, October). Measuring the effectiveness of public health nursing service. *Nurs. Outlook,* 9:605–607.

Freeman, R., & Heinrich, J. (1981). *Community Health Nursing Practice* (2nd ed.). Philadelphia, W.B. Saunders.

Gebbie, K., & Lavin, M. (Eds.) (1975). *Classification of Nursing Diagnoses.* St. Louis, C. V. Mosby.

Giovannetti, P. (1988). Compatibility of existing patient classification systems with the nursing minimum data set. In Werley, H., & Lang, N. (Eds.), *Identification of the Nursing Minimum Data Set* (pp. 103–111). New York, Springer.

Gleit, C., & Tatro, S. (1981, October). Nursing diagnoses for healthy individuals. *Nurs. Health Care,* 11:456–457.

Gordon, M. (1987). *Nursing Diagnosis: Process and Application* (2nd ed.). New York, McGraw-Hill.

Gordon, M, Sweeney, M., & McKeehan, K. (1980, April). Nursing diagnoses: Looking at its use in the clinical area. *Am. J. Nurs.,* 80:672–674.

Gough, H. (1971, February). Some reflections on the meaning of psychodiagnosis. *Am. Psychol.,* 26:160–167.

Grobe, S. (1989, January). *Nursing's Language: Implications for Practice and Scientific Discovery.* Paper presented at the Seventh Annual Conference on Research in Nursing Education, San Francisco, CA.

Hagey, R., & McDonough, P. (1984, May/June). The problem of professional labeling. *Nurs. Outlook,* 32:151–157.

Halloran, E. (1985, December). Nursing workload, medical diagnosis related groups, and nursing diagnoses. *Res. Nurs. Health,* 8:421–433.

Haussmann, R., Hegyvary, S., & Newman, J. (1976). *Monitoring Quality of Nursing Care, Part II, Assessment and Study Correlates.* Bethesda, MD, DHEW Bureau of Health Manpower, Division of Nursing.

Hays, B. (1990). *Relationships Among Nursing Care Requirements, Selected Patient Factors, Selected Nurse Factors, and Nursing Resource Consumption in Home Health Care.* Unpublished doctoral dissertation, Cleveland, OH, Case Western Reserve University.

Horn, B., & Swain, M. (1977). *Development of Criterion Measures of Nursing Care:* Vol. I. Ann Arbor, MI, University of Michigan.

Hoskins, L., McFarlane, E., Rubenfeld, M., et al. (1986, April). Nursing diagnosis in the chronically ill: Methodology for clinical validation. *Adv. Nurs. Sci.,* 8:80–89.

Januska, C., Engle, J., & Wood, J. (1976). *Status of Quality Assurance in Public Health Nursing.* [Mimeograph]. Public Health Nursing Section, American Public Health Association.

Jenny, J. (1987, Winter). Knowledge deficit: Not a nursing diagnosis. *Image,* 19:184–185.

Kramer, M. (1972, September/October). Nursing care plans . . . power to the patient. *J. Nurs. Admin.,* 12:34–39.

Kuhn, T. (1970). *The Structure of Scientific Revolutions* (2nd ed., enlarged). Chicago, University of Chicago Press.

Lalonde, B. (1988, January). Assuring the quality of home care via the assessment of client outcomes. *Caring,* 12:20–24.

Lang, N. (1976). Issues in quality assurance in nursing. *Issues in Evaluation Research* (pp. 45–56). Kansas City, MO, American Nurses' Association.

Laros, J. (1977, May) Deriving outcome criteria from a conceptual model. *Nurs. Outlook,* 25:333–336.

Leavell, H., & Clark, E. (1965). *Preventive Medicine for the Doctor in His Community* (3rd ed.). New York, McGraw-Hill.

Lunney, M. (1986). The PES system: A time for change. In Hurley, M. (Ed.), *Classification of Nursing Diagnoses: Proceedings of the Sixth National Conference* (pp. 215–225). St. Louis, C. V. Mosby.

Maas, M., Hardy, M., & Craft, M. (1990, January–March). Some methodologic considerations in nursing diagnosis research. *Nurs. Diagnosis,* 1:24–30.

Marek, K. (1989). Classification of outcome measures in nursing care. *Classification Systems for Describing Nursing Practice.* Kansas City, MO, American Nurses' Association.

Mayers, M. (1983). *A Systematic Approach to the Nursing Care Plan* (3rd ed.). Norwalk, CT, Appleton-Century-Crofts.

McKibbin, R., Brimmer, P., Clinton, J., et al. (1985). *DRGs and Nursing Care.* Kansas City, MO, American Nurses' Association.

McLane, A., & Fehring, R. (1984). Nursing diagnosis: A review of the literature. In Kim, M., McFarland, G., & McLane, A. (Eds.), *Classification of Nursing Diagnoses: Proceedings of the Fifth National Conference* (pp. 529–540). St. Louis, C. V. Mosby.

Mundt, M. (1988, May). An analysis of nurse recording in family health clinics of a county health department. *J. Commun. Health Nurs.*, 5:3–10.

Nichols, E., & Barstow, R. (1980, May). Do nurses really use standard care plans? *J. Nurs. Admin.*, 10:27–31.

Nightingale, F. (1859). *Notes on Nursing: What it is and What it is Not.* London, Harrison.

Ozbolt, J., McHugh, M., Schultz, S., et al. (1985). Designing the cybernurse system: A proposed information system to support nursing practice, administration, research and quality assurance. In Hannah, K., Guillemin, F., & Conklin, D. (Eds.), *Nursing Uses of Computers and Information Science.* Amsterdam, North-Holland.

Pender, N., & Pender, A. (1986, January/February). Attitudes, subjective norms, and intentions to engage in health behaviors. *Nurs. Res.*, 35:15–18.

Perry, A. (1982). Analysis of the components of the nursing process. In Carlson, J., Corft, C., & McGuire, A. (Eds.), *Nursing Diagnosis* (pp. 41–45). Philadelphia, W.B. Saunders.

Peters, D. (1988). Classifying patients using a nursing diagnosis taxonomy. In Harris, M. (Ed.), *Home Health Administration* (pp. 311–322). Owings Mills, MD, Rynd Communications.

Peters, D. (1989, March). An overview of current research relating to long-term outcomes. *Nurs. Health Care*, 10:133–136.

Phaneuf, M. (1976). *The Nursing Audit Self-regulation in Nursing Practice* (2nd ed.). New York, Appleton-Century-Crofts.

Pigg, J., & Schroeder, P. (1984, December). Frequently occurring problems of patients with rheumatic diseases. *Nurs. Clin. North Am.*, 19:697–708.

Roberts, D. (1962, July). How effective is public health nursing? *Am. J. Public Health*, 52:1077–1083.

Roy, C. (1984). Framework for classification systems development: Progress and issues. In Kim, M., McFarland, G., & McLane, A. (Eds.), *Classification of Nursing Diagnoses: Proceedings of the Fifth National Conference* (pp. 26–45). St. Louis, C. V. Mosby.

Schmele, J. (1986, July/August). Teaching nurses how to improve their documentation. *Home Healthcare Nurse*, 5:6–10.

Schultz, P., & Meleis, A. (1988, Winter). Nursing epistemology: Traditions, insights, questions. *Image*, 20:217–221.

Shaffer, F. (Ed.) (1986). *Patients and Purse Strings: Patient Classification and Cost Management.* New York, National League for Nursing.

Shamansky, S., & Yanni, C. (1983, Spring). In opposition to nursing diagnosis: A minority opinion. *Image*, 15:47–50.

Shoemaker, J. (1984). Essentials of a nursing diagnosis. In Kim, M., McFarland, G., & McLane, A. (Eds.), *Classification of Nursing Diagnoses: Proceedings of Fifth National Conference* (pp. 104–115). St. Louis, C. V. Mosby.

Snyder, M. (1985). *Independent Nursing Interventions.* New York, John Wiley & Sons.

Stanhope, M., & Lancaster, J. (1988). *Community Health Nursing: Process and Practice for Promoting Health.* St. Louis, C. V. Mosby.

Tanner, C. (1988). Curriculum revolution: The practice mandate. In National League for Nursing (Ed.), *Curriculum Revolution: Mandate for Change* (pp. 201–216). New York, National League for Nursing.

Taylor, D. (1989). Interventions. *Classification Systems for Describing Nursing Practice.* Kansas City, MO, American Nurses' Association.

Tinkham, C., Voorhies, E., & McCarthy, N. (1984). *Community Health Nursing: Evolution and Process in the Family and Community* (3rd ed.). New York, Appleton-Century-Crofts.

Urwick, L. (1943). *The Elements of Administration.* New York, Harper and Brothers.

Visiting Nurse and Home Care (1987). Self management outcome criteria (SMOC) record form. In Rinke, L., & Wilson, A. (Eds.), *Outcome Measures in Home Care: Volume II, Service* (pp. 255–260). New York, National League for Nursing.

Walter, J., Pardee, G., & Malbo, D. (1976). *Dynamics of Problem Oriented Approaches: Patient Care and Documentation.* Philadelphia, J. B. Lippincott.

Weed, L. (1968, March 14–21). Special article: Medical records that guide and teach. *New Engl. J. Med.*, 278:593–600, 652–657.

Weidmann, J., & North, H. (1987, December). Implementing the Omaha classification system in a public health agency. *Nurs. Clin. North Am.*, 22:971–979.

Werley, H., & Lang, N. (1988). *Identification of the Nursing Minimum Data Set.* New York, Springer.

Yura, H., & Walsh, M. (1988). *The Nursing Process: Assessing, Planning, Implementing, Evaluating.* Norwalk, CT, Appleton & Lange.

BIBLIOGRAPHY

American Nurses' Association (1977). *Guidelines for Review of Nursing Care at the Local Level.* Kansas City, MO.

American Nurses' Association (1986). *Standards of Community Health Nursing Practice.* Kansas City, MO.

Ballard, S., & McNamara, R. (1983, July/August). Quantifying nursing needs in home health care. *Nurs. Res.*, 32:236–241.

Boesch, D. (Ed.) (1990, January). CHAP develops consumer-oriented outcome standards. *Hosp. Home Health*, 7:1.

Brand, L., Chisholm, S., Hoelzel-Seipp, L., et al. (1987, December). A new nursing diagnosis system. *Home Healthcare Nurse*, 5:12–16.

Carnevali, D. (1983). *Nursing Care Planning: Diagnoses and Management* (3rd ed.). Philadelphia, J. B. Lippincott.

Carnevali, D., Mitchell, P., Woods, N., et al. (1984). *Diagnostic Reasoning in Nursing.* Philadelphia, J. B. Lippincott.

Carpenito, L. (1989). *Nursing Diagnosis: Application to Clinical Practice* (3rd ed.). Philadelphia, J. B. Lippincott.

Carroll-Johnson, R. (Ed.) (1989). *Classification of Nursing Diagnoses: Proceedings of Eighth National Conference.* St. Louis, C. V. Mosby.

Deniston, O. (1976). A model for program evaluation. *Community Health Agency Evaluation* (pp. 1–7). New York, National League for Nursing.

Dickoff, J., James, P., & Wiedenbach, E. (1968a, September/October). Theory in a practice discipline: Part I. Practice oriented theory. *Nurs. Res.*, 17:415–435.

Dickoff, J., James, P., & Wiedenbach, E. (1968b, November/December). Theory in a practice discipline: Part II. Practice oriented research. *Nurs. Res.*, 17:545–554.

Dickoff, J., & James, P. (1989). Theoretical pluralism for nursing diagnosis. In Carroll-Johnson, P. (Ed.), *Classification of Nursing Diagnoses: Proceedings of Eighth National Conference* (pp. 98–125). St. Louis, C. V. Mosby.

Diers, D. (1990, January). The art and craft of nursing. *Am. J. Nurs.*, 90:65–66.

Donabedian, A. (1984, May/June). Quality, cost, and cost containment. *Nurs. Outlook*, 32:142–145.

Durand, M., & Prince, R. (1966, April). Nursing diagnosis: Process and decision. *Nurs. Forum*, 5:50–64.

Gould, E., & Wargo, J. (1987). *Home Health Nursing Care Plans.* Rockville, MD, Aspen.

Hannah, K., Reimer, M., Mills, W., et al. (Eds.) (1987). *Clinical Judgement and Decision Making: The Future with Nursing Diagnosis.* New York, John Wiley & Sons.

Kritek, P. (1978, June). The generation and classification of nursing diagnoses: Toward a theory of nursing. *Image*, 10:33–40.

Maas, M., & Hardy, M. (1988, March). A challenge for the future. *J. Gerontol. Nurs.*, 14:8–13.

Mackay, C., & Ault, L. (1977, January). A systematic approach to individualizing nursing care. *J. Nurs. Admin.*, 7:39–48.

Marriner, A. (1983). *The Nursing Process: A Scientific Approach to Nursing Care* (3rd ed.). St. Louis, C. V. Mosby.

Martin, K., Scheet, N., Crews, C., et al. (1986). *Client Management Information System for Community Health Nursing Agencies: An Implementation Manual.* Rockville, MD, Division of Nursing, US DHHS, PHS, HRSA.

McCloskey, J., & Grace, H. (Eds.) (1990). *Current Issues in Nursing* (3rd ed.). St. Louis, C. V. Mosby.

McFarland, G., & McFarlane, E. (1989). *Nursing Diagnosis and Intervention: Planning for Patient Care.* St. Louis, C. V. Mosby.

Meisenheimer, C. (1989). *Quality Assurance for Home Health Care.* Rockville, MD, Aspen.

Miller, J., Steele, K., & Boisen, A. (1987, December). The impact of nursing diagnosis in a long-term care setting. *Nurs. Clin. North Am.*, 22:905–915.

Nursing Development Conference Group (1973). *Concept Formalization in Nursing: Process and Product.* Boston, Little, Brown.

Pinnell, N., & de Menses, M. (1986). *The Nursing Process.* Norwalk, CT, Appleton-Century-Crofts.

Porter, E. (1986, Winter). Critical analysis of NANDA nursing diagnosis taxonomy I. *Image, 18*:136–139.

Rinke, L. (Ed.) (1987). *Outcome Measures in Home Care: Volume I, Research.* New York, National League for Nursing.

Rinke, L., & Wilson, A. (Eds.) (1987). *Outcome Measures in Home Care: Volume II, Service.* New York, National League for Nursing.

Scherman, S. (1990). *Community Health Nursing Care Plans* (2nd ed.). Albany, NY, Delmar.

Simmons, D. (1975). Quality assurance in a home health agency. *Quality Assurance — A Joint Venture* (pp. 7–11). New York, National League for Nursing.

Stainton, M. (1987). Nursing process: Is that how nurses think! In Hannah, K., Reimer, M., Mills, W., et al. (Eds.), *Clinical Judgement and Decision Making: The Future with Nursing Diagnosis* (pp. 273–277). New York, John Wiley & Sons.

Strickland, O., & Waltz, C. (Eds.) (1988). *Measurement of Nursing Outcomes Vol. 2, Measuring Nursing Performance: Practice, Education, and Research.* New York, Springer.

Ulrich, S., Canale, S., & Wendell, S. (1986). *Nursing Care Planning Guides.* Philadelphia, W.B. Saunders.

Waltz, C., & Strickland, O. (Eds.) (1988). *Measurement of Nursing Outcomes Vol. 1, Measuring Client Outcomes.* New York, Springer.

Werley, H., & Grier, M. (Eds.) (1981). *Nursing Information Systems.* New York, Springer.

Ziegler, S., Vaughan-Wrobel, B., & Erlen, J. (1986). *Nursing Process, Nursing Diagnosis, Nursing Knowledge: Avenues to Autonomy.* Norwalk, CT, Appleton-Century-Crofts.

Zimmer, M. (1976). *Manual: Nursing Quality Assurance.* [Mimeograph]. Madison, WI, University of Wisconsin Hospitals.

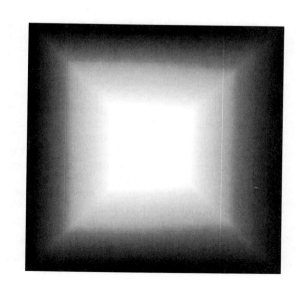

CHAPTER FOUR

*A*t the inception of this initial contract, it was stated that it has ". . . become evident that a method of documentation that was uniform, precise, and accepted by the profession must be developed and implemented" (Simmons, 1980, p. iv). While it was evident at our inception, it is imperative to the point of crisis in today's environment. Indeed, the success or failure of home health agencies can be directly related to the timeliness, the accuracy, and the specificity of documentation. (Simmons in Martin, Scheet, Crews, et al., 1986a, p. iv)

The management and supervisory staff at the VNA of Omaha began to address documentation issues as early as 1970. Their interest arose not only from increasingly restrictive documentation regulations but also from a concern that staff members were not adequately using their full range of professional skills in the provision of nursing care. A committee of the management and supervisory staff was formed to develop the Systematic Guide to Observation that was used by nursing staff to complete an initial and ongoing assessment of each client admitted to service.

Concurrently, references to a problem-oriented system began to appear in medical literature. This method of organizing and documenting health care, developed by Lawrence Weed, a physician at the University of Vermont, was gaining acceptance for use in acute care settings and in physicians' offices. The Omaha committee of management and the supervisory staff who had developed the assessment tool were joined by service delivery staff. They were given the task of adapting Weed's problem-oriented record to the community health setting. The committee began by developing a defined data base to be used as a guide in collection of data. VNA of Omaha's earlier Systematic Guide to Observation, which included physiologic data only, was expanded to include data relative to environmental and psychosocial factors as well as health behaviors. A defined data base guide was completed in 1972, and testing was begun. It rapidly became apparent that, although a good beginning step, this data base would not suffice. The primary difficulty was that it focused on the individual client and did not adequately reflect the family as the focus of nursing intervention. Through continuing committee efforts, a family data base evolved and was integrated into the recording system.

Collection of defined data was the first step in the problem-oriented method proposed by Weed. Identification and recording of problems on a problem list was the second step. The problem list was described as the index used by service providers to plan, deliver, and record care. It became apparent to VNA of Omaha supervisors and staff that the goal of simplifying and standardizing recording would not be realized until tools were developed to systematically identify and record problems, plans, outcomes, and interventions. It was at this point that VNA of Omaha staff decided to seek external funding for development of a comprehensive uniform system.

RESEARCH

The Omaha System was developed during a series of three research contracts between the VNA of Omaha and the Division of Nursing, Public Health Service, US Department of Health and Human Services (DHHS). Terms of the first contract were fulfilled between October, 1975, and May, 1976. Work focused on development and preliminary testing of the Problem Classification Scheme (VNA of Omaha, 1976). Field testing of the Problem Classification Scheme and development of an Expected Outcome-Outcome Criteria Scheme were accomplished during the second contract. This phase of development occurred from September, 1977, to September, 1980 (Simmons, 1980; VNA of Omaha, 1980). Terms of the third contract were met between July, 1984, and November, 1986. They included testing and revision of the Problem Classification Scheme, as well as development and testing of the Problem Rating Scale for Outcomes and the Intervention Scheme (Martin, et al., 1986a, 1986b; Martin, 1988). Developing and conducting such research within a service setting were viewed by VNA of Omaha staff and others throughout the country as unique.

Development of the Omaha System

Participants

Many people with experience in various areas contributed their expertise during the development, testing, and completion of the Omaha System. They are cited in Table 4–1. The management, supervisory, and service delivery staff at the VNA of Omaha were involved throughout the research process. In addition, four community health nursing agencies served as test sites during the second and third contracts. These agencies were selected to reflect the diversity of settings in which community health nurses practice. Differences among the agencies included their (1) geographic location, (2) type and organization, and (3) focus of services provided. The Public Health Nursing Association of Des Moines (IA) represented combined official and voluntary community health agencies. This agency provides homes health care to acutely ill and chronically ill clients and, as the Division of Public Health Nursing of the local Health Department, offers preventive services in home and clinic settings. The Division of Public Health, Bureau of Nursing, State of Delaware was representative of official agencies that provide preventive services in home and clinic settings. The Visiting Nurse Association of Dallas (TX) represented voluntary agencies. This private, nonprofit agency offers primarily home health services. During the third contract, the Dallas agency was replaced by the Visiting Nurse Service of Indianapolis (IN). This agency is also a private, nonprofit agency providing home health services.

Approximately 500 staff nurses participated in various phases of research during the three projects. Because the goal was to produce a system useful to all community health staff, members of other disciplines were also included in group discussion and other means of data collection. Conscious effort was made to include staff with diverse educational preparation, length of employment, and clinical experience.

Guidelines

The three studies were designed to incorporate the same basic guidelines throughout the research process. These guidelines provided the basis for development of research methods and procedures, for analysis of research data, and for revision of clinical components. The guidelines were formulated as follows:

- Empirical data — actual client data gathered and recorded by practicing community health nurses, along with users' experiences, would serve as the basis of the clinical components.
- Inductive reasoning — specific observations would be used to develop generalizations regarding data.
- Simplicity — the clinical components would be organized into Schemes that would be simple and easy to use.
- Reliability and validity — testing and retesting would continue until these research issues appeared to be satisfactorily resolved.
    Reliability — attention to measures of stability or consistency, homogeneity, and equivalence.
    Validity — attention to content, concurrent, construct, and predictive issues.
- Practicality — the clinical components would have value for users in organizing and documenting their practice.
- Unity — the clinical components would complement one another to produce a meaningful practice and recording framework.
- Relevance — the clinical components would be con-

TABLE 4–1 ■ Contributors to the Development of the Omaha System, 1975 to 1986

CONTRIBUTOR	PLACE OF EMPLOYMENT	ROLE
Felice Armignacco	Monroe County Department of Health Rochester, NY	Advisory Committee #1
Gary Bargstadt	VNA of Omaha Omaha, NE	Project Staff #2
Violet Barkauskas	University of Michigan Ann Arbor, MI	Consultant #3
Michael Branson	Oklahoma State University Stillwater, OK	Advisory Committee #3
Sr. M. Consilia Buka	College of Allied Health Services St. Louis, MO	Advisory Committee #1
Joan Caserta	National League for Nursing New York, NY	Advisory Committee #1 and #2
Marjorie Corrigan	University of NE Medical Center Omaha, NE	Consultant #1, #2, & #3
Carli Crews	VNA of Omaha Omaha, NE	Project Staff #3
Ken Dennert	VNA of Omaha Omaha, NE	Project Staff #3
Jean Denton	Visiting Nurse Service Indianapolis, IN	Advisory Committee #3 Test Agency #3
Avedis Donabedian	University of Michigan Ann Arbor, MI	Advisory Committee #3
R.K. Dieter Haussmann	Medicus Systems Corporation Chicago, IL	Advisory Committee #1 & #2
O. Marie Henry	Division of Nursing, USPHS, DHHS Rockville, MD	Contracting Officer #3
Marion Highriter	University of North Carolina Chapel Hill, NC	Advisory Committee #2
Barbara Horn	University of Washington Seattle, WA	Advisory Committee #3
William Kehl	Peat, Marwick & Mitchell Omaha, NE	Consultant #3
Patricia Kelly	Medical Center Hospital of Vermont Burlington, VT	Advisory Committee #1
Prudence Kobasa	State of Delaware, DPH Dover, DE	Advisory Committee #3 Test Agency #3
Alice Kruszon	American Nurses' Association Kansas City, MO	Advisory Committee #1
William Lake	Information Management Services Bethesda, MD	Subcontractor #2
Norma Lang	University of Wisconsin Milwaukee, WI	Advisory Committee #3
Eugene Levine	Division of Nursing, USPHS, DHHS Rockville, MD	Contracting Officer #1
Robert Lindner	Peat, Marwick & Mitchell Kansas City, MO	Consultant #3
Karen Martin	VNA of Omaha Omaha, NE	Project Staff #2 & #3
Frances McVey	VNA of Brooklyn New York, NY	Advisory Committee #3
Sr. Patricia Miller	University of NE Medical Center Omaha, NE	Consultant #3
Cheryl Moore	DE Department of Health & Social Service Dover, DE	Advisory Committee #2 Test Agency #2
Cheryl Muck	Dallas VNA Dallas, TX	Advisory Committee #2 Test Agency #2
Dorothea Orem	Orem & Shields, Inc. Chevy Chase, MD	Advisory Committee #1
J. V. Petty	ConAgra, Inc. Omaha, NE	Advisory Committee #3
Suzanne Resner	Division of Nursing, USPHS, DHHS Rockville, MD	Contracting Officer #3
Rovia Rich	VNA of Omaha Omaha, NE	Project Staff #1 & #2
Edward Roberts	Peat, Marwick & Mitchell Kansas City, MO	Consultant #3
Virginia Saba	Division of Nursing, USPHS, DHHS Rockville, MD	Contracting Officer #1 & #2
Nancy Scheet	VNA of Omaha Omaha, NE	Project Staff #1, #2, & #3

TABLE 4–1 ■ Contributors to the Development of the Omaha System, 1975 to 1986 *Continued*

CONTRIBUTOR	PLACE OF EMPLOYMENT	ROLE
Rose Marie Serra	Public Health Nursing Association Des Moines, IA	Advisory Committee #2 & #3 Test Agency #2 & #3
DeLanne Simmons	VNA of Omaha Omaha, NE	Project Dir. #1, #2 & #3
Lillian Wagner	DE Department of Health & Social Service Dover, DE	Advisory Committee #2 Test Agency #2
Una Beth Westfall	American Nurses' Association Kansas City, MO	Advisory Committee #2
Richard Wikoff	University of NE at Omaha Omaha, NE	Consultant #3
Lois Young	National League for Nursing New York, NY	Advisory Committee #2
Rita Zielstorff	Massachusetts General Hospital Boston, MA	Advisory Committee #3

gruent with community health practice and recording.

- Framework—the clinical components would provide a comprehensive framework for practicing and documenting community health nursing.
- Computer compatibility—the clinical components would be structured for computerization.
- Taxonomic principles—organization of the clinical components would be based on principles including comparable levels of specificity and mutual exclusivity.

PROBLEM CLASSIFICATION SCHEME

Development of the Omaha System began with identification and classification of client problems addressed by community health nurses. Development, testing, and revision of the Problem Classification Scheme (PCS) began in October, 1975, and continued throughout the three research contracts. The PCS was completed in November, 1986. The principal steps in the research process related to the PCS are shown in Figure 4–1.

Pilot Study and Problem Classification Scheme Draft

Development of the Problem Classification Scheme (PCS) began with a 3-month pilot study. Community health nurses employed by the VNA of Omaha functioned as data collectors as they admitted families to agency service. Data were collected on all of the 338 families admitted during the study time. Preventive services were the focus of care provided to 57% of the sample population, whereas 43% of the sample had physical problems requiring home health nursing care. The raw data showed a mixture of nursing problems, medical diagnoses, causes of problems, results of prob-

lems, risk factors, and interventions for problems. The 61 nurses who participated identified a total of 1,341 client problems, or 3.97 problems per family, each with descriptors or defining characteristics. Medical diagnoses comprised 4% of the data, and 4% of the data were unusable. Therefore, 8% of the data was discarded.

Project staff used a process of sorting and collapsing data to identify 49 problem labels, each with mutually exclusive descriptors. The more ill-defined the problem name, the less consensus there was regarding the descriptors. For example, a mixture of several different

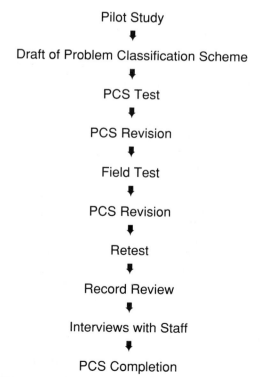

FIGURE 4–1 ■ Development of the Problem Classification Scheme.

problems was described under the problem name "Emotional Stress," with 51 accompanying descriptors. Nurses demonstrated little agreement regarding descriptors for the problems of Dependency, Emotional Instability, Disruption of Family Mental Health, Parenting, Inadequate Income, and Growth and Development Lag.

Research project staff examined the problem labels and descriptors for similarities and differences. This data analysis suggested problem categories related to the sections of the VNA of Omaha's defined data base. The categories were as follows: Life Style and Living Resources, Family Dynamics and Structure, Current Health Status and Deviations, and Patterns and Knowledge of Health Maintenance. The modifiers Actual or Potential could be used with all the 49 problems.

PCS PILOT STUDY

Dates: March to June, 1976
Location: VNA of Omaha
Data Collectors: 61 staff nurses
Data Source: 338 families admitted to service during the study
Data Description: 1,341 client problems, each with descriptors
Data Analysis: Data sorted and collapsed
Results: Problem Classification Scheme: 4 categories, 49 problems with mutually exclusive descriptors, modifiers—actual or potential

PCS Test and Revision

The next phase of development involved testing the PCS. The agency caseload was analyzed in relation to (1) client age and (2) assignment to a preventive or home health agency program. A sample of 99 current records was selected. Each record contained one family member representative by age and diagnosis of the total agency caseload. A total of 16 home health and public health nurses used the newly developed PCS to list problems they identified from a review of the data bases in the sample. The nurses were encouraged to add or delete problem names and accompanying descriptors.

Research staff analyzed the problem lists generated by the nurse testers. All of the problem names from the Scheme were used in the testing phase. A comparison was made of the number of problems identified in the records and the number of problems identified by the nurse testers. The testers identified a total of 1,341 problems, or 3.97 per family. In every record, a greater number of client problems was found on the problem list generated for the test than on the problem list in the record. It appeared that the nurse could more clearly define the focus of nursing due to the specificity of the problem labels. In contrast to the pilot study, no medical diagnoses, causes of problems, results of problems, or risk factors were identified as problems. The results

of this test were used to further refine and revise the PCS by adding and subdividing problems and by clarifying the language of signs and symptoms. The revised PCS was integrated into the VNA of Omaha recording system and used by all service delivery staff during the following 2 years. This represented the first attempt to implement a system of nursing diagnoses in a community health agency.

PCS TEST

Date: November, 1976
Location: VNA of Omaha
Data Collectors: 16 staff nurses
Data Source: 99 current family records
Data Description: Client problems, each with descriptors
Data Analysis: Comparison of problems identified by data collectors with (a) problems in the record and (b) problems in the PCS
Results: All problems used; all data collectors identified more problems than were identified in the records. PCS revisions made.

Field Test and PCS Revision

During the second contract, the PCS was field tested at the Public Health Nursing Association of Des Moines; the Division of Nursing, Delaware State Department of Health and Social Services; and the Visiting Nurse Association of Dallas. The objectives of the field test were to:

- Determine the completeness of the categories, problem labels, modifiers, and descriptors that comprised the PCS
- Determine the usefulness of the PCS for community health nursing practice in diverse settings
- Determine the effectiveness of the PCS as a tool for use in community health nursing agencies

The test procedures at each agency were similar. Variation was introduced purposely to explore the ease of using non-VNA of Omaha instructors. At the Des Moines agency, orientation was provided by research staff from the VNA of Omaha; at the Delaware agency, orientation was provided jointly by the VNA of Omaha and Delaware staff; at the Dallas agency, orientation was provided by the Dallas staff with the VNA of Omaha staff available for questions.

The nursing staff at each agency completed a data base and problem list on newly admitted clients. The Des Moines sample contained 93 clients with 487 problems; the Delaware sample contained 91 clients with 572 problems, and the Dallas sample contained 86 clients with 411 problems. The PCS was used by the nurses to identify and record problems. Using the data base generated by admitting nurses, the project staff at the VNA of Omaha also completed problem lists on all

93 Des Moines clients and a random sample of 31 Delaware and 31 Dallas clients. The problem lists were then statistically compared. Average percentage of agreement between the Omaha research project staff and the Des Moines, Delaware, and Dallas staff nurses was 78%, 66%, and 66%, respectively. The different percentage of agreement between the three test sites could be attributed to differences in orientation methods and to sample size. After analysis was completed, consultants indicated that this level of agreement was very acceptable for the particular test design.

The PCS was again revised based on field test results, suggestions from project Advisory Committee members, and input from the staff at the VNA of Omaha who had been using the PCS for 3 years. The PCS was revised in five principal ways. First, the four categories of the PCS were changed to four domains that more precisely delineated areas addressed by community health nurses. The domains were named Environmental, Psychosocial, Physiological, and Health Related Behaviors. Second, risk factors and laboratory tests included as descriptors in the original Scheme were deleted; the final descriptors were sufficiently refined to be considered signs and symptoms. Third, some problems were combined, strengthening the Scheme by eliminating redundancy and creating mutually exclusive problems. Fourth, seven problem labels were added to the Scheme. These additions were suggested by the staff who had used the PCS in their practice. Finally, four problem labels were deleted. The signs and symptoms associated with these problem labels were subsumed into other problems.

The revisions resulted in a Scheme of four domains and 38 problems, each having mutually exclusive signs/symptoms. Each problem could be designated as (1) Actual or Potential and (2) Family or Individual. Data within each level of the PCS showed a comparable level of specificity. The domains were viewed as exhaustive and mutually exclusive; the problems and signs/symptoms were non-exhaustive. The label "Other" appeared within each domain and within each grouping of signs/symptoms to allow for additions to the Scheme.

PCS FIELD TEST

Dates: July, 1978 to February, 1989
Location: Test agencies in Des Moines, Delaware, and Dallas
Data Collectors: Nurses at each test agency
Data Source: 270 records
Data Description: Problem lists generated at test agencies and problem lists generated from same data bases by research project staff
Data Analysis: Comparison of problems identified by test agency staff and research project staff. Des Moines 93 records; Delaware and Dallas samples of 31 records each
Results: Percentage of agreement — Des Moines 78%; Delaware 66%, Dallas 68%. PCS revised: 4 domains, 38 problems, mutually exclusive signs/symptoms

Retest

The refinements made to strengthen the PCS warranted retesting. Home health and public health nurses from the VNA of Omaha and the three test agencies participated in retesting. At the VNA of Omaha, each of eight staff nurses reviewed four randomly selected current records for a total sample of 32 records. The nurses generated a new problem list for each record in the sample. The nurses were encouraged to record and label signs/symptoms or problems not included in the revised PCS. No new problem labels were identified and only two labels were not used.

Retesting at the four agencies was conducted like the original field testing. The sample consisted of 31 randomly selected open records from each agency for a total sample of 93 records. Sample size was based on the recommendation of project consultants. Nursing staff at the test agencies and research project staff at the VNA of Omaha used the same 93 data bases to generate problem lists. Percentage of agreement from the retest was compared with the original field test results. The Des Moines agency percentage of agreement for the field test was 78%; for the retest it was 90%. The Delaware agency percentage of agreement for the field test was 66%, compared to 73% for the retest. The Dallas agency had 66% agreement for the field test and 77% for the retest. This comparison indicated that the average percentage of agreement for each agency increased. The improvement was attributed to refinement of the PCS, increased user experience with the Scheme, and revised test design. The greater degree of agreement between the Omaha and Des Moines results may be attributed to the similarities in agency organization, client mix, and staff. No changes were made in the Scheme as a result of the retest.

The revised PCS was integrated into the recording system at the VNA of Omaha. The PCS also became a mandatory component of the record systems at each of the three tests agencies.

PCS RETEST

Date: April, 1979
Location: VNA of Omaha and test agencies in Des Moines, Delaware, and Dallas
Data Collectors: Staff nurses at each agency
Data Source: Randomly selected current records; 32 in Omaha, 31 at each test agency
Data Description: List of problems with descriptors identified by testers and lists of problems with descriptors identified by research project staff
Data Analysis: Omaha — comparison of problems identified by testers with PCS. Test agencies — comparison of problems identified by testers with problems identified by research project staff.
Results: Omaha — 36 to 38 problems in PCS were identified; no new problem labels identified. Test agencies — percentage of agreement for Des Moines was 90%, for Delaware 73%, and Dallas 77%.

Record Review

The PCS was reviewed again as part of the third contract. The objective of this phase of the research project was to determine the validity, reliability, and usefulness of the PCS. The review consisted of two processes. The first process focused on data collection in relation to three major variables.

1. Frequency of occurrence of domains, problems, and signs/symptoms from the existing PCS and frequency of occurrence of additional problems and signs/symptoms
2. Consistency with which problems and signs/symptoms were selected from similar data by multiple nurses
3. Clustering of problems around medical diagnoses

A tool was designed to collect data ranging from simple and objective through complex and subjective; also the tool was to produce meaningful frequencies. Data collection categories included (1) domains, problems, and signs/symptoms; (2) other problems and signs/symptoms; (3) consistency of problem selection by multiple nurses; (4) clustering of problems around medical diagnoses; and (5) appropriateness of problem selection relative to clients' data bases.

The initial sample consisted of 25 records each from the VNA of Omaha and the Indianapolis, Des Moines, and Delaware agencies. Preliminary review of data collection tools revealed insufficient data. Therefore, an additional 75 records from the VNA of Omaha were added to the sample. Based on data assessment, it was determined that bias introduced by selecting additional Omaha records was not significant. Independent review of a 15% randomly chosen sample of records was completed by two VNA of Omaha research staff. Total interrater agreement was established above 98%.

Analysis of collected data revealed relatively similar consistency of problem usage within and among the four agencies, with variations in frequency of usage. The number of problems per record varied from 4.9 in the Omaha sample to 2.7 in the Delaware sample. Physiologic problems constituted the largest percentage of the total problems identified by staff at each agency, with Environmental problems accounting for the smallest percentage. The percentage of problems in Psychosocial and Health Related Behavior Domains ranked second and third respectively in Omaha and Delaware; the rankings were reversed in Des Moines and Indianapolis. Data were not found in any of the records to support additional problems. All identified problems were appropriately delineated as Actual or Potential and Individual or Family.

A total of 86 medical diagnoses was found within the record sample. No consistent relationships were found between medical diagnoses and client problems. Therefore, investigation was not continued.

RECORD REVIEW

Dates: September to October, 1984
Location: VNA of Omaha and test agencies in Des Moines, Delaware, and Indianapolis
Data Collector: VNA of Omaha research assistant
Data Source: 175 records
Data Description: Worksheet for each record
Data Analysis: (1) Appropriateness of problem selection, (2) comparison of average number of problems per record and by domain for each agency, (3) comparison of medical diagnoses and nursing problems
Results: 98% problems supported by data; 100% of modifiers used correctly; 2.7 to 4.9 average problems per record. Number of problems by domain highest for Physiological, lowest for Environmental. Eighty-six medical diagnoses, only some related to nursing problems. PCS revised—4 domains; 40 problems; modifiers—Actual, Potential, Health Promotion

---

Interviews with Staff

The second data collection process focused on subjective data. At each agency, an agency representative conducted tape-recorded interviews with all supervisors and over 50% of staff nurses. A discussion guide was used to facilitate consistency among agencies. Staff and supervisors were encouraged to suggest Scheme improvements and share their personal opinions and experiences while using the PCS. The comments were generally positive, although several staff identified difficulties in using the Scheme with certain medical diagnoses, such as diabetes and cancer, and with healthy clients. Staff identified benefits and deficiencies that they had experienced in using the PCS. Project staff and Advisory Committee members determined that these difficulties were not deficiencies in the PCS. Instead, these difficulties were attributed to using a nursing rather than the more familiar medical model and lack of experience with a problem-oriented system. Benefits were identified as follows:

- Promoted understanding of other nurses' records
- Distinguished between medical and nursing diagnoses
- Simplified problem identification
- Directed nurses' thought processes
- Promoted consistency among agency branch offices
- Encouraged the nurse to think about the entire family
- Helped organize care

STAFF INTERVIEWS

Date: November, 1984
Location: VNA of Omaha and test agencies in Des Moines, Delaware, and Indianapolis
Data Collectors: VNA of Omaha research staff and one agency liaison person in each of the three test agencies
Data Source: Informal group interviews using a discussion guide with all supervisors and at least 50% of the staff nurses in each agency
Data Description: Tape recordings of interviews
Data Analysis: Compilation of comments
Results: Lists of benefits, deficiencies, and suggestions for improvement of the PCS provided subjective data for revision of the Scheme.

PCS Completion

The PCS was revised, based on (1) the objective and subjective data previously gathered and (2) suggestions from consultants and Advisory Committee members. Data analysis indicated that validity, reliability, and usefulness of the PCS were established satisfactorily. No changes in the basic organization of the scheme were suggested by the data. No additional domains were suggested. Analysis of data did suggest revising the labels and signs/symptoms of certain problems and adding, deleting, and combining certain problems and signs/symptoms. In addition, the problem modifier Health Promotion was added to enhance usability of the PCS with preventive or public health clients.

The final PCS consisted of 40 problems organized in four domains. Each problem could be modified as Health Promotion, Potential, or Actual, and Family or Individual. The actual state of each problem was defined by a cluster of mutually exclusive signs and symptoms. The Problem Classification Scheme is illustrated and described in detail in Chapter 5.

PROBLEM RATING SCALE FOR OUTCOMES

The second tool developed during the research study at the VNA of Omaha was designed to measure client outcomes of community health nursing care. Development, testing, and revision of the second component of the Omaha was initiated in September, 1977, continued throughout the second and third research contracts, and was completed in November, 1986. Important steps in development, testing, and revision of the Problem Rating Scale for Outcomes are shown in Figure 4–2.

Pilot Study and Draft of Expected Outcome-Outcome Criterion (EO-OC) Schemes

Development of the outcome component of the Omaha System began with a pilot study conducted at the VNA of Omaha during a 3-month period in 1978. The objective of this phase of the research project was to develop expected outcomes and outcome criteria to be used by home health and public health nurses in conjunction with the Problem Classification Scheme. The EO-OC Schemes would enhance the effectiveness, accountability, and documentation of community health nursing services. All clients admitted to service by nurses at four of the eight nursing offices constituted the sample that contained 211 family records and 376 clients. Each nurse used the defined data base to conduct an assessment of the family unit and individual members and then identified nursing problems using

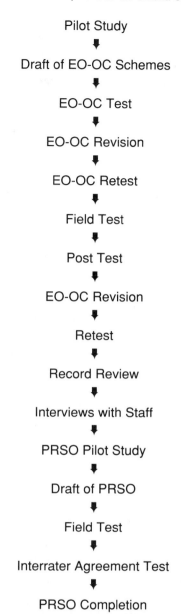

Pilot Study
↓
Draft of EO-OC Schemes
↓
EO-OC Test
↓
EO-OC Revision
↓
EO-OC Retest
↓
Field Test
↓
Post Test
↓
EO-OC Revision
↓
Retest
↓
Record Review
↓
Interviews with Staff
↓
PRSO Pilot Study
↓
Draft of PRSO
↓
Field Test
↓
Interrater Agreement Test
↓
PRSO Completion

FIGURE 4–2 ■ Development of the Problem Rating Scale for Outcomes.

the PCS. The nurse also listed one expected outcome and one or more outcome criteria for each problem.

The raw data generated during the pilot study varied in quantity and quality. The data contained 580 problems, each with one expected outcome. In addition, a total of 2,125 outcome criteria, or 3.66 per problem, was generated. The highest number of times any problem was identified was 84. One problem was not identified, and five problems were identified fewer than five times. Research staff examined expected outcomes and outcome criteria for similarity in terminology and ideas. Similarity among the 580 expected outcomes enabled the research staff to develop five basic expected outcome statements that could be applied to all problems. Comprehensive clusters of four to eight outcome criteria were identified for each problem using 2,075 of the outcome criteria. Time frames from problem identification to outcome ranged from 1 day to 2 years, with the most frequently identified frames in the 2- to 6-month range. No trends between time frames and expected outcomes for a given problem or for the problems as a whole could be determined. Therefore, the expected outcomes were open-ended as to time.

The expected outcomes and outcome criteria were organized into schemes that were compatible to the organization of the PCS. The Expected Outcome-Outcome Criterion (EO-OC) Scheme had two hierarchical levels that preceded the level of expected outcomes. The first level corresponded with the four categories of the PCS. The second level corresponded with the problem. The Expected Outcomes were designed for use with all problems, and the Outcome Criteria were organized in problem-specific clusters. Each outcome criterion had two levels of specificity. First, a statement described how a client would look, feel, or behave in observable and measurable terms. Second, parentheses included more specific examples of client behavior. The Expected Outcomes were exhaustive and mutually exclusive. The Outcome Criteria were neither exhaustive nor mutually exclusive.

EO-OC PILOT STUDY

Dates: July to October, 1978
Location: VNA of Omaha
Data Collectors: 31 staff nurses
Data Source: 376 clients admitted to service during the study
Data Description: 580 expected outcomes and 2,125 outcome criteria (3.66 outcome criteria per problem)
Data Analysis: Data sorted, condensed, and collapsed
Results: Five expected outcomes applicable to all problems; clusters of problem-specific outcome criteria with total of 230 statements; open-ended time frame

Expected Outcome-Outcome Criterion Test and Revision

The EO-OC Schemes were tested by 11 community health nurses employed at the VNA of Omaha using records of families currently receiving services. The records were purposively selected to yield at least three examples of each problem in the PCS. Each nurse was given five to seven records, and each used the recently developed Schemes to identify one expected outcome and one or more outcome criteria for each problem, using a time frame of 3 months. Assignments were made so that the nurse who received the record had neither visited the family nor read the record previously. Each record was independently reviewed by two nurses.

The expected outcomes and outcome criteria generated by the pairs of nurses were analyzed using quantitative and qualitative methods. Percentages of agree-

ment were calculated by problem for expected outcomes and outcome criteria and arbitrarily divided into high, medium, and low ranges. The mean percentage of agreement for expected outcomes was 54% with a median of 50%. The mean percentage of agreement for outcome criteria was 42.5% with a median of 35%. The project staff reviewed rank-ordered matches of expected outcomes and outcome criteria prior to refinement and revision of the Schemes. Particular attention was given to those expected outcomes and outcome criteria that ranked in the low range. Because the five expected outcomes were not found to be mutually exclusive and exhaustive statements, they were modified into three statements: Prevention, Improvement and Maintenance. The 230 outcome criteria were refined and revised into 237 outcome criteria. For example, an outcome criterion cluster was developed for the problem Hearing. Two of the five outcome criteria were (1) uses persons, assistive devices, and/or techniques (e.g., low tone, slow speech, touch visual materials, hearing aid), and (2) reports changes in hearing status to health personnel (e.g., less/more difficulty hearing, tinnitus).

EO-OC TEST

Date: July, 1979
Location: VNA of Omaha
Data Collectors: 11 staff nurses
Data Source: Sample of 35 family records admitted to service in 2 months preceding the test; selected to include at least three examples of each problem on the PCS
Data Description: One expected outcome and one or more outcome criteria for each problem using a time frame of 3 months; each record reviewed by two nurses
Data Analysis: Percentage of agreement for expected outcomes and outcome criteria calculated, rank ordered, and arbitrarily divided into high, medium, and low ranges
Results: Schemes revised into three mutually exclusive expected outcomes applicable to all problems of the PCS and 237 outcome criteria organized into nonmutually exclusive, problem-specific clusters

Retest

The revised EO-OC Schemes were tested on a limited basis at the VNA of Omaha. A sample record was distributed to eight community health nurses and three research staff, each of whom identified an expected outcome and one or more outcome criteria for each of the four problems identified in the record. Results were compared for percentage of agreement. Data analysis revealed an increase in agreement among testers using the revised schemes with a 100% agreement on expected outcomes.

EO-OC RETEST

Date: Fall, 1979
Location: VNA of Omaha
Data Collectors: Eight staff nurses; three research staff
Data Source: Sample record containing four problems
Data Description: 11 sets of one expected outcome and one or more outcome criteria for each problem
Data Analysis: Agreement between data collectors
Results: 100% agreement on expected outcomes for all problems; an increase in agreement on outcome criterion for all problems in comparison with previous test results

Field Test

The EO-OC Schemes were field tested at the VNA of Omaha and the three test agencies that had previously participated in the PCS field test. The testers were 40 randomly selected staff nurses, 10 from each agency. Following orientation, each nurse was given four sample records designed to collectively contain all the problems from the PCS. Working independently, each nurse identified one expected outcome and one or more outcome criteria for each problem. They were instructed to base their selections on the assumption that the client would be visited six times over a 3-month period.

Data for expected outcomes and outcome criteria were examined within and between the four test sites. Statistical analysis and subjective review revealed consistently high agreement among the staff nurses. The four sample records contained a total of 46 problems. Degree of concordance for expected outcomes was computed by problem, using percentage of agreement among the 40 staff nurses. The results were: 100%—20 problems, 90% to 99%—15 problems, 80% to 89%—six problems, 70% to 79%—two problems, 60% to 69%—two problems, and 55%—one problem. No changes were made in the EO Scheme.

Outcome criterion concordance was considered using two statistical tests. First, Kendall's coefficient of concordance was used to analyze outcome criteria selected from all problem-specific clusters by the total test group. In the total distribution, the 46 coefficients ranged from .95 to .56 with a mean of .82. A statistically significant degree of concordance was found with all outcome criterion clusters, the majority at the .01 level or less. Second, Spearman rank correlation coefficient was computed for five problem-specific outcome criterion clusters. The five clusters were chosen because their Kendall's coefficient of concordance scores were below .70. The score of .70 was selected because few or no intergroup differences were noted with clusters scoring above that level. Differences were greatest between Omaha and Delaware for four clusters and between Dallas and Delaware for one cluster. Outcome criteria clusters with low agreement scores were re-

vised. The resulting OC Scheme contained 188 outcome criterion statements in nonmutually exclusive, problem-specific clusters.

EO-OC FIELD TEST

Dates: December, 1979–January, 1980
Location: VNA of Omaha and test agencies in Des Moines, Delaware, and Dallas
Data Collectors: 10 staff nurses from each agency
Data Source: Four family records designed to include at least one example of each problem of the PCS
Data Description: Problem-specific worksheets containing one expected outcome and one or more outcome criteria
Data Analysis: Expected outcome: percentage of agreement by problem by agency. Outcome criteria—Kendall's coefficient of concordance (by problem); Spearman rank correlation coefficient (for five problems)
Results: Expected outcomes—high agreement among the nurses; no changes in EO Scheme. Outcome Criteria—Outcome criterion clusters with low agreement were revised. The resulting Outcome Criterion Scheme contained 188 outcome criterion statements in nonmutually exclusive, problem-specific clusters.

Post Test and EO-OC Revision

A post test was designed to assess reliability of the Expected Outcome-Outcome Criterion Schemes over time. Two community health nurses who had participated in the field test were randomly selected from each agency. One record containing 13 problems was used for the post test; procedures were identical to those in the field test. Each nurse selected one expected outcome and one or more outcome criteria for each problem. The nurses selected the same expected outcome in both tests with only six exceptions. Percentage of agreement was 100% for five nurses; the remaining three nurses scored 92%, 85%, and 77%.

The outcome criteria selected during the post test were compared with the outcome criteria identified by the same nurses during the field test. There was a tendency to select more outcome criteria in the post test. Out of 104 possible matches, the nurses selected identical outcome criteria for the post test 19 times. Only five times were none of the outcome criteria selected on the field test repeated on the post test. The nurses repeated all criteria previously selected on the field test and identified additional outcome criteria 40 times. The nurses repeated at least one but not all of the field test choices 45 times.

Statistical analysis and subjective review of field test and post test data provided the basis for completing the Expected Outcome-Outcome Criterion Scheme. The high degree of agreement in use of expected outcomes by many nurses and by the same nurses over time suggested that revision of the Expected Outcome Scheme was not indicated. Based on the significant agreement demonstrated by the nurses during the two tests, no revisions in the format of the Outcome Criteria Scheme were indicated. Some individual outcome criterion clusters were altered. Following revision, the Outcome Criteria Scheme was subjectively examined and standardized in relation to language use.

EO-OC POST TEST

Dates: January to February, 1980
Location: VNA of Omaha and test agencies in Des Moines, Delaware, and Dallas
Data Collectors: Two staff nurses from each agency
Data Source: One record selected at random from the four records used in the field test
Data Description: Problem-specific worksheets containing one expected outcome and one or more outcome criterion completed by each nurse
Data Analysis: Comparison by individual nurses of expected outcome-outcome criteria selections on field test and post test
Results: Expected outcomes—77 to 100% agreement. Outcome criteria—6 nurses selected more outcome criteria on the post test, one chose the same number and one chose fewer. Of 104 possible matches, the same individual outcome criteria were selected 19 times; the same plus additional outcome criteria 40 times; one or more but not all the same outcome criteria 45 times; none of the same outcome criteria 5 times. Results appeared to indicate relatively consistent use of expected outcomes and outcome criterion over time.

Retest

The revised Scheme was submitted to four VNA of Omaha staff nurses for limited retesting. The nurses were selected from among staff who had not participated in the field test. Each nurse independently reviewed the four field test records and selected one expected outcome and one or more outcome criteria for each problem. Percentage of agreement for selection of expected outcomes was computed for each of the 46 problems with the results as follow: 100% or all four nurses agreed on 25 problems, 75% or three nurses agreed on 15 problems, 50% or two nurses agreed on six problems. Of the 240 possible outcome criterion selections, 82 were selected by all nurses, 61 were selected by no nurses, 40 were selected by three nurses, 37 were selected by two nurses, and 20 were selected by one nurse. The nurses' comments indicated that the expected outcomes were mutually exclusive, exhaustive, and useful when applied to the four records. In addition, the nurses indicated that most outcome criterion clusters were complete and useful when applied to the four records. Following the retest, the EO-OC Schemes were integrated into the recording systems at the Omaha and Delaware agencies.

EO-OC RETEST

Date: April, 1980
Location: VNA of Omaha
Data Collectors: Four staff nurses
Data Source: Four records used in the previous EO-OC field test
Data Description: Problem-specific worksheet with one expected outcome and one or more outcome criteria
Data Analysis: Percentage of agreement for expected outcomes; number of times each individual outcome criteria was selected by four data collectors
Results: Nurses were relatively consistent in selection of expected outcomes and outcome criteria. Expected outcomes were determined to be exhaustive, mutually exclusive, and useful. Most outcome criterion clusters were felt to be complete and useful.

Record Review

During the third contract, the Expected Outcome-Outcome Criterion Schemes were again examined. Data were generated through a review of records and interviews with the staff. A tool was designed to gather data from a sample of client records at the VNA of Omaha and the three test agencies. Data collection categories included: (1) expected outcomes, outcome criteria, and time frames from the EO-OC Schemes; (2) other expected outcomes, outcome criteria, and time frames; (3) consistency of selection by multiple nurses; and (4) appropriateness of selection relative to client data. In the sample of 175 client records, 762 problems were identified; 333 of the problems also had expected outcomes. The lower number of expected outcomes was attributed to limited or no use of the EO Scheme at some of the test agencies as well as use of the Scheme with only certain problems. When the three expected outcomes were tabulated, Prevention was used 89 times, Improvement 203 times, and Maintenance 41 times. Of the total expected outcomes, 97% were supported by data in the record. Data were not found to support any more or any fewer expected outcomes or outcome criteria in 100% of the records.

RECORD REVIEW

Dates: September to October, 1984
Location: VNA of Omaha and test agencies in Des Moines, Delaware, and Indianapolis
Data Collector: VNA of Omaha Research Assistant
Data Source: 175 records
Data Description: Worksheet completed by research assistant for each record
Data Analysis: Appropriateness of EO-OC selections; frequency of use of each expected outcome
Results: 97% of expected outcomes/time frames was supported by data in records; data were not found to support more or less expected outcomes or outcome

criterion in 100% of the records. Of 762 identified problems, 333 had expected outcomes—Prevention 89 times, Improvement 203 times, and Maintenance 41 times. Results were one source of data for scheme revision.

Data were also collected by interviewing community health nursing supervisors and staff at each of the four participating agencies. Conducted in the same manner as interviews related to the PCS, the discussions yielded benefits of using the Schemes, deficiencies in the Schemes, and suggestions for improvement. The staff identified the following five benefits:

- Provided a starting point and showed progress
- Useful in developing a specific plan
- Provided guidelines for evaluation
- Helped to measure what the client is to demonstrate
- Provided excellent information

Many staff identified significant difficulties involved in using the EO-OC Schemes. These included repetition between the outcome criteria and the plan, excessive time required to use the Schemes, and redundancy. Major revisions in the Schemes appeared to be necessary. Although the concepts of the Schemes still appeared correct and reasonable, application to the practice setting was a problem, especially in relation to clinical records. The research project staff, advisory committee members, and consultants considered modifying the Schemes, especially in relation to the three identified difficulties. Because none of the alternatives appeared adequate, the research staff reviewed the literature extensively, communicated with staff at other agencies who were interested in the concept of outcomes, and consulted many experts. These efforts provided the rationale for discontinuing further research on or use of the EO-OC Scheme. Instead, a rating scale for measuring outcomes was developed, grounded on the principles of content validity. Literature review and consultation with experts in the fields of evaluation and community health identified Knowledge, Behavior, and Status as concepts that could provide the basis for the rating scale.

STAFF INTERVIEWS

Date: November, 1974
Location: VNA of Omaha and test agencies in Des Moines, Delaware, and Indianapolis
Data Collectors: VNA of Omaha research staff and one agency liaison person in each of three test agencies
Data Source: Informal group interviews using a discussion guide with all supervisors and at least 50% of the staff nurses in each agency
Data Description: Tape recordings of interviews
Data Analysis: Compilation of comments
Results: Lists of benefits, deficiencies, and suggestions for improvement in the EO-OC Schemes provided subjective data for revision of the Schemes.

Pilot Study and PRS for Outcomes Draft

The purposes of the pilot study were to (1) develop a scale that could be used in measuring outcomes and (2) examine the concepts of Knowledge, Behavior, and Status as a basis for the rating scale. A data collection tool was devised, evaluated by 11 VNA of Omaha staff nurses, and refined. The problem-specific tool was used by 35 VNA of Omaha staff nurses to collect data. A total of 283 tools were completed. Each nurse developed a problem-specific Likert-type scale indicating the most positive to the most negative state of the problem. The current status of the client, a time frame, and an anticipated status were also recorded. At the end of the time frame, the nurse recorded the actual rating of the problem. Each nurse also completed a composite tool, considering the aggregate of the client's problems. When data from the composite tools were analyzed, it became apparent that client-focused ratings tended to cluster at the midpoint of the scale as high ratings for some problems and low ratings for other problems were averaged. Therefore, a composite rating was not deemed valuable.

Problem-specific tools were also analyzed for similarities and differences. Although domain-specific trends were not evident, trends that appeared applicable to all problems did occur. Therefore, the data supported using a five-point Likert-type scale to rate the three discrete concepts of Knowledge, Behavior, and Status. The Scale was viewed as applicable to all problems of the Problem Classification Scheme. Staff at the VNA of Omaha then used the Scale for a 2-week period. Findings from this limited test were used to further refine the definitions of the Scale.

PRS FOR OUTCOMES PILOT STUDY

Date: May, 1985
Location: VNA of Omaha
Data Collectors: 38 staff nurses
Data Source: Records of clients admitted during the study period
Data Description: One composite rating for each client in the sample; 283 problem-specific scales and client ratings
Data Analysis: Compared similarities and differences between problem-specific scales for each problem and similarities and differences between composite rating and problem-specific ratings for each client; data were sorted, collapsed, and reorganized
Results: Composite tool did not provide meaningful ratings; problem-specific tools provided meaningful ratings applicable to all problems of the PCS and were used to develop the Problem Rating Scale for Outcomes

Field Test and Interrater Agreement

The Problem Rating Scale (PRS) for Outcomes was field tested by home health and public health nurses employed by the Omaha, Des Moines, Delaware, and Indianapolis agencies. A preliminary review of the Scale involved 36 staff nurses and supervisors in the four agencies. Staff indicated that the concepts of Knowledge, Behavior, and Status were understandable and that the Scale provided a tool to accurately describe the severity of client problems. Participants offered no major format revisions but did suggest changes in definitions and other terminology. In addition, they required clarification regarding application of the Scale to client and caregiver.

The second phase of the field test involved five staff nurses purposively selected from each of the four test agencies. The 20 nurses attended a 2.5-hour structured orientation session at the beginning of the field test. During the following 2 months, each nurse selected four representative client admissions with expected visit frequency of not less than every other week. The nurse used the PRS for Outcomes to rate each priority problem that was expected to require intervention over the following 2 months. In addition, the nurse selected expected outcome ratings. Actual outcome ratings were recorded at dismissal, following 60 days of nursing service, or at the end of the field test.

Interrater agreement was addressed using four randomly selected nurses from each of the four test sites. The nurses were paired and given two records randomly selected from records generated by another nurse in their agency. Each nurse independently developed admission ratings for each identified problem. Percentages of agreement were computed in a variety of ways. Using a very stringent standard with only exact matches as the criterion for agreement, the nurse who generated the record was compared with each nurse who rerated the record and with the reraters as a pair. Percentage of agreement for the staff nurse with both raters was: Knowledge 21.1%, Behavior 11.7%, and Status 23.4%. When the staff nurse was compared with one or the other of the raters, the percentage of agreement was: Knowledge 46.1%, Behavior 53.9%, and Status 64.8%. Similarly, the reraters were compared with each other. The percentage of agreement was: Knowledge 51.6%, Behavior 38.3%, and Status 41.4%. The same comparisons were computed defining agreement less stringently. The criterion for agreement was an exact match or a match with a difference of one. Percentage of agreement for the staff nurse compared to both raters was: Knowledge 87.5%, Behavior 92.2%, and Status 96.1%. The percentage of agreement between the two raters was: Knowledge 83.6%, Behavior 82.6%, and Status 82.8%. Results of data analysis and comments from the nurses were used to make final modifications in the Scale. It was determined that the Scale was most effective when used at admission, at defined intervals, and at dismissal. This determination was based on the opinions of the staff nurses and supervisors who participated in the field tests as well as the advisory committee members.

PRS FOR OUTCOMES FIELD TEST

Dates: January to March, 1985
Location: VNA of Omaha and test agencies in Des Moines, Delaware, and Indianapolis
Data Collectors: Five staff nurses from each agency
Data Source: 80 representative admissions with expected visit frequency of not less than every other week selected by each data collector
Data Description: One worksheet for each identified priority problem containing admission rating, expected rating with time frame, and actual rating at dismissal or end of study period; 16 records given to two other data collectors from the same agency who independently completed admission ratings for each problem
Data Analysis: Percentage of agreement between staff nurse and raters and between raters was computed for exact matches and for difference of one
Results: Exact matches—range of 11.7% to 64.8%; exact matches/differences of one—range of 82.6% to 96.1%

PRS for Outcomes Completion

The final Problem Rating Scale for Outcomes consisted of a five-point Likert-type scale measuring the concepts of Knowledge, Behavior, and Status. The Scale was designed for use with all the problems and all the modifiers of the PCS. Further, it was designed for use at admission, at periodic intervals during provision of service, and at dismissal. The PRS for Outcomes is depicted in detail in Chapter 7.

INTERVENTION SCHEME

The final clinical component of the Omaha System is the Intervention Scheme, designed to classify nursing activities and actions. Development, testing and revision of this component were begun in July, 1984, and completed in November, 1986. Principal steps of the research process relative to the Intervention Scheme are shown in Figure 4–3.

Data Collection and Intervention Scheme Draft

The objective of the intervention data collection phase of the research project was to develop a scheme of interventions that would be valid, reliable, and useful to the practicing community health nurse. Sources of data were the sample of 175 Omaha, Des Moines, Delaware, and Indianapolis records previously acquired for field testing the PCS and EO-OC Schemes and approxi-

Data Collection

Draft of Intervention Scheme

Pilot Study

Intervention Scheme Revision

Field Test

Interrater Agreement Test

↓

Intervention Scheme Completion

FIGURE 4–3 ■ Development of the Intervention Scheme.

mately 100 additional Omaha records. Data were collected until at least five interventions per problem were identified. The data ranged from very broad, general statements to extremely specific information relative to the particular client. The same ideas appeared in plans and in reports of visits. Extensive literature review and consultation were used to identify seven general intervention categories. Working independently, two research staff nurses sorted the intervention statements derived from the 275 record sample into these seven categories. Interrater agreement was found to be adequate. Data from client records and discussions with staff suggested reducing the number of categories to four. The categories were:

- Health Teaching, Guidance, and Counseling
- Treatment and Procedures
- Case Management
- Observation

These general interventions could be used to address each problem of the PCS. The second level of the Scheme contained an alphabetic listing of targets for each intervention category. These targets provided more specific intervention information. Examples of targets were Coping skills, Signs/symptoms—physical, and Support group. A third level of intervention information was found to be so specific to the client that it could not be addressed by a classification scheme. This level was felt, however, to be essential in delineating client-specific interventions. Therefore, the third level of the Intervention Scheme allowed the nurse to include narrative data specific to the client.

INTERVENTION DATA COLLECTION

Dates: September, 1984 to January, 1985
Location: VNA of Omaha and test agencies in Des Moines, Delaware, and Indianapolis

Data Collector: VNA of Omaha research assistant
Data Source: Plans and progress notes from 200 VNA of Omaha records and 25 records from each of the test agencies
Data Description: List of interventions with at least five intervention statements for each problem on the PCS
Data Analysis: Intervention statements categorized into seven general interventions; later condensed into four categories
Results: Intervention Scheme of four mutually exclusive general intervention categories, each with a listing of nonmutually exclusive targets specific to that intervention

---

Pilot Study and Intervention Scheme Revision

Data collectors were 38 staff nurses employed in the preventive and home health care programs of the VNA of Omaha. The nurses used problem-specific data collection tools to record intervention data at client admission. Data included general interventions, more specific intervention information or targets, and a narrative explanation. At the conclusion, at least five tools had been completed on all 40 problems, for a total of 283 tools.

Data analysis and discussion with nurses suggested that the four general intervention categories were logical and usable. Based on subjective data from the staff nurses and literature review, the category of Observation was retitled "Surveillance." Based on suggestions of the staff who had participated in testing, the targets were reorganized into an alphabetic listing that was applicable to all problems of the PCS. A total of 59 targets or objects of interventions was identified. The listing was later expanded to include 62 targets at approximately the same level of abstraction. Each target could be used with each intervention category and with each problem.

INTERVENTION PILOT STUDY

Date: May, 1985
Location: VNA of Omaha
Data Collectors: 38 staff nurses
Data Source: One data collection tool for each identified problem for all clients admitted to service during study period
Data Description: Problem-specific planned interventions including a general intervention, a target, and client-specific narrative data; interviews were conducted with participating staff nurses
Data Analysis: Data and the nurses' comments reviewed
Results: General interventions were unchanged; Observation relabeled Surveillance; targets refined and arranged in an alphabetic listing, applicable to all general interventions

---

Field Test and Interrater Agreement

The field test of the Intervention Scheme was conducted in conjunction with testing of the PCS and PRS for Outcomes. A preliminary review of the Scheme and discussion were conducted in each of the four field test sites. Staff nurses indicated that the Intervention Scheme was a valuable tool for planning and describing nursing activities or actions. No major format changes were suggested; however, some alterations in terminology and definitions were recommended. The actual testing involved five nurses from each of the test agencies. During the 2-month test period, each nurse selected four representative client admissions with expected visit frequency of at least every other week. A sample of 80 records resulted. Each nurse used the Intervention Scheme to record an initial plan and to document nursing care provided on each home visit during the 2 months.

Interrater agreement was addressed using four randomly selected nurses from each of the test sites. The nurses were paired and given two records to review. The records had been completed by another nurse from their agency. Working independently, they used the general intervention categories from the Intervention Scheme to develop a general plan for each problem identified in the records. Data were analyzed in three ways using percentage of agreement between:

- The nurse who had completed the record with each of the other two secondary record reviewers
- The nurse who had completed the record with both of the other two secondary record reviewers
- The two secondary record reviewers

Percentages ranged from a low of 42.2% to a high of 96.9%; 8 of 12 percentages of agreement were at or above 80%. These results were found to be supported by nursing publications.

INTERVENTION FIELD TEST

Dates: January to March, 1986
Location: VNA of Omaha and test agencies in Des Moines, Delaware, and Indianapolis
Data Collectors: Five staff nurses from each agency
Data Source: 80 records
Data Description: Problem-specific plan and progress note of each visit using Intervention Scheme, 16 records given to two other data collectors from the same agency who independently completed plans for each priority problem
Data Analysis: Percentage of agreement between the staff nurse and the nurse testers and between the testers computed for each general intervention
Results: Percentages of agreement ranged from 42.2% to 96.9% with 8 of the 12 percentages at or above 80%

Intervention Scheme Completed

Final modifications of the Intervention Scheme were based on statistical analysis of field test results and con-

sultation. The Scheme consisted of four broad intervention categories accompanied by targets or objects of nursing action. The Scheme was designed for use with client-specific information generated by the home health or public health nurse. The Intervention Scheme was incorporated into the recording system at the VNA of Omaha. The Scheme is described in detail in Chapter 6

SUMMARY

The three clinical components that comprise the Omaha System are the Problem Classification Scheme, the Problem Rating Scale for Outcomes, and the Intervention Scheme. These Schemes were developed between 1975 and 1986 in a series of three complex, interrelated projects. The research was funded by the Division of Nursing, Public Health Service, USDHHS and conducted at the VNA of Omaha and five test agencies. Each of the clinical components was developed inductively using empirical data. Approximately 1,000 client records were included in the sample of the three projects. Testing of each component and of the System as a whole provided the basis for revisions and for establishment of reliability and validity of the components. Throughout the three projects, 500 nurses at the four sites participated by generating client records and providing suggestions. The same nurses were involved in implementing the Omaha System in their respective agencies.

REFERENCES

Martin, K., Scheet, N., Crews, C., et al. (1986a). *Client Management Information System for Community Health Nursing Agencies: An Implementation Manual,* No. HRP-0907023. Rockville, MD, US DHHS, Public Health Service (PHS), Health Resources Administration (HRSA).

Martin, K., Scheet, N., Crews, C., et al. (1986b) *Client Management Information System for Community Health Nursing Agencies: Final Report.* [Unpublished.]

Martin, K. (1988, June). Research in home care. *Nurs. Clin. North Am. 23*:373–385.

Simmons, D. (1980). *A Classification Scheme for Client Problems in Community Health Nursing.* Hyattsville, MD, DHHS, Bureau of Health Professions, Division of Nursing.

Visiting Nurse Association of Omaha (1976). *Development of a Problem Classification Scheme, a Methodology for its Use and a System Designed to Computerize the Scheme for Community Health Nursing Services.* [Unpublished.]

Visiting Nurse Association of Omaha (1980). *Field Testing of a Problem Classification Scheme and Development and Field Testing of Expected Outcome-Outcome Criterion Schemes with a Methodology for Use.* [Unpublished.]

BIBLIOGRAPHY

Dickoff, J., James, P., & Wiedenbach, E. (1968a, September/October). Theory in a practice discipline: Part I. Practice oriented theory. *Nurs. Res., 17*:415–435.

Dickoff, J., James, P., & Wiedenbach, E. (1986b, November/December). Theory in a practice discipline: Part II. Practice oriented research. *Nurs. Res., 17*:545–554.

Giovannetti, P. (1979, February). Understanding patient classification systems. *J. Nurs. Admin., 9*:4–9.

Glaser, B., & Strauss, A. (1967). *The Discovery of Grounded Theory.* Chicago, Aldine.

Hurst, J. (1971, January). Ten reasons why Lawrence Weed is right. *New Engl. J. Med., 284*:51–52.

Phillips, L. (1986). *A Clinician's Guide to the Critique and Utilization of Nursing Research.* Norwalk, CT, Appleton-Century-Crofts.

Polit, D., & Hungler, B. (1987). *Nursing Research Principles and Methods* (3rd ed.). Philadelphia, J. B. Lippincott.

Schmid, E., Schall, D., & Morrison, C. (1974, April). Computerized problem-oriented medical records for ambulatory practice. *Med. Care, 12*:316–327.

Selltiz, C., Wrightsman, L., & Cook, S. (1973). *Research Methods in Social Relations* (3rd ed.). New York, Holt, Rinehart & Winston.

Treece, E., & Treece, Jr., J. (1986). *Elements of Research in Nursing* (4th ed.). St. Louis, C. V. Mosby.

Waltz, C., Strickland, O., & Lenz, E. (1984). *Measurement in Nursing Research.* Philadelphia, F. A. Davis.

Weed, L. (1968, March 14–21). Special article: Medical records that guide and teach. *New Engl. J. Med., 278*:593–600, 652–657.

SECTION II

DESCRIPTION AND IMPLEMENTATION OF THE OMAHA SYSTEM

CHAPTER FIVE

*W*henever the scientific method is used, it is essential to explicitly define the presenting problem in order for the subsequent steps of the problem-solving process to become clear. The steps should follow in logical sequence. When the statement of the problem is ambiguous, vague, or rambling, the remaining steps of the problem-solving process will also be unclear and indefinite. An unclear problem statement cannot provide the basis for a relevant and effective plan. (Mayers, 1983, p. 29)

The Problem Classification Scheme is a taxonomy of nursing diagnoses valuable to community health nurses, other community health providers, supervisors, and administrators. Since it has been developed from actual client data by practicing community health nurses during extensive research and testing, it provides the language and structure to define the practice of nursing in the community setting. Originating in 1970 with a VNA of Omaha nursing supervisor and her staff and continuing with the agency's three research projects, the Scheme has evolved into a holistic approach to community health client concerns. As a practice-based model, the Problem Classification Scheme is a framework of client-focused problems amenable to nursing intervention. A community health nurse uses the Problem Classification Scheme to collect data according to a selective, defined data base, ensuring that collected data relate to specific nursing diagnoses and interventions. The Problem Classification Scheme does not represent new community health nursing knowledge. The Scheme systematically organizes what compassionate community health nurses know about their clients as individuals, families, and groups. Understanding the importance of environmental, psychosocial, physiologic, and health-related behavior factors to a client is the foundation of sound community health nursing practice (see pp. 67 to 74).

The Problem Classification Scheme provides a comprehensive method for collecting, sorting, classifying, documenting, and analyzing client data for the staff nurse, supervisor, and agency administrator. Use of the Scheme enables community health nurses to (1) sort essential from nonessential data objectively and efficiently, and (2) identify patterns in the data. Medical diagnoses, laboratory tests, and etiologic or causation factors are not included in the Problem Classification Scheme. It does not replace other specialized frameworks but is compatible with and complementary to medical diagnoses and other such frameworks. Thus, the Problem Classification Scheme provides community health nurses with precise language vital to nursing practice. Such language furnishes a diagnostic bridge between the client data base and client care, and can enhance the science of nursing. The relationships among the Problem Classification Scheme, Omaha System, and family nursing process are shown in Figure 5–1.

ORGANIZATION

The purpose of the Problem Classification Scheme is to offer community health nurses an orderly method for identifying, labeling, and organizing concerns addressed during professional practice. These concerns may be communicated to others through oral and written methods. The Problem Classification Scheme has been designed to contain a manageable number of domains, problems, modifiers, and signs/symptoms and to follow the rules of a taxonomic system.

According to Rasch (1987), a taxonomy must be logically consistent by virtue of its development and organization. It must have criteria for classes and subclasses; those classes must be exhaustive and mutually exclusive (Aydelotte & Peterson, 1987).

A taxonomic structure is analogous to the hierarchic or descending levels of an outline. Similar to an outline, the levels of a taxonomy range from general to specific. Through such groupings, the Scheme organizes the "knowing" rather than the "doing" of nursing (Warren, 1987). The language of a taxonomy defines relationships and transmits meaning across the barriers of habit, place, time, and distance (Levine, 1989). A taxonomy involves a purpose, a principle of order, and discrete categories for classification of entities as pre-

Problem Classification Scheme

requisites; using a taxonomy facilitates understanding of its entities and clarifies similarities, differences, and relationships (Porter, 1986).

Artistic as well as scientific skills are required to develop the Problem Classification Scheme and other taxonomies (Avant, 1990; Kritek, 1989). Artistic skills include knowledge, appreciation, and understanding of the phenomena being classified. Expert nurses with such high level intuitive and language skills participated in developing the taxonomic structure of the Problem Classification Scheme. At the first level are the four domains: Environmental, Psychosocial, Physiological, and Health Related Behaviors. The domains represent major categories, or taxa, providing the structural and relational framework for client problems that concern practicing community health nurses.

Taxonomic Principles

The ordering of problems within the domains is based on three principles of classification. First, terms within each level of the classification are stated at the same degree of abstraction. The levels descend from domains that are general and broad categories through problem-specific clusters of signs/symptoms. Definitions of each level determine the placement of individual entities into the classification.

    Level 1: Domain
        Level 2: Problem
            Level 3: Modifier
                Level 4: Sign/Symptom

Second, the Problem Classification Scheme is comprehensive at the levels of domains and modifiers and nonexhaustive at the levels of problems, signs/symptoms, and risk factors. The four domains represent the full spectrum of community health nursing practice and make a statement about the holistic, community-based concerns of community health nurses. The modifiers identify the problem in terms of ownership as well as presence or absence of risk factors and signs/symptoms. Within the levels of problems and signs/symptoms, a flexible coding structure allows for expansion.

The same principles of classification should govern such expansion, however. As the Scheme evolved and was validated by practicing nurses, the number of problem labels was altered through the processes of dividing and collapsing in order to develop more functional entities. Each problem represents a discrete area of concern narrow enough to be easily identified and differentiated from other problems and broad enough to represent an area addressed by practitioners. The problems are not listed in hierarchical order; each is of equal importance.

Each of the four domains includes an available problem called "Other" to allow for additions. Because the Problem Classification Scheme has been extensively tested and revised over time, it is expected that few problems need be added. This is especially true if suggestions described in this chapter's Summary are followed. Furthermore, clusters of signs and symptoms are designed to include a workable number of entities identified through research as most commonly representing the actual state of the problem. However, each problem includes an available sign/symptom entitled Other to allow for additions. While the staff nurses who were initially involved in developing the Problem Classification Scheme did not want the final product to be cumbersome, Other is provided as a sign/symptom when legitimate need arises.

Third, terms are mutually exclusive both within and across the four levels. Limiting duplication of terminology facilitates use of the Scheme by practitioners. Together with standard nomenclature, mutually exclu-

65

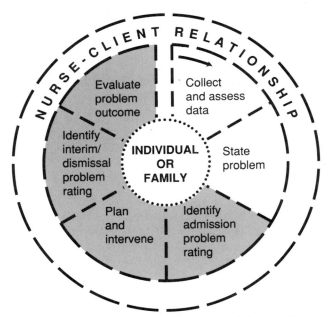

FIGURE 5 – 1 ■ Using the Problem Classification Scheme facilitates collecting and assessing client information and stating client problems — the initial steps of the family nursing process.

sive terms facilitate communication among users of the Scheme. Historically, diversity within and among community health agencies has made consistent and comparable measurement of client data difficult or impossible. Because the Scheme consists of discrete entities rather than overlapping or redundant categories, the Scheme meets the necessary prerequisite for computer application and generation of meaningful statistics. The specific, unique terms of problems and signs/symptoms make possible automated, uniform data storage and retrieval. In turn, comprehensive, multi-format, client-focused reports can be generated. Reports that suggest and document specific client trends, developments or changes in service programs, and costs of services are increasingly important to health care administrators. Furthermore, uniformity in data and ease of retrieval are becoming more desirable, especially given the progress in developing minimum data sets within nursing and the rest of the health care community.

Both the format and the numbering system of the Problem Classification Scheme are congruent and consistent with four distinct, hierarchical levels. These levels are domain, problem, modifiers, and signs/symptoms. At each level, the words or phrases are designed to be of equal importance; order in the Scheme does not mean priority or value. The domains provide an organizing framework for the Problem Classification Scheme. The problem statement consists of three parts: the problem; the family or individual modifier; and the health promotion, potential, or actual modifier. Signs and symptoms are used only with the actual state of the problem.

Definitions

Problem Identification. A clinical judgment about environmental, psychosocial, physiologic, and health-related behavior data that is of interest or concern to the client. Problem identification is closely related to nursing diagnosis, which is defined as "a clinical judgment about individual, family, or community responses to actual and potential health problem/life processes. Nursing diagnoses provide the basis for selection of nursing interventions to achieve outcomes for which the nurse is accountable" (Carroll-Johnson, 1990, p. 50).

Domains. The four general areas that represent community health practice and provide organizational groupings for client problems. Domains represent the first level of the Problem Classification Scheme (i.e., Environmental, Psychosocial, Physiological, Health Related Behaviors).

Client Problems. The 40 nursing diagnoses that represent matters of difficulty and concern that historically, presently, or potentially adversely affect any aspect of the client's well-being. Client problems represent health-related matters that nurses are licensed to diagnose and treat; problems are amenable to nursing intervention. Accurate identification of client problems enables the professional to focus interventions. Problems are: (1) stated from the client's perspective, (2) accompanied by two of five modifiers, and (3) represent the second level of the Problem Classification Scheme (e.g., 01. Income, 08. Role Change, 28. Respiration, and 40. Family Planning).

Modifiers. Two sets of terms used in conjunction with problems. The first set of modifiers represents the three stages of a continuum. These modifiers describe degree of severity in relation to client interest, risk factors, and signs/symptoms (i.e., Health Promotion, Potential, and Deficit/Impairment/Actual). The second set of modifiers allows a nurse to identify ownership of a problem (i.e., Family or Individual). Modifiers appear at the third level of the Problem Classification Scheme.

Risk Factors. Environmental, psychosocial, or physiologic events and/or health-related behaviors that occur in the past, present, or future and increase the client's exposure or vulnerability to the development of an actual problem. Risk factors are used only in conjunction with the modifier Potential. Terms that describe risk factors are *not* included in the Problem Classification Scheme. Instead, risk factors are identified by the community health nurse at the fourth level of the Scheme.

Signs. The objective evidence of a client's problem observed by a community health nurse or other health care providers (e.g., Problem 02. Sanitation: 02. *inadequate food storage/disposal*; 03. *insects/rodents*). Both signs and symptoms are used in conjunction with the modifier Actual; they are not used in conjunction with Health Promotion or Potential problems. Signs and symptoms appear at the fourth level of the Problem Classification Scheme.

Symptoms. The subjective evidence of a client's problem reported by the client or by significant others (e.g., Problem 02. Sanitation: 02. *inadequate food storage/*

disposal; 03. *insects/rodents*). These examples were selected as data that can be signs on some occasions *and* symptoms on other occasions. In contrast, some data are consistently signs *or* symptoms. For example, a sign develops when the community health nurse observes (1) purulent wound drainage or (2) a new mother who does not handle her newborn with affection. A symptom occurs when the client describes the location and sensation of pain.

Modifiers

Modifiers, which follow domains and problems, appear at the third level of the Problem Classification Scheme. The two sets of modifiers are applicable to and further delineate all 40 problems. Thus, a community health nurse or other professional records one modifier from each set in relation to a given problem, expediting use of the Problem Classification Scheme with the Problem Rating Scale for Outcomes and the Intervention Scheme.

The first set of modifiers includes Health Promotion, Potential Deficit/Impairment, and Deficit/Impairment/Actual. These modifiers can be viewed as forming a health-illness continuum. Starting at one end of the continuum, Health Promotion defines a positive state. Anticipatory guidance and other preventive interventions are applicable. Next, Potential Deficit/Impairment is less positive than Health Promotion but more positive than the third modifier. This means due to historic or current factors, the client is at greater risk to develop a problem. More aggressive educative and therapeutic interventions are required. At the far end of the continuum is Deficit/Impairment/Actual, the most negative of the three modifiers. Signs and symptoms are always present when this modifier is used. Severity can range from one relatively mild sign or symptom to several severe signs and symptoms. Interventions are directed toward resolution or control of the signs/symptoms. The modifiers are defined as follow:

Health Promotion. Client interest in increasing knowledge, behavior, and health expectations as well as developing resources that maintain or enhance well-being in the absence of risk factors, signs, or symptoms.
Potential Deficit/Impairment. Client status characterized by the absence of signs/symptoms and the presence of certain health patterns, practices, behaviors, or risk factors that may preclude optimal health.
Deficit/Impairment/Actual. Client status characterized by one or more existing signs and/or symptoms that may preclude optimal health.

The second set of modifiers are Family and Individual. Using one of these two modifiers with a problem enables the professional to clarify ownership and acknowledge involvement of one or more significant others. Significant others may or may not be related biologically or by marriage. During the VNA of Omaha research projects to date, the term "Group" was not investigated as a modifier. For this reason, it is not included in the Scheme. It has been suggested that "Group" would be a useful addition to the Problem Classification Scheme. For example, graduate students have successfully used the Scheme at the community level when they considered the Boston geographic area as a client (Chambers, 1990). The second set of modifiers are defined as follows:

Family. A social unit or related group of individuals who live together and who experience a health-related problem.
Individual. A person who lives alone or a single family member who experiences a health-related problem.

Environmental Domain

The Environmental Domain of the Problem Classification Scheme is defined as the material resources, physical surroundings, and substances both internal and external to the client, home, neighborhood, and broader community. The four problems included in this domain focus on critical factors that affect the health status, health behavior, and lifestyle of the client. A cluster of problem-specific signs/symptoms provide the diagnostic clues to problem identification. Signs and symptoms of problems in the Environmental Domain, as well as the other three domains, must be considered in relation to all other client data.

PROBLEM 01.
Income. Monies from wages, interest, dividends, or other sources available to family for living and health care expenses
MODIFIER

Health Promotion	Family
Potential Deficit	Individual
Deficit	

SIGNS/SYMPTOMS
01. low/no income
02. uninsured medical expenses
03. inadequate money management
04. able to buy only necessities
05. difficulty buying necessities
06. other

PROBLEM 02.
Sanitation. Environmental conditions pertaining to or affecting health with reference to cleanliness, precautions against infection or disease, and promotion of health
MODIFIER

Health Promotion	Family
Potential Deficit	Individual
Deficit	

SIGNS/SYMPTOMS
01. soiled living area
02. inadequate food storage/disposal
03. insects/rodents
04. foul odor

05. inadequate water supply
06. inadequate sewage disposal
07. inadequate laundry facilities
08. allergens
09. infectious/contaminating agents
10. other

PROBLEM 03.
Residence. Place where individual/family lives
MODIFIER

Health Promotion	Family
Potential Deficit	Individual
Deficit	

SIGNS/SYMPTOMS
01. structurally unsound
02. inadequate heating/cooling
03. steep stairs
04. inadequate/obstructed exits/entries
05. cluttered living space
06. unsafe storage of dangerous objects/substances
07. unsafe mats/throw rugs
08. inadequate safety devices
09. presence of lead-based paint
10. unsafe gas/electrical appliances
11. inadequate/crowded living space
12. homeless
13. other

PROBLEM 04.
Neighborhood/workplace safety. Freedom from injury or loss as it relates to the community/place of employment
MODIFIER

Health Promotion	Family
Potential Deficit	Individual
Deficit	

SIGNS/SYMPTOMS
01. high crime rate
02. high pollution level
03. uncontrolled animals
04. physical hazards
05. unsafe play areas
06. other

PROBLEM 05.
Other. Identified problem not in the classification
SIGNS/SYMPTOMS
01. other

Psychosocial Domain

The Psychosocial Domain is defined as patterns of behavior, communication, relationships, and development. The effects of situational and developmental crisis or stress are evident in the Psychosocial Domain. The domain includes 12 problems that address the relationships between the client as an individual or family and other persons. These persons may be immediate or extended family members, significant others, neigh-

bors, acquaintances, or community workers. Thus, the problems and signs/symptoms of the second domain often reflect difficulty or inability of the client to interact positively with persons inside or outside the family unit.

PROBLEM 06.
Communication with community resources. The interaction between the individual/family and social agencies in regard to information and services
MODIFIER

Health Promotion	Family
Potential Impairment	Individual
Impairment	

SIGNS/SYMPTOMS
01. unfamiliar with options/procedures for obtaining services
02. difficulty understanding roles/regulations of service providers
03. unable to communicate concerns to service provider
04. dissatisfaction with services
05. language barrier
06. inadequate/unavailable resources
07. other

PROBLEM 07.
Social contact. Communication or interactions between individual or family and people outside the immediate household
MODIFIER

Health Promotion	Family
Potential Impairment	Individual
Impairment	

SIGNS/SYMPTOMS
01. limited social contact
02. uses health care provider for social contact
03. minimal outside stimulation/leisure time activities
04. other

PROBLEM 08.
Role change. Movement from or addition of one set of expected behavioral characteristics to another
MODIFIER

Health Promotion	Family
Potential Impairment	Individual
Impairment	

SIGNS/SYMPTOMS
01. involuntary reversal of traditional male/female roles
02. involuntary reversal of dependent/independent roles
03. assumes new role
04. loses previous role
05. other

PROBLEM 09.
Interpersonal relationship. Association or connection between or among people

MODIFIER

Health Promotion	Family
Potential Impairment	Individual
Impairment	

SIGNS/SYMPTOMS
01. difficulty establishing/maintaining relationships
02. minimal shared activities
03. incongruent values/goals
04. inadequate interpersonal communication skills
05. prolonged, unrelieved tension
06. inappropriate suspicion/manipulation/compulsion/aggression
07. other

PROBLEM 10.

Spiritual distress. Discomfort related to religious, intellectual, or cultural concerns

MODIFIER

Health Promotion	Family
Potential	Individual
Actual	

SIGNS/SYMPTOMS
01. expresses spiritual concerns
02. disrupted spiritual rituals
03. disrupted spiritual trust
04. conflicting spiritual beliefs and medical regimen
05. other

PROBLEM 11.

Grief. Keen mental suffering or distress over affliction or loss

MODIFIER

Health Promotion	Family
Potential Impairment	Individual
Impairment	

SIGNS/SYMPTOMS
01. fails to recognize normal grief responses
02. difficulty coping with grief responses
03. difficulty expressing grief responses
04. conflicting stages of grief process among family/individual
05. other

PROBLEM 12.

Emotional stability. Reliable steadiness of temperament

MODIFIER

Health Promotion	Family
Potential Impairment	Individual
Impairment	

SIGNS/SYMPTOMS
01. sadness/hopelessness/worthlessness
02. apprehension/undefined fear
03. loss of interest/involvement in activities/self-care
04. narrowed perceptual focus
05. scattering of attention
06. flat affect
07. irritable/agitated
08. purposeless activity
09. difficulty managing stress
10. somatic complaints/chronic fatigue

11. expresses wish to die/attempts suicide
12. other

PROBLEM 13.

Human sexuality. Developmental state that focuses on attitudes, feelings, and behaviors related to male/female roles

MODIFIER

Health Promotion	Family
Potential Impairment	Individual
Impairment	

SIGNS/SYMPTOMS
01. difficulty recognizing consequences of sexual behavior
02. difficulty expressing intimacy
03. sexual identity confusion
04. sexual value confusion
05. dissatisfied with sexual relationships
06. other

PROBLEM 14.

Caretaking/parenting. Providing support, nurturance, stimulation, and physical care for dependent adult or child

MODIFIER

Health Promotion	Family
Potential Impairment	Individual
Impairment	

SIGNS/SYMPTOMS
01. difficulty providing physical care/safety
02. difficulty providing emotional nurturance
03. difficulty providing cognitive learning experiences and activities
04. difficulty providing preventive and therapeutic health care
05. expectations incongruent with stage of growth and development
06. dissatisfaction/difficulty with responsibilities
07. neglectful
08. abusive
09. other

PROBLEM 15.

Neglected child/adult. Child or adult deprived of minimally accepted standards of food, shelter, clothing, and care

MODIFIER

Health Promotion	Family
Potential	Individual
Actual	

SIGNS/SYMPTOMS
01. lacks adequate physical care
02. lacks emotional nurturance/support
03. lacks appropriate stimulation/cognitive experiences
04. inappropriately left alone
05. lacks necessary supervision
06. inadeqaute/delayed medical care
07. other

PROBLEM 16.

Abused child/adult. Child or adult subjected to nonaccidental physical, or emotional injury

MODIFIER

Health Promotion	Family
Potential	Individual
Actual	

SIGNS/SYMPTOMS

01. harsh/excessive discipline
02. welts/bruises/burns
03. questionable explanation of injury
04. attacked verbally
05. fearful/hypervigilant behavior
06. violent environment
07. consistent negative messages
08. assaulted sexually
09. other

PROBLEM 17.

Growth and development. Progressive physical development and gradual maturation or progression as the individual moves through childhood to old age

MODIFIER

Health Promotion	Family
Potential Impairment	Individual
Impairment	

SIGNS/SYMPTOMS

01. abnormal results of development screening tests
02. abnormal weight/height/head circumference in relation to growth curve/age
03. age-inappropriate behavior
04. inadequate achievement/maintenance of developmental tasks
05. other

PROBLEM 18.

Other. Identified problem not in the classification

SIGNS/SYMPTOMS

01. other

Physiological Domain

The Physiological Domain is defined as functional status of processes that maintain life. The 15 problems focus on physical health status. Therefore, problems in this domain are usually associated with the client as an individual rather than a family unit. Signs and symptoms of this domain may be observed, identified, or elicited through the practice skills of community health nurses.

PROBLEM 19.

Hearing. The perception of sound by the ears

MODIFIER

Health Promotion	Family
Potential Impairment	Individual
Impairment	

SIGNS/SYMPTOMS

01. difficulty hearing normal speech tones
02. absent/abnormal response to sound
03. abnormal results of hearing screening test
04. other

PROBLEM 20.

Vision. The act or power of sensing with the eyes

MODIFIER

Health Promotion	Family
Potential Impairment	Individual
Impairment	

SIGNS/SYMPTOMS

01. difficulty seeing small print/calibrations
02. difficulty seeing distant objects
03. difficulty seeing close objects
04. absent/abnormal response to visual stimuli
05. abnormal results of vision screening test
06. squinting/blinking/tearing/blurring
07. difficulty differentiating colors
08. other

PROBLEM 21.

Speech and language. Articulated vocal sounds, symbols, signs, or gestures used as a means of communication

MODIFIER

Health Promotion	Family
Potential Impairment	Individual
Impairment	

SIGNS/SYMPTOMS

01. absent/abnormal ability to speak
02. absent/abnormal ability to understand
03. lacks alternative communication skills
04. inappropriate sentence structure
05. limited enunciation/clarity
06. inappropriate word usage
07. other

PROBLEM 22.

Dentition. The kind, number, and arrangement of teeth

MODIFIER

Health Promotion	Family
Potential Impairment	Individual
Impairment	

SIGNS/SYMPTOMS

01. abnormalities of teeth
02. sore/swollen/bleeding gums
03. ill-fitting dentures
04. malocclusion
05. other

PROBLEM 23.

Cognition. The act or process of knowing, perceiving, or remembering

MODIFIER

Health Promotion	Family
Potential Impairment	Individual
Impairment	

SIGNS/SYMPTOMS

01. diminished judgment
02. disoriented to time/place/person

03. limited recall of recent events
04. limited recall of long past events
05. limited calculating/sequencing skills
06. limited concentration
07. limited reasoning/abstract thinking ability
08. impulsiveness
09. repetitious language/behavior
10. other

PROBLEM 24.
Pain. A feeling of distress, suffering, or agony caused by stimulation of specialized nerve endings

MODIFIER

Health Promotion	Family
Potential	Individual
Actual	

SIGNS/SYMPTOMS
01. expresses discomfort/pain
02. elevated pulse/respirations/blood pressure
03. compensated movement/guarding
04. restless behavior
05. facial grimaces
06. pallor/perspiration
07. other

PROBLEM 25.
Consciousness. Awareness of sensations, feelings/emotions, and actions

MODIFIER

Health Promotion	Family
Potential Impairment	Individual
Impairment	

SIGNS/SYMPTOMS
01. lethargic
02. stuporous
03. unresponsive
04. comatose
05. other

PROBLEM 26.
Integument. The natural covering of the body; the skin

MODIFIER

Health Promotion	Family
Potential Impairment	Individual
Impairment	

SIGNS/SYMPTOMS
01. lesion
02. rash
03. excessively dry
04. excessively oily
05. inflammation
06. pruritus
07. drainage
08. ecchymosis
09. hypertrophy of nails
10. other

PROBLEM 27.
Neuro-musculo-skeletal function. Ability of nerves, muscles, and bones to perform or coordinate specific activities

MODIFIER

Health Promotion	Family
Potential Impairment	Individual
Impairment	

SIGNS/SYMPTOMS
01. limited range of motion
02. decreased muscle strength
03. decreased coordination
04. decreased muscle tone
05. increased muscle tone
06. decreased sensation
07. increased sensation
08. decreased balance
09. gait/ambulation disturbance
10. difficulty managing activities of daily living
11. tremors/seizures
12. other

PROBLEM 28.
Respiration. The exchange of oxygen and carbon dioxide in the body.

MODIFIER

Health Promotion	Family
Potential Impairment	Individual
Impairment	

SIGNS/SYMPTOMS
01. abnormal breath patterns
02. unable to breathe independently
03. cough
04. unable to cough/expectorate independently
05. cyanosis
06. abnormal sputum
07. noisy respirations
08. rhinorrhea
09. abnormal breath sounds
10. other

PROBLEM 29.
Circulation. The movement of blood through the heart and blood vessels by which food, oxygen, and internal secretions are carried to and wastes are carried from the body tissues

MODIFIER

Health Promotion	Family
Potential Impairment	Individual
Impairment	

SIGNS/SYMPTOMS
01. edema
02. cramping/pain of extremities
03. decreased pulses
04. discoloration of skin/cyanosis
05. temperature change in affected area
06. varicosities
07. syncopal episodes
08. abnormal blood pressure reading
09. pulse deficit
10. irregular heart rate
11. excessively rapid heart rate
12. excessively slow heart rate
13. anginal pain

14. abnormal heart sounds/murmurs
15. other

PROBLEM 30.
Digestion-hydration. Converting food into substances suitable for absorption and assimilation into the body/ supplying water to maintain adequate body fluids
MODIFIER

Health Promotion	Family
Potential Impairment	Individual
Impairment	

SIGNS/SYMPTOMS
01. nausea/vomiting
02. difficulty/inability to chew/swallow/digest
03. indigestion
04. reflux
05. anorexia
06. anemia
07. ascites
08. jaundice/liver enlargement
09. decreased skin turgor
10. cracked lips/dry mouth
11. electrolyte imbalance
12. other

PROBLEM 31.
Bowel function. Ability of the intestine to digest food and evacuate waste
MODIFIER

Health Promotion	Family
Potential Impairment	Individual
Impairment	

SIGNS/SYMPTOMS
01. abnormal frequency/consistency of stool
02. painful defecation
03. decreased bowel sounds
04. blood in stools
05. abnormal color
06. cramping/abdominal discomfort
07. incontinent of stool
08. other

PROBLEM 32.
Genito-urinary function. Ability of the sexual organs to reproduce and of the kidneys, ureters, bladder, and urethra to produce and excrete urine
MODIFIER

Health Promotion	Family
Potential Impairment	Individual
Impairment	

SIGNS/SYMPTOMS
01. incontinent of urine
02. urgency/frequency
03. burning/painful urination
04. difficulty emptying bladder
05. abnormal urinary frequency/amount
06. hematuria
07. abnormal discharge
08. abnormal menstrual pattern
09. abnormal lumps/swelling/tenderness of male/female reproductive organs

10. dyspareunia
11. other

PROBLEM 33.
Antepartum/postpartum. Before or after parturition
MODIFIER

Health Promotion	Family
Potential Impairment	Individual
Impairment	

SIGNS/SYMPTOMS
01. difficulty coping with pregnancy/body changes
02. inappropriate exercise/rest/diet/behaviors
03. discomforts
04. complications
05. fears delivery procedure
06. difficulty breast-feeding
07. other

PROBLEM 34.
Other. Identified problem not in the classification
SIGNS/SYMPTOMS
01. other

Health Related Behaviors Domain

The Health Related Behaviors Domain is defined as activities that maintain or promote wellness, promote recovery, or maximize rehabilitation. The nine problems and their accompanying signs/symptoms address health-seeking actions that have the potential to improve the quality of a client's life. Personal motivation is especially critical to improving or resolving problems in this domain because a client must curtail or improve behavior appropriately, often without rapid or visible benefits.

PROBLEM 35.
Nutrition. Nourishment of body with food including the processes by which food is used to provide energy, maintenance, and growth
MODIFIER

Health Promotion	Family
Potential Impairment	Individual
Impairment	

SIGNS/SYMPTOMS
01. weighs 10% more than average
02. weighs 10% less than average
03. lacks established standards for daily caloric/fluid intake
04. exceeds established standards for daily caloric/ fluid intake
05. unbalanced diet
06. improper feeding schedule for age
07. nonadherence to prescribed diet
08. unexplained/progressive weight loss
09. hypoglycemia
10. hyperglycemia
11. other

PROBLEM 36.

Sleep and rest patterns. A natural, regularly recurring condition of decreased or suspended activity for the mind and body

MODIFIER

Health Promotion	Family
Potential Impairment	Individual
Impairment	

SIGNS/SYMPTOMS
01. sleep/rest pattern disrupts family
02. frequently wakes during night
03. somnambulism
04. insomnia
05. nightmares
06. insufficient sleep/rest for age/physical condition
07. other

PROBLEM 37.

Physical activity. State or quality of body actions in daily living

MODIFIER

Health Promotion	Family
Potential Impairment	Individual
Impairment	

SIGNS/SYMPTOMS
01. sedentary life style
02. inadequate/inconsistent exercise routine
03. inappropriate type/amount of exercise for age/physical condition
04. other

PROBLEM 38.

Personal hygiene. Individual practice conducive to health and cleanliness

MODIFIER

Health Promotion	Family
Potential Impairment	Individual
Impairment	

SIGNS/SYMPTOMS
01. inadequate laundering of clothing
02. inadequate bathing
03. body odor
04. inadequate shampooing/combing of hair
05. inadequate brushing/flossing/mouth care
06. other

PROBLEM 39.

Substance use. Inappropriate consumption of medicines, drugs, or other materials including prescription, over-the-counter or street drugs, alcohol, and tobacco

MODIFIER

Health Promotion	Family
Potential	Individual
Actual	

SIGNS/SYMPTOMS
01. abuses over-the-counter/street drugs
02. abuses alcohol
03. smokes
04. difficulty performing normal routines
05. reflex disturbances

06. behavior change
07. other

PROBLEM 40.

Family planning. The practice of birth control measures within the context of family values, attitudes, and beliefs

MODIFIER

Health Promotion	Family
Potential Impairment	Individual
Impairment	

SIGNS/SYMPTOMS
01. inappropriate/insufficient knowledge of family planning methods
02. inaccurate/inconsistent use of family planning methods
03. dissatisfied with present family planning method
04. other

PROBLEM 41.

Health care supervision. Management of the treatment plan by a health care professional

MODIFIER

Health Promotion	Family
Potential Impairment	Individual
Impairment	

SIGNS/SYMPTOMS
01. fails to obtain routine medical/dental evaluation
02. fails to seek care for symptoms requiring medical/dental evaluation
03. fails to return as requested to physician/dentist
04. inability to coordinate multiple appointments/regimens
05. inconsistent source of medical/dental care
06. inadequate prescribed medical/dental regimen
07. other

PROBLEM 42.

Prescribed medication regimen. A regulated course for the use or application of medicine ordered by the physician

MODIFIER

Health Promotion	Family
Potential Impairment	Individual
Impairment	

SIGNS/SYMPTOMS
01. deviates from prescribed dosage/schedule
02. demonstrates side-effects
03. inadequate system for taking medication
04. improper storage of medication
05. fails to obtain refills appropriately
06. fails to obtain immunizations
07. other

PROBLEM 43.

Technical procedure. A mode of action for tasks requiring professional nursing skill

MODIFIER

Health Promotion	Family
Potential Impairment	Individual
Impairment	

SIGNS/SYMPTOMS
01. unable to demonstrate/relate procedure accurately
02. does not follow/demonstrate principles of safe/ aseptic techniques
03. procedure requires nursing skill
04. unable/unwilling to perform procedure without assistance
05. unable/unwilling to operate special equipment
06. other person(s) unable/unavailable to assist
07. other

PROBLEM 44.

Other. Identified problem not in the classification
SIGNS/SYMPTOMS
01. other

ASSUMPTIONS

Application of the Problem Classification Scheme is based on general assumptions. The following four assumptions are particularly important:

■ The community health nurse genuinely cares about the client as an individual or family and has developed interpersonal and interview skills sufficient to obtain valid and reliable client data. Clients encompass the age and health-illness spectra and represent diverse cultural and religious values.

■ A problem or nursing diagnosis is stated from the client's perspective. Problems are owned by the client, not the nurse or another health care provider. Ideally, a client acknowledges the problem and is willing to become involved in change. The professional's ability to identify problems and set priorities may be different from that of the client.

■ A community health nurse or other health care provider has the knowledge and skills to differentiate between health promotion, potential, actual, family, and individual problems. Forty problem-specific clusters of signs and symptoms help nurses define the active state of the problems. In addition, a user of the Scheme must have a knowledge base of risk factors and the ability to elicit client interest in relation to the Problem Classification Scheme.

■ Each nursing diagnosis is amenable to intervention. As the initial component of the Omaha System, the Problem Classification Scheme is integrated into the Conceptualization of the Family Nursing Process shown in the diagrams in Chapters 3 and 5. (Fig. 5–1). The Scheme provides the bridge or mechanism to suggest appropriate interventions by community health nurses.

BENEFITS

The Problem Classification Scheme encompasses the essence of community health nursing through a ho-listic approach to the client as an individual or family. The Scheme can serve as part of a paradigm or tool to organize the puzzle of relationships among data. The Scheme can be used to explain the complex, comprehensive, and independent nature of community health nursing to newly employed staff, to students, and to other nurses as well as to clients and the general public. Use of the Scheme acknowledges, values, and enriches theoretical pluralism. The Problem Classification Scheme offers a method for contributing to theory-building and limitless opportunities for practice-oriented research — activities that are needed to advance nursing science. Thus, the Scheme is an example of a taxonomic tool, relevant to the specialty of community health nursing.

Practice Guide

Community health nurses use the Problem Classification Scheme as a system of clues and cues to guide practice. The Problem Classification Scheme is a tool that facilitates decision-making in relation to client assessment and nursing diagnosis, a critical component of professional practice. It helps the nurse to process client information and make conclusions. The Scheme enables a nurse to position a family on a problem continuum ranging from Health Promotion to Actual, an imaginary line that ranges from an acceptable to an unacceptable client situation. Hypothesis formulation and information processing are basic skills that a nurse uses constantly to narrow the data collection field (Arnold, 1988). The skills used to group data into patterns and to narrow the data field are essential as the nurse sets priorities. Because the Problem Classification Scheme incorporates a portion of the nursing process, community health nurses who apply the Scheme validate their ability to use and apply theory to human problems. Simultaneously, nurses are participating in a theory-building process. The identification of problems, modifiers, and signs/symptoms is a process referred to as "factor isolation" or "generation of first level theory."

The use of the Problem Classification Scheme requires the nurse to make decisions. The skills involved in decision-making vary along a continuum from simple to complex. Three general aspects of skilled performance were identified by Dreyfus and elaborated upon by Benner (1984). The aspects are: (1) reliance on past concrete experiences rather than abstract principles, (2) synthesis of a situation into a whole, and (3) conversion from a detached observer to an involved performer. Benner has incorporated aspects of performance or skill into a five-stage continuum of nursing practice. The stages are: novice, advanced beginner, competent, proficient, and expert. As a community health nurse begins employment, that nurse may be at any of Benner's stages. The goal is to facilitate a nurse's independent decision-making abilities and movement along Benner's continuum toward higher levels of competence and performance as quickly as possible.

In addition, epidemiologic trends within groups of clients can be examined. When nurses consider the relationships among the problems, modifiers, and signs/symptoms, they have moved to the second and third levels of theoretical complexity, referred to as descriptive and explanatory. The Problem Classification Scheme is useful to a nurse who is practicing at any of Benner's five stages because it enables the nurse to accurately identify patterns in client data. The community health nurse's information base must include knowledge about the natural history of client problems and diseases as well as factors associated with high risk. Applying the science of epidemiology based on the Leavell and Clark model (1965) helps the nurse to identify causes of illness as well as to predict the course of illness. Leavell and Clark developed a widely accepted model that illustrates the course of illness through the interactions of the agent of illness, the human host, and the environmental factors. As depicted by the model, the interactions occur during stages of primary, secondary, and tertiary prevention. Significant epidemiologic findings are important to both the community health administrator and staff nurse. Often, the administrator benefits from aggregate data, whereas the staff nurse is interested in individual client data. Since the administrator has access to data from many staff nurses and other professionals, such data can be used to identify patterns or trends that develop throughout the entire community.

In order to adequately use the Problem Classification Scheme and generate accurate data, the community health nurse must use a sound information base and thoughtfully complete the initial phase of data collection. Completed prior to planning and intervening, the collection, sorting, and synthesizing step is an essential phase of the nursing process; therefore, the Problem Classification Scheme provides an orderly, organized framework for nursing practice by enabling the nurse to:

- Sort extraneous from pertinent data
- Integrate the nursing process into practice
- Utilize a holistic approach
- Become more efficient

Documentation Guide

The Problem Classification Scheme serves as a documentation and coding framework, facilitating the naming and organization of individual and family data. Use of the Scheme helps the nurse to identify and focus on pertinent data. The four domains encompass the practice of community health nursing and provide a structure for the assessment phase of the nursing process. Collection and assessment of pertinent subjective and objective data within each domain result in an accurate portrayal of the diverse factors that affect client health status and service delivery. Included are: (a) strengths, (b) interests, (c) risk factors, (d) signs/symptoms. This information enables a nurse to complete the diagnostic process and generate a problem list. The list consists of systematic language to describe actual, potential, and health promotion problems for a family and individual. Signs and symptoms accompany actual problems.

The problem list, the product resulting from use of the Problem Classification Scheme, is intended to provide a concise index of a client's health-related interests or concerns as well as potential and actual problems. The problem list provides structure for implementing and documenting the steps of the nursing process in an agency's legal clinical record (Martin & Scheet, 1989). Therefore, it is essential that a nurse use sound judgement to sort and establish priorities within initial client data. Information contained in a client record needs to be complete and comprehensive, and the quantity of information must be controlled in order for it to be practical and efficient. Too many or too few problems and signs/symptoms make the ensuing steps of the nursing process unworkable.

Communication Guide

The Problem Classification Scheme facilitates interdisciplinary communication and continuity in the community health practice setting. Two goals were delineated. The first goal was to achieve clarity and brevity by using direct, concise, widely accepted parlance. The second goal was to decrease confusion for the two groups who are responsible for using the client record, but in dissimilar ways. One group includes novice and experienced staff nurses, other community health professionals, and students who document care they provide to clients or exchange with other direct delivery staff. The second group includes supervisors, administrators, educators, quality assurance coordinators, utilization review members, other record auditors, school personnel, and clients who examine and trace client care by reading a description of the health care professional's chain of thinking and action. Thus, efficiency and continuity increase when all use and understand the same language (Henry & LeClair, 1987).

Although community health nurses are the most frequent users of the Problem Classification Scheme, it may also be implemented by other direct delivery staff who function in the community health setting. Included are: physical therapists, occupational therapists, nutritionists, social workers, and speech pathologists. For example, a community health nurse may identify and address Problem 27. Neuro-Musculo-Skeletal Function. The nurse's interventions are in accord with nursing practice. A physical therapist, however, usually documents detailed subjective and objective data in relation to Problem 27. Most of physical therapists' interventions and evaluations are directed toward that problem, although they may address other problems such as 03. Residence, 24. Pain, and 35. Nutrition. In any case, use of these problems facilitates collection of data and direction of interventions and evaluation for the physical therapist. Often, a physical therapist recognizes that a client's problems involving Environmental, Psychosocial, or Health Related Behaviors Domains must be resolved along with Problem 27. Neuro-Musculo-Skeletal Function.

Data Management Guide

Others who use the client record vary in their purposes and methods. The supervisor, educator, and quality assurance coordinator are among those who monitor the skills of staff nurses and students, looking for written evidence of their ability to identify and address priority problems. Sometimes, client record data are compared and contrasted with shared visit observations. Utilization review members examine client records for evidence of appropriate admission to and dismissal from agency service; they also are interested in the fit between a family's problems and agency staff assigned to a home. Other record auditors focus on reimbursement issues, noting if care is provided in relation to the reason for referral. Many of these reviewers are concerned about individual clients, although some are also interested in aggregate data. Information regarding trends in the number and types of problems in geographic areas, over time, can serve as valuable data on which to base staffing and program decisions. Furthermore, as research on the Problem Classification Scheme and other components of the Omaha System continues, progress is being made toward establishing a system that is capable of identifying community health nursing costs. The goal is to provide community health nurses with a tool that more precisely describes and prices their services. (Martin & Scheet, 1985).

The Problem Classification Scheme provides an agency director with a precise framework for analyzing aggregate data. Analysis can be done manually, but clinical data analysis is a critical capability of an automated management information system. "To take advantage of the computer's data processing capabilities, the user must define precisely all elements of the data, all possible responses must be accounted for, and all contingencies must be planned" (Zielstorff, 1988, p. 67). The Problem Classification Scheme defines those elements that are of concern to community health nurses and their clients. The data produced are valuable to agency directors for programming, personnel administration, accreditation, and strategic planning as well as public relations and resource utilization management. Efforts to clarify the contributions of nurses and itemize nursing costs are gaining momentum because of managers' requests; ultimately, there is the potential for direct third-party reimbursement for nurses.

SUMMARY

When using the Problem Classification Scheme, certain suggestions and precautions need to be considered. Primary among the suggestions are the following:

- **Do** assume that nursing judgement will always be important. While the Scheme serves as a tool for sorting and organizing client data, a high level of skill is required for determining data priority and for using the Scheme with the nursing process. There are no "right" answers.
- **Do** approach the Scheme as a tool for practice and documentation. The need to increase practice expertise and efficiency of recording becomes more critical every year.
- **Do** recognize that it takes time and commitment to learn correct use of the Scheme.
- **Do** review the entire Scheme, definitions, and guidelines for use regularly. Discuss applications with others. Everyone profits from occasional review.
- **Do** remember that a problem consists of three parts: a problem label and two modifiers.
- **Do** view signs/symptoms in relation to their severity; and in relation to total client information. For instance, the Problem Classification Scheme identifies *missing or broken teeth* as a sign/symptom of Dentition: Impairment. Since a client with missing teeth may not need nursing intervention, the presence of a single sign/symptom may *or* may not be sufficient cause for recording it on the problem list.
- **Do** use signs/symptoms with actual problems only. One *or* more signs/symptoms may be appropriate to identify an actual problem.
- **Do not** add to the Scheme indiscriminately. Specify terms when the sign/symptom *Other* is used. Likewise, be specific when adding a problem with its cluster of signs/symptoms to any of the four domains. It is essential that additions to the Problem Classification Scheme be (1) nursing focused, (2) amenable to nursing interventions, and (3) parallel to and not duplicates of the ideas of existing signs/symptoms or problems. Taxonomic principles of mutual exclusivity, order, and comparable levels are incorporated into the Scheme.
- **Do not** confuse nursing diagnoses with medical diagnoses. Both are important and serve different purposes. Community health client records, especially those in home health agencies, require identification of nursing and medical diagnoses. For example, community health nurses do not treat diabetes mellitus. Client problems associated with this medical diagnosis may include Nutrition and Technical Procedures.
- **Do not** confuse interventions with signs/symptoms or problems. For example, the presence of a Foley catheter is an intervention to address the problem of Genito-Urinary Function: Impairment.
- **Do not** confuse the cause or etiology of a problem with the problem itself. For example, a fractured limb may erroneously be considered a problem

when, in fact, the real problem is Neuro-Musculo-Skeletal Function: Impairment.

- **Do not** confuse risk factors with the signs/symptoms of a problem. For example, "first experience with parenting" is a risk factor and not a sign/symptom of Parenting: Impairment. Risk factors are used only with the modifier *Potential*. Signs and symptoms are used only with the modifier *Actual*.
- **Do not** list a physical abnormality as a problem if it does not interfere with the client's ability to function or if adequate correction has been made by external devices such as glasses or prostheses.
- **Do not** identify problems or signs/symptoms indiscriminately. More is not necessarily better.

Further recommendations related to planning, instruction, and continuation for the Problem Classification Scheme and other components of the Omaha System are described in Chapter 8. Use of the Problem Classification Scheme by specific types of staff and within various programs and recording systems are described and illustrated in Chapters 9 through 13.

REFERENCES

Arnold, J. (1988). Diagnostic reasoning protocols for clinical simulations in nursing. In Strickland, O., & Waltz, C. (Eds.), *Measurement of Nursing Outcomes, Vol. 2, Measuring Nursing Performance: Practice, education, and research* (pp. 53–87). New York, Springer.

Avant, K. (1990, April–June). The art and science in nursing diagnosis development. *Nurs. Diagnosis, 1*:51–56.

Aydelotte, M., & Peterson, K. (1987). Keynote address: Nursing taxonomies—state of the art. In McLane, A. (Ed.), *Classification of Nursing Diagnoses: Proceedings of the Seventh Conference* (pp. 1–16). St. Louis, C. V. Mosby Company.

Benner, P. (1984). *From Novice to Expert.* Menlo Park, CA, Addison-Wesley.

Carroll-Johnson, R. (1990, April–June). Editorial: Reflections on the 9th biennial conference. *Nurs. Diagnosis, 1*:49–50.

Chambers, B. (1990, May). [Graduate student experiences with the Omaha System.] Personal communication regarding unpublished data.

Henry, B., & LeClair, H. (1987, January). Language, leadership, and power. *J. Nurs. Admin., 17*:19–25.

Kritek, P. (1989). An introduction to the science and art of taxonomy. *Classification Systems for Describing Nursing Practice* (pp. 6–12). Kansas City, MO, American Nurses' Association.

Leavell, H., & Clark, E. (1965). *Preventive Medicine for the Doctor in His Community* (3rd. ed.). New York, McGraw-Hill.

Levine, M. (1989, Spring). The ethics of nursing rhetoric. *Image, 21*:4–6.

Martin, K., & Scheet, N. (1985). The Omaha system: Implications for costing community health nursing. In Shaffer, F. (Ed.), *Costing Out Nursing: Pricing our Product* (pp. 197–206). New York, National League for Nursing.

Martin, K., & Scheet, N. (1989). Nursing diagnosis in home health: The Omaha system. In Martinson, I., & Widmer, A. (Eds.), *Home Health Care Nursing* (pp. 67–72). Philadelphia, W.B. Saunders.

Mayers, M. (1983). *A Systematic Approach to the Nursing Care Plan* (3rd ed.). Norwalk, CT, Appleton-Century-Crofts.

Porter, E. (1986, Winter). Critical analysis of NANDA nursing diagnosis taxonomy I. *Image, 18*:136–139.

Rasch, R. (1987, Fall). The nature of taxonomy. *Image, 19*:147–149.

Warren, J. (1987). A proposal for testing the nursing diagnosis: Taxonomy I. In Hannah, K., Reimer, M., Mills, W., et al. (Eds.), *Clini-*

cal Judgement and Decision Making: The Future with Nursing Diagnosis (pp. 111–114). New York, John Wiley & Sons.

Zielstorff, R. (1988). Considerations in data capture, storage, and retrieval for the nursing minimum data set. In Werley, H., & Lang, N. (Eds.). *Identification of the Nursing Minimum Data Set* (pp. 67–76). New York, Springer.

BIBLIOGRAPHY

Bloom, B. (1956). *Taxonomy of Educational Objectives: The Classification of Educational Goals Handbook I: Cognitive Domain.* New York, David McKay.

Brown, M. (1974). The epidemiologic approach to the study of clinical nursing diagnoses. *Nurs. Forum, 13*:346–359.

Carnevali, D. (1983). *Nursing Care Planning: Diagnoses and Management* (3rd ed.). Philadelphia, J. B. Lippincott.

Carnevali, D. (1987). Diagnostic reasoning: Nursing and medicine compared. In Hannah, K., Reimer, M., Mills, W., et al. (Eds.), *Clinical Judgement and Decision Making: The Future With Nursing Diagnosis* (pp. 29–32). New York, John Wiley & Sons.

Crawford, G. (1982, October). The concept of pattern in nursing: Conceptual development and measurement. *Adv. Nurs. Sci., 5*:1–6.

Dickoff, J., James, P., & Wiedenbach, E. (1968a, September/October). Theory in a practice discipline: Part I. Practice oriented theory. *Nurs. Res., 17*:415–435.

Dickoff, J., James, P., & Wiedenbach, E. (1968b, November/December). Theory in a practice discipline: Part II. Practice oriented research. *Nurs. Res., 17*:545–554.

Dickoff, J., & James, P. (1989). Theoretical pluralism for nursing diagnosis. In Carroll-Johnson, R. (Ed.), *Classification of Nursing Diagnoses: Proceedings of Eighth National Conference* (pp. 98–125). St. Louis, C. V. Mosby.

Douglas, D., & Murphy, E. (1985). Nursing process, nursing diagnosis, and emerging taxonomies. In McCloskey, J., & Grace, H. (Eds.), *Current Issues in Nursing* (2nd ed.) (pp. 63–72). Boston, Blackwell.

Douglas, D., & Murphy, E. (1990). Nursing process, nursing diagnosis, and emerging taxonomies. In McCloskey, J., & Grace, H. (Eds.), *Current Issues in Nursing* (3rd ed.) (pp. 17–22). St. Louis, C. V. Mosby.

Fleishman, E. (1982, July). Systems for describing human tasks. *Am. Psychol., 37*:821–834.

Gebbie, K., & Lavin, M. (Eds.) (1975). *Classification of Nursing Diagnoses.* St. Louis, C. V. Mosby.

Gordon, M. (1990, January–March). Toward history-based diagnostic categories. *Nurs. Diagnosis, 1*:5–11.

Hays, B. (1990). *Relationships Among Nursing Care Requirements, Selected Patient Factors, Selected Nurse Factors, and Nursing Resource Consumption in Home Health Care.* [Unpublished doctoral dissertation.] Cleveland, OH, Case Western Reserve University.

Hinshaw, A. (1989). Keynote address: Nursing diagnosis: Forging the link between theory and practice. In Carroll-Johnson, R. (Ed.), *Classification of Nursing Diagnoses: Proceedings of Eighth National Conference* (pp. 3–10). St. Louis, C. V. Mosby.

Hoskins, L., McFarlane, E., Rubenfeld, M., et al. (1986, April). Nursing diagnosis in the chronically ill: Methodology for clinical validation. *Adv. Nurs. Sci., 8*:80–89.

Jenny, J. (1989). Classification of nursing diagnosis: A self-care approach. In Carroll-Johnson, R. (Ed.), *Classification of Nursing Diagnoses: Proceedings of Eighth National Conference* (pp. 152–157). St. Louis, C. V. Mosby.

Jewell, M., & Peters, D. (1989, September/October). An assessment guide for community health nurses. *Home Healthcare Nurse, 7*:32–36.

Kuhn, T. (1962). *The Structure of Scientific Revolutions.* Chicago, University of Chicago Press.

Levine, M. (1987). Approaches to the development of a nursing diagnosis taxonomy. In McLane, A. (Ed.), *Classification of Nursing Diagnoses* (pp. 45–52). St. Louis, C. V. Mosby.

Martin, K. (1988). Nursing minimum data set requirements for the community setting. In Werley, H., & Lang, N. (Eds.), *Identification of the Nursing Minimum Data Set* (pp. 214–222). New York, Springer.

McCloskey, J. (1989, January). Implications of costing out nursing services for reimbursement. *Nurs. Manag.*, 20:44–49.

Mehmert, P. (1987, December). A nursing information system: The outcome of implementing nursing diagnoses. *Nurs. Clin. North Am.*, 22:971–979.

Peters, D. (1988). Classifying patients using a nursing diagnosis taxonomy. In Harris, M. (Ed.), *Home Health Administration* (pp. 311–322). Owings Mills, MD, Rynd Communications.

Phillips, L. (1987). Critical points in decision making. In Hannah, K., Reimer, M., Mills, W., et al. (Eds.), *Clinical Judgement and Decision Making: The Future With Nursing Diagnosis* (pp. 63–67). New York, John Wiley & Sons.

Pinnell, N., & de Menses, M. (1986). *The Nursing Process.* Norwalk, CT, Appleton-Century-Crofts.

Roy, C. (1987). The influence of nursing models on clinical decision making II. In Hannah, K., Reimer, M., Mills, W., et al. (Eds.), *Clinical Judgement and Decision Making: The Future with Nursing Diagnosis* (pp. 42–47). New York, John Wiley & Sons.

Simpson, G. (1961). *Principles of Animal Taxonomy.* San Francisco, Freeman.

Stanhope, M., & Lancaster, J. (1988). *Community Health Nursing: Process and Practice for Promoting Health.* St. Louis, C. V. Mosby.

Strickland, O., & Waltz, C. (Eds.) (1988). *Measurement of Nursing Outcomes, Vol. 2, Measuring Nursing Performance: Practice, Education, and Research.* New York, Springer.

Tanner, C. (1988, October). Curriculum revolution: The practice mandate. *Nurs. Health Care,* 9:427–430.

Warren, J. (1983, October). Accountability and nursing diagnosis. *J. Nurs. Admin.,* 10:34–37.

Weidmann, J., & North, H. (1987, December). Implementing the Omaha classification system in a public health agency. *Nurs. Clin. North Am.,* 22:971–979.

Werley, H., & Lang, N. (Eds.) (1988). *Identification of the Nursing Minimum Data Set.* New York, Springer.

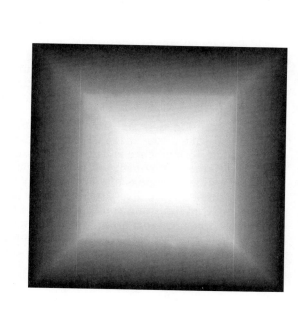

CHAPTER SIX

*F*or the first time in a century of organized nursing, nurses are defining an autonomous role. To this end we have seen in the past decade more specialization, changes in licensure laws, and the movement for nursing diagnosis. The key to an autonomous profession is a clearly defined base of knowledge. While nursing will continue to use knowledge from other disciplines, it must define what it is that nurses do and whether what they do makes a difference. (Bulechek & McCloskey, 1985, p. 1)

The Intervention Scheme is a systematic arrangement of nursing actions or activities. As such, it does not represent new community health nursing knowledge but clarifies critical nursing decisions and strategies that are planned and completed in a community health practice setting. The Intervention Scheme is designed to help a community health nurse and other community health personnel document both plans and interventions.

The Intervention Scheme is a framework of nursing actions designed for use with nursing diagnoses. It represents an initial research-based effort to link the effectiveness of interventions with diagnoses, an effort not yet accomplished within the nursing profession. Stevenson (1990) completed a review of quantitative research related to interventions and categorized studies into 30 nursing care activities and foci. The review documents both the extent of interest and need for further investigation. In 1985, Douglas and Murphy suggested ". . . that the profession should not feel compelled to 'finish' work on nursing diagnoses before proceeding to other critical investigations, such as those into nursing interventions and their impact" (p. 70). "Nurses are also reporting the development of individual diagnoses and the interventions associated with them" (Aydelotte & Peterson, 1987, p. 12).

The Intervention Scheme provides a community health nurse with a tool that includes standard language to guide both practice and documentation in relation to the other components of the nursing process. The Intervention Scheme is of value not only to staff nurses and other direct delivery staff members but also to supervisors, administrators, utilization review committee members, and other client record auditors. The relationships among the Problem Classification Scheme, the Omaha System, and the family nursing process are depicted in Figure 6–1.

ORGANIZATION

The purpose of the Intervention Scheme is to offer an organized, standard language to community health professionals for use during planning and intervening. The Intervention Scheme is designed to address all activities involved in community health nursing practice, including preventing illness and improving, maintaining, or restoring client health (Table 6–1).

Nurses in general have given much less attention to plans and interventions than to other components of the nursing process, especially nursing diagnosis. With less nursing intervention research comes more confusion in this area. As recently as 1985, Aydelotte noted that intervention knowledge is not systematically organized. Barnard (1985) described the need to develop the science of nursing, to discover what makes nursing effective, and to develop valid and reliable intervention measures. In comparison to other components of the nursing process, planning and intervening require as much or more talent and creativity from the professional and provide the greatest potential value for the client. Testing nursing interventions is the challenge of the 1990s (Barnard, 1985).

Those who have addressed nursing interventions have focused on diverse levels of abstraction. Many tend to emphasize single treatment methods (Taylor, 1989). Such methods are highly specific to certain age groups or to certain nursing or medical diagnoses. For example, Campbell (1984) suggested applying a hot water bottle to the abdomen for painful bladder spasms. In contrast, she suggested that the nurse approach the client unhurriedly, a broad category of intervention listed for most of the other client problems in her extensive book. Campbell organized general interventions into four categories: (1) nursing treatments, (2) nursing observations, (3) health teaching, and (4)

Intervention Scheme

medical treatments performed by nurses. Other nurses have approached nursing interventions from a broad frame of reference and have developed general intervention models. Their efforts are described in Chapter 3.

Criteria for Intervention Selections

The community health nurses involved in the VNA of Omaha research study were not willing to accept either the single treatment methods or the very broad interventions previously described. These nurses did not want to select interventions from extensive or standard problem-specific lists. The nurses wanted an Intervention Scheme to describe a series of functions or actions useful when providing individual care to clients of diverse ages and diagnoses. The Scheme needed to be adaptable to the wide range of time frames possible for setting goals and developing plans with clients. Thus, based on empirical data, the Intervention Scheme was designed to be an open, flexible system of cues and clues for use in conjunction with the Problem Classification Scheme and the Problem Rating Scale for Outcomes. Furthermore, the Scheme could accommodate primary nursing functions that are either autonomous or collaborative. As professionals who are increasingly well educated and competent, nurses work with diverse health, social, technical, and other professional groups. These working relationships require the "expansion of professional functions" (Mussallem, 1985, p. 60).

The Intervention Scheme is organized into three levels of abstraction or specificity to accommodate the needs of direct care delivery staff, supervisors, and administrators. The hierarchical levels are: (1) categories, (2) targets, and (3) client-specific information. According to the principles of taxonomy, each level of abstraction serves a specific, essential purpose and does not duplicate information at the other levels. The levels can be illustrated as:

Category
  Target
    Client-specific Information

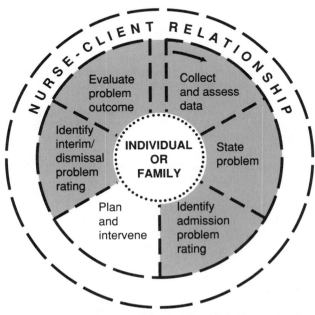

FIGURE 6 – 1 ■ Using the Intervention Scheme facilitates the planning and intervening step of the family nursing process.

TABLE 6-1 ■ Intervention Scheme

CATEGORIES

I. Health Teaching, Guidance, and Counseling
II. Treatments and Procedures
III. Case Management
IV. Surveillance

TARGETS

01. Anatomy/physiology
02. Behavior modification
03. Bladder care
04. Bonding
05. Bowel care
06. Bronchial hygiene
07. Cardiac care
08. Caretaking/parenting skills
09. Cast care
10. Communication
11. Coping skills
12. Day care/respite
13. Discipline
14. Dressing change/wound care
15. Durable medical equipment
16. Education
17. Employment
18. Environment
19. Exercises
20. Family planning
21. Feeding procedures
22. Finances
23. Food
24. Gait training
25. Growth/development
26. Homemaking
27. Housing
28. Interaction
29. Lab findings
30. Legal system
31. Medical/dental care
32. Medication action/side effects
33. Medication administration
34. Medication set-up
35. Mobility/transfers
36. Nursing care, supplementary
37. Nutrition
38. Nutritionist
39. Ostomy care
40. Other community resource
41. Personal care
42. Positioning
43. Rehabilitation
44. Relaxation/breathing techniques
45. Rest/sleep
46. Safety
47. Screening
48. Sickness/injury care
49. Signs/symptoms — mental/emotional
50. Signs/symptoms — physical
51. Skin care
52. Social work/counseling
53. Specimen collection
54. Spiritual care
55. Stimulation/nurturance
56. Stress management
57. Substance use
58. Supplies
59. Support group
60. Support system
61. Transportation
62. Wellness
63. Other

CLIENT-SPECIFIC INFORMATION
Generated and individualized by health care provider

CATEGORY DEFINITIONS

I. Health Teaching, Guidance, and Counseling
Health teaching, guidance, and counseling are nursing activities that range from giving information, anticipating client problems, encouraging client action and responsibility for self-care and coping, to assisting with decision-making and problem-solving. The overlapping concepts occur on a continuum with the variation due to the client's self-direction capabilities.

II. Treatments and Procedures
Treatments and procedures are technical nursing activities directed toward preventing signs and symptoms, identifying risk factors and early signs and symptoms, and decreasing or alleviating signs and symptoms.

III. Case Management
Case management includes nursing activities of coordination, advocacy, and referral. These activities involve facilitating service delivery on behalf of the client, communicating with health and human service providers, promoting assertive client communication, and guiding the client toward use of appropriate community resources.

IV. Surveillance
Surveillance includes nursing activities of detection, measurement, critical analysis, and monitoring to indicate client status in relation to a given condition or phenomenon.

TARGET DEFINITIONS

01. **Anatomy/physiology:** Structure and function of the human body.
02. **Behavior modification:** Activities designed to promote a change of habits.
03. **Bladder care:** Activities directed toward maintenance of urinary bladder function, including bladder retraining, catheter change, and catheter irrigation.
04. **Bonding:** Unique emotional, synchronized parent-child relationship.
05. **Bowel care:** Activities directed toward maintenance of bowel function, including enema, bowel training, diet, and medication.
06. **Bronchial hygiene:** Activities directed toward maintenance of respiratory or pulmonary function, incuding inhalation therapy, percussion, and cannula insertion.
07. **Cardiac care:** Activities directed toward maintenance of cardiac or circulatory function, including diet, medication, vital signs, and relief of edema.
08. **Caretaking/parenting skills:** Abilities necessary to maintain a dependent child or adult, including feeding, bathing, discipline, nurturing, and stimulation.
09. **Cast care:** Activities directed toward maintenance of an immobilized body part, including relief of pain, pressure, or constriction of circulation.
10. **Communication:** The exchange of verbal or nonverbal information.
11. **Coping skills:** Ability to deal with or gain control of existing problems, including family tasks, illness, and employment.

TABLE 6-1 ■ Intervention Scheme *Continued*

TARGET DEFINITIONS

12. **Day-care/respite:** Individual or institution providing child or adult supervision or care in the absence of the parent or caregiver.
13. **Discipline:** Activities designed to promote appropriate behavior, conduct, or action, including time out, limits, and controls.
14. **Dressing change/wound care:** Observing, cleansing, irrigating, or covering a wound, lesion, or incision.
15. **Durable medical equipment:** Nonexpendable articles primarily used for medical purposes in the presence of illness or injury, including hospital beds, respirators, walkers, and apnea monitors.
16. **Education:** Programs for development of special and general abilities, including Headstart, individualized study, GED, and vocational rehabilitation.
17. **Employment:** Occupation that provides income.
18. **Environment:** Aggregate of surrounding conditions or influences, including housing, community, and family.
19. **Exercises:** Therapeutic physical exertion, including active/passive range of motion, isometrics, and strengthening exercises.
20. **Family planning:** Practice of birth control measures within the context of family values, attitudes, and beliefs, including oral contraceptive, diaphragm, condom, and natural family planning.
21. **Feeding procedures:** Method of giving food or fluid, including breast, formula, intravenous, or tube.
22. **Finances:** Management of available economic resources in relation to family needs, including credit counseling, Assistance to Families with Dependent Children (AFDC), and Medicaid.
23. **Food:** Nourishing substance that is eaten or otherwise taken into the body to sustain life, provide energy, or promote growth.
24. **Gait training:** Systematic activities designed to promote walking with or without assistive devices.
25. **Growth/development:** Progressive physical, mental, emotional, and social maturation in relation to age, including developmental milestones and Erikson's developmental stages.
26. **Homemaking:** Management of the home, including cooking, cleaning, and laundry.
27. **Housing:** Place or type of residence.
28. **Interaction:** Reciprocal actions or influences among people, including mother-child, husband-wife, client-nurse, and parent-teacher.
29. **Lab findings:** Results of physiologic tests, including urinalysis and blood work.
30. **Legal system:** Connected with law or its administration, including legal aid, attorney, court, or Child Protective Services (CPS).
31. **Medical/dental care:** Diagnosis and treatment by a physician or dentist.
32. **Medication action/side effects:** Information regarding the purposes and positive or negative consequences of therapeutic drugs.
33. **Medication administration:** Applying, dispensing, or giving of drugs or medicines as prescribed by a physician.
34. **Medication set-up:** Organizing or arranging medicines for self-administration, including a Mediset.
35. **Mobility/transfers:** Movement of body or body parts, including activities of walking, swimming, and moving from one position or location to another.
36. **Nursing care, supplementary:** Therapeutic activities in addition to intermittent service, including private duty nursing and home health aide.
37. **Nutrition:** Nourishment of body with balanced food and fluid capable of providing energy, maintenance, and growth.
38. **Nutritionist:** A person who utilizes the science of nutrition to help individuals improve their health.
39. **Ostomy care:** Management of elimination through artificial openings, including colostomy and ileostomy.
40. **Other community resource:** An agency or group that offers goods or services not specifically identified in other targets, including day care/respite and education.
41. **Personal care:** Management of hygiene, including bathing, shampooing, shaving, nail trimming, and dressing.
42. **Positioning:** Placing the body into a particular position/alignment for a specified activity or response.
43. **Rehabilitation:** Process of restoring the ability to live and work as normally as possible after a disabling injury or illness, including physical, speech, and occupational therapy.
44. **Relaxation/breathing techniques:** Activities that relieve muscle tension, induce a quieting body response, and rebuild energy resources, including deep breathing exercises, imagery, and meditation.
45. **Rest/sleep:** Period of inactivity, repose, or mental calm with or without suspension of sensory activity.
46. **Safety:** A state of freedom from the risk or occurrence of injury or loss.
47. **Screening:** Individual or group testing procedures, including vision, hearing, height-weight, developmental, scoliosis, and blood pressure.
48. **Sickness/injury care:** Appropriate responses to illness or accidents, including first aid, taking temperature, and seeking medical care.
49. **Signs/symptoms—mental/emotional:** Objective or subjective evidence of a mental/emotional health problem, including depression, confusion, agitation, and suicidal threats.
50. **Signs/symptoms—physical:** Objective or subjective evidence of a physical health problem, including elevated temperature, failure to thrive, and statement of pain.
51. **Skin care:** Activities directed toward maintaining integrity of integument, including decubitus care and massage.
52. **Social work/counseling:** Plan designed by a social worker or counselor to promote the welfare of individual/families.
53. **Specimen collection:** Obtaining samples of body fluids, secretions, or excreta, including blood, urine, feces, sputum, or drainage.
54. **Spiritual care:** Activities directed toward management of religious concerns.
55. **Stimulation/nurturance:** Activities that promote healthy physical and emotional development.
56. **Stress management:** Physical and emotional activities that immunize the body from known stressors.
57. **Substance use:** Consumption of medicines, drugs, or other materials, including prescription drugs, over-the-counter or street drugs, alcohol, and tobacco.
58. **Supplies:** Articles necessary to the management of personal care or the treatment plan, including dressings, syringes, lotions, or baby bottles.
59. **Support group:** Regular planned gatherings designed to accomplish some compatible goal, including Alcoholics Anonymous, I Can Cope, or Pilot Parents.
60. **Support system:** The circle of friends, family, and associates that provide love, care, and need gratification, including church, school, and workplace.
61. **Transportation:** Method of travel, including car, bus, and taxi.
62. **Wellness:** Practices that promote health, including immunization, exercise, nutrition, and birth control.
63. **Other:** Nursing action not identified in this list.

Categories of Intervention

The four intervention categories represent the first level of the Intervention Scheme. They are Health Teaching, Guidance, and Counseling; Treatments and Procedures; Case Management; and Surveillance. The four categories are comprehensive, inclusive concepts used frequently by community health nurses. When viewed collectively, the categories are equated with the essence of community health nursing practice, thus describing a nurse's primary functions both in terms of importance and time. The four intervention categories are essentially discrete, not overlapping. One or more categories can be used by a community health nurse to develop a plan or document an intervention specific to a client problem. The categories represent the final results of the data collection and field testing procedures that were conducted at four community health agencies during the VNA of Omaha research project. In terms of hierarchical levels, the categories parallel the four domains of the Problem Classification Scheme.

Target Selection

The second level of the Intervention Scheme is an alphabetic listing of 62 targets. Targets are defined as objects of nursing interventions or nursing activities. The targets are used to delineate a problem-specific intervention category in terms of or in relation to which action or activity is addressed. The nurse selects one or more targets to further describe a plan or intervention category specific to a client problem. During the VNA research project, targets were organized in various ways, including domain-specific groupings. Participating community health nurses decided that an alphabetic listing was the most efficient and acceptable option. Because the target listing is not intended to be exhaustive, "Other" appears at the end of the list, enabling the nurse to document a word or words that describe a needed addition.

Client-specific Information

The third level of the Intervention Scheme is designed for client-specific information. Pertinent, concise words or short phrases are generated by community health nurses or other community health professionals as they develop plans or document care provided to a specific client. Based on the VNA of Omaha research project, completed during 1986, no narrative was written or organized at the third level. In contrast to the category and target levels the diversity and amount of data at the third level was too great to organize into the Intervention Scheme or into an automated management information system. The information at the third level of specificity is as important, however, as the category and target levels in relation to professional practice, documentation, communication, quality assurance, and legal issues. Therefore, VNA of Omaha staff organized a portion of the data at the third level into Care Planning Guides. (The Guides appear in *The Omaha System: A Pocket Guide for Community Health Nursing*, a companion to this book.)

The Intervention Scheme is designed for use with any client problem from the Problem Classification Scheme. The Intervention Scheme is organized into categories and targets and used to document plans and interventions.

Definitions

Plan. The action(s) or activity(ies) designed to establish a course of client care. This analytic process includes establishing priorities and selecting a course of action from identified alternatives. The plan always includes a category and target(s); it usually includes client-specific information.

Intervention. An action or activity implemented to address a specific client problem and to improve, maintain, or restore health or prevent illness. The intervention always includes a category and target(s); it usually includes client-specific information.

Categories. The four broad areas that provide a structure for describing community health nursing actions or activities (i.e., Health Teaching, Guidance, and Counseling; Treatments and Procedures; Case Management; Surveillance).

Targets. The 62 objects of nursing actions or activities that serve to further describe interventions (e.g., Coping skills, Mobility/transfers, Substance use).

Client-specific information. The detailed portion of a plan or intervention statement that is generated by the community health nurse or other health-care professional.

ASSUMPTIONS

Application of the Intervention Scheme is based on general assumptions. The following six assumptions are particularly important:

■ Community health nurses develop extensive nursing judgment as a result of sound educational preparation, personal experiences, and experience providing care to clients. Therefore, they recognize the benefits of practice and documentation systems that offer flexibility as well as clues and cues; they tend to reject exhaustive standardized plans as burdensome.

■ In collaboration with a client, a community health nurse identifies strengths and sets priorities among problems prior to developing plans and interventions. Priorities must take into account factors such as the urgency of client needs, family dynamics, and a comparison of costs versus benefits.

■ Community health nurses, other health care providers, and clients develop the plan and implement the interventions through mutual effort. Advances in a client's self-sufficiency and progress require considerable client action, as compared to client responsibilities in an acute care setting.

■ A nurse needs to develop plans and implement interventions carefully. This is especially important as a nurse assists a client to modify situations, environments, and/or behaviors.

■ Individuals and families have the right and the responsibility to make their own decisions. Such decisions reflect their social and cultural systems and personal values.

■ Nursing plans and interventions are closely linked and are often developed or completed simultaneously. As illustrated in the Conceptualization of the Family Nursing Process (see Fig. 6–1), use of the Intervention Scheme is dependent upon collection of client data and identification of client problems.

BENEFITS

Community health staff nurses, supervisors, and administrators need a method of organizing, documenting, and communicating the process of providing client care. They need a method of defining, quantifying, and reporting community health nursing practice for a wide range of clients. Community health care clients are diverse in relation to nursing and medical diagnoses as well as in age, socioeconomic status, education, ethnicity, and cultural values. Furthermore, nurses need a valid and reliable system that can be used to facilitate decision-making and discussion and to document services in legal client records.

The Intervention Scheme is a research-based tool that is congruent with the nursing process and clinical judgement. The Intervention Scheme is a relatively simple system of categories, targets, and client-specific information useful for organizing, documenting, and communicating the process of care. It is based on the premise that a community health nurse has autonomy in practice and functions as a competent professional.

Practice Guide

Community health nurses carry out extensive, highly complex, and skilled functions during the process of providing care to clients. These functions are both autonomous and collaborative and often occur simultaneously. The two types of functions are distinct yet interrelated. Such functions represent the comprehensive intervention skills of the practitioner and are purposeful, goal-directed nursing activities. The functions also define the practice of nursing and clarify how nursing is similar to and different from medicine and other disciplines.

The accuracy, variety, complexity, and speed used by a staff nurse to select and complete interventions increase proportionately as a nurse moves along a continuum of practice as described by Benner (1984). An increase in competence includes the ability to solve problems quickly; with experience, a nurse perceives a client's status and responds rapidly with precise nursing interventions or strategies. As nurses become more experienced, proficient, and flexible, they can apply their community health practice skills to assist clients of many ages and cultures who have various nursing and medical diagnoses. Experience enables nurses to assist profoundly troubled families or families with several problems more easily. A nurse becomes more familiar with family dynamics, with care that is available from other nurses and disciplines within the agency, and with services that are available and/or provided by

other community resources. Increased familiarity also assists a nurse to involve several family members or significant others in the process of care, involvement that increases the likelihood of client improvement and success.

Nursing plans and interventions are the most complex and important portions of the nursing process in certain respects. Nurses must accurately assess and diagnose client problems in order to identify and carry out appropriate plans and interventions. It is important for nurses to competently evaluate client progress. The sensitivity, skill, and sophistication, however, that truly expert nurses use for planning and intervening are phenomenal. Expert nurses are change agents as they

- Select the best combination of interventions
- Adapt them to meet a client's environmental, psychosocial, physiologic, and health-related behavior needs and wants, and
- time the implementation and repetition of the interventions.

Community health nurses must consider various perspectives as they select and carry out nursing functions. Included are (1) characteristics of the nursing diagnosis, (2) research base associated with the intervention, (3) feasibility of successfully implementing the intervention, (4) acceptability of intervention to the client, and (5) capabilities of the nurse.

The four categories of the Intervention Scheme incorporate the practice of community health nursing, the nursing process, clinical judgement theories, and the epidemiologic model. Use of the categories in conjunction with the targets and client-specific information enables the community health nurse to organize abstract ideas into specific, concrete plans and interventions. Throughout the process of client service, tools such as the Intervention Scheme assist the nurse to consider the entire client situation and set priorities for services. Using the Intervention Scheme can help the nurse differentiate care that must be done immediately from care that might be done at a later time. Community health professionals can also use the Scheme to document the complex clinical judgements made as they select and eliminate intervention options in relation to a specific client.

Many aspects of clinical intervention decisions made on a daily basis by practicing community health nurses are being investigated. Decisions made by nurses are extremely complex, similar to those made by other health care professionals. The diagnostic decision-making processes related to interventions are part of "the knowing how" or competence that a nurse develops (Benner, 1983). Benner (1984) used vignettes called "exemplars" to demonstrate how nursing competence evolves systematically along a novice-to-expert continuum. As community health nurses gain experience and competence, their use of the categories, targets, and client-specific information of the Intervention Scheme becomes more comprehensive and rapid.

Documentation Guide

The Intervention Scheme benefits an agency's client records and the nurses who keep them. First, use of the Scheme's systematic language decreases the volume of documentation. Nurses can develop plans and progress notes that are shorter and less rambling. Second, documentation consistency increases as the nurse uses the structure and patterns provided by the Intervention Scheme. Third, client record clarity is enhanced for individual nurses and agency personnel who review entries. Fourth, time needed to document and read client data is decreased through use of the Intervention Scheme, thus increasing the efficiency of agency personnel. All four benefits can be demonstrated when documentation for a specific visit includes not only the categories and targets but also client-specific information. By using this three-step process to document care, a nurse can communicate what care was provided and describe a client's response to care. Client response is indicated in various ways as verbal and nonverbal communication, repetition of a task, and return demonstration of a skill.

The Intervention Scheme is important for professional accountability, an area of concern that is closely related to documentation consistency and clarity. The process of developing care plans is a mechanism to demonstrate accountability. When community health nurses are considered primary nurses, they need to demonstrate professional autonomy, responsibility, and accountability.

Communication Guide

Community health nurses and members of other disciplines can examine their own patterns of care when they read their documentation on clients. Using the standard language of the Intervention Scheme facilitates communication of plans and interventions between the primary nurse and others who provide services to a specific client. Providers include after-hours nursing staff, weekend nursing staff, physical therapists, social workers, occupational therapists, nutritionists, and speech pathologists. Typically, the primary nurse is responsible for case management, which includes coordinating services of the agency's health care team and organizing the client record. Anticipated plans and completed interventions must be clearly and accurately recorded by the primary nurse to communicate vital information to the other team members. Likewise, documentation completed by each team member must be understandable to the entire team, especially the primary nurse. When several providers document client care, it is critical that anticipated plans and completed interventions be simultaneously concise and detailed. Attaining a sophisticated level of competence in relation to documentation requires commitment and tools like the Intervention Scheme.

Data Management Guide

Nursing supervisors, administrators, auditors, utilization review committee members, and third-party payors examine client records with increasing frequency. Although their purposes vary, they use client records as a means to track the accuracy and logic of professional practice.

Professional practice review through record audit can accomplish three equally important objectives. First, because use of the Intervention Scheme produces uniform, precise, and concise documentation, a reviewer can readily identify the worth and value of specific interventions. Disseminating such knowledge can improve client services and reduce the cost of providing those services. Second, a reviewer can recognize readily omissions or mistakes. Corrections can be accomplished through individual or individual and supervisory efforts. Improvements in documentation can result in improvement in the quality of client care. Third, individual practitioners, teams of staff, and entire agencies can receive positive reinforcement for excellence in practice. Especially in today's complex and often frustrating health care delivery arena, success needs to be celebrated.

Administrators value two types of intervention data: that which is client-specific and that which represents client aggregates. Interventions are another essential component of an automated, client-focused management information system. Aggregate data offer the administrator benefits similar to those described in relation to the Problem Classification Scheme (see Chapter 5). McCloskey (1989) noted that answers are needed to the following five cost-benefit questions:

1. What nursing diagnoses are associated with what medical diagnoses (DRGs)?
2. What nursing interventions provide the best outcomes for specific nursing diagnoses?
3. What are the costs of different nursing interventions?
4. What conditions exist wherein (a) nurses are inadequately prepared to diagnose and treat and thus, need more educational preparation or (b) nurses have an inadequate knowledge base?
5. What is the cost of achieving a specific outcome for a particular nursing diagnosis? (p. 44)

These benefits are closely related to reimbursement and costing issues. These issues and the relationships among nursing diagnoses, client outcomes, and nursing interventions are the basis for the 1989 to 1991 VNA of Omaha research project.

The value of a simple, systematic method of organizing and documenting plans and interventions has been described in relation to clients, nurses, administrators, and community health agencies. In addition, Bulechek and McCloskey (1985) have delineated more global client-nurse benefits for identifying nursing diagnoses and interventions. These benefits include the ability to (1) increase the number of problems that are identified and treated appropriately, (2) standardize nursing care, because care of today's client will benefit the client of tomorrow, (3) increase the value of nursing through increased nurse autonomy and satisfaction, and (4) develop a body of knowledge that is uniquely nursing.

SUMMARY

When using the Intervention Scheme, certain suggestions and precautions need to be considered. The following represents a summary of such advice; note that some suggestions are similar to those given for the Problem Classification Scheme in Chapter 5 and the Problem Rating Scale for Outcomes in Chapter 7.

- **Do** assume that nursing judgement will always be important in determining what, when, and how client care is provided. In a legal sense, care that is not documented has not been provided.
- **Do** approach the Scheme as a tool for practice and documentation. The need to increase practice expertise and efficiency of recording becomes more critical every year.
- **Do** use the language of the Intervention Scheme in two ways. First, use it to develop a plan defined as a set of anticipated interventions. Second, use it to document interventions that have occurred.
- **Do** document plans and interventions in three parts: category, target(s), and client-specific information.
- **Do** recognize that the time frame for the plan can vary with the client, nurse, and agency.
- **Do** recognize that it takes time and commitment to learn correct use of the Scheme.
- **Do** review the entire Scheme, definitions, and guidelines for use regularly, and discuss application with others. Everyone profits from review.
- **Do not** confuse objective and subjective data with interventions. For example, the numeric blood pressure reading is objective information, not an intervention; comparing the current and previous blood pressure readings and reporting significant differences to a physician is an intervention.
- **Do not** be repetitious or verbose. Be brief and concise. When developing plans, document type and number of categories, targets, and client-specific information that are most likely to be applicable. When recording interventions, select information that is most relevant and pertinent. The choice of categories and targets should be as specific as possible. More is still not necessarily better.

Further recommendations related to planning, instruction, and continuation for the Intervention Scheme and other components of the Omaha System are described in Chapter 8. Use of the Intervention Scheme by specific groups of staff and within various programs and recording systems are described and illustrated in Chapters 9 through 13.

REFERENCES

Aydelotte, M., & Peterson, K. (1987). Keynote address: Nursing taxonomies—state of the art. In McLane, A. (Ed.), *Classification of Nursing Diagnoses: Proceedings of the Seventh Conference* (pp. 1–16). St. Louis, C. V. Mosby.

Barnard, K. (1985, January/February). Blending the art and the science of nursing. *Matern. Child Nurs.*, 10:63.

Benner, P. (1983, Spring). Uncovering the knowledge embedded in clinical practice. *Image*, 15:36–41.

Benner, P. (1984). *From Novice to Expert*. Menlo Park, CA, Addison-Wesley.

Campbell, C. (1984). *Nursing Diagnosis and Intervention in Nursing Practice* (2nd ed.). New York, John Wiley & Sons.

Douglas, D., & Murphy, E. (1985). Nursing process, nursing diagnosis, and emerging taxonomies. In McCloskey, J., & Grace, H. (Eds.), *Current Issues in Nursing* (2nd ed.) (pp. 63–72). Boston, Blackwell.

McCloskey, J. (1989, January). Implications of costing out nursing services for reimbursement. *Nurs. Manag.*, 20:44–49.

Mussallem, H. (1985). Political issues and professional associations. In Stewart, M., Innes, J., Searl, S., et al. (Eds.), *Community Health Nursing in Canada* (pp. 49–69). Toronto, Ontario, Gage.

Scherman, S. (1982). *Community Health Nursing Care Plans*. [Mimeograph]. Hoboken, NJ, Hoboken Public Health Nursing Service.

Stevenson, J. (1990). Quantitative care research: Review of content, process, and product. In Stevenson, J., & Tripp-Reimer, T. (Eds.), *Knowledge about Care and Caring* (pp. 97–118). Kansas City, MO, American Academy of Nursing.

Taylor, D. (1989). Interventions. *Classification Systems for Describing Nursing Practice* (pp. 31–36). Kansas City, MO, American Nurses' Association.

BIBLIOGRAPHY

Arnold, J. (1988). Diagnostic reasoning protocols for clinical simulations in nursing. In Strickland, O., & Waltz, C., (Eds.), *Measurement of Nursing Outcomes, Vol. 2, Measuring Nursing Performance: Practice, Education, and Research* (pp. 53–87). New York, Springer.

Barnard, K. (1984). *Newborn Nursing Models: Final report of project supported by grant no. RO1 NU-00719*. Division of Nursing, Bureau of Health Manpower, Health Resources Administration, DHHS. Seattle, WA, University of Washington.

Benner, P., & Tanner, C. (1987, January). Clinical judgement: How expert nurses use intuition. *Am. J. Nurs.*, 87:23–31.

Benner, P., & Wrubel, J. (1989). *The Primacy of Caring*. Menlo Park, CA, Addison-Wesley.

Bennis, W., Benne, K., & Chin, P. (1969). *The Planning of Change* (2nd ed.). New York, Holt, Rinehart & Winston.

Benoliel, J., Ellison, E., Kogan, H., et al. (1985). Report of the clinical therapeutics task force. Seattle, University of Washington, School of Nursing.

Braden, C. (1984). *The Focus and Limits of Community Health Nursing*. Norwalk, CT, Appleton-Century-Crofts.

Bulechek, G., & McCloskey, J. (1985). *Nursing Interventions: Treatments for Nursing Diagnosis*. Philadelphia, W.B. Saunders.

Bulechek, G., & McCloskey, J. (1990). Nursing intervention taxonomy development. In McCloskey, J., & Grace, H. (Eds.), *Current Issues in Nursing* (3rd ed.) (pp. 23–28). St. Louis, C. V. Mosby.

Carnevali, D. (1983). *Nursing Care Planning: Diagnoses and Management* (3rd ed.). Philadelphia, J. B. Lippincott.

Carpenito, L. (1983). *Nursing Diagnosis: Application to Clinical Practice*. Philadelphia, J. B. Lippincott.

Doenges, M., Jeffries, M., & Moorhouse, M. (1989). *Nursing Care Plans: Guidelines for Planning*. Philadelphia, F. A. Davis.

Douglas, D., & Murphy, E. (1990). Nursing process, nursing diagnosis, and emerging taxonomies. In McCloskey, J., & Grace, H. (Eds.), *Current Issues in Nursing* (3rd ed.) (pp. 17–22). St. Louis, C. V. Mosby.

Elkins, C. (1984). *Community Health Nursing: Skills and Strategies.*. Bowie, MD, Brady.

Gettrust, K., Ryan, S., & Engelman, D. (Eds.) (1985). *Applied Nursing Diagnoses: Guides for Comprehensive Care Planning.* New York, John Wiley & Sons.

Grobe, S. (1989, January). *Nursing's Language: Implications for Practice and Scientific Discovery.* San Francisco, CA, Paper presented at the Seventh Annual Conference on Research in Nursing Education.

Gould, E., & Wargo, J. (1987). *Home Health Nursing Care Plans.* Rockville, MD, Aspen.

Hall, J., & Weaver, B. (1985). *Distributive Nursing Practice: A Systems Approach to Community Health* (2nd ed.). Philadelphia, J. B. Lippincott.

Henry, B., & LeClair, H. (1987, January). Language, leadership, and power. *J. Nurs. Admin.*, *17*:19–25.

Knollmueller, R. (1989, October). Case management: What's in a name? *Nurs. Manag.*, *20*:38–42.

Kuhn, T. (1970). *The Structure of Scientific Revolutions* (2nd ed., Enlarged). Chicago, University of Chicago Press.

Martin, K. (1988, June). Research in home care. *Nurs. Clin. North Am.*, *23*:373–385.

Martin, K. (1989). Omaha system. In *Classification Systems for Describing Nursing Practice* (pp. 43–47). Kansas City, MO, American Nurses' Association.

Mayers, M. (1983). *A Systematic Approach to the Nursing Care Plan* (3rd ed.). Norwalk, CT, Appleton-Century-Crofts.

Mehmert, P. (1987, December). A nursing information system: The outcome of implementing nursing diagnoses. *Nurs. Clin. North Am.*, *22*:943–953.

Melosh, B. (1982). *The Physician's Hand.* Philadelphia, Temple University Press.

Pender, N. (1982). *Health Promotion in Nursing Practice.* Norwalk, CT, Appleton-Century-Crofts.

Ryan, B. (1973, May/June). Nursing care plans: A systems approach to developing criteria for planning and evaluation. *J. Nurs. Admin.*, *3*:50–58.

Shuster, III, G., & Cloonan, P. (1989, September/October). Nursing activities and reimbursement in clinical case management. *Home Healthcare Nurse*, *7*:10–15.

Snyder, M. (1985). *Independent Nursing Interventions.* New York, John Wiley & Sons.

Stanhope, M., & Lancaster, J. (1988). *Community Health Nursing: Process and Practice for Promoting Health.* St. Louis, C. V. Mosby.

Stewart, M., Downe-Wamboldt, B., Lambie, E., et al. (1985). Educational strategies for primary health care nursing. In Stewart, M., Innes, J., Searl, S., et al. (Eds.), *Community Health Nursing in Canada* (pp. 567–578). Toronto, Ontario, Gage.

Ulrich, S., Canale, S., & Wendell, S. (1986). *Nursing Care Planning Guides.* Philadelphia, W.B. Saunders.

Weidmann, J., & North, H. (1987, December). Implementing the Omaha classification system in a public health agency. *Nurs. Clin. North Am.*, *22*:971–979.

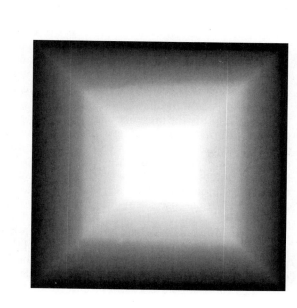

CHAPTER SEVEN

*T*he development of sound measurement practices is germane to the further development and advancement of nursing as a profession. Yet measurement, to date, has not been given the attention it warrants. Measurement per se has not been viewed as vital content in most nursing education programs, and too much of the measurement encountered in nursing practice and in the literature lacks rigor and precision. (Waltz, Strickland, & Lenz, 1984, p. v)

The Problem Rating Scale for Outcomes is designed to measure client progress in relation to specific client problems. Although the Rating Scale has been developed *by* practicing community health nurses *for* practicing community health nurses, it can serve also as a valuable tool for other health care disciplines. When used by a community health professional, the Problem Rating Scale for Outcomes provides both a guide for practice and a method of documentation.

The Problem Rating Scale for Outcomes offers a community health nurse a comprehensive, research-based evaluation method for use throughout the time of client service. Valid methods, ones that are capable of documenting the effectiveness of community health nursing service to clients, are definitely needed, especially those that demonstrate scientific rigor. Because the design of the Problem Rating Scale for Outcomes is simple, it is practical to implement and it can be completed quickly by a nurse or another health care professional. Thus, when establishing the initial ratings for client problems, a community health nurse creates an independent data baseline, capturing the condition and circumstances of the client at a given point in time. This admission baseline is used to compare and contrast the client's condition and circumstances with ratings completed at later intervals and at client dismissal.

The comparison or change in ratings over time can be used to identify the presence or absence of client progress in relation to nursing intervention. When used by a staff nurse, the comparison provides data to judge the effectiveness of the plan of care. The Problem Rating Scale for Outcomes provides a needed supervisory tool and a data set for agency management. Supervisors and administrators can use client data from individuals or aggregates to evaluate the impact of services and agency operations. The same data can be used by researchers to advance the science of nursing. Investigation of the implications of aggregate data generated from the Problem Rating Scale for Outcomes as well as the Problem Classification Scheme and Intervention Scheme is a primary objective of ongoing research at the VNA of Omaha. The relationship among the Problem Rating Scale for Outcomes, Omaha System, and family nursing process are depicted in Figure 7–1.

ORGANIZATION

The purpose of the Problem Rating Scale for Outcomes is to offer community health nurses a systematic, recurring way to measure client change. The Scale evolved through an ongoing, research-based process that is described in Chapter 4. Initial efforts to design and implement an evaluation tool were directed toward the concepts of expected outcomes and outcome criteria. The final Problem Rating Scale for Outcomes is designed for measuring change in relation to all 40 problems and three modifiers of the Problem Classification Scheme. Change can be communicated verbally among nurses and members of other disciplines or through a legal client record (Table 7–1).

The Problem Rating Scale for Outcomes has characteristics of a viable system, as described by Ryan (1973). When related to evaluation, such a system involves a dynamic, cyclic flow process and three specific elements. First, use of the Scale encourages a community health nurse or another health care professional to consider goals for client care. Second, use of the Problem Rating Scale for Outcomes helps a community health professional to consider intervention alternatives relative to a client's circumstances or need for change or adaptation. Third, feedback to a practitioner is enhanced through a method of information-gathering and regular review.

Measurement is quantified when the concepts of the Rating Scale are scored in relation to a specific client problem. Use of the Scale makes the measurement process possible by transforming abstract concepts into

Problem Rating Scale for Outcomes

those that are concrete. The three concepts of Knowledge, Behavior, and Status were selected during the third VNA of Omaha research project as representing essential client-nurse concerns. The concepts were based on (1) an exhaustive literature review, (2) discussion with people in other agencies who were interested in the concept of outcome measurement, and (3) consultation with experts in the field.

Outcome Model

A model that depicts nurse-client interactions relative to outcomes was developed in consultation with Avedis Donabedian (1985) (Figure 7–2). The model is based on the assumption that the interactions of a community health nurse and a client in relation to a problem affect what that client knows (Knowledge), does (Behavior), and is (Status). Nurse-client interactions lead to changes or various possible outcomes.

The first portion of the Outcome Model depicts the initial steps of the nursing process—those of problem identification and plan selection. As with all steps of the nursing process, positive nurse-client interaction is essential. Using the Problem Classification Scheme to identify problems or nursing diagnoses was described in Chapter 5. Quickly or simultaneously, the nurse and client initiate action. Within the framework of the Omaha System, nursing action or skilled interventions are classified as (1) Health Teaching, Guidance, and Counseling, (2) Treatments and Procedures, (3) Case Management, and (4) Surveillance. Those interventions were defined and described in Chapter 6. The three concepts of the Problem Rating Scale for Outcomes are viewed as a separate, time-related continuum. Knowledge involves what a client knows and understands about a specific health-related problem. Behavior involves what a client does—the client's practices, performances, and skills. Status involves

what a client is and how the client's conditions or circumstances improve, remain stable, or deteriorate. As depicted in the Outcome Model, the three continua run parallel before changing direction and merging at the ultimate goals of client adaptation and coping.

The potential for reaching the goals of adaptation and coping is increased by a high degree of client motivation and nurse-client collaboration. Motivation is especially important with the concepts of Knowledge and Behavior. A decrease in the degree of motivation or collaboration during the period of client service may be followed by a decrease in goal attainment. Principles of group dynamics and group effectiveness help explain health-related habits and client actions. Lewin's field theory (Deutsch & Krauss, 1965) includes concepts of group cohesiveness and group locomotion; the relationships among conformity, cohesiveness, and communication are always dynamic, never static. Events, circumstances, and people are among the dynamic forces that affect the client. It is crucial for a nurse to recognize whether forces are positive and driving or negative and restraining in order to develop appropriate intervention strategies. Confusion and even conflict may occur when a nurse does not accurately identify and respect forces, values, and goals.

Scaling Principles

The Problem Rating Scale for Outcomes is used to depict the most positive to the most negative client state in relation to a specific problem. The Scale is actually comprised of three summated or Likert-type ordinal scales: the first scale for Knowledge, the second for Behavior, and the third for Status. Whereas the three concepts of the Problem Rating Scale for Outcomes are interrelated, they represent three discrete dimensions of client outcomes. The three dimensions of the Problem Rating Scale for Outcomes are equal in

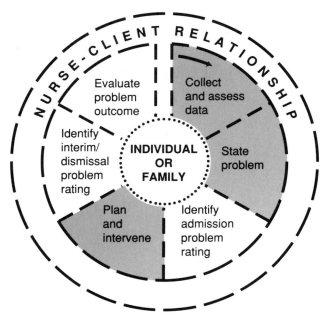

FIGURE 7–1 ■ Using the Problem Rating Scale for Outcomes enables identification of admission, interim, and dismissal problem ratings and facilitates evaluation of problem outcomes—the final step in the family nursing process.

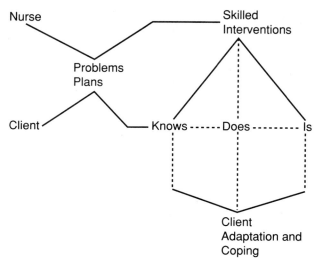

FIGURE 7–2 ■ The outcome model depicts how nurse-client interactions in relation to client problems affect client adaptation and coping.

importance, although they may not be equal when used with a specific client. For example, changes in the status rating of the child who has been abused are of extreme concern to a nurse; the nurse, however, may be much less concerned about the knowledge rating. In contrast, the knowledge rating of a client with a respiration problem may be of greater concern to a hospice nurse than the status rating.

The ratings have characteristics of ordinal scales: (1) five mutually exclusive classes or categories, (2) each continuum collectively exhaustive, and (3) categories that fit into a specific order or sequence. Based on the scaling pattern devised by Likert, the scale for each of the concepts has five categories or degrees for response. Unlike some Likert scales, the Problem Rating Scale for Outcomes does not include a formal set of questions that can be scored and summed to produce a final numeric rating. Instead, community health nurses and

other users are expected to have a knowledge base that allows them to arrive at a final score for each of the three concepts. Users are also expected to recognize that the continuum represents the universe of clients. The range within the continuum is not restricted to clients in one neighborhood or in one nurse's caseload.

Development of a community health nurse's knowledge base has already been described in relation to the Problem Classification Scheme and the Intervention Scheme in Chapters 5 and 6. Similarly, community health nurses accrue knowledge and expand their highly complex and sophisticated knowledge base related to client outcomes as they continue their nursing practice. They develop definitions of expected outcomes and unexpected outcomes in relation to individuals, families, and groups. As nurses develop clinical judgement, they increase their accuracy and speed as they distinguish between normal and abnormal trends in client changes. They become increasingly sensitive to positive or negative changes in Knowledge, Behavior, or Status, discriminating between actual differences and illusions of change. In addition, nurses use a process of constant comparison to evaluate for interre-

TABLE 7–1 ■ Problem Rating Scale for Outcomes

CONCEPT	1	2	3	4	5
Knowledge The ability of the client to remember and interpret information	No knowledge	Minimal knowledge	Basic knowledge	Adequate knowledge	Superior knowledge
Behavior The observable responses, actions, or activities of the client fitting the occasion or purpose	Never appropriate	Rarely appropriate	Inconsistently appropriate	Usually appropriate	Consistently appropriate
Status The condition of the client in relation to objective and subjective defining characteristics	Extreme signs/symptoms	Severe signs/symptoms	Moderate signs/symptoms	Minimal signs/symptoms	No signs/symptoms

lationships and collective change among the three concepts. As community health nurses move along a continuum from novice to expert, as described by Benner, they increase the ease, accuracy, and reliability with which they arrive at the final score for each of the concepts.

Formative and Summative Evaluation

The Problem Rating Scale for Outcomes provides a framework for evaluating the client's problem-specific Knowledge, Behavior, and Status at regular or predictable time intervals. "Formative evaluation" is the term used to describe the continuous, ongoing process of measuring client progress toward goals throughout the period of service. In contrast, "summative evaluation" is used to delineate the terminal process of measuring client progress toward goals completed at the end of service. Occasions suggested for using the Problem Rating Scale for Outcomes as a formative and summative measure include upon admission, at specific interim points, and on dismissal. The frequency of interim ratings should be established by agency staff and management personnel based on client needs and what is practical at a given agency. It is possible, even preferable, that different intervals be selected for dissimilar programs within a particular agency.

An example of a cycle established in certified home health agencies is the Medicare-mandated 60-day review of client records and physicians' orders. Thus, the staff and supervisors of the VNA of Omaha home health program decided that these regular intervals would be appropriate and convenient times to schedule interim review of clients' Knowledge, Behavior, and Status ratings. After expectations and responsibilities were delineated, a system was established whereby professional and clerical staff work together to complete the Medicare review and rerating process in a timely, efficient manner.

Ratings for each problem are intended to be reviewed independently, both initially and at later intervals. The initial rating for each concept can be compared and contrasted to ratings for that concept at later intervals; in addition, it can be compared to later ratings for the other two concepts. When the numeric ratings for Knowledge, Behavior, and Status are summed or averaged, they tend to lose their power of discrimination and become meaningless in many instances. This occurs as scores converge and markedly high scores are offset by markedly low scores during the averaging process. When all the client's ratings are either unusually high or low, the averaging process does not have the same detrimental effect.

Norm- and Criterion-referenced Instruments

The Problem Rating Scale for Outcomes has characteristics of both norm- and criterion-referenced instruments. The two types of instruments are briefly described in the following paragraphs.

Norm-referenced instruments are used to examine quality of performance or outcome in relation to (1) relative position held in a known group or some ideal model on the same measuring device, (2) degree of guidance needed, or (3) frequency with which the described behaviors occur (Krumme, 1975). A norm-referenced instrument should be constructed to measure a characteristic across a wide range of scores, usually spreading the subjects in a normal or bell-shaped curve (Waltz, et al., 1984). An example of a norm-referenced instrument is a rating scale with the following levels: superior, above average, average, below average, and unacceptable. Conventional grading by letters (A–F) or numbers (1–5) is a further example. Norm-referenced instruments have been widely used for many years in educational settings, where three advantages have been noted. First, valid and reliable norm-referenced instruments can be developed with relative ease. Second, users experience few difficulties implementing these instruments. Third, norm-referenced instruments can provide consistent, useful evaluation data.

In contrast to norm-referenced instruments, criterion-referenced instruments are used to examine outcomes in relation to specific behavioral criteria (Mayers, 1983). A criterion-referenced instrument should be constructed to discriminate between subjects who have and those who have not acquired specific target behaviors or skills (Waltz, et al., 1984). The outcomes are examined without reference to the performance of others. Criterion-referenced instruments are developed by stating the objectives of care in terms of client behaviors and defining the criteria of acceptable performance (Mager, 1972). Usually, the distribution of scores shows a cluster toward the high end of the scale; scores exhibit less variance than those from a norm-referenced instrument (Waltz, et al., 1984). The most significant advantage of a criterion-referenced instrument involves the control of subjectivity by clearly defining the ideal standard of achievement.

Norm- and criterion-referenced instruments have inherent disadvantages and limitations. Because a person's performance is generally judged in relation to the group, subjectivity is more likely within norm-referenced instruments. In comparison, more time and effort are required to develop valid criterion-referenced instruments because they involve specific behavior criteria. Criterion-referenced instruments also tend to be lengthy and cumbersome, characteristics that lead to rejection in a practice setting.

The Problem Rating Scale for Outcomes contains elements, and therefore advantages and disadvantages, of both a norm-referenced and a criterion-referenced instrument. As occurs with norm-referenced instruments, the nurse selects one of five categories or numeric ratings relating to the concepts of Knowledge, Behavior, and Status. Ratings are selected for only those problems that a nurse, in collaboration with a client, plans to address. The five numeric ratings form a continuum ranging from the most negative to the most positive state of the problem.

The Problem Rating Scale for Outcomes does have

characteristics of a criterion-referenced instrument. Definitions for each numeric rating provide a standard criterion against which a client's condition or circumstances can be measured, decreasing the subjectivity of the tool. Also, the tool was designed with a client as the unit of analysis, to facilitate evaluation of an individual client's performance over time, rather than in relation to other clients.

Definitions

Evaluation. Measurement of client progress by comparing client Knowledge, Behavior, and Status ratings at admission, at regular intervals, and at dismissal. The ratings reflect client change by indicating the client's response to nursing intervention and to many variables that are beyond a nurse's control (e.g., Knowledge — Client progress reflected by change from 2 to 4 during last 2 months).

Concepts. The three major areas that represent basic community health client issues of knowing, doing, and being. These areas provide a realistic and usable framework for measuring the effectiveness of care provided to a client in relation to specific problems.

Knowledge. The ability of the client to remember and interpret information.

Behavior. The observable responses, actions, or activities of the client fitting the occasion or purpose.

Status. The condition of the client in relation to objective and subjective defining characteristics.

Ratings. The five numeric levels representing continua depicting the most negative to most positive state of a problem. A verbal description defines each numeric rating.

Admission Rating for Outcomes. Problem-specific numeric ratings for the concepts of Knowledge, Behavior, and Status completed at the time of admission to community health service (e.g., Knowledge — 2 at admission).

Interim Rating for Outcomes. Problem-specific numeric ratings for the concepts of Knowledge, Behavior, and Status completed at periodic intervals during the course of community health service (e.g., Knowledge — 3 at 2 months).

Dismissal Rating for Outcomes. Problem-specific numeric ratings for the concepts of Knowledge, Behavior, and Status completed at the time of client discharge from community health service (e.g., Knowledge — 4 at dismissal).

ASSUMPTIONS

Application of the Problem Rating Scale for Outcomes is based on general assumptions. The following six assumptions are particularly important:

■ Client change is inevitable and especially desirable when it involves movement in a positive direction.

Most individual clients and families value improvements that increase their competence, enhance control over their own lives, and promote their functioning at the highest possible level.

■ Client change is influenced significantly by community health nurses and other health care providers, although cause-effect relationships can be proven on few occasions. Clients own their problems, develop unique value systems, and control some variables that affect change. In addition, some variables are beyond the control of clients, nurses, physicians, or any other health care providers.

■ Implementing measures of changes can occur in many ways, including the nurse's use of self as a change agent. Wilson (1988) has described basic criteria of successful outcome assessment by writing "(a) professionals need to understand the purpose of outcome measurement, (b) professionals need to value the purpose, [and] (c) the outcome measurement must be achievable within professional practice" (Wilson, 1988, pp. 15–16).

■ A community health nurse or another health care practitioner uses an extensive knowledge base to determine a specific numeric rating from among the available choices. The knowledge base includes information regarding client history and assessment, nursing practice, and disease pathology. It also includes the knowledge gained through the practitioner's experiences with others in similar circumstances, whether those others were family members, friends, or clients.

■ Subjectivity is involved in applying the Scale, even when the health care provider is thoughtful and follows the directions for use. "Evaluation is a process of judgment. Evolution pursues questions relative to client behavior, nursing behavior, goal adequacy, goal attainment factors, problem resolution, and overall changes" (Braden, 1984, p. 364).

■ Measurement of client outcomes is inherent in the nursing process as shown in the Conceptualization of the Family Nursing Process (Fig. 7–1). The Problem Rating Scale for Outcomes is intended for use with the Problem Classification Scheme and the Intervention Scheme.

BENEFITS

Community health nurses and other health care professionals have struggled for many years to devise methods of measuring client progress, to compare accomplishments with some acceptable standards. Client evaluation in the community health setting is elusive at best. Mortality and morbidity rates alone are not capable of providing necessary information to nursing supervisors or administrators. Community health nurses have actively searched for indices of achievement. They have pursued viable methods and criteria suitable for measuring or quantifying the impact of clinical performance on client progress and for measuring the effectiveness of interventions. Evidence of similar effort appears in Waltz and Strickland's (1988) extensive compilation of nursing practice and education-based tools. They describe measurement tools oriented toward specific disease conditions, community health issues, and clinical performance. A chapter by Feldman and Richard (1988) includes a tool based on the Problem Classification Scheme developed at the VNA of Omaha. "Once more, nurses, particularly community health nurses with their whole-population and multisystem-level orientation, are in an excellent position to contribute to the emerging knowledge associated with human services evaluation" (Braden, 1984, p. 375).

The search for evaluation measures by so many nurses has been based on the philosophy that progress of the client is a significant, or even ultimate, test of nursing care. Rising health care costs, federal legislation and regulation, and outcome effectiveness initiatives are encouraging the search. Brett (1989) noted that ". . . outcomes, experienced as a result of nursing practice, reflect one key aspect of quality nursing care" (p. 353). Because of the complexity inherent in developing adequate evaluation tools, however, the struggle to construct generally acceptable client outcome measurement tools is far from over.

The dilemmas faced by nurses were summarized by Lewis (1976) in an excellent editorial entitled, "Quantifying the Unquantifiable." Lewis described the necessity for the evaluation process to include both quantifiable, or objective, as well as qualitative, or subjective, data. According to Lewis, the good practitioner or evaluator can assess a client in a holistic manner, combining the parts into a meaningful whole, a process of almost automatic synthesis. Such expert, multidimensional, and practice-based skills, which may or may not be observable, are identical to those described by others; they represent one of the strongest values of nursing.

Some evaluation methods developed by academicians have been considered unacceptable in practice settings due to deficits that involve relevance, complexity, or length. Community health staff quickly reject tools that prove impractical, fail to show obvious benefits to a nurse and client, or take a long time to complete. Likewise, various evaluation approaches are rejected by academicians because the approaches are not based on sound measurement principles, are outside the conceptual framework of nursing, or are inadequately tested for reliability and validity. Thus, to be widely accepted, a tool must meet rigorous standards.

Practice and Documentation Guide

The Problem Rating Scale for Outcomes was developed as an integral portion of the total Omaha System. Nursing process and clinical judgement theories are the basis of the System. Community health nurses who have used the Rating Scale state that it provides a realis-

tic, focused, concrete tool for rapidly quantifying and expressing what they know about the client in relation to three essential dimensions or concepts. Likewise, nurses have determined that these concepts are clear, meaningful, and discrete. They note that application rules are explicit, yet flexible, to allow for use with widely differing client situations. Initial reliability and validity were established for the Rating Scale during the 1984 to 1986 Omaha research study; extensive additional research began in 1989.

The ratings produced by using the Scale serve three significant purposes. First, the initial ratings provide support for client admission to agency service, along with a baseline against which subsequent change can be compared and contrasted. Use of the Rating Scale in conjunction with the Problem Classification Scheme provides a concise yet comprehensive overview of the client as an individual or a family. The three concepts of Knowledge, Behavior, and Status represent areas of basic concern to community health professionals. In order for the ratings to be a true baseline measure and to reflect a client's condition prior to intervention, it is essential that they be completed within the first one or two nurse-client contacts. It is equally important that the nurse complete the ratings thoughtfully while following the established guidelines. The process of identifying problems and completing admission ratings enables a community health nurse to capture an accurate, composite picture of a client.

A second purpose is served by the Problem Rating Scale for Outcomes; the ratings are a guide for community health professionals when client care is planned and provided. Whereas the Intervention Scheme provides the structure and terminology for planning and intervening, the Problem Rating Scale for Outcomes drives the process by providing a framework that helps to focus nursing effort and selection of specific nursing interventions. Throughout the time of service, a community health nurse and a client make many complex decisions about client care. The nurse:

- Differentiates between problems of greater and lesser priority
- Judges the severity of client problems
- Assesses client perceptiveness and willingness to address specific problems
- Identifies others, such as health care and social service personnel, family members, and significant others, who can contribute to client improvement

Based on client data, the nurse applies the Problem Rating Scale for Outcomes and continues to make decisions and set priorities for nursing interventions. Use of the Problem Rating Scale for Outcomes enables the nurse to identify (1) those problems requiring immediate intervention regardless of the problem's Actual, Potential, or Health Promotion modifier, (2) those aspects of the problems needing initial attention, and (3) those interventions offering the greatest possibility of improving the client's situation. Tracking this decision-making process may be accomplished through review of documentation in the client record and discussions.

Supervisors and staff nurses have described the value of discussing ratings, especially for families with many severe problems. Documentation and discussion enhance accountability regarding nursing decisions.

A third purpose is served by implementing the Problem Rating Scale for Outcomes throughout the period of agency service. The Scale incorporates both continuous or formative and terminal or summative evaluation methods of measuring client progress.

As the nurse completes interim and dismissal ratings for client problems, the ratings develop two meanings. First, the changes in ratings for one concept of a given problem are significant and are an important method for examining client outcomes. Second, ratings are also significant when compared and contrasted to ratings for (1) other concepts of the same problem and (2) the same concepts of other problems.

Nurses must learn to celebrate large and small successes with clients rather than emphasize relapses or failures (Levine, 1989). When improvement occurs, the client, nurse, and agency should share a sense of success and pride. The Problem Rating Scale for Outcomes serves as a tool for identifying specific areas and amounts of change. The nurse and supervisor should use the Scale as one method to examine why positive change occurs.

1. Did both the client and the nurse identify similar problems?
2. Was the client highly motivated?
3. Were the client's and the nurse's goals and expectations similar?
4. Were the benefits of change greater than the barriers?
5. Were the nurse's selection and timing of specific interventions critical to success?

Client change in a negative direction is also a reality of community health nursing practice. The staff nurse and supervisor should examine why such negative change occurs.

1. Did the client and nurse identify dissimilar problems and/or goals?
2. Did the client lack motivation?
3. Were barriers to change greater than benefits?
4. Did the nurse consider why families fail to understand, accept, or act upon health problems?

Data Management Guide

The amount and direction of changes in the ratings as well as the rating patterns are beneficial to staff, supervisors, and administrators. These data provide practitioners with a basis for judging the success or effectiveness of nursing interventions and for making needed modifications in the care plan during the ensuing period of service. In addition, examination of rating changes assists the practitioner, supervisor, and administrator to make decisions about appropriate frequency of client visits and the continuation of service. Agency administrators can examine aggregate rating data produced by an automated management information system. Both professional practice and internal agency management are improved when the staff consider reasonable alternatives and make sound decisions regularly. Likewise, agencies reap benefits involving energy, time, and money when they can quantify and demonstrate the impact of services to third party payors. Examining rating changes and modifying client services increase the potential for improving the quality of client care, client-nurse success, and agency viability.

Through use of the three concepts, each rated on a five-point scale, client progress is measured and becomes tangible. Progress can be articulated and communicated to other nurses, administrators, auditors, and reimbursement sources. As measures of client outcome or progress, the three concepts of Knowledge, Behavior, and Status represent understandable concepts. Outcome measures must be commonly understood and valued to be meaningful to the public (Barnard, 1984). When the Problem Rating Scale for Outcomes is used in a client record system, a nurse can document the benefits of care. With an automated management information system, the Rating Scale offers an important evaluation data element for aggregates. These evaluation data are a source of meaningful information beyond the traditional measures of number and length of visits. In addition, Problem Rating Scale for Outcomes data can establish initial rationale for developing a much needed, logical community health reimbursement system.

SUMMARY

When using the Problem Rating Scale for Outcomes, certain suggestions and precautions need to be considered. The following statements represent a summary of such advice; note that suggestions and precautions are similar to those given for the Problem Classification and Intervention Schemes.

■ **Do** assume that nursing judgement will always be important. Although the Scale serves as a tool for measuring client progress, a high level of skill is required for deciding which problems to rate, selecting the ratings, interpreting, and explaining change in the client record. There are no "right" ratings.

■ **Do** approach the Scale as a tool for practice and documentation. The need to increase practice expertise and efficiency of recording becomes more critical every year.

■ **Do** recognize that it takes time and commitment to learn effective and efficient use of the Scale. Although the Scale will always contain a degree of subjectivity, conscientious use increases reliability. Because nursing is both an art and a science, client evaluation will never be a totally objective process, regardless of the sophistication of the evaluation method.

- **Do** review the entire Scale, definitions, and guidelines for use regularly. Discuss application with others. Everyone profits from occasional review.
- **Do** select ratings thoughtfully while considering the universe of individuals who have a specific problem. Remember all your previous contacts with persons who had a given Health Promotion, Potential, or Actual problem. Include all (1) current community health clients, (2) previous community health clients, (3) clients from previous work/school settings, and (4) other relatives, friends, and neighbors.
- **Do** select one numeric rating for Knowledge, for Behavior, and for Status in relation to a specific problem. The ratings for each concept may or may not be identical.
- **Do** rate Knowledge, Behavior, and Status for all priority problems. For example, do not ignore the concept Knowledge when the care is provided to an infant, child, or dependent adult. Rate the knowledge of the caregiver.
- **Do** recognize that evaluation will not occur unless the nurse or other health care professional uses and documents evaluation methods.
- **Do not** develop ratings and plans for all problems identified on the problem list. Rank problems into those to be addressed now and those to be addressed later; develop ratings and plans for the former. No problem ranked Actual should automatically be considered a priority; some problems ranked Potential and Health Promotion should be considered priorities. More is still not necessarily better.
- **Do not** base ratings on desired or predicted change. Base the rating on existing client Knowledge, Behavior, and Status.
- **Do not** view the ratings as a report card for community health nursing. If nurses experience pressure from others to document specific changes in the ratings, the ratings will not be accurate or reflect reality. No nurse can control all variables that affect client change.
- **Do not** select a range or a fraction of a rating. Limit selection to the five numeric choices.

Further recommendations related to planning, instruction, and continuation for the Problem Rating Scale for Outcomes and other components of the Omaha System are described in Chapter 8. Use of the Problem Rating Scale for Outcomes by specific types of staff and within various programs and recording systems are described in Chapters 9 through 13.

REFERENCES

Barnard, K. (1984, March/April). Commonly understood outcomes. *Matern. Child Nurs.*, 9:99.

Braden, C. (1984). *The Focus and Limits of Community Health Nursing*. Norwalk, CT, Appleton-Century-Crofts.

Brett, J. (1989). Outcome indicators of quality care. In Henry, B., Arndt, C., DiVincenti, M., et al. (Eds.), *Dimensions of Nursing Administration: Theory, Research, Education, and Practice* (pp. 353–369). Boston, Blackwell.

Deutsch, M., & Krauss, R. (1965). *Theories in Social Psychology*. New York, Basic Books.

Donabedian, A. (1985, April 30). [Consultation regarding Outcome model.] Ann Arbor, MI.

Feldman, J., & Richard, R. (1988). The measurement of nursing outcomes for home health care. In Waltz, C., & Strickland, O. (Eds.), *Measurement of Nursing Outcomes, Vol. 1, Measuring Client Outcomes* (pp. 475–495). New York, Springer.

Krumme, U. (1975, December). The case for criterion-referenced measurement. *Nurs. Outlook*, 23:764–770.

Levine, M. (1989, Spring). The ethics of nursing rhetoric. *Image*, 21:4–6.

Lewis, E. (1976, March). Quantifying the unquantifiable. *Nurs. Outlook*, 24:147.

Mager, R. (1972). *Goal Analysis*. Belmont, CA, Fearon.

Mayers, M. (1983). *A Systematic Approach to the Nursing Care Plan* (3rd ed.). Norwalk, CT, Appleton-Century-Crofts.

Ryan, B. (1973, May/June). Nursing care plans: A systems approach to developing criteria for planning and evaluation. *J. Nurs. Admin.*, 3:50–58.

Waltz, C., Strickland, O., & Lenz, E. (1984). *Measurement in Nursing Research*. Philadelphia, F. A. Davis.

Waltz, C., & Strickland, O. (Eds.) (1988). *Measurement of Nursing Outcomes, Vol. 1, Measuring Client Outcomes*. New York, Springer.

Wilson, A. (1988, November/December). Measurable patient outcomes: Putting theory into practice. *Home Healthcare Nurse*, 6:15–18.

BIBLIOGRAPHY

Benner, P. (1983, Spring). Uncovering the knowledge embedded in clinical practice. *Image*, 15:36–41.

Benner, P., & Wrubel, J. (1989). *The Primacy of Caring*. Menlo Park, CA, Addison-Wesley.

Bower, F. (1974, August). Normative—or criterion-referenced evaluation? *Nurs. Outlook*, 22:499–502.

Decker, F., Stevens, L., Vancini, M., et al. (1979, April). Using patient outcomes to evaluate community health nursing. *Nurs. Outlook*, 27:278–282.

Donabedian, A. (1984, May/June). Quality, cost, and cost containment. *Nurs. Outlook*, 32:142–145.

Elkins, C. (1984). *Community Health Nursing: Skills and Strategies*. Bowie, MD, Brady.

Elwood, P. (1988, June 9). Outcomes management: A technology of patient experience. *New Engl. J. Med.*, 318:1549–1556.

Freeman, R. (1961, October). Measuring the effectiveness of public health nursing service. *Nurs. Outlook*, 9:605–607.

Freeman, R., & Heinrich, J. (1981). *Community Health Nursing Practice* (2nd ed.). Philadelphia, W.B. Saunders.

Henry, B., & LeClair, H. (1987, January). Language, leadership, and power. *J. Nurs. Admin.*, 17:19–25.

Kritek, P. (1979). Commentary: The development of nursing diagnosis and theory. *Adv. Nurs. Sci.*, 2:73–79.

Lohn, K. (Ed.) (1990). *Medicare: A Strategy for Quality Assurance*, Vol. I. Washington, DC, National Academy Press.

Marek, K. (1989). Classification of outcome measures in nursing care. In *Classification Systems for Describing Nursing Practice* (pp. 37–42). Kansas City, MO, American Nurses' Association.

Martin, K. (1988, June). Research in home care. *Nurs. Clin. North Am.*, 23:373–385.

Martin, K. (1989). Omaha system. In *Classification Systems for Describing Nursing Practice* (pp. 43–47). Kansas City, MO, American Nurses' Association.

McCloskey, J. (1989, January). Implications of costing out nursing services for reimbursement. *Nurs. Manag.*, 20:44–49.

Meisenheimer, C. (1989). *Quality Assurance for Home Health Care*. Rockville, MD, Aspen.

Oda, D. (1989, March/April). Home visits: Effective or obsolete nursing practice? *Nurs. Res.*, 38:121–123.

Oda, D., & Boyd, P. (1988, December). The outcome of public health nursing service in a preventive child health program: Phase 1, health assessment. *Public Health Nurs.*, 5:209–213.

Olds, D., Henderson, Jr., C., Tatelbaum, R., et al. (1986a, June). Improving the delivery of prenatal care and outcomes of pregnancy: A randomized trial of nurse home visitation. *Pediatrics*, 77: 16–28.

Olds, D., Henderson, Jr., C., Chamberlin, R., et al. (1986b, July). Preventing child abuse and neglect: A randomized trial of nurse home visitation. *Pediatrics*, 78:65–78.

Olds, D., Henderson, Jr., C., Tatelbaum, R., et al. (1988, November). Improving the life-course development of socially disadvantaged mothers: A randomized trial of home nurse visitation. *Am. J. Public Health*, 78:1436–1445.

Peters, D. (1988, July/August). Development of a community health intensity rating scale. *Nurs. Res.*, 37:202–207.

Rinke, L. (Ed.) (1987). *Outcome Measures in Home Care: Vol. I, Research.* New York, National League for Nursing.

Rinke, L., & Wilson, A. (Eds.) (1987). *Outcome Measures in Home Care: Vol. II, Service.* New York, National League for Nursing.

Rooks, J., Weatherby, N., Ernst, E., et al. (1989, December 28). Outcomes of care in birth centers. *New Engl. J. Med.*, *321*:1804–1811.

Selltiz, C., Wrightsman, L., & Cook, S. (1973). *Research Methods in Social Relations* (3rd ed.). New York, Holt, Rinehart & Winston.

Sienkiewicz, J. (1984, November/December). Patient classification in community health nursing. *Nurs. Outlook*, *32*:319–321.

Starfield, B. (1974, Winter). Measurement of outcome: A proposed scheme. *Milbank Memorial Fund Q.*, *52*:39–50.

Stewart, M., Downe-Wamboldt, B., Lambie, E., et al. (1985). Educational strategies for primary health care nursing. In Stewart, M., Innes, J., Searl, S., et al. (Eds.), *Community Health Nursing in Canada* (pp. 567–578). Toronto, Ontario, Gage.

Strickland, O., & Waltz, C. (Eds.) (1988). *Measurement of Nursing Outcomes, Vol. 2, Measuring Nursing Performance: Practice, Education, and Research.* New York, Springer.

Tanner, C. (1988). Curriculum revolution: The practice mandate. In *Curriculum Revolution: Mandate for Change* (pp. 201–216). New York, National League for Nursing.

Treece, E., & Treece, Jr., J. (1986). *Elements of Research in Nursing* (4th ed.). St. Louis, C. V. Mosby.

Werley, H., & Lang, N. (Eds.) (1988). *Identification of the Nursing Minimum Data Set.* New York, Springer.

Wold, S. (Ed.) (1990). *Community Health Nursing: Issues and Topics.* Norwalk, CT, Appleton & Lange.

Woolley, A. (1977, May). The long and tortured history of clinical evaluation. *Nurs. Outlook*, *25*:308–315.

Zimmer, M. (1974, June). Quality assurance for outcomes of patient care. *Nurs. Clin. North Am.*, *9*:305–315.

Zimmer, M. (1976). *Manual: Nursing Quality Assurance.* [Mimeograph]. Madison, WI, University of Wisconsin Hospitals.

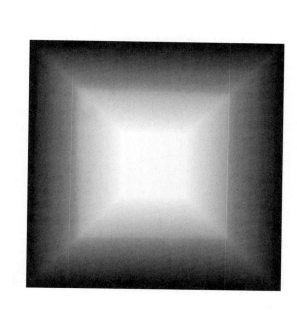

CHAPTER EIGHT

*C*hanges that are conscious, deliberate, and intended—at least on the part of one or more agents of change—are planned changes. One of the advantages of planned change is the use of valid knowledge and information as a basis for plans and programs of change. The planned change process involves a change agent, a client system, and the collaborative attempt to apply valid knowledge to clients' problems. Benne, Chin, and Bennis (1976) acknowledge that the outcome of any planned change attempt depends to a great extent on the relationship between the change agent and the client system (Simms, Price, & Ervin, 1985, p. 87).

Implementation of the Omaha System should occur in a systematic manner. Whether implementation is being considered in community health agencies, other community-based settings, or educational institutions, the first step of the implementation process must be investigation. All benefits and possible consequences need to be considered; likewise, any disadvantages or potential problems should be identified (Hays, 1990; Jorgensen & Young, 1989; Martin & Scheet, 1988; Schmele, 1986; Weidmann & North, 1987). After making a decision to implement, the steps of planning, instruction, and continuation need to be completed to ensure success. The requirements for each step are described below.

Planning. Requires the active participation of agency staff and management prior to and during implementation of the clinical components.

Instruction. Requires discussion of philosophy and objectives as well as details and application.

Continuation. Requires that personnel monitor agency activities to ensure that the clinical components are being used as intended.

The three steps of the implementation process must be tailored to fit specific user needs. These needs vary depending on type of setting, target populations, programs, personnel, resources, and constraints. Consideration should be given to the number of people involved and the amount of time devoted to each of the three steps.

PLANNING

The ease with which the clinical components can be introduced within an agency or educational setting is directly related to the planning process. Incorporated into the process should be (1) the determination to help personnel feel good about change and (2) knowledge about the dynamics of change and resistance. Change is typically described as a three-phase process of unfreezing, changing, and refreezing (Lewin, 1951). The aim of unfreezing is to prepare the participant to change. Once a person is motivated to change, that person is ready to accept new patterns of behavior. Refreezing is defined as the integration of the newly patterned behavior into the person's personality and emotional relationships. It is inevitable that agency personnel will resist changing their usual client record and adopting the Omaha System. Resistance, frustration, and other negative emotions can be decreased if personnel actively participate in an organized planning process and become committed to the effort.

The planning process is described in relation to implementation in a middle- to large-size community health agency. Adaptations in the process are necessary for implementation in very small agencies and in other service or educational settings, particularly in relation to the number of people involved in the planning, instruction, and continuation processes.

Steering Committee

A nurse coordinator should be designated to be responsible for the steering committee and total implementation plan. The coordinator directs the instruction process; if possible, the coordinator should serve as one of the principal instructors. Commitment of agency staff, management, and resources should be evident through the support given to the coordinator dur-

The Process
of Implementation

ing the planning and implementation process. The creativity, determination, patience, and understanding of the nurse coordinator are tested repeatedly throughout the processes. Qualifications of the coordinator should be carefully considered. Especially important are:

- Leadership skills with individuals and groups
- Sensitivity to the needs of adult learners
- Familiarity with community health practice and agency procedures
- Understanding of the nursing process
- Proficiency in use of the recording system of the agency
- Working knowledge of problem-oriented recording
- Creativity
- Determination
- A sense of humor

An agency steering committee should be formed as early as possible and should continue to function throughout the entire implementation process. Ideally, four to six agency representatives work with the nurse coordinator. They serve as a core group capable of informing other staff, generating commitment and acceptance, and bringing staff concerns or suggestions back to the committee for action. Included should be:

- Administrative and management staff
- Nursing supervisors
- Nursing staff
- Clerical staff
- Physical, speech, and occupational therapists
- Medical social workers
- Other agency disciplines

Developing a realistic schedule for instruction and implementation is essential early in the planning process. The steering committee must decide whether nursing, other professional, and clerical staff will receive separate or combined instruction and materials. Projected effectiveness and cost of each alternative are important considerations.

Many agency personnel do not view participation in efforts to modify the record system as an opportunity. Most community health nurses and members of other disciplines were not attracted to their professions because of documentation issues. Few describe completing the client record as either exciting or rewarding. If given a choice, many staff would eliminate client records from their job responsibilities. Often, it is advantageous to include staff members with neutral or even negative attitudes on the agency steering committee and in the pilot test group. If these individuals develop positive attitudes, they may become the strongest advocates of the Omaha System.

Implementation Questions

The steering committee needs to address specific questions about use of the Problem Classification Scheme, the Intervention Scheme, and the Problem Rating Scale for Outcomes in the agency. Committee decisions about the clinical components must be communicated to staff as part of the instruction process. Some of these questions are listed below:

1. Which clinical components of the Omaha System will be implemented?
2. Which disciplines will use the clinical components?
3. What will the implementation schedule be? Who will decide?

4. What procedures will be followed to phase in the new clinical record system?
5. Which staff will be involved in a pilot test prior to full implementation?
6. Do the current clinical record forms need to be revised? By whom?
7. Will agency rules governing recording need to be changed?
8. Will the new records be used on all clients or only on certain categories of clients?
9. How will data about multiple family members be managed?
10. Will both family and individual problems be recorded?
11. Will actual, potential, and health promotion problems be recorded?
12. Will all problems be noted on the problem list or only those for which plans are developed?
13. How will additions, resolutions, or other changes in the problem list be recorded?
14. Where will medical diagnoses be recorded?
15. Will pre-established time frames for outcome ratings be used?
16. What will be the content and format of the progress notes?
17. How will client-specific information be handled in relation to the Intervention Scheme?
18. How will staff document the evaluation of client care, explaining client ratings over time?
19. What methods will be used to obtain feedback from staff regarding successes and problems with the new record system?
20. What methods will be used to maintain staff support?
21. How will documentation and data management problems be controlled or resolved?
22. How will the cost-effectiveness of having a manual, word-processed, computerized, or combined client documentation system be evaluated?
23. How will information about each of the clinical components be transmitted from the record to the computer if agency personnel decide to automate?
24. How can aggregate client data be integrated cost-effectively with personnel and financial data as a part of a management information system?

Record Revision

Steering committee members need to think creatively about all aspects of the client record at the time questions are being addressed. Narratives, case examples, and forms included in Chapters 9 through 13 illustrate use of the Problem Classification Scheme, the Problem Rating Scale for Outcomes, and the Intervention Scheme in client records. An agency steering committee may consider adapting some of these materials without revision; others require tailoring to an agency's programs and staff needs.

Steering committee members should consider more efficient alternatives to the client record content, organization, and forms. Committee members need to consider data entry and record management options. Sovie (1989) stated a strong case for nurses to lead a "revolutionary transformation" in documentation systems. The statement, "more is not necessarily better," should guide steering committee members' decisions.

The Omaha System was developed to incorporate the philosophy of problem-oriented records. Thus, the Omaha System is easily adapted to various types of problem-oriented records. It is possible, although difficult, to implement the Omaha System with a narrative record. The following list includes suggested sections or pages of an agency record congruent with the Omaha System. The information found in the first six sections is basic to all records, but agency staff may organize that information in various ways. For example, agency staff may elect to develop one form that incorporates the problem list, problem ratings, and plans.

- Referral form — the client's presenting health problems and initial plan of treatment identified during the intake process
- Client data/face sheet — demographic and financial information
- Data base — detailed environmental, psychosocial, physiologic, health-related behavior, and health history information
- Problem list — a summary of individual, family, health promotion, potential, and actual problems
- Problem Rating Scale for Outcomes/Plans form — Knowledge, Behavior, and Status ratings as well as a brief plan for priority problems
- Visit reports/Progress notes — description of services provided and client responses from various disciplines

Agency staff, programs, and services must be considered when selecting additional forms for inclusion in the client record. The following is a list of eight possible forms. As with the first six sections, the information incorporated in these forms may be organized in various ways.

- Immunization record — list of inoculations received by a child
- Developmental screening forms — results of tests such as the Denver Developmental Screening Test, Washington Guide, and growth grid
- Physician's Orders — medical plan of care prescribed by a physician; may be synonymous with Health Care Financing Administration (HCFA) 485.
- Medication sheets — description of drugs taken by the client
- Consent, Patient Rights, and Service Agreement forms — diverse documents signed by the client as a method of authorization
- Other referral information — information forwarded by individuals, agencies, or institutions where the client received care previously
- Home Health Aide (HHA) service forms — notes completed by HHAs as they provide services
- Reports to others — descriptions of client services

distributed to other agencies as HCFA 486, discharge summaries, and reports to referral sources

Record forms that involve application of the Problem Classification Scheme, the Problem Rating Scale for Outcomes, and the Intervention Scheme require particular attention during the planning phase. Steering committee members should review all forms carefully to achieve unity and efficiency. Duplicating information on one or several forms not only wastes valuable professional time but also decreases secretarial productivity and consumes unnecessary supplies. Furthermore, redundancy hinders tracking of client needs, care provided, and client responses.

The data base and the problem list need to be congruent with the Problem Classification Scheme. The data base must be defined and structured to facilitate comprehensive data collection (see Chapter 5). It is essential to include both objective and subjective data on the data base. The format and content of the problem list need to flow from the data base, providing a link to the next component, the Problem Rating Scale for Outcomes.

Information appearing on the Problem Rating Scale for Outcomes/Plans form should be congruent with the data base and problem list. A community health nurse uses professional judgment to decide which problems are priorities and should, therefore, appear on this form (see Chapter 7). Recurring use of the Scale allows a nurse to evaluate the effects of planned, individual care and to revise interventions accordingly. Client data in the entire record needs periodic updating, but the Problem Rating Scale for Outcomes/Plans form must be adaptable to regular revision whenever new ratings and modified plans are completed. Ideally, re-evaluation and revision of ratings and plans could occur in conjunction with every visit. However, few if any agencies have adequate professional and support personnel or sufficiently sophisticated systems to require manual or automated revision that frequently.

Visit reports or progress notes are the final portion of the client record; these are especially relevant to the Omaha System. The Intervention Scheme should be used to document client care congruent with the problems and plans that were documented in earlier sections of the record (see Chapter 6). A logical flow of client information throughout the record provides individual community health nurses, members of other disciplines, or supervisors with important data and with a tool to make several complex decisions. These decisions involve individual clients, aggregates of clients, agency programs, and reimbursement issues.

Pilot Testing

A pilot test is the final task to be completed prior to the instruction phase. All proposed record revisions need to be tested by a sample of staff members who regularly document their services in the clinical record. Concurrently, any agency documentation protocols that require revision need to be discussed and written. Such protocols address client admission, the period of service, and dismissal.

Pilot testing serves three major purposes. First, staff frustration and agency expense can be decreased by identification and resolution of problems before the record system is completed and implemented. Second, the staff members who participate in the pilot test have a tendency to become positive ambassadors; they become committed to the record system and transmit their enthusiasm to other staff. Third, the coordinator and steering committee can develop and explain the total agency implementation plan, knowing that it is based on valuable information obtained during the pilot test.

INSTRUCTION

A formal instruction process should be designed to introduce the nursing, supervisory, and ancillary personnel to the Omaha System. To ensure success, the needs of adult learners and the principles of planned change must be recognized. Adults must be ready and willing to learn. Adult learners are motivated more by their own internal incentives than by external incentives. They tend to be self-directed learners. Adults expect relevant, well organized sessions. An instructor increases the participants' motivation by adopting the style of a facilitator or a role model rather than a lecturer, acknowledging that the instructional process provides an opportunity for the instructor to learn, too. Furthermore, an instructor who demonstrates enthusiasm, competence, and experience regarding documentation will gain the participants' confidence and increase their desire to learn.

A major focus of the instruction process involves new, special-purpose vocabulary. The enthusiasm of participants decreases if unfamiliar and pretentious terms are used by a nurse coordinator. Enthusiasm increases as interesting, practical examples and humor are introduced into the sessions (Matthis, 1974). The instructor's goal is to make learning the new words and their meanings easy and complete.

Orientation programs and internships are mechanisms for secondary socialization. Through these mechanisms, new information is internalized through new language, we learn a second language by building on our "mother tongue." Exposed for the first time to unfamiliar language, we consciously translate and integrate new words into our existing vocabulary to give the unaccustomed words meaning. As socialization proceeds, we increasingly forego translation and think in our newly acquired language. (Henry & LeClair, 1987, p. 21)

Participants need to practice applying the Omaha System to their agency's record system. Personnel should have ample time to relate the Omaha System to their own experiences and ask questions. Learning is enhanced when:

■ The group does not exceed 100 people; ideal group size is 20 to 30

- The instructor to participant ratio approximates 1 to 15
- Room arrangements and conditions are satisfactory
- Handouts are relevant
- Audiovisual materials are appropriate
- Client examples reflect familiar practice situations
- Those in attendance participate actively
- The instructor is well informed about the Omaha System
- The instructor is enthusiastic about the Omaha System and its documentation

The time required for the complete instruction process varies among agencies. For example, staff who are accustomed to a problem-oriented record system may learn to use the clinical components after one meeting; others with less experience may require several hours of instruction and discussion during a 1- or 2-week period. The availability of the coordinator or instructor to answer questions throughout the instruction phase and to monitor use of the Omaha System in agency records expedites learning and successful implementation.

Training materials include:

1. The Problem Classification Scheme, the Problem Rating Scale for Outcomes, and the Intervention Scheme (see Chapters 5, 6, and 7)
2. A glossary of terms (see Glossary)
3. A videotape of an admission visit and/or client records that include a data base
4. Blank record forms or overhead transparencies (see Appendix)
5. An entire sample client record (see Chapters 9, 10, and 11)

Initially, the instructor should discuss the objectives, the course plan, and the schedule by distributing a handout or using an overhead projector. At the conclusion of the instruction process, the participant will be able to:

1. Delineate the fundamental concepts within the nursing process
2. Describe the major components of the Omaha System: Problem Classification Scheme, Problem Rating Scale for Outcomes, and Intervention Scheme
3. Relate advantages and disadvantages of using the problem-oriented record and the schemes in manual or computerized systems
4. Practice using the Omaha System with client data
5. Identify steps necessary to implement the schemes in multiple settings

The following contains a description of the six course content areas. Approximation of the time needed for instruction is:

Nursing Process	30 minutes
Advantages and Disadvantages	15 minutes
Agency Record	30 minutes
Clinical Components of the Omaha System	2 hours
Group Discussion	15 minutes
Small Group Work	4 hours

Nursing Process

The instructor should define the nursing process as a rational, dynamic, problem-solving process by which a community health nurse or other professional implements systematic, individual, and comprehensive care. Such care is designed to assist the client to attain the highest possible level of functioning. The concepts of the nursing process are usually described as assessment, problem identification or diagnosis, planning, intervention, and evaluation (see Chapter 3). The recording system of the agency should be reviewed and related to the concepts of the nursing process. The benefits of using client examples and personal experiences as part of the record instruction process were described previously.

Advantages and Disadvantages

The instructor should briefly describe the advantages and disadvantages of the clinical components in relation to the nursing process and the agency's recording system.

Advantages are:

- Client information can be classified as significant or extraneous because the Problem Classification Scheme facilitates sorting and evaluating data related to problems.
- Planning and intervening are more precise because of the specificity of the problem labels, modifiers, and signs/symptoms.
- Use of the Intervention Scheme clarifies documentation of significant activities and allows the professional to complete the process more quickly.
- The Problem Rating Scale helps the professional to identify a client's admission status and potential interventions. The professional can use the interim and dismissal ratings to track client progress.
- Users can see their accomplishments more readily.
- Communication among agency staff is facilitated because all staff are using a standard system for recording.

Disadvantages are:

- Staff require time to become proficient in use of the Omaha System. The time, of course, varies with the experience and attitude of the staff.
- Staff who are accustomed to a medical-based model may have difficulty initially as they adapt to the nursing focus of the Omaha System.

Agency Record

The instructor should discuss the agency's client record, describing that record from (1) a historic perspective, (2) the current system, and (3) the future or anticipated goals. The time required for discussion of the record relates directly to the number and scope of planned revisions. Several areas for special emphasis during this portion of the instruction process include:

- Newly revised portions of the record
- The record as the sum of its parts
- Agency policies and expectations of staff
- Use of the record as a tool for client care

Discussion of the record will be organized in relation to the problem-solving process and use of the clinical components. As the first step in using the Omaha System, collection of pertinent data needs to be described thoroughly (see Chapter 5). Data base modifications may be few because any systematic method of organizing and recording data is adaptable for the data base used in conjunction with the Problem Classification Scheme. Similarly, the method of developing a problem list from the data base may change very little. The second step in implementing the Omaha System involves the Problem Rating Scale for Outcomes (see Chapter 7). If measurement of client progress is a new concept to participants, the Rating Scale requires careful attention, especially in relation to the Scale's value. The third step in implementing the Omaha System relates to the Intervention Scheme (see Chapter 6). The forms that will be used by agency participants can be reviewed while the instructor identifies similarities and differences to the previous methods of recording plans and interventions.

Clinical Components

The instructor should review and discuss the clinical components thoroughly (see Chapters 5, 6, and 7). Four assumptions are prerequisite to this discussion:

1. Community health staff have the skills necessary to identify client problems, use nursing interventions, and measure client progress.
2. Community health staff and clients must work together to identify mutual concerns, enabling staff members to use and record clinical components accurately and realistically.
3. Most individual clients and families are interested in increasing their competence, enhancing control over their own lives, and promoting their functioning at the highest possible level.
4. The health/illness status of a client is influenced by complex forces, often outside the control of community health staff.

The clinical components, the group discussion, and the small group work may be organized in either of two ways. One clinical component can be described, discussed by the total group, and practiced in small groups; the schedule would be repeated for the other two clinical components. An alternative is to describe two or three of the clinical components, then follow with discussion and practice. The former method may foster a more positive learning environment because it

alternates participant activities and physical movement and may be less overwhelming.

Group Discussion

The instructor needs to help the entire group consider the Omaha System in relation to actual or fictitious client data. Group discussion is enhanced if the instructor selects client data that are typical for an agency admission but are relatively simple and brief. Using data base materials and the four domains of the Problem Classification Scheme, the instructor can assist the participants to identify client problems, modifiers, and signs/symptoms. After consensus is reached on identification of problems, the participants should identify a priority problem. For that problem, participants should apply the Problem Rating Scale for Outcomes and select appropriate Knowledge, Behavior, and Status admission ratings. Finally, the participants should consider the categories and targets of the Intervention Scheme and list reasonable choices for initial planning and intervening activities.

Small Group Work

The purpose of small group work is to practice applying the Omaha System. Through practice, participants learn to identify client problems, admission ratings, and nursing interventions. A second example of client data can be introduced through role play, a videotape, use of overhead transparencies, or a handout. Although role play requires live actors, it offers an opportunity to create a bond between participants and instructors. Role play and videos also offer the opportunity to introduce humor into the instruction process, an important benefit.

One instructor can work satisfactorily with 20 to 30 participants. If the audience is larger, the participants should be divided into groups of 5 to 10 persons, separating the groups throughout the room. Personnel who attend an instruction session may differ in regard to professional disciplines, work responsibilities, and knowledge of the Omaha System. When participants are diverse, it is advantageous to ensure that each subgroup is as heterogeneous as possible. In this way, participants are exposed to experiences, opinions, and skills similar to their own as well as to those that differ markedly. Such exposure tends to hasten learning.

Practice is organized around the three segments that conform to the clinical components of the Omaha System. The first segment includes developing a data base and problem list using the Problem Classification Scheme. The second segment involves selecting ratings using the Problem Rating Scale for Outcomes. The third segment consists of identifying proposed and completed plans using the Intervention Scheme. Learning is enhanced if the complexity of the task is not overwhelming. It is important to control the amount of data to be considered and the length of time provided for each segment. For example, instructors may choose to limit problem identification to one domain and focus establishment of ratings and interventions on a selected problem or problems. Further, instructors should be available to clarify instructions and answer questions during small group work. Group decisions made during each segment should be recorded. Blank overhead transparencies may be used if an overhead projector is available.

Practice tasks should include:

1. Review the visit information provided through role play, videotape, transparency, and/or handout. Use the four domains and 40 problems of the Problem Classification Scheme as a data collection guide to develop the client data base. Establish the initial problem list. Referral, historic, and visit data are used to identify family and individual actual, potential, or health promotion problems. One or more signs/symptoms will accompany each actual problem. While risk factors and client interest are used to identify potential and health promotion problems, respectively, these data do not have to be recorded on the problem list.
2. Identify an admission Knowledge, Behavior, and Status rating for priority problems using the Problem Rating Scale for Outcomes.
3. Develop plans for priority problems using the Intervention Scheme. Record the interventions of initial and subsequent visits using the Intervention Scheme.

The benefits of practicing and discussing the Omaha System informally within a small group of peers should not be underestimated. Too often during formal, large group instruction, participants believe and indicate that they are grasping the details of the Omaha System. When they begin a small group practice session, they recognize that they do have questions and are able to share opinions within the group. If participants become actively involved in group discussion, they are likely to be more confident when they leave. They also become more confident as they use the Omaha System and instruct others.

Practice in applying the Omaha System will increase a user's accuracy. During the small group work, participants employ complex reasoning and clinical judgment skills to apply the Omaha System to hypothetical client data. Participants need to be told that no answer is "right" or "wrong." They must understand, however, that there are degrees of accuracy. Lunney (1990) defines accuracy as a "continuous variable and as such contrasts with the prevailing view of accuracy that diagnoses are either accurate or inaccurate" (p. 12). This definition of accuracy is made concrete by assigning numeric values to accuracy criteria (Table 8–1).

Small group sessions and later discussions serve to identify participants whose answers fall within an acceptable range of accuracy as well as those whose answers do not. If discussions are handled in a caring,

TABLE 8–1 ■ Ordinal Scale for Degrees of Accuracy

VALUE	CRITERIA
+5	Diagnosis is consistent with all of the cues, supported by highly relevant cues, and precise.
+4	Diagnosis is consistent with most or all of the cues and supported by relevant cues but fails to reflect one or a few highly relevant cues.
+3	Diagnosis is consistent with many of the cues but fails to reflect the specificity of available cues.
+2	Diagnosis is indicated by some of the cues but there are insufficient cues relevant to the diagnosis and/or the diagnosis is a lower priority than other diagnoses.
+1	Diagnosis is only suggested by one or a few cues.
0	Diagnosis is not indicated by any of the cues. No diagnosis is stated when there are sufficient cues to state a diagnosis. The diagnosis cannot be rated.
−1	Diagnosis is indicated by more than one cue but should be rejected based on the presence of at least two disconfirming cues.

From Lunney, M. (1990, January–March). Accuracy of nursing diagnoses: Concept development. *Nuras. Diagnosis, 1:*16.

courteous manner by the instructor, all participants gain insight into the process of using the Omaha System. Time should be allowed for participants to reconvene after small group sessions are completed. Representatives from some or all of the small groups are requested to describe their experiences and conclusions. Members of other small groups can ask questions or describe differing opinions. Participants are encouraged to develop and support their own opinions within the large group, just as they are expected to contribute to decision-making discussions that occur during the small group sessions. Often, different groups reach similar conclusions. The similarity validates the usefulness of the Omaha System and reinforces the accuracy and concreteness of the decision-making process in clinical practice.

Group work is focused initially on use of the Omaha System for admission documentation only. Therefore, participants need additional documentation instruction and sample materials about the procedures used to update and close a client record. Instruction must be tailored to meet the participants' and agency's needs. For example, additional instruction can be (1) part of the initial formal session, (2) a second formal session, or (3) incorporated into the continuation process.

All participants are not documentation experts at the conclusion of instruction, regardless of the skill of a nurse coordinator or the completeness of an orientation plan. It is important for the steering committee members and the nurse coordinator to maintain (1) realistic expectations of the learners, (2) a sense of humor, and (3) commitment to the followup process. The instruction process will be most successful when those involved:

■ Recognize that absolute answers are not congruent with the Omaha System. Answers must be considered in relation to a participant's judgment and rationale.

- Do not try to accomplish everything during formal instruction; sessions that are too long or too intense overwhelm participants.
- Expect that most staff will have a good documentation foundation at the conclusion of formal instruction; as participants apply their skills, they will increase those skills quickly.
- Recognize that some participants will profit more from the discussion with peers than from the instructor's presentation.
- Accept that at least one participant may try to understand the Omaha System during formal instruction but will not be successful then — or later.
- Accept that at least one participant may not try to understand the Omaha System during the instruction process — or ever.

CONTINUATION

Planning and instruction are important for successful implementation of the Omaha System. The work of the nurse coordinator and steering committee does not end when instruction is completed. Their interest and involvement must continue during the continuation phase. Successful implementation of the Omaha System requires consistent, planned followup with staff. The goal of the coordinator and steering committee is not just to educate other staff and management personnel to document correctly, applying the Omaha System in an automatic manner. The ultimate goals are socialization and attainment of higher cognitive levels in order for users to understand and integrate the System into their methods of practice. If personnel develop extensive understanding and mastery, they become committed to the Omaha System, internalize the concepts, and sustain their improved clinical practice and documentation skills. For example, monitoring is an essential component of followup in all agencies. However, the amount of effort and energy required to ensure that the clinical components are being used accurately, consistently, effectively, and in accordance with agency expectations varies between individuals and among agencies.

The nurse coordinator and steering committee should discuss different approaches to maintaining appropriate use of the Omaha System before instruction is completed. To enhance continuity, personnel previously involved in instruction should be included in the continuation process. The group can consider reasonable alternatives, selecting those that are the most practical and efficient. Some approaches, such as record orientation, may already be part of agency operations; little modification would then be needed. Approaches include but are not limited to:

- A documentation manual
- Orientation of new staff
- Supervisory record review

- Peer record review
- Utilization review
- Record audit
- Refresher and formal sessions
- Informal discussions

Of these eight approaches, four are described in Chapter 14. These are (1) supervisory record review, (2) peer record review, (3) utilization review, and (4) record audit. The remaining four approaches are discussed in the following paragraphs.

Documentation Manual

A reference manual that includes definitions of terms, instructions, and blank client record forms should be available in the agency office. In addition, some agencies include completed sample forms. The manual needs to be updated on a regular basis to ensure that it includes current materials.

Orientation of New Staff

A systematic orientation to the Omaha System and the agency's client record is essential for newly employed community health nurses and members of other disciplines. Orientation should be the ongoing responsibility of the nurse coordinator or another enthusiastic staffer. Such an orientation helps the staff (1) understand community health practice, (2) improve decision-making skills, (3) view the client record more positively, (4) increase documentation accuracy, and (5) decrease the time supervisors must devote to correcting errors.

Orientation to the Omaha System and the client record can be structured like the instruction section of this chapter. In addition, new employees should receive handouts, such as those developed during implementation. The potential for success increases when the nurse coordinator, supervisor, and peers incorporate the Omaha System into various orientation activities rather than a single session or approach. A comprehensive plan for new staff orientation includes:

1. Conduct several shared visits with experienced peers followed by record review and discussion
2. Present formal session
   a. History of agency record, agency philosophy, and nursing process — 30 minutes
   b. Introduction of the Problem Classification Scheme, Problem Rating Scale for Outcomes, and Intervention Scheme — 1 hour
   c. Review of the Omaha System in relation to a sample record — 30 minutes
   d. Practice in relation to another sample record — 3 hours
3. Complete and document a visit to a client open to service

4. Hold informal staff-supervisor discussion about the visit and documentation of that visit
5. Conduct several more visits, followed by a review and discussion of documentation
6. Complete and document a visit to a new client
7. Hold informal staff-supervisor discussion about the visit and documentation of that visit
8. Perform ongoing review of documentation as needed.

Refresher and Formal Sessions

Periodic documentation discussions should be scheduled for groups of staff and supervisors. The impetus may be (1) addition of a form to the client record, (2) revision of a form, (3) deletion of a form, and (4) completion of a record audit as well as supervisory, peer, and utilization review. The latter discussion is frequently scheduled when problems arise that involve many staff. It is equally important to schedule discussions when a record review has been completed and the results are positive and complimentary.

Informal Discussions

The nurse coordinator, steering committee members, supervisors, and staff should all feel a sense of re-

sponsibility concerning a client record. Such a feeling can promote spontaneous discussions and valuable sharing between individuals. If the discussion originates with someone asking a question, that person tends to benefit from the discussion. In addition, people who provide an answer tend to benefit as they consider their answer and other alternatives.

EXPERIENCES WITH IMPLEMENTATION

The systematic continuation activities that have been described, as well as the planning and instruction guidelines, increase the probability of successfully implementing the Omaha System. There are instances, however, when the guidelines are followed but implementation is not considered successful. The following description involving Florida community health nurses is such an example. What makes this narrative unique and rewarding is the perseverance exhibited by the authors. Rather than deciding to abandon their implementation plans, they applied a problem-solving approach and identified alternative strategies. Once these strategies were introduced in Florida agencies, successful implementation of the Omaha System occurred.

IMPLEMENTING THE OMAHA SYSTEM IN FLORIDA

by MARY JANE RUNNING, BSN, MPH, CNAA, Senior Executive Community Health Nursing Director, State Health Office, Florida Department of Health and Rehabilitative Services, Tallahassee, FL; and MARILYN MAUD, BSN, MHEd, Community Health Nursing Consultant, State Health Office, Florida Department of Health and Rehabilitative Services, Tallahassee, FL

Public health services in Florida are provided through contracts with the State Health Office, Florida Department of Health and Rehabilitative Service (HRS) and the 67 counties. The HRS county public health units are organizationally responsible to 11 district administrators, with technical assistance and monitoring provided by the districts and the state staff. Nursing services are provided in schools, homes, and other community locations, but clinics are the primary service setting.

Use of problem-oriented records in documentation of the provision of indigent medical care in the health units was mandated in 1987. The HRS Quality Assurance Unit was given primary responsibility to implement this mandate in conjunction with ongoing activities to standardize records and record management.

The Omaha System was introduced through statewide workshops beginning in November, 1985, but there had not been a method to encourage and support the staff in efforts to implement it. Adoption of the System was disappointing,

indicating that if lasting change was to occur, a closer relationship was needed between those who understood the System and those who were learning. Consequently, the decision was made to concentrate on four pilot counties, involving staff from those counties in developing training materials. District staff who were familiar with the Omaha System would serve as resources to gradually expand implementation through the entire state.

Planning

Planning for the pilot project began in April, 1988. A nurse was designated as the leader responsible for coordinating the project. She was knowledgeable about community health nursing practice and documentation, especially within the Florida system. Four units in different districts were selected, based on criteria that included commitments by the district nursing consultant and the administration of the local county public health unit. Representatives from the district and state units met to plan the training components and process. Nutrition consultants prepared a list of nutritional problems identified in clients seen at the health units. This list was compared to the Problem Classification Scheme. It was decided that nutritional concerns were encompassed by the latter, thus taking the first step toward interdisciplinary use of the Omaha System.

An interdisciplinary team from the state health office was established to provide all training. The team was composed of nurses, a physician, and a nutritionist. All physicians, nurses, advanced registered nurse practitioners, physician assistants, nutritionists, and social workers who wrote in the client clinical record were required to attend the training session. Training sessions were organized to include formal presentation, discussion, and small group work. Members of each discipline would comprise the small groups.

Implementation

Training was offered during the first quarter of 1989 in the Pasco, Citrus, Walton, and Martin health units. Followup visits were made at regular intervals by the project nurse who was usually accompanied by the district nursing or nutrition consultant. The purpose of the visits was to ensure use of the Omaha System, identify problem areas, and offer assistance in resolving concerns. The project nurse made a "crisis visit" to one county to address concerns regarding use of time and effort and duplication of recording.

An evaluation tool was developed for use in reviewing records during the followup visits. The tool enabled the team to measure progress. Nursing supervisors reviewed records and provided support and encouragement to the staff during the implementation process. All members of the interdisciplinary training team returned to the county health units 6 months after the training to evaluate progress.

Findings

Some of the nurses had a difficult time using the term "problem" when clients entered the health unit for preventive measures or health maintenance. For them a problem had been associated with an impairment or deficit. The nurses were encouraged to focus on client needs and reasons for coming to the health unit, which included well child, family planning, or prenatal care. In this way, the nurses were able to use the Problem Classification Scheme to document a wellness focus.

The staff expressed concern that the Problem Classification Scheme was too long for successful use during a busy clinic day. They found completion of documentation following the clinic session too time-consuming. They were advised to use a modified problem list that narrowed the focus for clients with specific health services. In one county, this list was laminated and a copy posted in each clinic area within the health unit. The list was refined after the training project was completed; it was referred to as Common Client Problems (Table 8–2).

There were concerns in one county that the physicians recognized only a medical diagnosis as a problem. The physician on the training team was very supportive of the interdisciplinary focus and assisted in working through this difficulty. Initially, some duplication in the progress notes by physicians, nurses, and nutritionists was identified. The proj-

TABLE 8–2 ■ Florida Department of Health and Rehabilitative Services, Common Client Problems

The following list contains client problems which could be commonly identified when health services are offered to clients. Each problem could be designed as health promotion, prevention or actual impairment. Additional problems contained in the Classification of Client Problems could also be identified. Problems from the physiologic domain may be addressed by identified medical diagnoses.

SEXUALLY TRANSMITTED DISEASE
Human sexuality:
Family planning:
Prescribed medication regimen:

TUBERCULOSIS
Communication with community
    resources:
Vision:
Nutrition:
Substance misuse:
Medical supervision:
Prescribed medication regimen:

FAMILY PLANNING
Human sexuality:
Family planning:
Prescribed medication regimen:

PRENATAL
Role change:
Caretaking/parenting:
Antepartum/postpartum:
Nutrition/WIC:
Substance misuse:
Medical supervision:
Low income: no medical insurance

CHILD HEALTH
Residence:
Neglected child:
Abused child:
Growth and development:
Hearing:
Vision:
Dentition:
Nutrition/WIC:
Sleep and rest patterns:
Physical activity:
Personal hygiene:
Substance misuse:
Medical/dental supervision:
Medication regimen:

ADULT HEALTH
Income:
Residence:
Dentition:
Nutrition:
Substance misuse/abuse:
Medical/dental supervision:
Medication regimen:
Abuse/neglect:

ect staff helped each member to focus on writing only new information regarding an identified problem.

Some staff, particularly the nurses and advanced registered nurse practitioners, tried to identify all client problems and record in the "SOAP" format (Subjective, Objective, Assessment, Plan) for each problem. This resulted in lengthy, time-consuming, duplicative progress notes. Project staff helped them to more selectively identify problems and record notes in a more concise fashion. For example, it was possible to address more than one problem in a single SOAP note when interventions were the same. The staff were also encouraged to use flow sheets when appropriate.

Examination of records at the conclusion of the pilot project revealed that client problems and problem-specific progress were clearly identified. We found better communication and coordination between providers and improved documentation of nursing practice. District and state personnel will monitor progress and provide assistance to ensure continuing success.

The authors wish to acknowledge the other members of the Florida Department of Health and Rehabilitative Services multidisciplinary team: Terrance Broadway, BSN, MSN, Community Health Nursing Consultant; James Conn, MD, Assistant Health Officer for Family Health Services; and Jane Van Wart, RD, MS, Public Health Nursing Consultant.

AUTOMATION

The Omaha System was designed as (1) an integrated practice and documentation system and (2) a method of organizing and entering client data into a manual or computerized management information system in small or large community health agencies. An organized, comprehensive approach is essential to implement a partially or completely automated management information system that incorporates the Omaha System. Many aspects of an organized approach are similar to the planning, implementing, and continuation processes described earlier in this chapter in relation to the clinical components and the client record. A comprehensive discussion of the steps necessary to revise or implement a management information system is beyond the scope of this book but is available in other references. A multiple-step implementation plan will be briefly described. Such a plan was developed in conjunction with the VNA of Omaha system design that was described in Chapter 2. Suggested steps of the automation plan included:

1. Organize a project team that includes nurses.
2. Analyze current agency information processing methods and identify needs.
3. Determine if the system will be manual, automated, or a combination of manual and automated.
4. If automated, investigate vendors and select software and hardware.
5. If manual, modify the system and develop appropriate forms.
6. Test the system and modify as necessary.
7. Conduct training.
8. Implement use of the system.
9. Evaluate system functioning and project team performance (Martin, Scheet, Crews, et al., 1986).

Although an automated information system has the potential to provide uniform and comprehensive service and financial data, it requires a major commitment of agency personnel and funds. If an agency does not already employ someone with extensive computer experience, it is wise to locate and retain a consultant to assist agency personnel as they make long-term decisions about expensive equipment. It is preferable, even essential, that the consultant be knowledgeable about community health agency information needs to ensure success of the entire system.

Information specific to hardware and software is available from various sources. Vendor advertisements in journals, vendor displays at conventions, and contact with other community health nursing agency administrators who purchased hardware and software are sources of information. Books and articles are other sources of information. Software vendors offer three basic types of systems:

- Service bureaus process agency data on their own computers. The data is compiled by the agency and sent by mail or transmitted via a terminal located at the agency. The service bureau is the most common type of automation currently used by community health agencies. It is relatively inexpensive because there are no hardware costs.
- Timesharing arrangements provide a linkage via a modem and telephone line to the vendor's host computer. Some hardware costs may be involved but the agency gains some flexibility and is able to process data more rapidly.
- Inhouse systems are available for microcomputers and smallframe or minicomputers. The agency can purchase software, contract with a vendor to develop software, or develop its own system. Inhouse systems offer the most flexibility but are more expensive because the agency must lease or purchase hardware and hire programming and operating staff (Martin, et al., 1986, p. 40).

The systematic and comprehensive methods of instruction used with implementation of the Omaha System are applicable to a management information system. A project team, especially the nurse members, must be involved with instruction; they must participate in writing a user manual. Such involvement ensures that the instruction process meets the needs of nurses and other service delivery staff. Furthermore, interdisciplinary collaboration ensures that the user manual is (1) complete, (2) practical, and (3) written in language understandable to the average user.

The most effective training method for direct users of a computer system is a workshop that combines theory and practice. Training materials should include the purpose of the software and hardware, significance to the user, and detailed operation procedures for pertinent software. Although some explanation of the technology may be useful, users are more interested in learning how the software operates. The training should provide the user with complete instructions in all functions performed by the system or software package and should include adequate practice in operating the computer.

The staff of various agencies have followed these automation guidelines and suggestions. Some have partially automated the Omaha System whereas others have completely automated it; some have had very successful experiences and others have been less successful. In the following excerpt, Rita Zielstorff describes a successful implementation.

USING THE OMAHA CLASSIFICATION SCHEME IN AN INTERDISCIPLINARY AUTOMATED RECORD SYSTEM*

by RITA ZIELSTORFF, RN, MS, Assistant Director, Laboratory of Computer Science, Massachusetts General Hospital, Boston, Massachusetts

In 1984, the staff of the Massachusetts General Hospital (MGH) founded the MGH Coordinated Care Program to meet the long-term care needs of the elderly. (The program is described in more detail in Chapter 12.) For this discussion, it is important to know that Coordinated Care Teams consisting of a nurse, a social worker, and a geriatric consultant monitored and coordinated the long-term care of selected elderly patients after hospital discharge. In addition, most patients were linked to one of three MGH health centers where physicians, nurse practitioners, and nutritionists provided primary care. All of these providers used a common automated record system for this project. Patients also received a variety of home care services from other agencies, all of which was coordinated by the Coordinated Care Teams.

A previously existing automated ambulatory record system called COSTAR (COmputer-STored Ambulatory Record) was enhanced and adapted for the special needs of this project (Zielstorff, et al., 1985; Zielstorff, et al., 1986a; Zielstorff, Jette, & Barnett, 1990). Because COSTAR is a directory-based system, it was necessary to have a coded vocabulary of problems, assessments, and interventions. COSTAR had a rich lexicon of medical diagnosis, laboratory tests, procedures, and medications, but the nurses and social workers found this to be inadequate for recording their observations and interventions. We adopted the Omaha Problem Classification Scheme, making some adjustments for (1) the structure of the automated system and (2) the specialized nature of the high-risk elders and the services that were being provided. In all, we added eight problem terms to the vocabulary, most of which were added within the first year of the project (see Chapter 12).

All team members used structured assessment forms pertinent to their discipline to establish the initial patient data base (Zielstorff, Jette, Gillick, et al., 1986b; Zielstorff, et al., 1990). Medical diagnoses were described using COSTAR's lexicon of medical terms; the Omaha Problem Classification Scheme was used to describe problems in the Environmental, Psychosocial, and Health Related Behaviors Domains. Physiologic problem terms from the Scheme were also used,

but since they were often duplicates of medical diagnoses, they were used less frequently in this project. Data recorded on the forms were entered into the automated record system by a data entry clerk. Progress notes reflecting each provider's encounter with the patient were produced by the system. In addition to producing visit-specific progress notes, the system integrated data from all disciplines to produce a Coordinated Care Plan organized according to Problems, Assessments, and Management.

After the initial data base was established, providers used the Coordinated Care Plan to record their encounters with the patients, updating information as needed. The Coordinated Care Plan reflected the most recent note about each problem, regardless of the discipline of the provider who created the note. An important feature of the system was that once a problem was defined with a specific term such as "Sleep and Rest Patterns: Impairment," all providers of all disciplines used that term to record their observations about that problem. These notes were also entered into the automated system by a data entry clerk, with the system producing the individual progress note as well as an updated Coordinated Care Plan. The system could be called upon at any time to produce a listing of all progress notes written for any problem, regardless of the provider who entered the note.

The Omaha Problem Classification Scheme proved to be invaluable for this research project. The availability of a valid, reliable vocabulary for recording nonmedical patient problems greatly facilitated the timely implementation of the automated record system. The structure of the Problem Classification Scheme was highly amenable to computerization. The three-tier nature of the Scheme with domains, problems, and signs/symptoms was compatible with the structure of the COSTAR directory. The actual and potential problem modifiers were handled as a COSTAR "status." The terms from the Environmental, Health Related Behaviors, and Psychosocial Domains were particularly useful to us. They added a dimension to the data base that might otherwise have only been incorporated as textual data recorded under medical diagnoses. Textual data is not nearly so amenable to analysis, quantification, and research. Thus, the Omaha Scheme enabled us to capture in structured format the full range of problems of frail elder patients in the community. This valuable data base is being used to answer many questions about the needs of the rapidly growing elderly population and the services that are required to meet their needs.

*The MGH Coordinated Care Program was supported by Grant #9991, Robert Wood Johnson Program for Hospital Initiatives in Long-Term Care.

The implementation and evaluation of the enhanced COSTAR system was supported by Grant 1 R18 HSO5261, National Center for Health Services Research, OASH.

SUMMARY

Thoughtful, realistic planning precedes successful implementation of a management information system or tools such as the Problem Classification Scheme, the

Intervention Scheme, and the Problem Rating Scale for Outcomes. Suggestions that apply to professional community health practice, the client record, and management information systems were included in Chapters 2 and 8. Details related to implementation in specific settings and community health programs are described in Chapters 9 through 13.

A step-wise implementation process needs to precede actual use of the Omaha System clinical components by community health staff professionals, student nurses, or educators. The planning, instruction, and followup processes should be adapted to be congruent with the skills of the specific learner. The processes must be flexible to allow for those who assimilate the information and skills quickly and those who have difficulties. Some people develop keen problem-solving skills before they begin their nursing careers. Although these staff members will require little guidance as they are introduced to the Omaha System, they should receive positive reinforcement for their proficiency and sustained, effective use. Other staff, regardless of age, educational background, or work experience, are slower to develop these skills.

A similar approach is required when agency personnel are introduced to a new management information system. Successful implementation is directly related to the commitment of agency leaders, the comprehensiveness of the implementation plan, and the quality of ongoing monitoring.

REFERENCES

Hays, B. (1990). *Relationships Among Nursing Care Requirements, Selected Patient Factors, Selected Nurse Factors, and Nursing Resource Consumption in Home Health Care.* Unpublished doctoral dissertation, Cleveland, OH, Case Western Reserve University.

Henry, B., & LeClair, H. (1987, January). Language, leadership, and power. *J. Nurs. Admin., 17*:19–25.

Jorgensen, C., & Young, B. (1989, May/June). The supervisory shared home visit tool. *Home Healthcare Nurse, 7*:33–36.

Lewin, K. (1951). *Field Theory in Social Science: Selected Theoretical Papers.* New York, Harper & Brothers.

Lunney, M. (1990, January-March). Accuracy of nursing diagnoses: Concept development. *Nurs. Diagnosis, 1*:12–17.

Martin, K., & Scheet, N. (1988, May/June). The Omaha system: Providing a framework for assuring quality of home care. *Home Healthcare Nurse, 6*:24–28.

Martin, K., Scheet, N., Crews, C., et al. (1986). *Client Management Information System for Community Health Nursing Agencies: An Implementation Manual.* Rockville, MD, Division of Nursing, US DHHS, PHS, HRSA.

Matthis, E. (1974). The problem-oriented system in public health nursing. In *The Problem-oriented System—A Multi-disciplinary Approach* (pp. 48–54). New York, National League for Nursing.

Schmele, J. (1986, July/August). Teaching nurses how to improve their documentation. *Home Healthcare Nurse, 4*:6–10.

Simms, L., Price, S., & Ervin, N. (1985). *The Professional Practice of Nursing Administration.* New York, John Wiley & Sons.

Sovie, M. (1989, March/April). Clinical nursing practices and patient outcomes: Evaluation, evolution, and revolution. *Nurs. Economics, 7*:79–85.

Weidmann, J., & North, H. (1987, December). Implementing the Omaha classification system in a public health agency. *Nurs. Clin. North Am., 22*:971–979.

Zielstorff, R., Barnett, G., Jette, A., et al. (1986a). A COSTAR-based multidisciplinary record system for long-term care practice and research. In Salamon, R., Blum, B., & Jorgensen, M. (Eds.), *Medinfo '86* (pp. 844–848). North Holland, Elsevier.

Zielstorff, R., Jette, A., & Barnett, G. (1990, December). Issues in designing an automated record system for clinical care and research. *Adv. Nurs. Sci., 13*:75–88.

Zielstorff, R., Jette, A., Barnett, G., et al. (1985). A COSTAR system for hospital-based coordination of long-term care for the elderly. In Ackerman, M. (Ed.), *Proceeding, Ninth Annual Symposium on Computer Applications in Medical Care* (pp. 17–21). New York, IEEE Press.

Zielstorff, R., Jette, A., Gillick, M., et al. (1986b). Functional assessment in an automated medical record system for coordination of long-term care. *Geriatr. Rehabil., 1*:43–57.

BIBLIOGRAPHY

Bennis, W., Benne, K., & Chin, P. (1969). *The Planning of Change* (2nd ed.). New York, Holt, Rinehart & Winston.

Birdsall, C., & Valoon, P. (1986). Management information systems. In Schweiger, J. (Ed.), *Handbook for First-line Nurse Managers* (pp. 343–375). New York, John Wiley & Sons.

Braden, C. (1984). *The Focus and Limits of Community Health Nursing.* Norwalk, CT, Appleton-Century-Crofts.

Brill, J. (1990, May). Handle medical records with care. *Am. Nurse, 47*:51.

Budd-Hoffman, C. (1989). The clinical nurse specialist: A catalyst in the nursing diagnosis evolution. In *Classification Systems for Describing Nursing Practice* (pp. 62–69). Kansas City, MO, American Nurses' Association.

Carroll-Johnson, R. (Ed.) (1989). *Classification of Nursing Diagnoses: Proceedings of the Eighth National Conference.* St. Louis, C. V. Mosby.

Caserta, J. (1987, September/October). People, not paper. *Home Healthcare Nurse, 2*:15–22.

Echols, J. (1984, April). The teacher-facilitator role of clinical nursing leaders. *Top. Clin. Nurs., 6*:28–40.

Elkins, C. (1984). *Community Health Nursing.* Bowie, MD, Brady.

Firlit, S. (1990). Nursing theory and nursing practice: Do they connect? In McCloskey, J., & Grace, H. (Eds.), *Current Issues in Nursing* (3rd ed.) (pp. 4–11). St. Louis, C. V. Mosby.

Freeman, R., & Heinrich, J. (1981). *Community Health Nursing Practice* (2nd ed.). Philadelphia, W. B. Saunders.

Gardner, M. (1917). *Public Health Nursing.* New York, Macmillan.

Hannah, K., Gullemin, E., & Conklin, D. (Eds.) (1985). *Nursing Uses of Computers and Information Science.* New York, North-Holland.

Harris, M. (1988). *Home Health Administration.* Owings Mills, MD, Rynd Communications.

Hendrickson, G., & Kovner, C. (1990, January/February). Effects of computers on nursing resource use: Do computers save nurses' time? *Comput. Nurs., 8*:16–22.

Hersey, P., & Blanchard, K. (1988). *Management of Organizational Behavior.* Englewood Cliffs, NJ, Prentice Hall.

Kanter, R. (1983). *The Change Masters.* New York, Simon & Schuster.

Knowles, M. (1975). *Self-directed Learning: A Guide for Learners and Teachers.* Chicago, Follett.

Lash, A. (1981). Nursing diagnosis: Some comments on the gap between theory and practice. In McCloskey, J., & Grace, H. (Eds.), *Current Issues in Nursing* (pp. 44–50). Boston, MA, Blackwell.

MacAvoy, S. (1989). Continuing education in nursing diagnosis: Issues, strategies, and trends. In Carroll-Johnson, R. (Ed.), *Classification of Nursing Diagnoses: Proceedings of the Eighth National Conference* (pp. 67–72). St. Louis, C. V. Mosby.

Mayers, M. (1983). *A Systematic Approach to the Nursing Care Plan* (3rd ed.). Norwalk, CT, Appleton-Century-Crofts.

Mehmert, P. (1987, December). A nursing information system: The outcome of implementing nursing diagnoses. *Nurs. Clin. North Am., 22*:943–953.

Meisenheimer, C. (1985). *Quality Assurance: A Complete Guide to Effective Programs.* Rockville, MD, Aspen.

Miller, S. (1986). *Documentation for Home Health Care: A Record Management Handbook.* Chicago, Foundation of Record Education of the American Medical Record Association.

Morrissey-Ross, M. (1988, June). Documentation: If you haven't written it, you haven't done it. *Nurs. Clin. North Am., 23*:363–371.

Mundt, M. (1988, May). An analysis of nurse recording in family health clinics of a county health department. *J. Community Health Nurs.*, 5:3–10.

National League for Nursing (1988). *Administrator's Handbook for Community Health and Home Care Services.* New York.

Pulliam, L., & Boettcher, E. (1989, November/December). A process for introducing computerized information systems into long-term care facilities. *Comput. Nurs.*, 7:251–257.

Saba, V., & McCormick, K. (1986). *Essentials of Computers for Nurses.* Philadelphia, J. B. Lippincott.

Secretary's Commission on Nursing (1988a, December). *Secretary's Commission on Nursing: Final Report*, Vol. I. Washington, DC, DHHS.

Secretary's Commission on Nursing (1988b, December). *Secretary's Commission on Nursing: Support Studies & Background Information*, Vol. II. Washington, DC, DHHS.

Simmons, D., & Hailey, R. (1988). Management information sys-tems. In Benefield, L. (Ed.), *Home Health Care Management* (pp. 39–51). Englewood Cliffs, NJ, Prentice Hall.

Stanhope, M., & Lancaster, J. (1988). *Community Health Nursing: Process and Practice for Promoting Health.* St. Louis, C. V. Mosby.

Wold, S. (Ed.) (1990). *Community Health Nursing: Issues and Topics.* Norwalk, CT, Appleton & Lange.

Zielstorff, R. (1988). Considerations in data capture, storage, and re-trieval for the nursing minimum data set. In Werley, H., Lang, N. (Eds.), *Identification of the Nursing Minimum Data Set* (pp. 67–76). New York, Springer.

Zielstorff, R., Abraham, I., Werley, H., et al. (1989, September/October). Guidelines for reporting innovations in computer-based information systems for nursing. *Comput. Nurs.*, 7:203–208.

Zielstorff, R., McHugh, M., & Clinton, J. (1988). *Computer Design Criteria for Systems That Support the Nursing Process.* Kansas City, MO, American Nurses' Association.

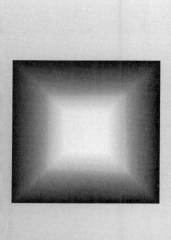

SECTION III

USING THE OMAHA SYSTEM

CHAPTER NINE

*T*he experience of the Waukesha County Health Department as the system continues to evolve has been a very positive one. The advantages previously listed have been realized since its [Problem Classification Scheme] introduction in 1983. The time saved by using a system with preselected labels has been worth the effort of implementation. The open-ended feature allows flexibility when necessary, the labels are comprehensive enough to be practicable, and the specificity of the signs and symptoms and criteria measures provide direction for planning care and closure with the client. (Weidmann & North, 1987, pp. 975, 978)

Public health and home health nursing programs deliver a preponderance of organized health care outside the hospital and nursing home. These programs employ the majority of contemporary community health nurses. When considered together, public health and home health care are the essence of community health nursing. Nearly 40,000 public health nurses and 54,000 home health nurses were employed in 1988, according to a national sample survey (Moses, 1990).

Community health nurses are concerned about the health of individuals, families, groups, and communities. The practice setting of home health and public health nurses is frequently the home, but public health nurses are found also in schools, clinics, ambulatory care centers, and businesses. According to Williams (1977, 1988), the specialty of community health nursing is linked to fundamental concepts and approaches, although functional inconsistencies and controversy about the specialty persist. "There is more to community health nursing than family-oriented care delivered outside the institutional setting; it's a matter of focus on group health problems, present and projected, in contrast to individual, clinically oriented care" (1977, p. 250). Population-based practice provides accessible, available, accountable, acceptable, comprehensive, coordinated, and cost-effective health services (Dreher, 1984). Therefore, factors central to community health practice are (1) a systems approach, incorporating individuals, families, groups, and the community, (2) concern for the health status of multiple, overlapping aggregates, (3) attention to the physical, social, political, and economic environment, and (4) use of preventive strategies.

PUBLIC HEALTH MILESTONES

Early US community health nursing services were provided by the staff of voluntary agencies; the staff were usually referred to as visiting nurses. Lillian Wald established standards for the practice and administration of public health nursing—a phrase she coined during her 40 years at the Henry Street Settlement. Her term appears to parallel Florence Nightingale's definition of health nursing as emphasizing prevention. Wald established procedures for assigning one nurse to one family. She wanted families to have direct access to nurses and nurses to families, a degree of freedom beyond that which was present in hospitals. She frequently described the importance of the professional nurse-client relationship. Nursing practice at Henry Street represented a major advance in nursing autonomy. Sound nursing judgment was essential as staff offered comprehensive preventive, curative, and social services. Families were referred to physicians, when appropriate, and staff accepted referrals from physicians. Services were available to all, regardless of ability to pay.

The Sheppard-Towner Act was a milestone for public health nursing practice, representing the beginning of tax support for client services. Between 1921 and 1929, this legislation provided massive federal aid to mothers and children. Prepared community health nurses were sent to local communities to establish maternity and infant programs. They made home visits, referred clients to physicians, and conducted classes for area nurses, midwives, and physicians.

The Social Security Act of 1935 was another significant legislative milestone; it was passed in direct response to the economic instability of the era. When the Act was amended in 1939 and 1945, the scope was ex-

Use in Public Health Settings

panded to provide financial assistance to vulnerable populations such as the unemployed, blind, elderly, and dependent and/or handicapped children. The Act also included funds for Public Health Service research and training activities and for local and state public health services. Under the direction of Pearl McIver, general public health nursing services were developed along with special programs for tuberculosis, maternal and child welfare, school children, industrial workers, insurance recipients, and home-bound sick. The number of public health agencies increased markedly during this era, but the number and complexity of practice and reimbursement issues also increased. (For a more complete discussion of the history of public health nursing, refer to Chapter 1.)

PUBLIC HEALTH ISSUES

Lillian Wald, Margaret Sanger, and other leaders struggled successfully to establish the practice of public health nursing at the beginning of the century. They championed a sound, preventive orientation for nursing services, a struggle that contemporary and future community health professionals must continue. The success nurses achieved in 1910 as they demonstrated the value of public health nursing practice is not sufficient to ensure success in the 1990s and beyond. Society changes constantly, as does health care, often in inequitable and unpredictable ways. Although some of the crises that staff and supervisory nurses face now are different from those of the past, the struggles are equally intense and the implications for public health and the nursing profession remain critical. Many skills and attributes are required of public health nurses who

wish to earn community trust and achieve success in the twenty-first century. Like the qualities demonstrated by former leaders, public health nurses of the future must exhibit political savvy and skillful leadership.

Some nursing leaders equate the present and future status of public health nursing with crisis. "The public health specialty has been declining insidiously since the late '60s and actively deteriorating for over a decade. Three factors that may have contributed to the present situation are fragmentation of services, problems in educational preparation, and role confusion of the public health nurse" (Chavigny & Kroske, 1983, p. 312). Public health practitioners and administrators must confront current problems that include: (1) less dramatic but more complex public health issues, (2) an increased number of vulnerable and dysfunctional families, (3) financial constraints, and (4) changing public expectations (Institute of Medicine, 1988; McCreight, 1989; Tinkham, Voorhies, & McCarthy, 1984).

PUBLIC HEALTH AND THE OMAHA SYSTEM

How does the Omaha System relate to the concerns of public health practitioners and administrators? Although use of the Omaha System cannot be expected to solve all public health problems, it does offer potential benefits. These benefits relate to improving practice, standardizing documentation, facilitating communication, increasing efficiency, enhancing effectiveness, and allowing public health practitioners and administrators to portray their services more precisely. Chapter 2 delineated benefits of the Omaha System for the community health setting at large. This chapter focuses on benefits of the Omaha System specific to public health practice, documentation, and data management in relation to home visit programs. Since the Omaha System is based on the nursing process, it is congruent with the ANA standards developed for public health nursing (1986a, 1986b). For the purpose of this book, a differentiation has been made between public health and home health nursing. Public health nurses focus, to a large degree, on clients who are physically well. In contrast, home health nurses focus, to a large degree, on clients with one or more physiologic problems.

There are many similarities between the practice of public health and home health, but significant differences do exist. Differences include the likelihood that public health nurses will serve a younger population whose members may be less receptive to services and more diverse in relation to values, culture, ethnicity, and language. Typically, home health clients recognize their need for service; public health nurses find, however, that they may recognize a client's needs long before the client. Some specific ways that public health professionals and their agencies can use the Omaha System include:

- To explain practice and documentation expectations during orientation of new professional personnel
- To provide a useful index of the client's health problems; it is not unusual for families who are served by public health professionals to have many members and many problems, generating voluminous data
- To provide cues and clues for a practice as well as a documentation guide; although public health nurses use all four domains, they address problems in the Physiological Domain less frequently because of the nature of the population they serve; thus, the third domain may be especially useful as a reminder system
- To identify client progress that occurs slowly and is often limited and difficult to measure
- To facilitate supervisor-staff conferences that involve evaluation and decisions about (1) client progress or lack of progress, (2) cost-benefit comparison of continuing public health service, and (3) client dismissal
- To help cope with requests for service to clients who

are admitted to and dismissed from service frequently; this phenomenon has increased due to diminished funding for continuous care
- To generate standard, aggregate data appropriate for use within an integrated management information system
- To articulate the essence of public health nursing to other nurses and to society at large; the Omaha System helps a public health nurse describe the universe of community health and nursing concerns, the scope of nursing practice, and the effectiveness of care provided

THE OMAHA SYSTEM

A variety of public health agencies are using the Omaha System as a practice and documentation framework within home visit programs. Authors have written about this application in Wisconsin, New Jersey, Saskatchewan, and New York (Cell, Peters, & Gordon, 1984; Helberg, 1988; Neufeld & Misselbrook, 1987; Weidmann & North, 1987). In this chapter, the description by Theresa DuPuis and Prudence Kobasa is representative of public health agency staff and management experiences as implementation evolves. Another description of experiences in a public health agency is written by Beverly Larson. Larson's contribution addresses practice and documentation issues specific to the problems 15. Neglected Child/Adult and 16. Abused Child/Adult.

Sharon Rolph has contributed an overview of her agency's experiences with the Omaha System, focusing on another client group—those with infectious diseases. In contrast to use of the System at the Delaware and Wisconsin agencies, Rolph and her staff have modified the Problem Classification Scheme to meet their unique needs. Although their addition of a problem produces a desirable benefit, they recognize that the signs and symptoms duplicate those of several other problems, reducing the discreteness of categories and the reliability of the Problem Classification Scheme in its entirety. But after thoughtful consideration of their circumstances, they concluded that the advantages of adding a problem exceeded the disadvantages.

USING THE OMAHA SYSTEM IN A STATE HEALTH DEPARTMENT

by THERESA DuPUIS, RN, MPH, MBA, Director, Bureau of Nursing, State of Delaware, Department of Health and Social Services, Dover, DE; and PRUDENCE KOBASA, RN, MSN, (formerly) Assistant Director, Bureau of Nursing, State of Delaware, Department of Health and Social Services, Dover, DE

The Division of Public Health of the State of Delaware shares with a small number of other states the distinction of having no county health departments. The Division is, therefore, responsible for the provision of all public health services in the state and is the sole funding source for these services.

In 1978, the Bureau of Nursing in the Division of Public Health became the official or tax-supported agency to participate in the research and development of the Omaha Problem Classification Scheme and remained a participant throughout the entire project. As all the various phases of the Omaha System were developed, the Bureau staff incorporated them into the record program throughout the state. The final phase of using the Intervention Scheme and the Problem Rating Scale for Outcomes is gradually being implemented.

From management's point of view, the Problem Classification Scheme provides uniformity of recording statewide so that transfer of the records or staff does not necessitate a great deal of time or effort to provide continuity of care. Additionally, the Scheme facilitates easy analysis of the types of problems public health nurses deal with and the time that the staff spend with family planning, prenatal, child health, and other programs.

Some of the other advantages are expressed in comments made by Delaware public health nurses who are using the Omaha System.

- "It provides succinct wording for problems and outcomes and the many choices reduce thinking time needed."
- "Use of the system results in uniformity and consistency in all clients' charts." (JoAnn Thomas, PHN)
- "System allows gathered facts and information to be funneled, sifted, and boxed for speedy recording." (Shirley Pettit, PHN)
- "System helps me when I am doing a home visit, especially on a client that isn't mine."
- "The system helps to organize the clients' problems and makes documentation of progress and findings easier. It is versatile enough to be easily used in all situations."
- "It is a systematic way of identifying and labeling problems, allowing continuity of service and understanding among health professionals utilizing the care plan." (Renata Wiley, PHN)
- "The specificity of the problem names provides the basis for planning intervention measures. Use of the classification system with expected outcomes enables the nurse to see accomplishments."
- "The classification system is clear, concise, and problems are easily identifiable."

The following comments reflect a supervisor's point of view.

- "The system is particularly well suited to the multidisciplinary team approach to family care. Any discipline, be it social work, nursing, nutrition, physical therapy, or speech and language, can utilize the system to identify potential and actual problems affecting the family unit as well as individuals within that unit. Short- and long-range plans for the resolution of problems can be formulated to achieve specific expected outcomes. Additionally, the system is a consistent and easily learned method of documentation requiring less time in new employee orientation." (Barbara DeBastiani, Nursing Supervisor)
- "When reviewing 'closing summaries' by problem, the system lends itself to quick evaluation." (Joan Bauer, Nursing Supervisor)

In addition to use by the public health nursing staff, two other disciplines have embraced the system. Within our own agency, the staff of the Nutrition/Women, Infant, and Children Program (WIC) use the Problem Classification Scheme to document services. This has created uniformity across disciplines, especially where cases are served by both disciplines. Our WIC and Child Health services use the same client record, so information is shared consistently with all providers within those services. Nutritionists did add signs/symptoms, but this was done while maintaining the integrity of the published system. For example, under 40 Family Planning, a descriptor was added for nutrition concerns related to birth control pills.

Outside our own Division of Public Health, the Division of Aging, which had recently begun an Adult Protective Services Unit, was searching for a recording system. The social work staff were familiar with the Omaha System because they employed public health nurses to evaluate health-related concerns of their clients. Training focused primarily on use of the Omaha System, but staff also required instruction on the problem-oriented structure of the record. This proved to be the most difficult concept for staff to understand. The supervisor of the unit summarized the adaptability of the system as follows:

- More precise. Ensures maximum standardization and makes identification of service needs easier between different disciplines.
- More holistic. Less cumbersome than working with a variety of tools.
- Universally applicable. A social worker or nurse can use the system, assessing needs and outcomes in the same way.
- Outcome oriented. Too often outcome goals have been identified in a very generic manner. The Omaha System ties specific outcomes to specific deficits.

- Flexibility of the system that allows for addition of signs and symptoms. This enables ongoing growth and adaptation. (Karen Michel, MSW)

Overall, the Omaha System has provided a positive tool for client management for staff and an evaluative tool for management at the Division of Public Health.

DOCUMENTATION FOCUSING ON ABUSE AND NEGLECT

by BEVERLY LARSON, RN, MPH, Director, Polk County Public Health Nursing Service,
Balsam Lake, WI

Supervisors in our agency, and other agencies as well, have noted that different nurses approach charting differently. The public health nursing staff of Polk County Public Health Nursing Service became acutely aware of differences in documentation when we modified our client record. Specifically, concern developed in relation to the documentation of home visits, use of the Intervention Scheme, and child abuse/neglect cases. The Intervention Scheme was designed to assist the nurse to write brief, concise notes that are client-specific. Nurses must have confidence that the categories and targets in conjunction with client-specific information adequately describe nurse-family interaction.

Our nurses have developed a high level of professional judgment through their experiences with high-risk families who are likely to be involved in future court action. When we implemented the Omaha System, some nurses became uncomfortable and were uncertain that they had adequate documentation to support testimony they would need to give in court regarding the parents' behavior or children's status. Overly brief client-specific notes would not capture the imminent danger children face. Extensive narrative documentation such as lengthy direct quotes from clients defeated the purpose of the Intervention Scheme, the Family Visit Record, and our goal to decrease recording time.

The supervisor must be able to recognize a nurse's personality characteristics in relation to documentation style. Does a nurse prefer to rely on senses and details? Does a nurse view the greater picture and leave out pertinent details? Is a nurse afraid of how the clients would feel about the assessment she/he is making of them? Is a nurse calm, objective, and firm with documentation? Is a nurse not satisfied until everything is in its place? Does a nurse not want to wrap something up, preferring to keep all the options open?

The Myers-Briggs Type Indicator (MBTI) is one tool that supervisors can use to help them understand why nurses are approaching charting tasks in different ways and how they can best assist them in reaching a common goal (Kroeger & Thuesen, 1988; McCaulley, 1981; Myers, 1980; Myers & McCaulley, 1985). The MBTI is a classification system developed by Katharine Briggs and Isabel Briggs Myers. The idea behind this tool is that it can be used to establish individual preferences and then promote a more constructive use of the differences between people. Although very few managers will have knowledge of the personality type of the staff nurses, a basic working knowledge of the MBTI can help them make a good estimate of the way an individual nurse is viewing the world and operating accordingly.

The MBTI is based on the theory that you are born with a predisposition for certain personality preferences. You are:

- Extraverted or introverted
- Sensing or intuitive
- Thinking or feeling
- Judging or perceiving

There are 16 combinations of these four alternates. The extraverted nurse gains energy from outwardly interacting with people. These nurses often conduct their thinking processes out loud. The introverted nurse, although able to deal with people, needs time alone to recharge. This nurse often requires time to mentally process data before being able to respond to a situation. The sensing nurse will insist on details gathered through the five senses, whereas the intuitive nurse would rather look at the larger picture. The thinking nurse will lend credence to things that are logical and scientific, but the feeling nurse will rely on what feels right and try not to hurt feelings by making value judgments. The judger wants everything in its place and thrives on order. The perceiver finds order a bore and would rather rely on creativity, spontaneity, and responsiveness. These different preferences can greatly influence how a nurse approaches charting responsibilities.

The supervisor must attempt to see the charting goal from the perspective of the nurse and then provide guidance to find a middle ground that will satisfy documentation requirements while still using the Intervention Scheme to its full potential. This may mean supporting the nurse in a professional judgment that a particular court-bound family may require more detailed client-specific notes, including some pertinent quotes. It may also mean setting boundaries on the desire to document extensively and repetitively just to be sure all the bases are covered. The supervisor may need to continue to reassure nurses that they are able to use the categories, targets, and client-specific information to describe what nursing practice has done for the client, even to outside professionals.

An adjustment process should be expected for nurses who are changing from traditional narrative nursing notes to the use of the Intervention Scheme and streamlined documentation. Such an adjustment can be facilitated by an awareness that different nurses will view the Intervention Scheme and the changes in the client record in different ways. Adapting orientation and continuing guidance to differences among nurses will increase success both for the individual nurse and the agency as a whole.

USING THE OMAHA SYSTEM WITH AN INFECTIOUS DISEASE PROGRAM

by SHARON ROLPH, RN, BSN, MPA, Director of Public Health Nursing, Yolo County Public Health Department, Woodland, CA

Use of the Omaha System in Yolo County Public Health Nursing was the result of considerable thought and research. The staff wanted a system that provided efficiency, standardization, and a method of articulating what public health nurses do. Furthermore, we were concerned that we were lagging behind our nursing colleagues in other settings by not using nursing diagnosis in a systematic manner. In the face of dwindling resources despite increasing needs of dysfunctional families and demands of complex issues, we needed to be extremely efficient. Discussion of cases among field and supervisory staff and transfer of cases between staff members required standard terminology that was immediately recognizable. The issues of describing what a public health nurse does and conveying that information for reimbursement of services required a system that could be easily understood by both professional and lay persons. The Omaha Problem Classification Scheme appeared to best meet our concerns and requirements.

The staff nurses were involved in discussions and preparation for implementation. They adapted to the Scheme readily and willingly due to its ease of use coupled with common-sense domains, problems, modifiers, and signs/symptoms. There was one exception. As an official agency, we have a mandate for control of infectious diseases. After trying to fit epidemiology concerns into the existing categories, it was decided to add one problem to the Physiological Domain, that of Infection Management: Communicable Disease. We were aware that some of the signs and symptoms we developed for this problem related to other client problems or nursing diagnoses. However, we wanted the efficiency and specificity for our clients with communicable disease. As public health nurses, we are able to use the entire Problem Classification Scheme more readily since we have added the problem. Our problem with its associated signs and symptoms is listed as follows:

Infection Management: Communicable Disease
    Health Promotion
    Potential Impairment
    Impairment
        01. infection with disease (case)
        02. exposure to disease (contacts and reactors)
        03. lacks understanding of disease process
        04. lacks knowledge/motivation to prevent disease transmission
        05. fails to take/obtain medication as recommended
        06. fails to provide required specimens
        07. fails to attend medical appointments
        08. abnormal weight loss/gain
        09. adverse reaction/intolerance to medication
        10. other

Application — Bell Family

Application of the Omaha System in a public health home visit program is illustrated through two case studies: the Bell case and the Mullen case. The data collection, data assessment, and problem identification steps of the diagnostic process are demonstrated by applying the Problem Classification Scheme to client data. Steps in developing plans and implementing interventions are described in relation to the Intervention Scheme. The process of evaluation is described through application of the Problem Rating Scale for Outcomes.

The clients described in the two case studies and in other chapters are fictitious, although the information about the clients represents the compilation of actual data. The names of staff members and the description of the services they provide are factual and reflect actual public health practice. The examples depict a method of applying the nursing process in public health practice, and the forms shown are offered as examples, not requirements.

The Bell case study (pp. 123–140) includes (1) a description of the referral process, (2) dialogue between a nurse and client, and (3) the following VNA of Omaha forms:

Figure 9–1, Public Health Referral (p. 122)
Figure 9–2, Patient Information Record (pp. 124–125)
Figure 9–3, Data Base (p. 128)
Figure 9–4, Data Base (Adult) (p. 129)
Figure 9–5, Data Base (Child) (p. 130)
Figure 9–6, Problem List (p. 131)
Figure 9–7, Problems/Ratings/Plans Data Input Form (pp. 133–136)
Figure 9–8, Problem Ratings/Plans (pp. 137–138)
Figure 9–9, Family Visit Report (p. 140)

Bell Family Case Example

REFERRAL PROCESS

Ann and Alex Bell, featured in the first case study, can be considered representative of many clients referred for public health nursing service. When a hospital staff nurse called to refer Ann to the VNA of Omaha, an intake nurse completed a Public Health Referral

FOR VNA USE ONLY   **THE VISITING NURSE ASSOCIATION OF OMAHA**   **FOR VNA USE ONLY**

DATE: 4/05/90   H/HOLD #: 33514   CT: 29

ACCOUNT #: 33514

NOTIFIED HEALTH DEPT.   Yes   STATION: VNCHS

VNAM ☐   VNHR ☐   VNCHS ☒   Payment Discussed Y ☐ N ☒   HV program

FAX Y ☐ N ☒

SOURCE NAME: UNMC 4 West, B. Jones, RN

RELATIONSHIP: _____   PHONE 559-4441

Previous VNA Record N ☒   Y ☐   DATE FROM _____ TO _____

REJECTED? ☐   ON _____

URGENT VISIT _____ REASON _____

S.S.# 328-17-4652

MEDICAID # 328-17-4652-02 VERIFIED Y ☒

INS. _____

POLICY # _____

OTHER # _____

IS CLIENT AWARE OF REFERRAL? yes

HEAD OF HOUSEHOLD (Last Name, First) Bell, Ann   BIRTH DATE 3/03/73   SEX M ☐ F ☒   MARITAL STATUS S ☒ M ☐ W ☐ D ☐ SEP ☐

STREET ADDRESS: 2605 "Q" St.   CITY Omaha   ZIP 68107   PHONE 731-2978

VNA#	NAME	BIRTH DATE	SEX	VISITS	DATE
33514	Bell, Ann	3/03/73	F		
33515	Bell, Alex	4/01/90	M		

EMERGENCY CONTACT NAME: Cynthia Bell   RELATIONSHIP: Mother   PHONE: 731-6508

REASON FOR REFERRAL: Inexperienced, adolescent mother with many questions about baby care. Birth weight 7 lbs. 8 oz. Length 19½ in. Small support system. Receptive to having PHN.

EXPLANATION OF CARE REQUESTED: TREATMENTS, DRESSINGS, INJECTIONS, TEACHING, OBSERVATIONS, EVALUATIONS, OTHER _____

Health guidance for PP/NB

Evaluate needs

Referral and advocacy

MOTHER	**INFANT**

DIAGNOSIS: Postpartum

PHYSICIAN: James Brown
ADDRESS: UNMC OB Clinic
PHONE: 559-7102
HOSPITAL UNMC   DATES: 4/01 TO 4/03

E.D.C. 4/01/90   BREAST FEEDING: No

DELIVERY DATE: 4/01/90   TYPE Vaginal with midline episiotomy
BONDING: Strong

B.P.: 116/74   MENTAL STATUS alert and interested

MEDICATION & DOSAGE: None

M.D. SIGNATURE: _____

DIAGNOSIS: Newborn

PHYSICIAN: _____
ADDRESS: UNMC Pediatric Clinic
PHONE: 559-2345
HOSPITAL UNMC
BIRTH WEIGHT: 7 lbs. 8 oz.
APGAR: _____ 1 MIN 8 5 MIN 9
GESTATION: 40 weeks

FORMULA TYPE: Enfamil with Fe   AMT. _____

MEDICATIONS & DOSAGE: _____

RETURN APPOINTMENT _____

R.N. SIGNATURE: Karen Connolly, RN

ADDITIONAL INFORMATION
ATTACHED SHEET Y ☐ N ☐

FIGURE 9–1 ■ The Public Health Referral is the initial document used to gather data before client service is initiated.

and initiated a Patient Information Record (Figs. 9–1 and 9–2). The referral form and Patient Information Record, essential to the process of gathering and disseminating client data, were transmitted to the public health nursing supervisor who assigned the Bell family to a staff nurse. Following agency policy, the staff nurse was expected to contact Ann or visit the Bell family within 24 hours.

USING THE PROBLEM CLASSIFICATION SCHEME

The public health nurse, Jane Allen, called the Bell residence to schedule a visit for the following day. Based on the referral information and the phone conversation with Ann Bell, the nurse began to plan an agenda for the visit and think about the client data she expected to obtain. As an experienced public health nurse, Jane knew that she would use an agenda as a guide but would conduct her visit in a flexible manner, responding to Ann's needs and questions at the moment. Jane planned to have a copy of the agency's Data Base forms beside her during the visit, using the forms to remind her of data collection topics and to take notes. The Data Base forms included certain problems and clues selected from all 40 problems of the Problem Classification Scheme. These problems were used frequently by Jane and her public health nursing peers as they received referrals for service to antepartum and postpartum women. In addition, they served infants and children who had difficulties associated with the birth process, developmental delays, or handicaps. Because Jane recognized that review of all 40 problems and the clusters of signs/symptoms was necessary for less typical referrals and for maintaining her high standards of data collection and assessment, she carried a copy of the entire Problem Classification Scheme in her notebook. Included on Jane's agenda for the Bell visit were:

- Observe the physical environment
- Observe the physical appearance of Ann and Alex
- Elicit verbal and nonverbal information from Ann about her physical and emotional status in relation to pregnancy and delivery
- Elicit verbal and nonverbal information from Ann about Alex's feeding, sleeping, and elimination patterns
- Observe bonding between Ann and Alex
- Solicit Ann's positive and negative reactions to parenting
- Complete physical assessments on Ann and Alex
- Assess Ann's self-motivation for enhancing her parenting and daily living skills
- Provide encouragement and positive reinforcement for Ann's successes
- Provide postpartum and infant care instruction as appropriate
- Initiate referrals to other community resources as needed
- Gather any missing demographic data for the client data/face sheet

- Document visit data on appropriate client record and agency forms
- Plan the next visit with Ann

The public health nurse, Jane Allen, arrived at her scheduled time and was met at the door by Ann Bell, who had forgotten about the appointment. During the next 45 minutes, the conversation focused on (1) Ann's limited opportunities to develop parenting skills prior to her baby's birth, (2) questions about newborn development and care, (3) the changes in Ann's lifestyle, (4) her weight gain during pregnancy, (5) her physiologic responses to delivery, and (6) her current diet. As the conversation proceeded, Jane reflected on the visit agenda that she had planned. Ann requested that Jane not awaken her sleeping newborn and Jane agreed to examine the baby when she returned in several days. Jane did observe the infant as he slept; he appeared to be normal. As a skilled public health nurse, Jane gathered diverse data, assessed that data, and implemented nursing interventions throughout the visit.

The entire dialogue of the visit is included here. It is impossible to convey the crucial nonverbal, sensory, and environmental cues that are apparent to a community health nurse during an actual visit, but re-creating the dialogue serves two purposes. First, it can be used as a script to develop a role play session or videotape for orientation to the Omaha System (see Chapter 8). The length, content, and complexity of the visit are applicable to public health orientation. Second, for the reader who is unfamiliar with the practice of community health nursing, the dialogue offers an example of the interpersonal and technical skills that an expert clinician applies during a visit.

The Bell Family Home Visit

JANE: Hi, are you Ann? I'm Jane Allen, the public health nurse who called you yesterday. May I come in?

ANN: Oh (hesitantly). Forgot you were coming. So I just got up—and the baby's still asleep. You aren't going to get him up, are you?

JANE: No, why don't you just show Alex to me? I want to check him over and weigh him but I can do that on my next visit unless he wakes up today.

(Ann and Jane walk into the bedroom quietly.)

JANE: Alex is really a beautiful baby, Ann. How do you feel about being a mom?

ANN: Well, okay, I suppose. But he doesn't act right. He's spoiled.

JANE: What do you mean by that, Ann?

ANN: Well, he doesn't smile and he wakes up *all* the time. He sleeps 3 or 4 hours, then wants another bottle. He's so greedy.

(Jane follows Ann as she walks out of the bedroom and sits down in the living room.)

JANE: Is it okay if I turn the TV off, Ann? I'm having trouble hearing you.

ANN: Yeah.

JANE: You described Alex's behavior a minute ago. Those are pretty normal patterns for newborns, Ann. Most babies don't

```
-------------------------------------------------------------------------
                    PATIENT   INFORMATION   RECORD                 PAGE   1
-------------------------------------------------------------------------

Household #:   33514                     Station: VHCHS-NORTH
Address 1:   2605 "Q" ST.                  Phone: 402 731-2978
Address 2:                          Census Tract: 29.00
City/St/Zip: OMAHA      NE 68107   Monthly Income:    293
Directions:
Case Manager:   JANE ALLEN

                     ACCOUNTS IN HOUSEHOLD
Patient's Name:              Account #:   Birth Date:    Rel. to HH:
BELL, ANN                      33514      3/03/1973      HEAD OF HOUSEHOLD
BELL, ALEX                     33515      4/01/1990      SON
                                                  -------------------------
-------------------------------------------------------------------------
Patient's Name:              Account #:
BELL, ANN                      33514


** EMERGENCY INFORMATION     Relation:  Address:              Phone:
   BELL, CYNTHIA              MOTHER     2019 VINTON       402 731-6508

** ADMISSION INFORMATION
   Soc Sec #:   328-17-4652         Rel. to HH: HH- HEAD OF HOUSEHOLD
   Birth Date:    3/03/1973           Religion: 2- PROTESTANT
   Admit Date:    4/06/90        Referral Code: UNIVERSITY OF NE HOSPITAL
   Refer Date:    4/05/90             Program: 240 - PRV HM CARE OTHER/DC
   1st Contact:   4/05/90                Race: 01- CAUCASIAN
   Care Started:  4/06/90                 Sex: FEMALE
   Plan Establ.:  4/06/90         Marital Sts: SINGLE
   Discharged:    0/00/00      Discharge Reason:
   Special Instructions:
   ICDA Diagnosis:


** DIAGNOSIS INFORMATION
   420       POSTPARTUM

** FUNDING SOURCES           Billing #:     Comment:        Effect Date:
   25- MEDICAID              328-17-4652-02                    4/06/90

** EMPLOYER - 32/ STUDENT

** OTHER AGENCIES            Contact:                      Phone:
   ADC                       MARY MORRIS               402 444-6000
   MD                        JAMES BROWN               402 559-7102

                                                     Orders Cover
** PHYSICIAN INFORMATION                       From Date:   To Date:
   UNMC, OB CLINIC                   888888
   42ND & DEWEY AVE
   OMAHA          NE 68105
A
```

FIGURE 9–2 ◼ (*A and B*) The Patient Information Record is a computer-generated facesheet that includes information obtained during the referral and admission process.

sleep all night until they're a month—or even 2 months—old. They don't respond to attention by smiling until 2 or 3 months.

ANN: That's so?

JANE: That's right. Babies are a lot of work and take a lot of care, as you're finding out. It really does look like you're doing a good job with him—he looks so contented, so clean, and has such a nice bed. Had you taken care of many babies before?

ANN: No. My sister in Chicago has a baby. But I don't see her much. I never babysat for others or at home.

JANE: If it's okay with you, I'd like to visit regularly and talk with you about infant care and normal growth. I'll come again this week and then we'll decide together when I should return. Usually, I expect to visit less often as Alex grows and you gain experience caring for him.

ANN: I guess you can come. Did you bring formula?

JANE: Yes, I brought some Enfamil with Iron. How much does Alex drink at a time?

ANN: Well—here's the last three bottles. He drinks about this much each time. Then he sleeps for 3 to 4 hours. Then he *cries*.

```
----------------------------------------------------------------------------
                      PATIENT   INFORMATION   RECORD                 PAGE    2
----------------------------------------------------------------------------
Household #:    33514                          Station: VHCHS-NORTH

----------------------------------------------------------------------------
----------------------------------------------------------------------------
Patient's Name:                  Account #:
BELL, ALEX                          33515


** EMERGENCY INFORMATION        Relation:  Address:                    Phone:

** ADMISSION INFORMATION
   Soc Sec #:    0                   Rel. to HH:  S - SON
   Birth Date:    4/01/1990            Religion:  2- PROTESTANT
   Admit Date:    4/06/90         Referral Code:  UNIVERSITY OF NE HOSPITAL
   Refer Date:    4/05/90               Program:  242 - DCHD PRV HM CARE/VST
   1st Contact:   4/05/90                  Race:  01- CAUCASIAN
   Care Started:  4/06/90                   Sex:  MALE
   Plan Establ.:  4/06/90           Marital Sts:  SINGLE
   Discharged:    0/00/00       Discharge Reason:
   Special Instructions:
   ICDA Diagnosis:


** DIAGNOSIS INFORMATION
   450       HEALTH SUPERVISION-INFANT

** FUNDING SOURCES              Billing #:      Comment:            Effect Date:
   30- D.C. HEALTH DEPT.        90-00000-00                          4/06/90

** EMPLOYER -   /

** OTHER AGENCIES               Contact:
   WIC                                                      Phone:
   MD                                                   402 698-1234
                                                        402 559-2345

                                                     Orders Cover
** PHYSICIAN INFORMATION                       From Date:   To Date:
   UNMC PEDIATRIC, CLINIC              777777
   42ND & DEWEY AVE
   OMAHA            NE 68105
```

B

FIGURE 9-2 Continued

JANE: That's a real normal amount for his age and size. One of the things you can do to keep Alex healthy is to pour the leftover milk out after he finishes a feeding, rinse out the bottle, and put cold water in it until you're ready to wash the bottles.

ANN: Why do that?

JANE: Because germs grow so quickly in warm milk. If you don't get the bottles real clean, those bacteria could give Alex diarrhea.

ANN: Yeah, the hospital said something about that. I sure didn't know it was such a big deal.

JANE: Did they explain the WIC program to you?

ANN: Yeah.

JANE: Have you gone to WIC yet?

ANN: No. My mom takes me to get stuff. I guess I can go to WIC this week. Will you bring more milk?

JANE: No, this is part of my emergency supply. You can go to WIC each month and get what Alex needs. Do you have the phone number and address?

ANN: Yeah, right here in my purse.

JANE: Are you getting along okay with Alex's cord?

ANN: Yeah, kinda.

JANE: You don't sound too sure.

ANN: Well, I use alcohol on it and stuff. When's it gonna drop off?

JANE: Probably not until next week. You want it to stay clean and heal completely before it falls off. How are you doing with his circumcision?

ANN: Okay. Does it hurt him?

JANE: I don't really know. Most doctors and nurses believe that it doesn't hurt much. I do know that it's important to keep it clean, too, and to apply Vaseline regularly.

ANN: I put Vaseline on it when I change his diaper.

JANE: That's great, Ann. You *are* doing a good job. How are you adjusting to motherhood?

ANN: Well, fine, I suppose. I miss seeing my friends. I'm used to going out a lot. They were here last night. We played cards 'til 2:00. I'm used to living with my mom, too. I've never lived by myself. I don't have much money left—I haven't paid the rent yet.

JANE: It will take time for you to adjust to all of these things, Ann. That's a lot of change for any person to deal with. Where do you get your income?

ANN: ADC. 'Bout $293 a month.

JANE: How do you think that will work out?

ANN: Don't know. I don't think it's enough money.

JANE: Are you getting food stamps?

ANN: Yeah, about $80.

JANE: And what about transportation for that?

ANN: I think it's okay. Like I said, my mom and my friends. They go, too.

JANE: During my next visit, would you like to spend some time going over your expenses? Maybe we can talk about budgets.

ANN: That might help.

JANE: Now, Ann, I'd like to take your blood pressure and check you over a little bit. Could we switch back to your bedroom if we're very quiet?

ANN: I suppose.

(Takes blood pressure.)

JANE: Your blood pressure is 118/68. That's very good. Did you have problems with high blood pressure or swelling during your pregnancy?

ANN: No.

JANE: Your breasts. Are they bothering you?

ANN: Not much. A little sore. The hospital sent home some pills. They worked.

JANE: Tell me about your bleeding. Are you still flowing much or having clots?

ANN: Not much now. It's kinda pink.

JANE: And your stitches. How are they?

ANN: Not bad. They hurt some.

JANE: I don't think I need to check your breasts but I'd like to check your stomach and take a look at your episiotomy, that's your stitches. Please lie down for a minute. That's fine. Your womb is in just the right place. Your episiotomy looks like it is healing very well. It will be tender for a while. Do you soak in the tub?

ANN: I don't have a tub. My mom would let me use hers if I said I needed it.

JANE: I really think that would be a good idea. Or did you bring home that little blue basin from the hospital?

ANN: Yeah.

JANE: You can use that basin to soak at least once a day for the rest of this week *or* you can bend over in the shower every day and let the water run over your episiotomy. Either will help your episiotomy heal faster. Let's go back to your living room.

ANN: Okay.

JANE: Do you have trouble urinating or passing your water?

ANN: No, I don't have to go to the bathroom so much anymore. Not like when I was carrying him.

JANE: And your bowels?

ANN: Better now, too.

JANE: Are you having any pain in the backs of your legs if you lift them like this?

(PHN demonstrates.)

ANN: No. (As she flexes her toes upward.)

JANE: Now that you have Alex, what are your plans for other babies?

ANN: I don't want any for a long time.

JANE: Did anyone at the hospital talk to you about this?

ANN: Well, the hospital gave me some pills. I didn't take any yet.

JANE: Do you know when you're supposed to start?

ANN: They wrote some stuff on a paper with the pills.

JANE: If you get the paper and pills, we'll see what it says.

(Ann gets the instructions.)

ANN: Says I should start in 2 weeks.

JANE: Have you ever used Norinyl before?

ANN: Yeah. Looks like the same kind I used to have.

JANE: How did you get along?

ANN: Okay. But I ran out. Then I got pregnant. I'm going to try harder this time.

JANE: The last things I want to ask about are how well you're eating and feeling. How much weight did you gain during pregnancy?

ANN: (Pause) About 75 pounds.

JANE: How is your appetite now?

ANN: Okay. I'm not as hungry as I was.

JANE: What did you have for breakfast today?

ANN: I just got up when you came. I've got these chips from last night and can of pop.

JANE: Can you tell me what you ate yesterday, Ann?

ANN: Umm. I had more chips, pop, and pizza when everyone was here. I had a bologna sandwich and some brownies earlier.

JANE: It sounds like you don't eat many fruits, vegetables, or milk products.

ANN: No, I'm not good at cooking. I buy easy foods at the convenience store across the street.

JANE: Do you use cigarettes, alcohol, or other drugs, Ann?

ANN: Not when I was pregnant. I don't like the taste of beer. A wine cooler sometimes.

JANE: Has your dentist talked to you about foods and your teeth?

ANN: I don't have a dentist.

JANE: You would benefit from a check-up—and Alex will need preventive care when he's older. Also, you need to begin eating a more balanced diet to help yourself heal from your pregnancy, to keep yourself healthy, and to get ready for feeding Alex. Could we talk about nutrition on the next visit? I can bring some menu plans and describe foods that will require very little cooking.

ANN: Sure. But I never liked that class.

JANE: Well, it isn't the most exciting topic! I'll just ask you to think about what you are eating—and what you want your body to be able to do in the future. I didn't bring any information on foods today but I will next time. I would like for you to scan this book about new babies before I return and tell me what looks interesting. Will you, Ann?

ANN: I will.

JANE: If it's okay with you, I'd like to return on Friday. How is 10 o'clock?

ANN: Well. (hesitantly)

JANE: Is that too early?

ANN: Yeah.

JANE: Then, let's make it 1 o'clock. Here is my card with my name and the VNA's phone number. Please call me if your plans change and you can't be here so we can schedule another appointment. Also, please call me if anything comes up about you or Alex that worries you. If I'm not in the office, I'll call you back as soon as possible.

ANN: Okay.

JANE: Do you think you can get formula before I return?

ANN: Yeah. I'm sure I can.

JANE: It was nice to meet you, Ann. Keep up the good work with Alex. I'll see you Friday. Goodbye.

ANN: Goodbye.

Jane was very pleased with the initial home visit to Ann Bell and with the opportunities for future visits. Clients are more receptive on later visits when the (1) initial visit is not long or overly structured and (2) the nurse does not offend the family's sense of privacy and control. Expertise in establishing rapport with clients was demonstrated during the home visit. Although still a new practitioner, Jane had recognized the value of developing interpersonal skills, a process that requires commitment, time, and energy.

All community health nurses know, or learn quickly, that clients control a nurse's entrance into the home and the direction of the visit. Furthermore, the client rather than the nurse controls what happens following the nurse's visit and if change and improvement occur. These realities of community health practice relate to both public health and home health clients. A home health client is likely to have one or more physiologic problems and perceives a nurse as one who possesses the skills to improve these problems. The client and the client's family may be receptive to service because they may have already made the decision to work with a nurse even before the initial home visit. In contrast, clients of public health nurses are likely to have more problems in the Environmental, Psychosocial, and Health Related Behaviors Domains of the Problem Classification Scheme (see Chapter 5). Often, a nurse must invest time and energy to help a client recognize these problems; only later in the relationship is the client ready to establish mutual goals with the nurse and to initiate problem-solving behavior.

Jane referred to copies of the Data Base forms at convenient times during the Bell home visit (Figs. 9–3, 9–4, and 9–5). The forms, based on the Problem Classification Scheme, have been organized to meet the

public health nurse's needs with typical referrals. In this way, the forms served as (1) guides for the visit, (2) reminders of needed data collection areas, and (3) methods for taking notes. Without distracting Ann or herself, Jane was able to complete portions of the Data Base during the visit. This technique eliminated recopying notes, and was, therefore, timesaving. Immediately after the first visit, Jane recorded the remaining objective and subjective data that she had obtained; those data appear on the three Data Base forms. Positive findings and information on areas of concern or problems should be recorded on the data base.

Public health nurses must make a conscious effort to record actual data and to make reasonable, not excessive, nursing assessments. Nurses must use the Scheme objectively and nonjudgmentally. They must not identify problems by imposing their own values upon clients; they must not, however, avoid identifying problems that could place a negative connotation on the client. It is appropriate for nurses to anticipate what data are needed in the future and what potential client problems may be. The nurse must identify those problems that are supported by current data.

During the second home visit, Jane planned to conduct a physical assessment on Alex and complete his Data Base. Furthermore, she intended to observe Ann's handling of and interacting with Alex. She planned to collect data about Ann's high school status, education and work plans, spiritual support, exercise patterns, and medical history as well as Ann's parents' medical history. With this information recorded, she will complete the initial data base; the three Data Base forms will be inserted in the Bell family folder.

The initial Data Base forms that Jane used did not have space for recording information collected during subsequent visits. Thus, a blank Data Base Update page is available for describing pertinent additions or family changes (see p. 358). During the first visit, Ann did not mention concerns about neighborhood safety. However, Jane was aware of recent drug activity in the area and planned to discuss Ann's feelings and security precautions in the near future. Furthermore, Jane planned to reintroduce the topic of substance abuse to elicit additional data on Ann's history.

The structure, content, and numbering system incorporated in the Data Base provide the information needed for developing the Problem List (Fig. 9–6). The use of a Problem List allows the nurse to narrow the data field from the broad domains of the Problem Classification Scheme and the Data Base. The nurse considers the problems, modifiers, risk factors, and signs/symptoms for a specific client. Then, the nurse records the appropriate problems, modifiers, and signs/symptoms. The Problem List represents an accurate, concise index of the client's health-related interests or concerns as well as problems that vary in severity or degree of intensity. Problems or concerns are identified by public health nurses during the complex process of sorting and setting data priorities, the initial steps of clinical judgment and the nursing process (see Chapter 5).

Jane began the three Data Base forms during the first

VISITING NURSE COMMUNITY HEALTH SERVICES: DATA BASE   Date _4-6-90_

Review entire *PCS; then check or fill in the blanks as needed to describe the situation and circle problem numbers.

HH Acct.# _3351/4_   Client Name _Bell, Ann_   Nurse _Jane Allen, PHN_

DOMAIN I.   ENVIRONMENTAL

(01) **INCOME:** Amount from Sources: Employment_____ ADC _$293/mo_
SSI_____ Other_____ Food Stamps _$80/mo_ WIC _yes_
Medicaid_____ Health Insurance_____

02. **SANITATION:** Adequate cleanliness _✓_____ Unsafe storage _—_____
Insects/Rodents _—_____

03. **RESIDENCE:** Type _Apartment_____ Stability of residency _< 1 month_____
Adequate space _yes_____ Utilities _yes_____
Hazards/Child Safety_____ Phone _yes_____ Rent _?_

04. **NEIGHBORHOOD/WORKPLACE SAFETY:** Safe _?_____ Hazards _drug activity in area_

OTHER PROBLEMS/DATA: _____

ASSESSMENT: _Environment adequate. Ann needs help with budgeting to meet expenses and may need help getting along in neighborhood._

DOMAIN II.   PSYCHOSOCIAL

06. **COMMUNICATION WITH COMMUNITY RESOURCES:** Transportation: Public_____ Walks _✓_
Owns reliable car_____ Depends on others (specify) _mom and friends have cars_
Accessible services: Groceries _✓_ Laundry_____ Pharmacy_____ Medical care_____
Language barrier_____ Literate _yes_
School yr. completed: K-12 _9_ College_____ Now attending_____

07. **SOCIAL CONTACT:** Lives with: Parents_____ Spouse/Significant other_____ Siblings_____
Children _Alex_ Others_____ Network/Support System Outside Household: Parents _mom-Omaha_
Spouse/Significant other_____ Siblings _Chicago_ Children_____ Friends _✓_ Church_____
Others_____ Frequency/manner of contact _phone & freq. visits_

(08) **ROLE CHANGE:** _First time parent; lack of child care experience; concerned about changes in lifestyle_

09. **INTERPERSONAL RELATIONSHIP:** Basic cooperation _some interest in follow up_
Decision making _may need some help_ Tension _appears WNL_
Relationship with husband/father of children_____

11. **GRIEF:**

13. **HUMAN SEXUALITY:** Recognizes consequences of behavior _has BCP_
Satisfaction with relationships _not assessed_

OTHER PROBLEMS/DATA: _Ann's mom takes her on errands weekly_

ASSESSMENT: _Unsure of new role, support systems available. May require assistance with problem solving and advocacy_

SIGNIFICANT PLANNING FACTORS: _visit late am or in PM_

*PCS = Problem Classification Scheme

FIGURE 9-3 ■ The Data Base is an assessment tool for obtaining and documenting general family information, especially that involving the initial portion of the Problem Classification Scheme; this tool was designed for use in the public health setting.

VISITING NURSE COMMUNITY HEALTH SERVICES: DATA BASE (ADULT)   Date _4-6-90_
Review entire PCS; then check or fill in the blanks as needed to describe the situation and
circle problem numbers.
Pt. Acct.# _33514_   Client Name _Bell, Ann_   Nurse _Jane Allen, PHN_
DOMAIN II. PSYCHOSOCIAL (con't)
(14.) CARETAKING/PARENTING: Primary Caregiver _Ann_   Other caregivers/helpers _____
      Physical care skills _____   Emotional/Nurturing skills _____
      Bonding _____ Appropriate expectations _no_   Discipline _____
      Satisfaction/comfort _Questionable_   Other _____

15. NEGLECTED CHILD/ADULT:

16. ABUSED CHILD/ADULT:
OTHER PROBLEMS/DATA: _____
ASSESSMENT: _Will require teaching about normal G+D_
DOMAIN III. PHYSIOLOGICAL
23. COGNITION: Problem solving ability _moderate_   Recall ability _WNL_

28. RESPIRATION: Rate/Quality _N/A_

29. CIRCULATION: Temp _____ BP _118/68_   Pulse/Quality _____ Edema _____

32. GENITO-URINARY FUNCTION: Urination _WNL_   Menstruation _____

(33.) ANTEPARTUM/POSTPARTUM: AP: EDC _____   *TPAL _1001_
      Date OB Care _____   Fetal Act/FHR _____
      L&D Prep _____   Abn Lab. _____
      Danger Sig _____   Preterm Labor _____
      PP: Del. Date _4-1-90_   Bonding _talks about baby appropriately_
      8 point check _WNL episiotomy intact and healing. Fundus firm and below_
      umbilicus
OTHER PROBLEMS/DATA: _negative Homan_

ASSESSMENT: _normal postpartum course_

*TPAL = Term(36–42 wk), Preterm(under 36 wk), Abortions, Living Children
DOMAIN IV. HEALTH RELATED BEHAVIORS
(35.) NUTRITION: Ht. _____ Wt. _151b_ Diet _high fat, high carb, low vitamin/mineral/fiber,_
                                                          much pop
36. SLEEP/REST PATTERNS: _fatigued_ _altered but still adequate_

37. PHYSICAL ACTIVITY: Usual _?_

38. PERSONAL HYGIENE: _adequate_

39. SUBSTANCE MISUSE: Cigarettes _no_   Alcohol _no_   Drugs _?_

(40.) FAMILY PLANNING: Method/Follow through _has Norinyl – to start in 2 wks; does not want_
                                             another pregnancy soon
(41.) HEALTH CARE SUPERVISION: MD _? adequate prenatal care – Dr. Brown_
      DDS _none_   Emergency _____ Other _____

42. ASSESSMENT: _Nutrition poor, needs guidance about more healthy lifestyle_

FIGURE 9–4 ■ The Data Base (Adult) is an assessment tool for obtaining and documenting information specific to an adult client, especially that involving the latter portion of the Problem Classification Scheme; this tool was designed for use in the public health setting.

home visit; these forms are included in this chapter. She completed the forms after the second visit. Based on the Data Base, Jane identified eight problem areas in the Bell family: 01. Income, 08. Role Change, 14. Caretaking/Parenting, 17. Growth and Development, 33. Antepartum/Postpartum, 35. Nutrition, 40. Family Planning, and 41. Health Care Supervision. Problems noted on the Problem List have Health Promotion, Po-

tential, or Actual Modifiers, as well as Individual or Family Modifiers. In the example, five problems were Actual and three were Potential. Actual problems have one or more signs and symptoms. Risk factors are associated with Potential problems. Six of the eight problems were Individual. The two Family problems involved both Ann and Alex.

Data collected on the first two visits were sufficient

VISITING NURSE COMMUNITY HEALTH SERVICES: DATA BASE (CHILD)   Date _4-6-90_

Review entire PCS; then check or fill in the blanks as needed to describe the situation and circle problem numbers.

Pt. Acct.# _33515_   Client Name _Bell, Alex_   Nurse _Jane Allen, PHN_

Birth Order _1_   Age _5 days_

DOMAIN II. PSYCHOSOCIAL (con't)

15. NEGLECTED CHILD/ADULT:

16. ABUSED CHILD/ADULT:

(17) GROWTH AND DEVELOPMENT OF CHILD/ADULT:Wt._____ Ht._____ HC._____

Newborn PA_____

Appearance/activity/personality _Ok_____ School/preschool day care_____

Parent interaction_____ Sibling interaction_____

OTHER PROBLEMS/DATA: _____

ASSESSMENT: _____

DOMAIN III. PHYSIOLOGICAL

19. HEARING:

20. VISION:

21. SPEECH AND LANGUAGE:

22. DENTITION:

23. COGNITION:

26. INTEGUMENT:Mongolian Spots_____

27. NEURO–MUSCULO–SKELETAL FUNCTION:Reflexes_____

28. RESPIRATION:Rate/Quality_____ Apnea Monitor_____

29. CIRCULATION:Temp_____ BP_____ Pulse/A/R/F_____

30. DIGESTION–HYDRATION:Colic_____ Indigestion/Reflux_____

31. BOWEL FUNCTION:No. of stools/day_____ Color_____ Consistency_____

32. GENITO–URINARY FUNCTION:

OTHER PROBLEMS/DATA: _____

_____

ASSESSMENT: _____

_____

DOMAIN IV. HEALTH RELATED BEHAVIORS

35. NUTRITION:Breast _NA_____ Formula/Type/24 hour _Enfamil c̄ Fe 3 oz q̄ 3-4 hr._

Solids __—_____ Eating habits_____

FIGURE 9–5 ■ The Data Base (Child) is an assessment tool for obtaining and documenting information specific to an infant or child, especially that involving the latter portion of the Problem Classification Scheme; this tool was designed for use in the public health setting. (The complete form is shown in the Appendix.)

```
                            PROBLEM LIST

Family Name:  Bell                        Household #: 33514
Date          Individual   Problem   Problem Titles              Date
Noted         Name         Number    (with descriptors)          Resolved/
                                                                  Inactivated

4/06/90       Family       01        INCOME:  Deficit
                                     01. low/no income
                                     03. inadequate money management

04/06/90      Family       41        HEALTH CARE SUPERVISION:  Impairment
                                     05. inconsistent source of medical/dental
                                         care

04/06/90      Ann          08        ROLE CHANGE:  Impairment
                                     03. assumes new role

04/06/90      Ann          14        CARETAKING/PARENTING:  Impairment
                                     05. expectations incongruent with stage of
                                         growth and development

04/06/90      Ann          33        ANTEPARTUM/POSTPARTUM:  Potential
                                     Impairment

04/06/90      Ann          35        NUTRITION:  Impairment
                                     01. weighs 10% more than average
                                     04. exceeds established standards for
                                         daily caloric/fluid intake
                                     05. unbalanced diet

04/06/90      Ann          40        FAMILY PLANNING:  Potential Impairment

04/06/90      Alex         17        GROWTH AND DEVELOPMENT:  Potential
                                     Impairment
```

FIGURE 9–6 ■ The Problem List is a computer-generated index of the client's health-related interests, concerns, and problems and is based on the Problem Classification Scheme.

for Jane to feel comfortable with the initial Data Base and Problem List. The forms reflected the objective and subjective data available at that time. She planned to be alert for additional data, especially for data that would suggest the following problem areas: 04. Neighborhood/Workplace Safety, 06. Communication With Community Resources, 36. Sleep and Rest Patterns, and 39. Substance Use. Because the Data Base and the Problem List are intended to be dynamic forms in the client record, the public health nurse is responsible for adding to or deleting from the forms during the period of time that services are provided. For example, changes in the Bell family situation that occur during the next weeks or months may prompt Jane to edit the Problem List as follows:

■ Add or resolve a sign/symptom of a problem
■ Change a modifier of a problem
■ Add a problem with its modifier and signs/symptoms (signs/symptoms for Actual problem only)
■ Resolve a problem with its modifier and signs/symptoms (signs/symptoms for Actual problem only)

USING THE PROBLEM RATING SCALE FOR OUTCOMES

The Problem Rating Scale for Outcomes provides a framework for measuring client progress in relation to problems of the Problem Classification Scheme. The framework incorporates the three concepts of Knowledge, Behavior, and Status with a five-point Likert-type scale (see Chapter 7). When using the Problem Rating Scale for Outcomes, the public health nurse reviews client data specific to priority problems and documents these data. Determining problem priorities is based on clinical expertise and judgment about client need and willingness to address specific problems. It is completed without regard to the specified problem modifier, since Actual, Potential, and Health Promotion problems all may be considered priorities.

Numeric ratings for the three concepts serve as one means for a nurse to evaluate a client's progress over time when ratings are completed at admission, at periodic intervals, and on dismissal. As part of the evaluation process, a public health nurse can compare and contrast client data as reflected by the ratings for the three concepts. For a given client, whether an individual or a family, the initial rating for each concept should be reviewed and evaluated in relation to (1) ratings for that concept at later time intervals and (2) ratings for the other two concepts. Thus, it is as important to consider the correlation between each concept and a client's change over time as it is to consider the correlations between the concepts.

Jane Allen narrowed the data field as she developed the Problem List from the Data Base after the second home visit to the Bell family. Similarly, she narrowed the field even more as she set priorities for problems before completing admission client ratings. Initially, Jane identified eight problem areas for Ann and Alex Bell. Of those, she decided that 01. Income, 08. Role Change, 14. Caretaking/Parenting, 35. Nutrition, and 17. Growth and Development were priorities. She decided that 33. Antepartum/Postpartum, 40. Family Planning, and 41. Health Care Supervision were not priorities. The decisions Jane made about problem priorities were based on clinical judgment and family cues regarding needs and interests. The distinctions were not based on which of the modifiers Jane had documented in relation to the eight problems. For example, it may be as important for a nurse to work with a family on a Health Promotion or a Potential problem as on an Actual problem. In the Bell family case study, four priority and one nonpriority problems were modified by Actual; one priority and two nonpriority problems were modified by Potential. Jane planned to be alert for data that would suggest a change in the priority of problems throughout the time of client service. In addition, she recognized that she might address one or more additional problems after progress or resolution occurred with the priority problems.

The process of establishing ratings specific to a problem is the same for the Bell family as for all other clients. Simultaneously, the process is simple and difficult. It is simple in that Jane or any other public health nurse can quickly write one number for the Knowledge, Behavior, and Status ratings of all priority problems. With two exceptions, a rating from 1 to 5 may be selected for all problems and their modifiers. When the problem modifier is Actual, signs/symptoms exist so that the Status rating cannot be 5; when a problem modifier is Potential or Health Promotion, signs/symptoms do not exist, so that the Status rating will be a 5.

Completing the rating process does require time and concentration if the nurse adheres to the principles associated with the Scale and completes the ratings thoughtfully. A careful, consistent, and accurate approach requires that the nurse follow a logical, problem-solving, nursing-focused process. The prerequisites for use of the Scale are (1) collecting a realistic quantity of comprehensive, accurate data and (2) identifying client problems from that data. During the process of establishing ratings, the nurse must consider two important questions or principles:

■ What is the total universe or continuum for Knowledge, Behavior, and Status in relation to a specific problem? To increase consistent use of the Scale by many nurses, this universe or total population must

be drawn from the nurse's educational background and work experiences as well as from exposure to friends, neighbors, and family members.

■ Where does this individual or family best fit on the Knowledge, Behavior, or Status continuum in relation to a specific problem? Although variability among nurses is inevitable and no individual nurse will always be right, thoughtful consideration has been associated with acceptable levels of interrater agreement during the VNA of Omaha research projects and examinations of reliability.

To begin documenting the Knowledge, Behavior, and Status ratings for the five priority problems, Jane used the Problems/Ratings/Plans Data Input Form (Fig. 9–7). This form serves as a worksheet for the nurse to write both the ratings and plans; the computer-generated Problem Ratings/Plans, developed from the worksheet, becomes part of the permanent client record (Fig. 9–8). Although the data input form in the Bell case study was destroyed according to VNA of Omaha procedures, it can serve as a permanent, handwritten form in another agency's record system when typing or computer recordkeeping is not available.

A public health nurse completes the first step toward accountability by completing initial ratings based on client data. Scheduling an appropriate date to review client data and the ratings is the nurse's next step. In the case study, Jane planned to review and complete Knowledge, Behavior, and Status ratings again in 3 months for the Bells' five priority problems. If Jane did not detect that the Bells were making progress as she expected, she intended to review the Data Base, Problem List, and interventions in relation to the ratings before 3 months elapsed. Jane would be especially concerned if lack of progress occurred in relation to the problem areas of 14. Caretaking/Parenting and 17. Growth and Development.

USING THE INTERVENTION SCHEME

Nurses are responsible for developing care plans as part of their public health practice. Furthermore, when nurses and other community health professionals make home visits to clients, they document the care they actually provide; this care reflects the implementation of plans. In order to standardize the language needed to describe the problem-specific planning and intervening processes, the categories and targets of the Intervention Scheme were developed (see Chapter 6). As the third component of the Omaha System, the Intervention Scheme was developed to use with the Problem Classification Scheme and the Problem Rating Scale for Outcomes. The three components provide the framework for organizing client data into a logical and orderly documentation system, a system that is driven by client problems.

Jane developed plans for Ann and Alex Bell based on the data collection and assessment process (Fig. 9–8). She completed the plans after the second home visit.

Text continued on page 140

PROBLEMS/RATINGS/PLANS
DATA INPUT FORM

ADMISSION ✓
UPDATE ___
DISCHARGE ___

HHACCT #: _33514_   HOUSEHOLD NAME: _Bell_   NURSE: _Jane Allen, PHN_

DATE: _4/9/90_   PACCT # _33514_   PACCT # _33514_

NAME _Bell_   NAME _Bell_

PROBLEM NO: _01 (F) I_					PROBLEM NO: _41 (F) I_			
HP	P	(A)			HP	P	(A)	

SIGNS/SYMPTOMS:

(01)	05	09	13		01	(05)	09	13
02	06	10	14		02	06	10	14
(03)	07	11	15		03	07	11	15
04	08	12	16		04	08	12	16

RATINGS:

KNOWLEDGE	1 (2) 3 4 5		1 2 3 4 5
BEHAVIOR	1 (2) 3 4 5		1 2 3 4 5
STATUS	1 (2) 3 4 5		1 2 3 4 5

REVIEW: (MONTHS) 1 2 (3) 4   1 2 3 4

INTERVENTIONS: (I) II III (IV)   I II III IV

CLIENT SPECIFIC COMMENTS   CLIENT SPECIFIC COMMENTS

TARGETS:								
ANATOMY/PHYSIOLOGY	01					01		
BEHAVIOR MODIFICATION	02					02		
BLADDER CARE	03					03		
BONDING	04					04		
BOWEL CARE	05					05		
BRONCHIAL HYGIENE	06					06		
CARDIAC CARE	07					07		
CARETAKING/PARENTING SKILLS	08					08		
CAST CARE	09					09		
COMMUNICATION	10					10		
COPING SKILLS	11					11		
DAY CARE/RESPITE	12					12		
DISCIPLINE	13					13		
DRESSING CHG/WOUND CARE	14					14		
DURABLE MEDICAL EQUIP	15					15		
EDUCATION	16	✓	✓	complete school		16		
EMPLOYMENT	17					17		
ENVIRONMENT	18					18		
EXERCISES	19					19		
FAMILY PLANNING	20					20		
FEEDING PROCEDURES	21					21		
FINANCES	22	✓	✓	Budgeting		22		
FOOD	23					23		
GAIT TRAINING	24					24		
GROWTH/DEVELOPMENT	25					25		
HOMEMAKING	26					26		
HOUSING	27					27		
INTERACTION	28					28		
LAB FINDINGS	29					29		
LEGAL SYSTEM	30					30		
MEDICAL/DENTAL CARE	31					31		
MED ACTN/SIDE EFFECTS	32					32		
MEDICATION ADMIN	33					33		
MEDICATION SETUP	34					34		
MOBILITY/TRANSFERS	35					35		
NURSING CARE, SUPPLEMENTARY	36					36		
NUTRITION	37					37		
NUTRITIONIST	38					38		
OSTOMY CARE	39					39		
OTHER COMMUNITY RESOURCE	40					40		
PERSONAL CARE	41					41		
POSITIONING	42					42		
REHABILITATION	43					43		
RELAXATION/BREATHING TECH	44					44		
REST/SLEEP	45					45		
SAFETY	46					46		
SCREENING	47					47		
SICKNESS/INJURY CARE	48					48		
SIGNS/SYMP-MENTAL/EMOTION	49					49		
SIGNS/SYMP-PHYSICAL	50					50		
SKIN CARE	51					51		
SOCIAL WORK/COUNSELING	52					52		
SPECIMEN COLLECTION	53					53		
SPIRITUAL CARE	54					54		
STIMULATION/NURTURANCE	55					55		
STRESS MANAGEMENT	56					56		
SUBSTANCE USE	57					57		
SUPPLIES	58					58		
SUPPORT GROUP	59					59		
SUPPORT SYSTEM	60					60		
TRANSPORTATION	61					61		
WELLNESS	62					62		
OTHER	63					63		

A

FIGURE 9–7 ■ (*A–D*) The Problems/Ratings/Plans Data Input Form is a data-gathering guide and worksheet to note both problem-specific client ratings and plans associated with the Problem Rating Scale for Outcomes and the Intervention Scheme.

PROBLEMS/RATINGS/PLANS
DATA INPUT FORM

ADMISSION ✓
UPDATE _____
DISCHARGE _____

HHACCT #: _33514_ HOUSEHOLD NAME: _Bell_ NURSE: _Jane Allen, PHN_

DATE: _4/9/90_ PACCT # _33514_ PACCT # _33514_

NAME _Ann_ NAME _Ann_

	PROBLEM NO: _08_ F ①				PROBLEM NO: _14_ F ①		
	HP P Ⓐ				HP P Ⓐ		
SIGNS/SYMPTOMS:	01 05 09 13				01 ⑤ 09 13		
	02 06 10 14				02 06 10 14		
	③ 07 11 15				03 07 11 15		
	04 08 12 16				04 08 12 16		
RATINGS:							
KNOWLEDGE	1 ② 3 4 5				1 ② 3 4 5		
BEHAVIOR	1 2 ③ 4 5				1 2 ③ 4 5		
STATUS	1 2 ③ 4 5				1 2 3 ④ 5		
REVIEW: (MONTHS)	1 2 ③ 4				1 2 ③ 4		
INTERVENTIONS:	① II Ⓘ Ⓘ Ⓘ Ⓘ Ⓥ				① II Ⓘ Ⓘ Ⓘ Ⓘ Ⓥ		

CLIENT SPECIFIC COMMENTS (Problem 08)
CLIENT SPECIFIC COMMENTS (Problem 14)

TARGETS:

TARGET	#	Problem 08	Comments 08	Problem 14	Comments 14
ANATOMY/PHYSIOLOGY	01				
BEHAVIOR MODIFICATION	02				
BLADDER CARE	03				
BONDING	04			✓	holding, talking
BOWEL CARE	05				
BRONCHIAL HYGIENE	06				
CARDIAC CARE	07			✓	physical, social tasks
CARETAKING/PARENTING SKILLS	08			✓	explore family history
CAST CARE	09			✓	
COMMUNICATION	10				
COPING SKILLS	11	✓	balance resp., problem solving	✓	finding sitter
DAY CARE/RESPITE	12				
DISCIPLINE	13				
DRESSING CHG/WOUND CARE	14				
DURABLE MEDICAL EQUIP	15				
EDUCATION	16	✓	complete school		
EMPLOYMENT	17				
ENVIRONMENT	18				
EXERCISES	19				
FAMILY PLANNING	20				
FEEDING PROCEDURES	21				
FINANCES	22				
FOOD	23				
GAIT TRAINING	24				
GROWTH/DEVELOPMENT	25				
HOMEMAKING	26				
HOUSING	27				
INTERACTION	28				
LAB FINDINGS	29				
LEGAL SYSTEM	30				
MEDICAL/DENTAL CARE	31				
MED ACTN/SIDE EFFECTS	32				
MEDICATION ADMIN	33				
MEDICATION SETUP	34				
MOBILITY/TRANSFERS	35				
NURSING CARE, SUPPLEMENTARY	36				
NUTRITION	37				
NUTRITIONIST	38				
OSTOMY CARE	39				
OTHER COMMUNITY RESOURCE	40				
PERSONAL CARE	41				
POSITIONING	42				
REHABILITATION	43				
RELAXATION/BREATHING TECH	44				
REST/SLEEP	45				
SAFETY	46				
SCREENING	47				
SICKNESS/INJURY CARE	48			✓	taking temp, recog.
SIGNS/SYMP-MENTAL/EMOTION	49	✓	her questions, feelings		S/S & fu
SIGNS/SYMP-PHYSICAL	50				
SKIN CARE	51				
SOCIAL WORK/COUNSELING	52				
SPECIMEN COLLECTION	53				
SPIRITUAL CARE	54				
STIMULATION/NURTURANCE	55				
STRESS MANAGEMENT	56				
SUBSTANCE USE	57				
SUPPLIES	58				
SUPPORT GROUP	59			✓	group @ school or
SUPPORT SYSTEM	60				neighborhood
TRANSPORTATION	61				
WELLNESS	62				
OTHER	63				

B

FIGURE 9-7 Continued

PROBLEMS/RATINGS/PLANS
DATA INPUT FORM

ADMISSION ✓
UPDATE _____
DISCHARGE _____

HHACCT #: _33514_   HOUSEHOLD NAME: _Bell_   NURSE: _Jane Allen, PHN_

DATE: _4/9/90_   PACCT # _33514_   PACCT # _33514_

NAME _Ann_   NAME _Ann_

	PROBLEM NO: 33 F ①					PROBLEM NO: 35 F ①			
	HP (P) A					HP P (A)			
SIGNS/SYMPTOMS:	01 05 09 13					⦰01 (05) 09 13			
	02 06 10 14					02 06 10 14			
	03 07 11 15					03 07 11 15			
	04 08 12 16					⦰04 08 12 16			
RATINGS:									
KNOWLEDGE	1 2 3 4 5					1 2 ③ 4 5			
BEHAVIOR	1 2 3 4 5					1 ② 3 4 5			
STATUS	1 2 3 4 5					1 ② 3 4 5			
REVIEW: (MONTHS)	1 2 3 4					1 2 ③ 4			
INTERVENTIONS:	I II III IV					① II ⦿III ⦿IV			

CLIENT SPECIFIC COMMENTS (Problem 33)
CLIENT SPECIFIC COMMENTS (Problem 35)

TARGETS:		Problem 33	Problem 35	Comments
ANATOMY/PHYSIOLOGY	01			
BEHAVIOR MODIFICATION	02			
BLADDER CARE	03			
BONDING	04			
BOWEL CARE	05			
BRONCHIAL HYGIENE	06			
CARDIAC CARE	07			
CARETAKING/PARENTING SKILLS	08			
CAST CARE	09			
COMMUNICATION	10			
COPING SKILLS	11			
DAY CARE/RESPITE	12			
DISCIPLINE	13			
DRESSING CHG/WOUND CARE	14			
DURABLE MEDICAL EQUIP	15			
EDUCATION	16			
EMPLOYMENT	17			
ENVIRONMENT	18			
EXERCISES	19			
FAMILY PLANNING	20			
FEEDING PROCEDURES	21			
FINANCES	22			
FOOD	23			
GAIT TRAINING	24			
GROWTH/DEVELOPMENT	25			
HOMEMAKING	26			
HOUSING	27			
INTERACTION	28			
LAB FINDINGS	29			
LEGAL SYSTEM	30			
MEDICAL/DENTAL CARE	31			
MED ACTN/SIDE EFFECTS	32			
MEDICATION ADMIN	33			
MEDICATION SETUP	34			
MOBILITY/TRANSFERS	35			
NURSING CARE, SUPPLEMENTARY	36			
NUTRITION	37		✓ ✓	modify intake, use booklet
NUTRITIONIST	38			
OSTOMY CARE	39			
OTHER COMMUNITY RESOURCE	40			
PERSONAL CARE	41			
POSITIONING	42			
REHABILITATION	43			
RELAXATION/BREATHING TECH	44			
REST/SLEEP	45			
SAFETY	46			
SCREENING	47			
SICKNESS/INJURY CARE	48			
SIGNS/SYMP-MENTAL/EMOTION	49			
SIGNS/SYMP-PHYSICAL	50			
SKIN CARE	51			
SOCIAL WORK/COUNSELING	52			
SPECIMEN COLLECTION	53			
SPIRITUAL CARE	54			
STIMULATION/NURTURANCE	55			
STRESS MANAGEMENT	56			
SUBSTANCE USE	57			
SUPPLIES	58			
SUPPORT GROUP	59		✓	group PRN
SUPPORT SYSTEM	60			
TRANSPORTATION	61			
WELLNESS	62			
OTHER	63			

C

FIGURE 9-7 *Continued*

PROBLEMS/RATINGS/PLANS
DATA INPUT FORM

HHACCT #: __33514__   HOUSEHOLD NAME: __Bell__   NURSE: __Jane Allen, PHN__

DATE: __4/9/90__   PACCT # __33514__   PACCT # __33515__

NAME __Ann__   NAME __Alex__

	PROBLEM NO: 40 F ①		PROBLEM NO: 17 F ①
	HP ⓟ A		HP ⓟ A
SIGNS/SYMPTOMS:	01 05 09 13		01 05 09 13
	02 06 10 14		02 06 10 14
	03 07 11 15		03 07 11 15
	04 08 12 16		04 08 12 16
RATINGS:			
KNOWLEDGE	1 2 3 4 5		1 ② 3 4 5
BEHAVIOR	1 2 3 4 5		1 2 ③ 4 5
STATUS	1 2 3 4 5		1 2 3 ⑤
REVIEW: (MONTHS)	1 2 3 4		1 2 ③ 4
INTERVENTIONS:	I. II III IV		① II III Ⓥ

TARGETS:		Ann cols	CLIENT SPECIFIC COMMENTS	Alex cols	CLIENT SPECIFIC COMMENTS
ANATOMY/PHYSIOLOGY	01			✓ ___ ___ ✓	normal stages, use booklets
BEHAVIOR MODIFICATION	02				
BLADDER CARE	03				
BONDING	04				
BOWEL CARE	05				
BRONCHIAL HYGIENE	06				
CARDIAC CARE	07				
CARETAKING/PARENTING SKILLS	08				
CAST CARE	09				
COMMUNICATION	10				
COPING SKILLS	11				
DAY CARE/RESPITE	12				
DISCIPLINE	13				
DRESSING CHG/WOUND CARE	14				
DURABLE MEDICAL EQUIP	15				
EDUCATION	16				
EMPLOYMENT	17				
ENVIRONMENT	18				
EXERCISES	19				
FAMILY PLANNING	20				
FEEDING PROCEDURES	21				
FINANCES	22				
FOOD	23				
GAIT TRAINING	24				
GROWTH/DEVELOPMENT	25				
HOMEMAKING	26				
HOUSING	27				
INTERACTION	28				
LAB FINDINGS	29				
LEGAL SYSTEM	30				
MEDICAL/DENTAL CARE	31				
MED ACTN/SIDE EFFECTS	32				
MEDICATION ADMIN	33				
MEDICATION SETUP	34				
MOBILITY/TRANSFERS	35				
NURSING CARE, SUPPLEMENTARY	36				
NUTRITION	37			✓ ___ ___ ✓	normal patterns
NUTRITIONIST	38				
OSTOMY CARE	39				
OTHER COMMUNITY RESOURCE	40				
PERSONAL CARE	41				
POSITIONING	42				
REHABILITATION	43				
RELAXATION/BREATHING TECH	44				
REST/SLEEP	45				
SAFETY	46			✓ ___ ___ ✓	basics in home
SCREENING	47				
SICKNESS/INJURY CARE	48				
SIGNS/SYMP-MENTAL/EMOTION	49				
SIGNS/SYMP-PHYSICAL	50				
SKIN CARE	51				
SOCIAL WORK/COUNSELING	52				
SPECIMEN COLLECTION	53				
SPIRITUAL CARE	54				
STIMULATION/NURTURANCE	55			✓ ___ ___ ✓	role model
STRESS MANAGEMENT	56				
SUBSTANCE USE	57				
SUPPLIES	58				
SUPPORT GROUP	59				
SUPPORT SYSTEM	60				
TRANSPORTATION	61				
WELLNESS	62				
OTHER	63				

D

FIGURE 9–7 Continued

```
-----------------------------------------------------------------------
          * * *   P R O B L E M   R A T I N G S/P L A N S   * * *      PAGE    1
HOUSEHOLD #:   33514    2605 "Q" ST.          STATION- VHCHS-NORTH
-----------------------------------------------------------------------
                        ACCOUNTS IN HOUSEHOLD
Patient's Name:              Account #:          From Date:
BELL, ANN                       33514            4/06/90
BELL, ALEX                      33515            4/06/90
-----------------------------------------------------------------------

* 04/09/90 FAMILY
              01
           INCOME

              K2
           KNOWLEDGE - Minimal knowledge

              B2
           BEHAVIOR - Rarely appropriate

              S2
           STATUS - Severe signs/symptoms

              3
           Re-Evaluate Three Months
PLAN:
1. HTGC, S:  education:  complete school.
2. HTGC, S:  finances:  budgeting.

* 04/09/90 BELL, ANN
              08
           ROLE CHANGE

              K2
           KNOWLEDGE - Minimal knowledge

              B3
           BEHAVIOR - Inconsistently appropriate

              S3
           STATUS - Moderate signs/symptoms

              3
           Re-Evaluate Three Months
PLAN:
1. HTGC: coping skills:  balance responsibilities, problem solving.
2. CM: education:  complete school.
3. S:  s/s - mental/emotional:  her questions, feelings.

* 04/09/90 BELL, ANN
              14
           CARETAKING/PARENTING

              K2
           KNOWLEDGE - Minimal knowledge

              B3

-----------------------------------------------------------------------
HTGC = Health Teaching , Guidance , & Counseling
T & P = Treatments & Procedures
CM = Case Management      S = Surveillance
```

A

FIGURE 9–8 ■ (*A and B*) The Problem Ratings/Plans is a computer-generated form developed from the Problems/Ratings/Plans Data Input Form.

```
------------------------------------------------------------------------
          * * *  P R O B L E M   R A T I N G S / P L A N S  * * *    PAGE   2
   HOUSEHOLD #:    33514     2605 "Q" ST.        STATION- VHCHS-NORTH
------------------------------------------------------------------------
           BEHAVIOR - Inconsistently appropriate

                S4
           STATUS - Minimal signs/symptoms

                3
           Re-Evaluate Three Months
PLAN:
1. HTGC, S:  caretaking/parenting skills:  physical, social tasks.
2. HTGC:  communication:  explore family history.
3. HTGC:  sickness/injury care:  take temp, recognize s/s, and
follow-up.
4. CM:  day care respite:  finding sitter.
5. CM:  support group:  group at school or neighborhood.
6. S:  bonding:  holding, talking.

 * 04/09/90 BELL, ANN
                35
           NUTRITION

                K3
           KNOWLEDGE - Basic knowledge

                B2
           BEHAVIOR - Rarely appropriate

                S2
           STATUS - Severe signs/symptoms

                3
           Re-Evaluate Three Months
PLAN:
1. HTGC, S:  nutrition:  modify intake, use booklet.
2. CM:  support group:  group p.r.n.

 * 04/09/90 BELL, ALEX
                17
           GROWTH AND DEVELOPMENT

                K2
           KNOWLEDGE - Minimal knowledge

                B3
           BEHAVIOR - Inconsistently appropriate

                S5
           STATUS - No signs/symptoms

                3
           Re-Evaluate Three Months
PLAN:
1. HTGC, S:  anatomy/physiology:  normal stages, use booklets.
2. HTGC, S:  nutrition:  normal patterns.
3. HTGC, S:  safety:  basics in home.
4. HTGC, S:  stimulation/nurturance:  role model.
                        Jane Allen, PHN
                        Jane Allen, PHN/rip

------------------------------------------------------------------------
HTGC = Health Teaching , Guidance , & Counseling
T & P = Treatments & Procedures
CM = Case Management      S = Surveillance
```

B

FIGURE 9–8 Continued

FAMILY VISIT REPORT

Household Number 33514
Client Name Bill, Ann # _____ Age _____
Alex

Date 4-6-90

INTERVENTION SCHEME

CATEGORIES

I. Health Teaching, Guidance, and Counseling
II. Treatments and Procedures
III. Case Management
IV. Surveillance

TARGETS

01 Anatomy/physiology
02 Behavior modification
03 Bladder care
04 Bonding
05 Bowel care
06 Bronchial hygiene
07 Cardiac care
08 Caretaking/parenting skills
09 Cast care
10 Communication
11 Coping skills
12 Day care/respite
13 Discipline
14 Dressing change/wound care
15 Durable medical equipment
16 Education
17 Employment
18 Environment
19 Exercises
20 Family planning
21 Feeding procedures
22 Finances
23 Food
24 Gait training
25 Growth/development
26 Homemaking
27 Housing
28 Interaction
29 Lab findings
30 Legal system
31 Medical/dental care
32 Medication action/side effects
33 Medication administration
34 Medication set-up
35 Mobility/exercise
36 Nursing care, supplementary
37 Nutrition
38 Nutritionist
39 Ostomy care
40 Other community resource
41 Personal care
42 Positioning
43 Rehabilitation
44 Relaxation/breathing techniques
45 Rest/sleep
46 Safety
47 Screening
48 Sickness/injury care
49 Signs/symptoms - mental/emotional
50 Signs/symptoms - physical
51 Skin care
52 Social work/counseling
53 Specimen collection
54 Spiritual care
55 Stimulation/nurturance
56 Stress management
57 Substance use
58 Supplies
59 Support group
60 Support system
61 Transportation
62 Wellness
63 Other (specify)

Nursing Problem/Assessment Parameter

		CAT	TAR	INTERVENTIONS
35 NUTRITION Ann - eats mainly chips, pizza, sandwiches, cookies, pop. Cooks little.		I	37	Initiated Basic 4
14 CARETAKING/PARENTING Ann - not used to infant care. See Data Base. Will get formula from WIC before 4/9		I	21	Basic Bottle care. Left phone # for questions/worries.
17 GROWTH AND DEVELOPMENT Alex - asleep. See Data Base. Ann reports cord still on, drying, circumcision OK, applying vaseline regularly.		I	01	Normals for newborn; provided encouragement
33 ANTEPARTUM/POSTPARTUM See Data Base, WNL		I	14	Needs to soak episiotomy daily.
40 FAMILY PLANNING See Data Base				
2 OTHER PROBLEM Income - see Data Base		I	22	Budgeting, initiated
08 Role change - see Data Base, experiencing major changes		I	11	Encouraged

ASSESSMENT: Young mom who needs assistance. Seems receptive. Many strengths noted.

PLAN: (REVISIT-WHEN, PURPOSE) RV 4/9 / pm.
Examine + weigh Alex; observe handling.
Discussion of nutrition; Complete D.B.
Nurse's Signature Jane Klein, PHN

FIGURE 9–9 ■ The Family Visit Report is a problem-specific guide that incorporates the Intervention Scheme; it is used to document public health services that are provided during each home visit.

Each plan consisted of the following three parts: (1) categories, (2) targets, and (3) client-specific information generated by the nurse. Jane developed a plan of care for the five priority problems, the same problems for which she had completed Knowledge, Behavior, and Status ratings. The plans were designed to serve as a guide to probable interventions for the Bell family during the next 3 months. That coincides with the schedule Jane had established for reviewing all client data and the Knowledge, Behavior, and Status ratings. As part of her review, Jane expected to delete or add to the plans as appropriate and to schedule a time for the next review.

Jane used the Intervention Scheme as a framework to document the initial home visit with the Bells. She had the blank copy of the Family Visit Report with her and completed part of the documentation before she left the Bells' home (Fig. 9–9). Jane expected to follow the same procedure during subsequent home visits.

To maintain the continuity of the entire client record, the care that was actually provided during a given visit should be recorded in conjunction with (1) a specific problem and (2) the most current subjective/objective data associated with that problem. Thus, the same three-part format was used to describe both interventions and plans. For each problem and Jane's interventions (1) the category suggested the general direction of the intervention, (2) the target or object of the category provided specificity, and (3) the client-specific information that Jane generated allowed her to describe pertinent details unique to the Bell family. Within this documentation system, Jane not only identified the care she had provided but also described the client's response to nursing service.

The Bell Family example illustrates use of the Omaha System as a guide for practice and documentation. The thought processes of the nurse in a public health home visit program are demonstrated through use of record forms designed to reflect the Omaha System.

1. Referral and visit data provided the public health nurse with information needed for the Data Base. In turn, the Problem List was generated from the Data Base. The Problem Classification Scheme provided the framework and nomenclature for both the Data Base and the Problem List.
2. The Data Base and the Problem List provided the information the public health nurse needed to complete a baseline client outcome assessment. The Problem Rating Scale for Outcomes was used as the framework for the initial Knowledge, Behavior, and Status ratings for priority problems.
3. The public health nurse integrated the home visit data with all other parts of the Bell record to establish a Plan form and complete the Family Visit Report. The Intervention Scheme was used as the framework to document both the nurse's planned activities and those that occurred during the home visit.

Application — Mullen Family

The Mullen case study represents a compilation of forms (pp. 140–166). It includes (1) a description of the referral process and (2) the following VNA of Omaha and Polk County (WI) forms:

Figure 9–10, Public Health Referral (p. 141)
Figure 9–11, Patient Information Record (pp. 142–144)
Figure 9–12, Data Base/Problem List Worksheet (pp. 145–154)
Figure 9–13, Data Base (pp. 155–156)
Figures 9–14 and 9–20, Problem List (pp. 157–158 and 164)
Figures 9–15, 9–18, and 9–22, Public Health Nurse Record of Service from the Midland County (MI) Health Department (pp. 159, 162, and 165)
Figures 9–16 and 9–21, Nursing Care Plan from the Polk County (WI) Public Health Nursing Service (pp. 160 and 165)
Figure 9–17, Problem Rating Scale for Outcomes from the Polk County (WI) Public Health Nursing Service (p. 161)
Figure 9–19, Data Base Update (p. 163)

Mullen Family Case Example

The Mullens represent a hypothetical family referred to the VNA of Omaha by the VNA hospital coordinator and the pediatrician. Their daughter, born on March 17, 1990, had a cleft lip and palate. The mother and baby were discharged from the hospital on the third day after delivery. The family members were John, age 33; Sue, age 31; Vickie, age 2; and Karen, newborn (Figs. 9–10 and 9–11).

Sue Mullen had a normal vaginal delivery. Her newborn, Karen, weighed 6 pounds 2 ounces at birth and 5 pounds 13 ounces at dismissal; her length was 19 inches. Apgar scores were 8 and 9. Prior to dismissal, the hospital coordinator had seen the newborn and visited briefly with the mother. On the referral form she indicated that the public nurse from the VNA was to call the Mullen family, scheduling the first visit at a time when both parents might be home. The Mullens' insurance policy would cover service initiated within 3 days of hospital discharge. The coordinator also noted that the mother had received instruction and had fed the baby regularly at the hospital. The father visited infrequently and was reluctant to feed the infant.

The Mullen family was assigned to Jane Sherratt, a clinical specialist for handicapped children. As requested on the referral, Jane called the Mullens and scheduled a home visit at a time acceptable to both parents. When Jane arrived, Sue was home with her two daughters. She explained that John was detained at work. Jane conducted the home visit, using the Data Base/Problem List Worksheet as a guide for collecting initial data (Fig. 9–12). Secretarial staff typed a permanent Data Base and Problem List from the worksheet (Figs. 9–13 and 9–14). During the initial and subse-

FOR VNA USE ONLY   **THE VISITING NURSE ASSOCIATION OF OMAHA**   **FOR VNA USE ONLY**

DATE: __3/19/90__   H/HOLD #: __55849__   CT: __74.18__   URGENT VISIT _____ REASON _____

ACCOUNT #: _____

NOTIFIED HEALTH DEPT. __Yes__ _____ STATION: __VNCHS__

VNAM ☐   VNHR ☐   VNCHS ☒   Payment Discussed Y ☒ N ☐   FAX Y ☒ N ☐   S.S.# __506-48-3201__

SOURCE NAME: __Pediatrician – Dr. Charles Mark__   MEDICAID # _____ VERIFIED Y ☐

RELATIONSHIP: _____ PHONE _____   INS. __through work__

Previous VNA Record N ☒ Y ☐ DATE FROM _____ TO _____   POLICY # __ins. covers within 3 days__

REJECTED? ☐ ON _____   OTHER # _____

IS CLIENT AWARE OF REFERRAL? __yes__

HEAD OF HOUSEHOLD (Last Name, First) __Mullen, Sue__   BIRTH DATE __6/23/58__   SEX M ☐ F ☒   MARITAL STATUS S ☐ M ☒ W ☐ D ☐ SEP ☐

STREET ADDRESS: __1422 N. Metcalf__   CITY __Omaha__   ZIP __68111__   PHONE __553-2323__

VNA#	NAME	BIRTH DATE	SEX	VISITS	DATE
55851	Mullen, Karen	3/17/90	F		
55852	Mullen, Vickie	9/18/87	F		
55849	Mullen, Sue (mother)	6/23/58	F		
55850	Mullen, John (father)	1/02/57	M		

EMERGENCY CONTACT NAME: __Don & Kelly Siebenthal__   RELATIONSHIP: __neighbors__   PHONE: __551-2982__

REASON FOR REFERRAL: __Newborn with cleft lip and cleft palate. Birth weight 6 lbs. 2 oz. Length 19 in. No family in area. Needs reassurance and instruction. Mother instructed and fed baby regularly. Father visited infrequently and was reluctant to feed baby.__

EXPLANATION OF CARE REQUESTED: TREATMENTS, DRESSINGS, INJECTIONS, TEACHING, OBSERVATIONS, EVALUATIONS, OTHER __PHN determine frequency of home visits. Teach regarding cleft lip and cleft palate care and feeding procedures. Teach regarding normal newborn growth and development. Check weight every home visit. Assess needs for community resources. Emotional support. Social work referral if indicated by the case manager.__

MOTHER	**INFANT**
DIAGNOSIS: __Postpartum__	DIAGNOSIS: __newborn with cleft lip and palate__
PHYSICIAN: __Dr. Bioh, OB__	PHYSICIAN: __Dr. Charles Mark, pediatrician__
ADDRESS: __2240 Brown St.__	ADDRESS: __3415 Marinda St.__
PHONE: __331-4680__	PHONE: __333-0482__
HOSPITAL __Immanuel__ DATES: __3/17__ TO __3/19__	HOSPITAL __Immanuel__
	BIRTH WEIGHT: __6 lbs. 2 oz.__
E.D.C. __3/25/90__ BREAST FEEDING: __No__	APGAR: _____ 1 MIN __8__ 5 MIN __9__
	GESTATION: __39 weeks__
DELIVERY DATE: __3/17/90__ TYPE __normal vaginal__	FORMULA TYPE: __Similac 20 with Iron__ AMT. __2 oz. q 2½-3 hours and p.r.n.__
BONDING: __Starting to bond__	
B.P.: __128/86__ MENTAL STATUS __appropriately concerned about care for newborn__	MEDICATIONS & DOSAGE: _____
MEDICATION & DOSAGE: __Ortho Novum, start date per doctors orders__	RETURN APPOINTMENT __10 days__
M.D. SIGNATURE: _____	R.N. SIGNATURE: _Andi Leo-Gofta RN_

ADDITIONAL INFORMATION ATTACHED SHEET Y ☐ N ☒

FIGURE 9-10 ■ The Public Health Referral is the initial document used to gather data before client service is initiated.

```
------------------------------------------------------------------------
                    PATIENT  INFORMATION  RECORD                  PAGE    1
------------------------------------------------------------------------

Household #:   55849                    Station: VHCHS-NORTH
Address 1:   1422 N. METCALF              Phone: 402 553-2323
Address 2:                          Census Tract: 74.18
City/St/Zip: OMAHA          NE 68111  Monthly Income: 5,844
Directions:
Case Manager:   JANE SHERRATT

                       ACCOUNTS IN HOUSEHOLD
Patient's Name:              Account #:   Birth Date:     Rel. to HH:
MULLEN, SUE                      55849    6/23/1958       WIFE
MULLEN, JOHN                     55850    1/02/1957       HEAD OF HOUSEHOLD
MULLEN, KAREN                    55851    3/17/1990       DAUGHTER
MULLEN, VICKIE                   55852    9/18/1987 -NA   DAUGHTER
------------------------------------------------------------------------
------------------------------------------------------------------------
Patient's Name:              Account #:
MULLEN, SUE                      55849


** EMERGENCY INFORMATION     Relation:  Address:             Phone:
   SIEBENTHAL, DON & KELLY   NEIGHBORS                    402 551-2982

** ADMISSION INFORMATION
   Soc Sec #:   506-48-3201        Rel. to HH: W - WIFE
   Birth Date:     6/23/1958         Religion: 1- CATHOLIC
   Admit Date:     3/22/90       Referral Code: PRIVATE PHYSICIAN
   Refer Date:     3/19/90             Program: 240 - PRV HM CARE OTHER/DC
   1st Contact:    3/19/90                Race: 01- CAUCASIAN
   Care Started:   3/22/90                 Sex: FEMALE
   Plan Establ.:   3/22/90         Marital Sts: MARRIED
   Discharged:     0/00/00      Discharge Reason:
   Special Instructions:
   ICDA Diagnosis:


** DIAGNOSIS INFORMATION
   420      POSTPARTUM

** FUNDING SOURCES           Billing #:    Comment:          Effect Date:
   30- D.C. HEALTH DEPT.                                        3/22/90

** EMPLOYER - 47/ W.R. MANUFACTURING CO.

** OTHER AGENCIES            Contact:                  Phone:
   MD-OB                     DR BIOH               402 331-4680

                                              Orders Cover
                                          From Date:  To Date:
** PHYSICIAN INFORMATION
   DR. BIOH, OB                       787878
   2240 BROWN ST
   OMAHA          NE 68122
```

A

FIGURE 9–11 ■ (A–C) The Patient Information Record is a computer-generated facesheet that includes information obtained during the referral and admission process.

quent visits, Jane also used a Record of Service to document her care and the family's responses (Fig. 9–15).

After the visit, Jane thought about her experiences with other newborns who had cleft lips and cleft palates. She decided to call Tim McElroy, VNA social worker, asking that he accompany her on a shared visit in 1 week; she called Mrs. Mullen, who indicated approval of Jane's suggestion.

Although Jane felt very positive about many aspects of the Mullen family, their resources, and their strengths, she did have concerns. First, John Mullen was providing little caretaking assistance or emotional support to his wife at a time when she needed help. This was in contrast to his involvement when their toddler was a newborn. Second, his absence during the visit appeared to be another possible clue about his reaction to his new daughter.

According to plan, the nurse and social worker made a shared visit on March 31. When the public health nurse was reviewing feeding procedures and the baby's

```
    ------------------------------------------------------------------------
    ------------------------------------------------------------------------
                     PATIENT    INFORMATION    RECORD              PAGE    2
    ------------------------------------------------------------------------
       Household #:    55849
                                                     Station: VHCHS-NORTH

    ------------------------------------------------------------------------
    ------------------------------------------------------------------------
       Patient's Name:                  Account #:
       MULLEN, JOHN                        55850


       ** EMERGENCY INFORMATION        Relation:  Address:              Phone:

       ** ADMISSION INFORMATION
          Soc Sec #:   0                Rel. to HH: HH- HEAD OF HOUSEHOLD
          Birth Date:    1/02/1957        Religion:  1- CATHOLIC
          Admit Date:    3/22/90      Referral Code: VNA
          Refer Date:    3/19/90           Program: 240 - PRV HM CARE OTHER/DC
          1st Contact:   3/19/90              Race: 01- CAUCASIAN
          Care Started:  3/22/90               Sex: MALE
          Plan Establ.:  3/22/90       Marital Sts: MARRIED
          Discharged:    0/00/00      Discharge Reason:
          Special Instructions:
          ICDA Diagnosis:


       ** DIAGNOSIS INFORMATION

       ** FUNDING SOURCES            Billing #:      Comment:          Effect Date:
          30- D.C. HEALTH DEPT.                                         3/22/90

       ** EMPLOYER - 47/ W.R. MANUFACTURING CO.

       ** OTHER AGENCIES             Contact:                       Phone:


       ** PHYSICIAN INFORMATION               Orders Cover
                                          From Date:  To Date:


    ------------------------------------------------------------------------
    ------------------------------------------------------------------------
       Patient's Name:                  Account #:
       MULLEN, KAREN                       55851


       ** EMERGENCY INFORMATION        Relation:  Address:           Phone:
          WR MANUFACTURING, MOM WORK #                             402 978-6444

       ** ADMISSION INFORMATION
          Soc Sec #:   0                Rel. to HH: D - DAUGHTER
          Birth Date:    3/17/1990        Religion:  1- CATHOLIC
          Admit Date:    3/22/90      Referral Code: PRIVATE PHYSICIAN
          Refer Date:    3/19/89           Program: 240 - PRV HM CARE OTHER/DC
          1st Contact:   3/19/89              Race: 01- CAUCASIAN
          Care Started:  3/22/90               Sex: FEMALE
          Plan Establ.:  3/22/90       Marital Sts: SINGLE
          Discharged:    0/00/00      Discharge Reason:
          Special Instructions:
          ICDA Diagnosis:


       ** DIAGNOSIS INFORMATION
```

B

FIGURE 9–11 Continued

intake, Mr. Mullen excused himself to have a cigarette. Tim followed him outside and was able to get the new father to begin expressing his feelings and grief regarding his newborn and her cleft lip and palate. Following the home visit, the public health nurse and the social worker completed the Data Base/Problem List Worksheet that Jane had begun during the first visit. In addition, they (1) completed the Problem List, (2) initiated the two parts of the Nursing Care Plan (Figs. 9–16 and 9–17), and (3) completed a Record of Service (Fig. 9–

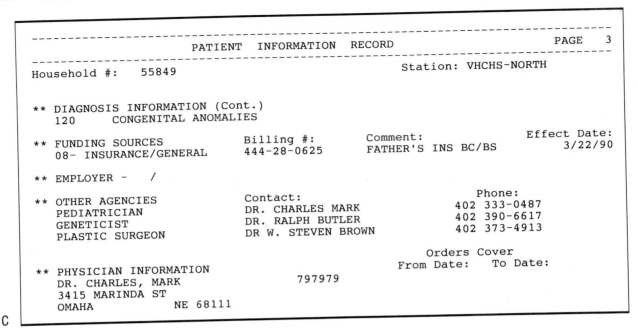

```
------------------------------------------------------------------
                 PATIENT   INFORMATION   RECORD          PAGE    3
------------------------------------------------------------------
                                       Station: VHCHS-NORTH
  Household #:    55849


  ** DIAGNOSIS INFORMATION (Cont.)
     120      CONGENITAL ANOMALIES

  ** FUNDING SOURCES          Billing #:     Comment:           Effect Date:
     08- INSURANCE/GENERAL    444-28-0625    FATHER'S INS BC/BS     3/22/90

  ** EMPLOYER -     /

  ** OTHER AGENCIES           Contact:                Phone:
     PEDIATRICIAN             DR. CHARLES MARK        402 333-0487
     GENETICIST               DR. RALPH BUTLER        402 390-6617
     PLASTIC SURGEON          DR W. STEVEN BROWN      402 373-4913

                                                 Orders Cover
                                           From Date:   To Date:
  ** PHYSICIAN INFORMATION
     DR. CHARLES, MARK                797979
     3415 MARINDA ST
     OMAHA        NE 68111
```
C

FIGURE 9–11 *Continued*

18). They agreed on most of the documentation, but they had a difference of opinion about the presence of 09. Interpersonal Relationship and 36. Sleep and Rest Patterns. They decided to observe two areas: the father's progress as he worked through his grief response, and the mother's return to their normal sleeping patterns. Adding data to the Data Base, problems to the Problem List, or problem-specific ratings and plans could be performed by either the public health nurse or social worker at any future date.

The public health nurse and the social worker made 12 more home visits during the next 4 months. Some visits they made individually; they shared others. Both professionals worked with all family members and their problems. The public health nurse assumed primary responsibility for (1) Sue in relation to caretaking, postpartum care, and sibling rivalry concerns, and (2) Karen in relation to infant care and physiologic problems. The social worker assumed primary responsibility for working with both parents in relation to grief and coordination of community resources, but the public health nurse was also directly involved in these efforts.

A Record of Service form was completed every time either professional made a home visit (See Fig. 9–18). Due to concern about Karen's development and her parents' coping abilities, the public health nurse and social worker discussed the Knowledge, Behavior, and Status ratings for the family's problems as well as their care plans. Because they were pleased with the family's progress, they waited to update the ratings and plans until after Karen's facial surgery was completed.

The oral surgeon repaired Karen Mullen's cleft lip in July when she was 4 months old. Jane scheduled a shared home visit for the first post-hospitalization day.

When she and Tim arrived, Sue was home with her two daughters. She explained that John had packed his clothes and moved out the evening before, having decided that the "entire situation was too much for him" and that he was unwilling to have so many family responsibilities. Because of the major changes in the family, the Data Base, Problem List, Problem Rating Scale for Outcomes, and Nursing Care Plan were updated (Figs. 9–19, 9–20, 9–17, and 9–21). A Record of Service was also completed (Fig. 9–22).

The nurse and the social worker changed the modifier for problem 01. Income from Health Promotion to Actual, based on the decrease in income caused by John leaving the home and Sue's knowledge of her financial situation. They identified 09. Interpersonal Relationship: Impairment due to the recent separation. Another problem area that they considered was 08. Role Change. However, they decided that data related to this problem could be subsumed in problem areas 06. Communication With Community Resources and 09. Interpersonal Relationship for the present.

The Bell and Mullen family records are not intended to be complete. Agency policy often requires additional documentation methods such as growth grids, immunization and medication records, Denver Developmental Screening Test (DDST) reports, interagency communication forms, and physician order forms. The Omaha System is compatible with a variety of forms. Some agencies use the Omaha System with a handwritten record, whereas others use it with a computerized record; some agencies use it with a record that is partially handwritten and partially computerized. The Bell and Mullen forms reflect that diversity.

Text continued on page 166

DATA BASE/PROBLEM LIST WORKSHEET

Instructions: Circle **one** choice (Adequate, Not Assessed, Not Applicable, Health Promotion, Potential **or** Deficit/Impairment/ Actual). CIRCLE F (Family) **or** I (Individual) **only** when using Health Promotion, Potential, or Deficit/Impairment/Actual. If Potential is circled, Risk Factors must be listed. If Deficit/Impairment is circled, one or more Signs/Symptoms (S/S) must be circled. If S/S are circled, elaboration must be included in the comments section. Starred (*) items on the worksheet must be completed.

Date Admitted _3/22/90_
Date Completed _3/31/90_
Nurse Name _J. Sherratt/T. McElroy_
Family Name _Mullen_
Household # _55849_
Account # _55849 Sue_
Account # _55850 John_
Account # _55851 Karen_

DOMAIN I. ENVIRONMENTAL

01. INCOME:
Adequate   Not Assessed   Not Applicable   (Health Promotion)
*Source _John-systems analyst; Sue-chemist @ W.R._
Manufacturing Co. _____ Amount _adequate_
(F)
I   **Potential**, Risk Factors:_____
Deficit, S/S: 1) low/no income 2) uninsured medical expenses
3) inadequate money management 4) able to buy only
_____ necessities 5) difficulty buying necessities 6) other _____

Medical insurance through employer; unsure about coverage for future expenses. Sue - 6 wk. maternity leave w/ pay

02. SANITATION:
(Adequate)   Not Assessed   Not Applicable   Health Promotion
F   **Potential**, Risk Factors:_____
I   **Deficit**, S/S: 1) soiled living area 2) inadequate food storage/
disposal 3) insects/ rodents 4) foul odor 5) inadequate water
supply 6) inadequate sewage disposal 7) inadequate laundry
facilities 8) allergens 9) infectious/contaminating agents
_____ 10) other _____

03. RESIDENCE:
(Adequate)   Not Assessed   Not Applicable   Health Promotion
*Type _4 bedroom, 2 story_
(Own)   Rent
F   **Potential**, Risk Factors:_____
I   **Deficit**, S/S: 1) structurally unsound 2) inadequate heating/
cooling 3)steep stairs 4)inadequate/obstructed exits/entries
5) cluttered living space 6) unsafe storage of dangerous
objects/substances 7) unsafe mats/throw rugs 8) inadequate
safety devices 9) presence of lead-based paint 10) unsafe
gas/electrical appliances 11) inadequate/crowded living space
_____ 12) homeless 13) other _____

Baby's rm. newly decorated. Many toys for baby and Vickie. Well cared for home.

04. NEIGHBORHOOD/WORKPLACE SAFETY:
(Adequate)   Not Assessed   Not Applicable   Health Promotion
F   **Potential**, Risk Factors:_____
I   **Deficit**, S/S: 1) high crime rate 2) high pollution level
3) uncontrolled animals 4) physical hazards 5) unsafe play
_____ area 6) other _____

05. OTHER: S/S: 1) other

*Environmental Assessment: _Adequate environment. Pursue ins. benefits vs. anticipated bills later. May need ref. to Medically Handicapped Children's Program._

A

FIGURE 9–12 ■ (A–J) The Data Base/Problem List Worksheet is an assessment tool for obtaining family and individual information related to the entire Problem Classification Scheme; the tool was designed for use in public health and home health settings.

DOMAIN II. PSYCHOSOCIAL

06. COMMUNICATION WITH COMMUNITY RESOURCES:

Adequate Not Assessed Not Applicable Health Promotion

*Transportation Resources _2 cars_

(F) **Potential**, Risk Factors: _____

I (**Impairment**) S/S: (1) unfamiliar with options/procedures for obtaining services 2) difficulty understanding roles/regulations of service providers 3) unable to communicate concerns to

service provider 4) dissatisfaction with services 5) language

_____ barrier 6) inadequate/unavailable resources 7) other _____

07. SOCIAL CONTACT:

(Adequate) Not Assessed Not Applicable Health Promotion

*Support System _No immediate or extended family in area. Moved to Omaha 6 mos. ago_

F **Potential**, Risk Factors: _____

I **Impairment**, S/S: 1) limited social contact 2) uses health care

provider for social contact 3) minimal outside stimulation/

_____ leisure time activities 4) other _____

08. ROLE CHANGE:

(Adequate) Not Assessed Not Applicable Health Promotion

F **Potential**, Risk Factors: _____

I **Impairment**, S/S: 1) involuntary reversal of traditional male/

female roles 2) involuntary reversal of dependent/independent

_____ roles 3) assumes new role 4) loses previous role 5) other

09. INTERPERSONAL RELATIONSHIP:

(Adequate) Not Assessed Not Applicable Health Promotion

F **Potential**, Risk Factors: _____

I **Impairment**, S/S: 1) difficulty establishing/maintaining relationships 2) minimal shared activities 3) incongruent values/goals 4) inadequate interpersonal communication skills

5) prolonged, unrelieved tension 6) inappropriate suspicion/

_____ manipulation/compulsion/aggression 7) other _____

10. SPIRITUAL DISTRESS:

(Adequate) Not Assessed Not Applicable Health Promotion

F **Potential**, Risk Factors: _____

I **Actual**, S/S: 1) expresses spiritual concerns 2) disrupted

spiritual rituals 3) disrupted spiritual trust 4) conflicting

_____ spiritual beliefs and medical regimen 5) other _____

11. GRIEF:

Adequate Not Assessed Not Applicable Health Promotion

(F) **Potential**, Risk Factors: _____

I (**Impairment**) S/S: 1) fails to recognize normal grief responses

(2) difficulty coping with grief responses 3) difficulty expressing

grief responses (4) conflicting stages of grief process among

_____ family/individual 5) other _____

birth, not ready to feed Karen; in denial; often works late.

Household # _55849_

Has no resource or support grp info other than oral surgeon.

Neighbor willing to help w/ child care. Had pvt. sitter for Vickie. Couple have numerous friends through work.

Couple seem to have warm relationship

Attending St. John's Catholic Church

Both parents "shocked" in delivery rm by cleft lip/palate. Sue-OB & RNs very supportive, asked if she could be "responsible." Eager to learn everything she can to help infant. No family hx. John fed Vickie soon p̄

B

FIGURE 9-12 Continued

12. EMOTIONAL STABILITY:

(Adequate) Not Assessed   Not Applicable   Health Promotion

F   **Potential**, Risk Factors: _____

I   **Impairment**, S/S: 1) sadness/hopelessness/worthlessness
2) apprehension/undefined fear 3) loss of interest/involvement
in activities/self-care 4) narrowed perceptual focus 5) scattering
of attention 6) flat affect 7) irritable/agitated 8) purposeless

\#   activity 9) difficulty managing stress 10) somatic complaints/
chronic fatigue 11) expresses wish to die/attempts suicide
_____ 12) other _____

13. HUMAN SEXUALITY:

Adequate (Not Assessed) Not Applicable   Health Promotion

F   **Potential**, Risk Factors: _____

I   **Impairment**, S/S: 1) difficulty recognizing consequences of
sexual behavior 2) difficulty expressing intimacy 3) sexual

\#   identity confusion 4) sexual value confusion 5) dissatisfied with
_____ sexual relationships 6) other_____

14. CARETAKING/PARENTING:

Adequate   Not Assessed   Not Applicable   Health Promotion
*Primary Caregiver: _Sue_____

(F)   **Potential**, Risk Factors: _____

I   (Impairment) S/S: (1) difficulty providing physical care/safety
(2) difficulty providing emotional nurturance 3) difficulty providing
cognitive learning experiences and activities 4) difficulty
providing preventive and therapeutic health care 5) expectations
incongruent with stage of growth and development

\#   6) dissatisfaction/difficulty with responsibilities 7) neglectful
_____ 8) abusive 9) other _____

Birth defect, special fdg. needs
John participating little in child
care ; says baby "just eats &
sleeps." Vickie –very active,
healthy toddler.

15. NEGLECTED CHILD/ADULT:

(Adequate) Not Assessed   Not Applicable   Health Promotion

F   **Potential**, Risk Factors: _____

I   **Actual**, S/S: 1) lacks adequate physical care 2) lacks emotional
nurturance/support 3) lacks appropriate stimulation/cognitive

\#   experiences 4) inappropriately left alone 5) lacks necessary
_____ supervision 6) inadequate/ delayed medical care 7) other ____

16. ABUSED CHILD/ADULT:

(Adequate) Not Assessed   Not Applicable   Health Promotion

F   **Potential**, Risk Factors: _____

I   **Actual**, S/S: 1) harsh/excessive discipline 2) welts/bruises/
burns 3) questionable explanation of injury 4) attacked
verbally 5) fearful/hypervigilant behavior 6) violent

\#   environment 7) consistently negative messages 8) assaulted
_____ sexually 9) Other _____

C

FIGURE 9-12 Continued

17. GROWTH AND DEVELOPMENT OF CHILD/ADULT:
Adequate   Not Assessed   Not Applicable   Health Promotion
Height _19"_ Weight _6#2_ Head Circumference _13 3/8 "today_
Feeding _Similac 20 w/ Fe 2 oz q 2½-3 hr_
Newborn PA _WNL except for cleft lip/palate_

F   **Potential,** Risk Factors: _____
(I)   (Impairment,) S/S: 1) abnormal results of development
      screening tests 2) abnormal weight/height/head circumference
      in relation to growth curve/age 3) age inappropriate behavior
(4)) inadequate achievement/maintenance of developmental
Karen tasks 5) other _____

18. OTHER: S/S: 1) Other

*Psychosocial Assessment: _Need to determine impact of Karen's cleft lip/palate on couple's_
relationship. Need ref. to parent support grp & school. Parents not in same stage of grief. Karen-
otherwise normal infant.   Vickie — normal toddler.

DOMAIN III. PHYSIOLOGICAL

19. HEARING:
      Adequate   Not Assessed   Not Applicable   Health Promotion
      Correction _____
F   (Potential,) Risk Factors: _Hearing loss 2° URIs & OM_
(I)   Impairment, R _____ L _____ S/S: 1) difficulty hearing normal
speech tones 2) absent/abnormal response to sound
Karen 3) abnormal results of hearing screening test 4) other _____

20. VISION:
      (Adequate) Not Assessed   Not Applicable   Health Promotion
      Correction _____
F   **Potential,** Risk Factors: _____
I   Impairment, R _____ L _____ S/S: 1) difficulty seeing small print/
      calibrations 2) difficulty seeing distant objects 3) difficulty
      seeing close objects 4) absent/abnormal response to visual
      stimuli 5) abnormal results of vision screening test
6) squinting/blinking/tearing/blurring 7) difficulty differentiating
_____ colors 8) other _____

21. SPEECH AND LANGUAGE:
      Adequate   Not Assessed   Not Applicable   Health Promotion
F   (Potential,) Risk Factors: _for delayed & distorted speech_
(I)   Impairment, S/S: 1) absent/abnormal ability to speak
      2) absent/abnormal ability to understand 3) lacks alternative
      communication skills 4) inappropriate sentence structure
5) limited enunciation/clarity 6) inappropriate word usage
Karen 7) other _____

22. DENTITION:
      Adequate   Not Assessed   Not Applicable   Health Promotion
      Correction _____
F   (Potential,) Risk Factors: _likely to have abnormally placed teeth_
(I)   Impairment, S/S: 1) abnormalities of teeth 2) sore/swollen/
      bleeding gums 3) ill-fitting dentures 4) malocclusion 5) other
#
Karen

Household # ___55849___

wt 6#1 oz today T 98.4 R AP120
R 40. Unable to create negative
sucking pressure. Falls asleep
during fdg. No quiet-alert
state.

Vickie — no URI now. Sue
anxious for warm weather

D

FIGURE 9-12 *Continued*

23. **COGNITION:**

F
I

(Adequate) Not Assessed   Not Applicable   Health Promotion
Potential, Risk Factors: _____
Impairment, S/S: 1) diminished judgment 2) disoriented to time/place/person 3) limited recall of recent events 4) limited recall of long past events 5) limited calculating/sequencing skills 6) limited concentration 7) limited reasoning/abstract thinking ability 8) impulsiveness 9) repetitive language/

\#

behavior 10) other _____

_____

24. **PAIN:**

F
I

Adequate   Not Assessed (Not Applicable) Health Promotion
Potential, Risk Factors: _____
Actual, Description _____

Relieved by: _____
S/S: 1) expresses discomfort/pain 2) elevated pulse/respirations/blood pressure 3) compensated movement/guarding 4) restless behavior 5) facial grimaces 6) pallor/

\#

perspiration 7) other _____

_____

25. **CONSCIOUSNESS:**

F
I

Adequate   Not Assessed (Not Applicable) Health Promotion
Potential, Risk Factors: _____
Impairment, S/S: 1) lethargic 2) stuporous 3) unresponsive 4) comatose 5) other _____

\#

_____

26. **INTEGUMENT:**

F
(I)
\#
Karen

Adequate   Not Assessed   Not Applicable   Health Promotion
(Potential) Risk Factors: _exposed mucosa likely to be traumatized_
Impairment, S/S: 1) lesion 2) rash 3) excessively dry 4) excessively oily 5) inflammation 6) pruritus 7) drainage 8) ecchymosis 9) hypertrophy of nails 10) other _____

_____

27. **NEURO-MUSCULO-SKELETAL FUNCTION:**

(Adequate) Not Assessed   Not Applicable   Health Promotion
Assistive Devices _____

_____

F
I

Potential, Risk Factors: _____
Impairment, S/S: 1) limited range of motion 2) decreased muscle strength 3) decreased coordination 4) decreased muscle tone 5) increased muscle tone 6) decreased sensation 7) increased sensation 8) decreased balance

\#

9) gait/ambulation disturbance 10) difficulty managing activities of daily living 11) tremors/seizures 12) other _____

_____

Mucous membrane moist & intact.
Sleeps in prone part of the time.

E

FIGURE 9–12 *Continued*

28. **RESPIRATION:**
   (Adequate) Not Assessed   Not Applicable   Health Promotion
   Rate _18_ Assistive Devices _____
   _____Sue_____

F **Potential**, Risk Factors:_____
I **Impairment**, S/S: 1) abnormal breathing patterns 2) unable to
   breathe independently 3) cough 4) unable to cough/
   expectorate independently 5) cyanosis 6) abnormal sputum
7) noisy respirations 8) rhinorrhea 9) abnormal breath sounds
   _____ 10) other _____

29. **CIRCULATION:**
   (Adequate) Not Assessed   Not Applicable   Health Promotion
   Temp _98.6_ Assistive Devices _____
   _____Sue_____
   BP: sitting R _____ L $^{122}/_{82}$; standing R _____ L _____ ;
   lying R _____ L _____
   Pulses: apical _____ radial_____ peripheral _____

F **Potential,** Risk Factors: _____
I **Impairment,** S/S: 1) edema 2) cramping/pain of extremities
   3) decreased pulses 4) discoloration of skin/cyanosis
   5) temperature change in affected area 6) varicosities
   7) syncopal episodes 8) abnormal blood pressure reading
   9) pulse deficit 10) irregular heart rate 11) excessively rapid
heart rate 12) excessively slow heart rate 13) anginal pain
   _____ 14) abnormal heart sounds 15) other _____

30. **DIGESTION-HYDRATION:**
   Adequate   Not Assessed   Not Applicable   Health Promotion
   Assistive Devices _____

F **Potential**, Risk Factors: _____
(I) (Impairment) S/S: 1) nausea/vomiting (2) difficulty/inability to
   chew/swallow/digest 3) indigestion/reflux 4) anorexia
   5) anemia 6) ascites 7) jaundice/liver enlargement
8) decreased skin turgor 9) cracked lips/dry mouth
   Karen 10) electrolyte imbalance 11) other _____

Taking 1-1½ oz. at some fdgs - esp. at night. Fdgs. take 45-60 min. c̄ reg. bottle/nipple. Some nipples cross cut & some c̄ holes.

Sue - soft, daily BM

31. **BOWEL FUNCTION:**
   (Adequate) Not Assessed   Not Applicable   Health Promotion
   Assistive Devices _____

F **Potential**, Risk Factors: _____
I **Impairment**, S/S: 1) abnormal frequency/consistency of stool
   2) painful defecation 3) decreased bowel sounds 4) blood in
   stools 5) abnormal color 6) cramping/abdominal discomfort
_____ 7) incontinent of stool 8) other _____

F

FIGURE 9-12 *Continued*

32. GENITO-URINARY FUNCTION:

(Adequate) Not Assessed   Not Applicable   Health Promotion

Assistive Devices _____

F   **Potential**, Risk Factors: _____

I   **Impairment**, S/S: 1) incontinent of urine 2) urgency/frequency
3) burning/painful urination 4) difficulty emptying bladder
5) abnormal urinary frequency/amount 6) hematuria
7) abnormal discharge 8) abnormal menstrual pattern

\#   9) abnormal lumps/swelling/tenderness of male/female
reproductive organs 10) dyspareunia 11) other _____

Household # _55849_

Sue — no hx UTIs

33. ANTEPARTUM/POSTPARTUM:

(Adequate) Not Assessed   Not Applicable   Health Promotion

AP: *TPAL _2002_ ___ EDC _____ Date OB Care _2nd mo_
Fetal Act/FHR _____
L&D Prep _____ Abn Lab _____
Danger Sig _____ Preterm Labor _____

PP: Del Date _3/17/90_ Bonding _Mom starting to bond_
8-point check _WNL; ↓ serosa lochia, fundus non-palpable_

F   **Potential**, Risk Factors: _____

I   **Impairment**, S/S: 1) difficulty coping with pregnancy/body
changes 2) inappropriate exercise/rest/diet/behaviors

\#   3) discomforts 4) complications 5) fears delivery procedure
6) difficulty breast-feeding 7) other _____

*TPAL = Term (36–42 wk), Preterm (under 36 wk), Abortions, Living
Children

_Dad rarely looks @ infant, did
not hold during hosp. stay_

34. OTHER: S/S: 1) other _____

*Physiological Assessment: _Sue- normal PP course. Noted no other physiological probs. in HH except
Karen. Doesn't have appropriate bottles/nipples; exhausted by fdg; risk for wt. loss & dev.
delays._

DOMAIN IV. HEALTH RELATED BEHAVIORS

35. NUTRITION:

(Adequate) Not Assessed   Not Applicable   Health Promotion

Sue Height _5'2"_ Weight _130#_ Diet _reg._

F   **Potential**, Risk Factors: _____

I   **Impairment**, S/S: 1) weighs 10% more than average
2) weighs 10% less than average 3) lacks established
standards for daily caloric/fluid intake 4) exceeds established
standards for daily caloric/fluid intake 5) unbalanced diet
6) improper feeding schedule for age 7) nonadherence to

\#   prescribed diet 8) unexplained/progressive weight loss
9) hypoglycemia 10) hyperglycemia 11) other _____

_AP wt 118#_

Karen - see probs # 17 & 30

36. SLEEP AND REST PATTERNS:

(Adequate) Not Assessed   Not Applicable   Health Promotion

F   **Potential**, Risk Factors: _____

I   **Impairment**, S/S: 1) sleep/rest pattern disrupts family
2) frequently wakes during night 3) somnambulism

\#   4) insomnia 5) nightmares 6) insufficient sleep/rest for age/
physical condition 7) other _____

_Sue doing nighttime fdgs. &
napping when toddler naps
except when fdg. baby._

G

FIGURE 9–12 Continued

37. PHYSICAL ACTIVITY:

(Adequate) Not Assessed   Not Applicable   Health Promotion

F   **Potential**, Risk Factors:_____

I   **Impairment**, S/S: 1) sedentary life style 2) inadequate/
inconsistent exercise routine 3) inappropriate type/amount of

exercise for age/physical condition 4) other _____

_____

38. PERSONAL HYGIENE:

(Adequate) Not Assessed   Not Applicable   Health Promotion

F   **Potential**, Risk Factors:_____

I   **Impairment**, S/S: 1) inadequate laundering of clothing
2) inadequate bathing 3) body odor 4) inadequate

shampooing/combing of hair 5) inadequate brushing/flossing/

_____ mouth care 6) other _____

Trying to quit smoking.
Neither parent uses other drugs.

39. SUBSTANCE USE:

Adequate   Not Assessed   Not Applicable   Health Promotion

F   **Potential**, Risk Factors:

(I) (Impairment) S/S: 1) abuses over-the-counter/street drugs

2) abuses alcohol (3) smokes 4) difficulty performing normal

John   routines 5) reflex disturbances 6) behavior change 7) other

40. FAMILY PLANNING

(Adequate) Not Assessed   Not Applicable   Health Promotion

Methods *will resume Ortho-Novum. Used*
satisfactorily before

F   **Potential**, Risk Factors: _____

I   **Impairment**, S/S: 1) inappropriate/insufficient knowledge of
family planning methods 2) inaccurate/inconsistent use of

family planning methods 3) dissatisfied with present family

_____ planning method 4) other _____

Karen – Dr. Mark, pediatrics
Has appt. in 10 days. Already
seen by oral surgeon & geneticist
Lip surgery not planned until
wt 8-10#; palate surgery p̄
1 yr.

41. HEALTH CARE SUPERVISION:

(Adequate) Not Assessed   Not Applicable   Health Promotion

*Routine care plans *Sue- Dr. Bioh, OB Will return*
for 6 wk exam
*Emergency care plans *911, neighbors*

f   **Potential**, Risk Factors:_____

I   **Impairment**, S/S: 1) fails to obtain routine medical/dental
evaluation 2) fails to seek care for symptoms requiring
medical/dental evaluation 3) fails to return as requested to
physician/dentist 4) inability to coordinate multiple
appointments/regimens 5) inconsistent source of medical/

dental care 6) inadequate prescribed medical/dental regimen

_____ 7) other _____

42. PRESCRIBED MEDICATION REGIMEN:

Adequate   (Not Assessed)   Not Applicable   Health Promotion

F   **Potential**, Risk Factors: _____

I   **Impairment**, S/S: 1) deviates from prescribed dosage/
schedule 2) demonstrates side effects 3) inadequate system
for taking medication 4) improper storage of medication 5)fails

to obtain refills appropriately 6) fails to obtain immunizations

_____ 7) other _____

Household # __55849__

H
FIGURE 9-12 *Continued*

43. TECHNICAL PROCEDURE:
        Adequate (Not Assessed) Not Applicable   Health Promotion

F   **Potential**, Risk Factors: _____

I   **Impairment**, S/S: 1) unable to demonstrate/relate procedure
      accurately 2) does not follow/demonstrate principles of safe/
      aseptic techniques 3) procedure requires nursing skill

4) unable/unwilling to perform procedure without assistance
   ——5) unable/unwilling to operate special equipment 6) other ____
   _____

Household # _55849_

_____

_____

_____

_____

_____

44. OTHER: S/S: 1) Other

***Health Behavior**
Assessment: _Family nutrition adequate; discuss Vickie's diet in future_ _____

_____

_____

_____

_____

Significant Planning Factors: _____

_____

_____

_____

***Homebound Status:** _____

_____

_____

_____

HEALTH HISTORY
Significant Medical History of Client(s)

Hospitalizations:

_____

_____

_____

_____

Pregnancies: _Sue_

2nd — both normal _____

_____

_____

Surgeries:

_____

_____

_____

Injuries:

_____

_____

_____

FIGURE 9–12 _Continued_

MEDICAL HISTORY OF CLIENT AND FAMILY MEMBERS

Complete column(s) below indicating client's name(s) and relationship of other pertinent family members. Focus on specific family history as it contributes to client care.

Diagnosis	Name/Relationship					
Diabetes						
Epilepsy						
Cardiac Disease						
Hypertension						
CVA						
Arthritis/Gout						
Cancer						
Frequent Headaches/Migraines						
Asthma/Allergies						
Respiratory Disease						
SIDS						
GI Problems/Ulcers						
Kidney/Bladder Problems						
Phlebitis/Varicose Veins						
Drug/Alcohol Abuse						
Mental Retardation						
Mental Illness						
Other *no hx cleft lip/palate or other birth defects*						

ASSESSMENT/COMMENTS: *No significant hx; gather additional data on following visits*

J

FIGURE 9-12 *Continued*

154

```
------------------------------------------------------------------
              * * * D A T A  B A S E * * *                 PAGE   1
HOUSEHOLD #:    55849    1422 N. METCALF     STATION- VHCHS-NORTH
------------------------------------------------------------------
                    ACCOUNTS IN HOUSEHOLD
Patient's Name:           Account #:       From Date:
MULLEN, SUE                 55849          3/22/90
MULLEN, JOHN                55850          3/22/90
MULLEN, KAREN               55851          3/22/90
MULLEN, VICKIE              55852          3/22/90 - NOT ADMITTED
------------------------------------------------------------------
```

DATE ADMITTED: 03/22/89

ENVIRONMENTAL DOMAIN: All areas assessed with significant findings as
follows: INCOME: Source: John - Systems Analyst; Sue - Chemist at
W.R. Manufacturing Co. Amount: Adequate. Medical insurance through
employer. Unsure about coverage for future expenses. Sue - 6 week
maternity leave with pay. RESIDENCE: Type: 4-bedroom, 2-story/own.
Baby's room newly decorated. Many toys for baby and Vickie. Well
cared for home.

A: ADEQUATE ENVIRONMENT. PURSUE INSURANCE BENEFITS VERSUS ANTICIPATED
BILLS LATER. MAY NEED REFERRAL TO MEDICALLY HANDICAPPED CHILDREN'S
PROGRAM.

PSYCHOSOCIAL DOMAIN: All areas assessed with significant findings as
follows: COMMUNICATION WITH COMMUNITY RESOURCES: Transportation
Resources: 2 cars. Has no resource or support group information other
than oral surgeon. SOCIAL CONTACT: Support System: No immediate or
extended family in area. Moved to Omaha 6 months ago. Neighbor
willing to help with child care. Had private sitter for Vickie.
Couple have numerous friends through work. INTERPERSONAL RELATIONSHIP:
Couple seem to have warm relationship. SPIRITUAL DISTRESS: Attending
St. John's Catholic Church. Not certain if will continue. GRIEF:
Both parents "shocked" in delivery room by cleft lip/palate. Sue - OB
and nurses were very supportive; asked if she could be "responsible".
Eager to learn everything she can do to help infant. No family
history. John fed Vickie soon after birth, not ready to feed Karen; in
denial; often works late. CARETAKING/PARENTING: Primary Caregiver:
Sue. Birth defect, special feeding needs. John participating little
in child care; says baby "just eats and sleeps". Vickie very active,
healthy toddler. GROWTH AND DEVELOPMENT OF CHILD/ADULT: Height 19
in., weight 6 lbs. 2 oz. at birth, head circumference 13 3/8 in.
(today). Feeding: Similac 20 with Iron 2 oz. q 2 1/2-3 hours.
Newborn PA: WNL except for cleft lip/palate. Weight 6 lbs. 1 oz.
today. Temp. 98.4 rectally, AP 120, R 40. Unable to create negative
sucking pressure. Falls asleep during feeding. No quiet-alert state.
Areas Not Assessed: Human Sexuality.

A: NEED TO DETERMINE IMPACT OF KAREN'S CLEFT LIP/PALATE ON COUPLE'S
RELATIONSHIP. NEEDS REFERRAL TO PARENT SUPPORT GROUP AND SCHOOL.
PARENTS NOT IN SAME STAGE OF GRIEF. KAREN - OTHERWISE NORMAL INFANT.
VICKIE - NORMAL TODDLER.

PHYSIOLOGICAL DOMAIN: All areas assessed with significant findings as
follows: HEARING: Hearing loss secondary to URIs and OM. Vickie - no

```
------------------------------------------------------------------
```

A

FIGURE 9-13 ■ (*A and B*) The Data Base is a computer-generated form developed from the Data Base/Problem List Worksheet.

```
-------------------------------------------------------------------------------
       * * *  D A T A   B A S E  * * *                     PAGE   2
   HOUSEHOLD #:   55849    1422 N. METCALF      STATION- VHCHS-NORTH
-------------------------------------------------------------------------------
```

URI now. Sue anxious for warm weather. SPEECH AND LANGUAGE: Risk
Factors for delayed and distorted speech. DENTITION: Likely to have
abnormally placed teeth. INTEGUMENT: Exposed mucosa likely to be
traumatized. Mucous membranes moist and intact. Sleeps in prone part
of the time. RESPIRATION: SUE: Rate 18. CIRCULATION: SUE: Temp
98.6, BP sitting left 122/82. DIGESTION-HYDRATION: Talung 1-1 1/2 oz.
at some feedings, especially at night. Feedings take 45-60 min. with
regular bottle and nipple. Some nipples crosscut and some with holes.
BOWEL FUNCTION: SUE: Soft, daily BM. GENITO-URINARY FUNCTION: SUE:
No history UTIs. ANTEPARTUM/POSTPARTUM: TPAL 2002. Date OB Care:
2nd month. Delivery date: 3/17/90. Bonding: Mother starting to
bond. Father rarely looks at infant; did not hold during visit. 8
point check: WNL including diminished serosa lochia; fundus
non-palpable.

A: SUE - NORMAL PP COURSE. NOTED NO OTHER PHYSIOLOGICAL PROBLEMS
IN HOUSEHOLD EXCEPT KAREN. DOESN'T HAVE APPROPRIATE BOTTLE/NIPPLE;
EXHAUSTED BY FEEDINGS; AT RISK FOR WEIGHT LOSS AND DEVELOPMENTAL DELAY.

HEALTH RELATED BEHAVIORS DOMAIN: All areas assessed with significant
findings as follows: NUTRITION: SUE: Height 5 ft. 2 in., weight 130
lbs. Regular diet. AP weight 118 lbs. KAREN: See G&D and
Digestion-Hydration. SLEEP AND REST PATTERNS: Sue is doing nighttime
feedings and napping when toddler naps unless feeding baby. SUBSTANCE
MISUSE: John trying to quit smoking. Neither parent uses other drugs.
FAMILY PLANNING: Methods: Will resume Ortho-Novum. Used
satisfactorily before. HEALTH CARE SUPERVISION: Routine care plans:
SUE: Dr. Bioh, OB. Will return for 6 week exam. Emergency care
plans: 911, neighbors. KAREN: Dr. Mark, pediatrician; has
appointment in 10 days. Already seen by oral surgeon and geneticist.
Lip surgery not planned until weight 8-10 lbs.; palate surgery after 1
year. Areas Not Assessed: Prescribed Medication Regimen, Technical
Procedure.

A: FAMILY NUTRITION ADEQUATE. DISCUSS VICKIE'S DIET IN FUTURE.

HEALTH HISTORY: Significant Medical History of Client

Pregnancies:
SUE: 2nd - both normal

Medical History of Client and Family Members

No history of cleft lip/palate or other birth defects.

ASSESSMENT/COMMENTS: NO SIGNIFICANT HISTORY; GATHER ADDITIONAL DATA ON
FOLLOWING VISITS
        Jane Sherratt, RN
        Jane Sherratt, RN, Clinical Specialist/rip
        Tim McElroy, MSW
        Tim McElroy, MSW/rip

```
-------------------------------------------------------------------------------
```

B

FIGURE 9-13 *Continued*

```
------------------------------------------------------------------------
            * * *  P R O B L E M   L I S T  * * *              PAGE   1
HOUSEHOLD #:    55849     1422 N. METCALF        STATION- VHCHS-NORTH
------------------------------------------------------------------------
                    ACCOUNTS IN HOUSEHOLD
Patient's Name:              Account #:        From Date:
MULLEN, SUE                     55849          3/22/90
MULLEN, JOHN                    55850          3/22/90
MULLEN, KAREN                   55851          3/22/90
MULLEN, VICKIE                  55852          3/22/90 - NOT ADMITTED
------------------------------------------------------------------------

* 03/31/90 FAMILY
            01A
        Income: Health Promotion

* 03/31/90 FAMILY
            06C
        Communication With Community Resources: Impairment

            0601
        Unfamiliar With Options/Procedures For Obtaining
        Services

* 03/31/90 FAMILY
            11C
        Grief: Impairment

            1102
        Difficulty Coping With Grief Responses

            1104
        Conflicting Stages Of Grief Process Among Family/
        Individual

* 03/31/90 FAMILY
            14C
        Caretaking/Parenting: Impairment

            1401
        Difficulty Providing Physical Care/Safety

            1402
        Difficulty Providing Emotional Nurturance

* 03/31/90 MULLEN, JOHN
            39C
        Substance Misuse: Actual

            3903
        Smokes

* 03/31/90 MULLEN, KAREN
            17C
        Growth And Development: Impairment

            1704

------------------------------------------------------------------------
            **
            **
            **
```

A

FIGURE 9-14 ■ (*A and B*) The Problem List is a computer-generated index of the client's health-related interests, concerns, and problems and is based on the Problem Classification Scheme.

```
--------------------------------------------------------------------------------
                  * * * P R O B L E M   L I S T * * *              PAGE  2
  HOUSEHOLD #:   55849    1422 N. METCALF        STATION- VHCHS-NORTH
--------------------------------------------------------------------------------
            Inadequate Achievement/Maintenance Of
            Developmental Tasks

  * 03/31/90 MULLEN, KAREN
            19B
            Hearing: Potential Impairment

  * 03/31/90 MULLEN, KAREN
            21B
            Speech And Language: Potential Impairment

  * 03/31/90 MULLEN, KAREN
            22B
            Dentition: Potential Impairment

  * 03/31/90 MULLEN, KAREN
            26B
            Integument: Potential Impairment

  * 03/31/90 MULLEN, KAREN
            30C
            Digestion-Hydration: Impairment

            3002
            Difficulty/Inability To Chew/Swallow/Digest
```
Jane Sherratt, RN
```
            Jane Sherratt, RN, Clinical Specialist/rip
```
Tim McElroy, MSW
```
            Tim McElroy, MSW/rip
```

```
--------------------------------------------------------------------------------
            **
            **
            **
```

B

FIGURE 9–14 *Continued*

MIDLAND COUNTY (MI) HEALTH DEPARTMENT
PUBLIC HEALTH NURSE RECORD OF SERVICE

NAME ___Mullen___

FF# ___55849___

Page ___1___

CODES:

Site:

HV = Home
OV = Office
SV = School
TC = Phone
NAH = Not at Home

Care Provided/Interventions:

Assmt = Assessment
HTG&C = Teaching
CAR = Coordination, Advocacy, and Referral
SUV = Surveillance

DATE	SITE	PROB. NO.	CARE PROVIDED	NARRATIVE	REVISIT DATE
3/22/90	HV	30	See Data Base HTGC: supplies HTGC: positioning	Gave Mead-Johnson disposable ch # p bottles w/lang premie cross cut nipple & demonstrated use. Demonstrated high sitting for fdg. & burping. Rinse mouth w/H₂0, clean nose PRN.	3/30/90
		11	HTGC: coping skills	Allowed to cry. Stages of grief & different ways couples react. Also freq. of chg.	
		17	See Data Base HTGC: Anatomy/physio.	Emphasized normals & similarity to Vickie. Need for mobile, cuddling, stimulation, etc. Kiss on top of head, not on face or hands. Avoid URIs.	
		06	HTGC, CAR: support group HTGC: education	Gave ph.# of Cleft Palate Grp @ BTNRI & Pilot Parents Support Grp. Will ask MD for reference to school program ō next HV. Discussed what each group offers.	
		14	See Data Base HTGC: coping skills	Many questions. Concerned about adequacy. Reassured, praised. Encouraged using neighbor who is willing to take Vickie several hrs. in AMs	
		33	See Data Base	Jane Sherrett, RN	

FIGURE 9–15 ■ The Public Health Nurse Record of Service reflects the Problem Classification Scheme, Intervention Scheme, and public health services that are provided during each home visit. (Courtesy of Midland Co. [MI] Health Department.)

POLK COUNTY PUBLIC HEALTH NURSING SERVICE

NURSING CARE PLAN

Original Nursing Office
Copy to RN

PATIENT NAME: Mullen
PATIENT NUMBER: 55849
PAGE: 2

PROBLEM NO.	PROBLEM TITLE	CATEGORY	TARGET	DATE OF PLAN	PATIENT SPECIFIC NURSING PLAN OF ACTION	DATE PROBLEM DC'D
06	Comm. w/comm. resources	1. Case mngt	16 education	3-31-90	Refer/coordinate w/school program	
		2. ↓	59 support grp	3-31-90	Refer/coord. w/Post Parents, Cleft Palate Grp @ BT-NRI	
		3. ↓	40 other comm res	3-31-90	Ref/coord. medically handicapped child program	
11.	Grief	1. HTG+C	11 coping skills	3-31-90	Analyze feelings	
		2. ↓	49 s/s ment/emot	3-31-90	norm. stages of grief, reactions of others	
		3. Surveillance	28 interaction	3-31-90	Active listening + support	
14	Caretaking/parenting	1. HTG+C	11 coping skills	3-31-90	Stress reduction, emphasize similarities w/1st child	
		2. ↓	21 fdg procedure	3-31-90	Ch+P bottle, cross cut nipples, hr sitting, enface position	
		3. ↓	41 personal care	3-31-90	protection of mucosa	
		4. Surveillance	See Categories 1,2,3	3-31-90		
17.	Growth + development	1. HTG+C	01 anatomy/phys.	3-31-90	causes, s/s, tx	
		2. ↓	49 s/s med./emot	3-31-90	normal development	
		3. ↓	50 s/s physical	3-31-90	"normal development"	
		4. ↓	55 stimulation	3-31-90	methods, s/s over-stim	
		5. Surveillance	49 s/s ment/emot	3-31-90	VDRT, Vidaro	
		6. ↓	50 s/s physical	3-31-90	ht, wt.	
30	Digestion hydration	1. HTG+C	58 supplies	3-31-90	methods/equip to improve fdg	
		2. ↓	21 feeding proc.	3-31-90	see prob 14, # 2	
39	Substance misuse	1. HTG+C	02 behavior mod	3-31-90	discontinue smoking	
		2. ↓	49 s/s med/emot.	3-31-90	s/s withdrawal (wt, sleep, agitation)	
		3. Case mngt	59 support group	3-31-90	ACS Stop Smoking Grp.	
		4. Surveillance	57 substance use	3-31-90	Behavioral change	

FIGURE 9 – 16 ■ The Nursing Care Plan serves as a tool to develop and document problem-specific client plans associated with the Intervention Scheme. (Courtesy of Polk Co. [WI] Public Health Nursing Service.)

NURSING CARE PLAN
PROBLEM RATING SCALE FOR OUTCOMES

Patient Name: Mullen
Patient Number: 55849

K = knowledge
B = behavior
S = status
C = caretaker

Problem Number and Name	Family 06 Comm w/comm. resources			Family 11 Grief			Family 14 Caretaking Parenting			Karen 17 G&D			Karen 30 Digestion Hydration			John 39 Subs. use			Family 01 Income			Family 09 Interpers. Relations			Nurse's Signature
Date	K	B	S	K	B	S	K	B	S	K	B	S	K	B	S	K	B	S	K	B	S	K	B	S	
3-31-90	2	3	3	3	3	2	3	3	3	3	4	3	2	3	2	3	3	3	—			—			Jane Sherratt / Tim McElroy
7-25-90	2	3	3	2	2	1	4	4	4	4	4	4	4	3	4				2	2	2	2	2	2	Jane Sherratt / Tim McElroy

CONCEPT	1	2	3	4	5
KNOWLEDGE: The ability of the client to remember and interpret information	(no knowledge)	(minimal knowledge)	(basic knowledge)	(adequate knowledge)	(superior knowledge)
BEHAVIOR: The observable responses, actions, or activities of the client	(never appropriate)	(rarely appropriate)	(inconsistently appropriate)	(usually appropriate)	(consistently appropriate)
STATUS: The condition of the client in relation to objective and subjective defining characteristics	(extreme signs/symp)	(severe signs/symp)	(moderate signs/symp)	(minimal signs/symp)	(no signs/symp)

FIGURE 9–17 ■ The Problem Rating Scale for Outcomes form serves as a tool to identify and document initial and interim problem-specific ratings; it is preferable that review and revision of ratings occur on an agency-wide schedule. (Courtesy of Polk Co. [WI] Public Health Nursing Service.)

MIDLAND COUNTY (MI) HEALTH DEPARTMENT
PUBLIC HEALTH NURSE RECORD OF SERVICE

NAME ___Mullen___

FF# ___55849___

Page ___2___

CODES:

Care Provided/Interventions:

Site:

HV	= Home
OV	= Office
SV	= School
TC	= Phone
NAH	= Not at Home

Assmt	= Assessment
HTG&C	= Teaching
CAR	= Coordination, Advocacy, and Referral
SUV	= Surveillance

DATE	SITE	PROB. NO.	CARE PROVIDED	NARRATIVE	REVISIT DATE
3/31/90	HV	30	SUV: fdg. procedure HTG-C: fdg. procedure CAR: fdg. procedure	Sue using new bottles satisfactorily, high sitting position. John still not fdg. Enc. on face position. Will become easier & quicker as baby grows. Reg. sitter will come during PHNs next HV—reluctant but willing to consider caring for baby when Sue returns to work.	4/6/90
		11	SUV: coping skills	Sue "wants school to begin," adjusting more, feeling more optimistic. John spent 2o "alone c̄ SW. Expressed feelings "can't believe this happened." Hopes he can "deal c̄ it." Hesitant but agreed to continue discussion c̄ SW & PHN.	
		39	HTG-C: S/S physical, S/S emotional CAR: substance misuse	John wanted to quit smoking on own. Very difficult, esp. now. Information & ph # of ACS Stop Smoking Program given. Appreciative	
				Jane Shirratt, PHN Tim McElroy, MSW	

```
-------------------------------------------------------------------------
                          * * * DATA BASE * * *              PAGE 2
 HOUSEHOLD #:    55849       1422 METCALF    STATION- VNCHS-NORTH
-------------------------------------------------------------------------
                          ACCOUNTS IN HOUSEHOLD
 Patient's Name:            Account #:            From Date:
 MULLEN, SUE                  55849                3/22/90
 MULLEN, JOHN                 55850                3/22/90
 MULLEN, KAREN                55851                3/22/90
 MULLEN, VICKIE               55852                3/22/90 - NOT ADM
-------------------------------------------------------------------------
```

DATA BASE UPDATE: 07/25/90

PSYCHOSOCIAL DOMAIN: John has moved out stating he cannot cope
with stress in the home. Sue concerned about future of their
relationship as well as her ability to manage on her own.

A: SUE IN CRISIS.

PHYSIOLOGICAL DOMAIN: Karen - successful surgical repair of
cleft lip 7/20/90.

Jane Sherratt, RN
Jane Sherratt, RN, Clinical Specialist/rip

```
    -------------------------------------------------------------------
```

FIGURE 9-19 ■ Additional participant data is documented by developing a Data Base Update entry (see Fig. 9-13).

```
------------------------------------------------------------
                    * * * PROBLEM LIST * * *         PAGE 1
  HOUSEHOLD #: 55849    1422 N. METCALF   STATION- VNCHS-NORTH
------------------------------------------------------------
                  ACCOUNTS IN HOUSEHOLD
  Patient's Name          Account #:        From Date:
  MULLEN, SUE                55849          3/20/90
  MULLEN, JOHN               55850          3/20/90
  MULLEN, KAREN              55851          3/20/90
  MULLEN VICKIE              55852          3/20/90-NOT ADM
------------------------------------------------------------


  *  03/31/90 MULLEN, JOHN
  07/25/90    RESOLVED
                  39C
              Substance Misuse:  Actual


                  3903
              Smokes


  *  07/25/90 FAMILY
                  09C
              Interpersonal Relationship:  Impairment


                  0901
              Difficulty Establishing/Maintaining Relationships


                  0903
              Incongruent Values/Goals


                  0905
              Prolonged, Unrelieved Tension

                  Jane Sherratt, RN
              Jane Sherratt, RN, Clinical Specialist/rip
                  Tim McElroy, MSW
                  Tim McElroy, MSW/rip




------------------------------------------------------------
```

FIGURE 9-20 ■ Additional problems and resolved problems are documented when appropriate (see Fig. 9-14).

POLK COUNTY PUBLIC HEALTH NURSING SERVICE
NURSING CARE PLAN

Original to Home Care Office
Copy to RN

PATIENT NAME: Mullen
PATIENT NUMBER: 55849
PAGE: 2

PROBLEM NO.	PROBLEM TITLE	CATEGORY	TARGET	DATE OF PLAN	PATIENT SPECIFIC NURSING PLAN OF ACTION	DATE PROBLEM DC'D
39	Substance misuse	1. HTG+C.	02 behavior mod	3-31-90	discontinue smoking	7-25-90
		2. ↓	49 s/s ment/emot	3-31-90	s/s withdrawal (wt, sleep, agitation)	
		3. Case mngt.	59 support group	3-31-90	ACS Stop Smoking Grp.	
		4. Surveillance	57 substance abuse	3-31-90	behavioral change	
01	Income	1. Case mngt.	30 legal system	7-25-90	obtain financial support from husband	
09	Interpersonal Relationships	1. HTG+C	11 coping skills	7-25-90	expression of feelings, support	
		2. Surveillance	49 s/s ment/emot.	7-25-90	pathological reactions	
30	Digestion/ Hydration	1. HTG+C	14 wound care	7-25-90	wrap finger w/ sterile gauze, cleanse in + outside suture line w/ 50% H2O2 soln; rinse w/ H2O pt.	
		2. Surveillance	50 s/s physical	7-25-90	healing of cleft lip repair, s/s infection	

FIGURE 9–21 ■ Pertinent changes in the Nursing Care Plan are documented when appropriate (see Fig. 9–16). (Courtesy of Polk Co. [WI] Public Health Nursing Service.)

PUBLIC HEALTH NURSE RECORD OF SERVICE

CODES:

Site:
HV = Home
OV = Office
SV = School
TC = Phone
NAH = Not at Home

Care Provided/Interventions:
Assmt = Assessment**
HTG&C = Teaching*
CAR = Coordination, Advocacy and Referral
SUV = Surveillance

NAME Mullen
FF# 55849
Page 13

*Reference: (1) Their Early Years; (2) Communicable Disease in Man
**Basis: (1) The Omaha System; (2) MCHD Post Partum Check List; (3) MDPH-CSHCS Nursing Assessment; (4) CD In Man

DATE	SITE	PROB. NO.	CARE PROVIDED	NARRATIVE	REVISIT DATE
7-25-90	HV	09	HTGC, coping skills, stress mngt.	John packed clothes and moved out 7/24. Entire situation was "too much for him." Sue's mother will arrive tomorrow to help and discuss options. Sue worried about financial support from John. Suggested she seek legal counsel soon.	8-1-90
		01	HTGC, CAR: finances, legal		
		11	HTGC, SUV: coping skills	Toys + clothes scattered, many dirty dishes in kitchen. Sue - "the house is a pit. I'm in shock again."	
		30	HTGC: anatomy/physiology, feeding procedure. SUV: s/s physical	Suture line intact, slightly red + swollen. Able to feed ā difficulty. Instructed to keep area clean + dry. Offer H2O after formula to rinse. Ret. appt w/ surgeon in 1 wk.	
				Jane Sherratt, PHN	

FIGURE 9–22 ■ The Public Health Nurse Record of Service is completed for each home visit. (Courtesy of Midland Co. [MI] Health Department.)

SUMMARY

The community health staff, supervisors, and administrators who provide home visit services and are employed by official agencies face many serious issues. One issue involves the ability to describe the value of public health nursing services to (1) fellow employees, (2) external accreditation and reimbursement auditors, (3) politicians, and (4) the general public. A tool that enables community health staff to efficiently and effectively document services is the Omaha System.

The Bell and Mullen case examples illustrate the application of the Omaha System in a public health home visit setting. Each family had unique needs and was visited by different staff members. The staff used various forms and methods of documentation. However, in both situations, the Omaha System provided the framework for guiding practice and documentation. With both families, the staff:

- Completed required demographic information forms
- Used the Problem Classification Scheme as an assessment guide
- Developed a problem list from the Data Base
- Set priorities and then rated and re-rated the client problems using the Problem Rating Scale for Outcomes
- Developed a problem-specific care plan and then revised that plan through identification of categories and targets from the Intervention Scheme and from client-specific comments
- Provided interdisciplinary services based on the care plan. The services were documented on visit entry forms that incorporated the Intervention Scheme. Using a problem-driven approach such as the Omaha System provides the public health nurse, supervisor, and administrator with a logical means of tracking client care and a method for implementing a quality assurance program.

The Omaha System has been implemented in various public health agencies. The experiences included in this chapter were written by nurses employed in California, Delaware, Wisconsin, and Nebraska. Although all agencies and their clients have unique characteristics and needs, many similarities are evident across the country.

REFERENCES

American Nurses' Association (1986a). *Standards of Community Health Nursing Practice.* Kansas City, MO.

American Nurses' Association (1986b). *Standards of Home Health Nursing Practice.* Kansas City, MO.

Cell, P., Peters, D., & Gordon, J. (1984, January/February). Implementing a nursing diagnosis system through research: The New Jersey experience. *Home Healthcare Nurse,* 2:26–32.

Chavigny, K., & Kroske, M. (1983, November/December). Public health nursing in crisis. *Nurs. Outlook,* 31:312–316.

Dreher, M. (1984, October). District nursing: The cost benefits of a population-based practice. *Am. J. Public Health,* 74:1107–1111.

Helberg, J. (1988, March). Reliability of a problem-classification index for well mothers and children in community health nursing. *Public Health Nurse,* 5:24–29.

Institute of Medicine (1988). *The Future of Public Health.* Washington, DC, National Academy Press.

Kroeger, O., & Thuesen, J. (1988). *Type Talk.* New York, Delacorte Press.

McCaulley, M. (1981). *Jung's Theory of Psychological Types and the Myers-Briggs Type Indicator.* Gainesville, FL, Center for Application of Psychological Type.

McCreight, L. (1989, September/October). The future of public health. *Nurs. Outlook,* 37:219–225.

Moses, E. (1990, March). [Survey of RNs in US] Personal communication regarding unpublished data.

Myers, I. (1980). *Gifts Differing.* Palo Alto, CA, Consulting Psychologists Press.

Myers, I., & McCaulley, M. (1985). *Manual: A Guide to the Development and the Use of the Myers-Briggs Type Indicator.* Palo Alto, CA, Consulting Psychologists Press.

Neufeld, A., & Misselbrook, C. (1987). Classification and use of nursing diagnosis in community health nursing. In Hannah, K., Reimer, M., Mills, W., et al. (Eds.), *Clinical Judgement and Decision Making: The Future With Nursing Diagnosis* (pp. 349–351). New York, John Wiley & Sons.

Tinkham, C., Voorhies, E., & McCarthy, N. (1984). *Community Health Nursing: Evolution and Process in the Family and Community* (3rd ed.). New York, Appleton-Century-Crofts.

Weidmann, J., & North, H. (1987, December). Implementing the Omaha classification system in a public health agency. *Nurs. Clin. North Am.,* 22:971–979.

Williams, C. (1977, April). Community health nursing: What is it? *Nurs. Outlook,* 25:250–254.

Williams, C. (1988). Population-focused practice: The basis of specialization in public health nursing. In Stanhope, M., & Lancaster, J. (Eds.), *Community Health Nursing: Process and Practice for Promoting Health* (pp. 292–303). St. Louis, C. V. Mosby.

BIBLIOGRAPHY

Andersen, E., & McFarlane, J. (1988). *Community as Client: Application of the Nursing Process.* Philadelphia, J. B. Lippincott.

Braden, C. (1984). *The Focus and Limits of Community Health Nursing.* Norwalk, CT, Appleton-Century-Crofts.

Buhler-Wilkerson, K. (1985). Public health nursing: In sickness or in health? *Am. J. Public Health,* 75:1155–1161.

Buhler-Wilkerson, K. (1987, January/February). Left carrying the bag: Experiments in visiting nursing, 1877–1909. *Nurs. Res.,* 36:42–47.

Chapman, C. (1988, June). Of mice and Merle. *Am. J. Nurs.,* 88:938.

Diers, D. (1988, Fall). On money . . . *Image,* 20:122.

Dolan, J., Fitzpatrick, M., & Herrmann, E. (1983). *Nursing in Society: A Historical Perspective* (15th ed.). Philadelphia, W. B. Saunders.

Donahue, M. (1985). *Nursing, the Finest Art: An Illustrated History.* St. Louis, C. V. Mosby.

Ervin, N. (1982, July/August). Public health nursing practice—an administrator's view. *Nurs. Outlook,* 30:390–394.

Gulino, C., & LaMonica, G. (1986, June). Public health nursing: A study of role implementation. *Public Health Nurs.,* 3:80–91.

Hall, J., & Weaver, B. (1985). *Distributive Nursing Practice: A Systems Approach to Community Health* (2nd ed.). Philadelphia, J. B. Lippincott.

Hamilton, D. (1988, Fall). Faith and finance. *Image,* 20:124–127.

Harris, M. (1988). *Home Health Administration.* Owings Mills, MD, Rynd Communications.

Josten, L. (1989, September/October). Wanted: Leaders for public health. *Nurs. Outlook,* 37:230–232.

Kalisch, P., & Kalisch, B. (1986). *The Advance of American Nursing* (2nd ed.). Boston, Little, Brown.

Kark, S. (1981). *Community-oriented Primary Care*. New York, Appleton-Century-Crofts.

Knollmueller, R. (1985, January). The growth and development of homecare: From no-tech to high tech. *Caring, 4*:3–8.

Laxton, C. (Ed.) (1988, December). Home care services—Past, present, and future. *Caring, 7*:4–7.

Lentz, J., & Myer, E. (1979, September). The dirty house. *Nurs. Outlook, 27*:590–593.

Magnan, M. (1989, February). Listening with care. *Am. J. Nurs., 89*:219–221.

Moore, P., & Williamson, G. (1984, June). Health promotion: Evolution of a concept. *Nurs. Clin. North Am., 19*:195–206.

Oda, D. (1989, March/April). Home visits: Effective or obsolete nursing practice? *Nurs. Res., 38*:121–123.

Oda, D., & Boyd, P. (1987, September). Documenting the effect and cost of public health nursing field services. *Public Health Nurs., 4*:180–182.

Petze, C. (1984, June). Health promotion for the well family. *Nurs. Clin. North Am., 19*:229–237.

Phillips, E., Fisher, M., MacMillan-Scattergood, D., et al. (1987, June). Home health care: Who's where? *Am. J. Nurs., 77*:733–734.

Roberts, D., & Heinrich, J. (1985, October). Public health nursing comes of age. *Am. J. Public Health, 75*:1162–1172.

Salmon, M. (1989, September/October). Public health nursing: The neglected specialty. *Nurs. Outlook, 37*:226–229.

Salmon, M., & Peoples-Sheps, M. (1989, January/February). Infant mortality and public health nursing: A history of accomplishments, a future of challenges. *Nurs. Outlook, 37*:6–7, 51.

Salmon, M., & Vanderbush, P. (1990). Leadership and change in public and community health nursing today: The essential intervention. In McCloskey, J., & Grace, H. (Eds.), *Current Issues in Nursing* (3rd ed.) (pp. 187–193). St. Louis, C. V. Mosby.

Smith, G. (1989, March). More power to you. *Am. J. Nurs., 89*:357–358.

Stanhope, M., & Lancaster, J. (1988). *Community Health Nursing: Process and Practice for Promoting Health*. St. Louis, C. V. Mosby.

Talbot, D. (1983). Public health nursing: Now and as it might be. In Chaska, N. (Ed.), *The Nursing Profession: A Time to Speak* (pp. 818–829). New York, McGraw-Hill.

Ward, D. (1989, December). Public health nursing and "The future of public health." *Public Health Nurs., 6*:163–168.

Wold, S. (Ed.) (1990). *Community Health Nursing: Issues and Topics*. Norwalk, CT, Appleton & Lange.

Worth, C. (1989, February). Handle with care. *Am. J. Nurs., 89*:197–198.

CHAPTER TEN

Documentation is an essential part of care. It is a vehicle for communicating from one professional to another about the status and needs of the patient. In fact, the chart is often the only means to demonstrate that professional standards, state regulations, and the criteria for reimbursement were met. However, to the extent that charting significantly interferes with the amount of time nurses can spend with patients, it must be limited. Agencies need to examine the documentation dilemma as it exists for them, and they must provide the necessary supports to allow nurses to both care for patients and write about what they have done. (Morrissey-Ross, 1988, pp. 370–371)

Organized home health care in the US began early in the 1800s when professionals employed by dispensaries initiated medical, surgical, and obstetric services in clinics and homes. During that century, the staff of settlement houses and visiting nurse associations provided the majority of home health care services. Donations were the primary source of support for these philanthropic organizations. Third-party reimbursement for home health care was virtually unknown. Although the primary emphasis was on home care of the sick, these organizations also provided preventive care, particularly in the area of maternal and child health. The nurses who worked for the settlement houses and visiting nurse associations were truly generalists. During the Depression years of the 1930s, there was an increasing emphasis on pubic health nursing and comprehensive care of the sick and the well.

The Social Security Amendments of 1965, which established the Medicare program and included home health care benefits, signaled the advent of the modern age of home health care. The growth of home health care was further stimulated by two changes in the Medicare program. First, the Social Security Amendments of 1972 expanded benefits. Second, the Omnibus Reconciliation Act of 1980 removed the restrictions on number of home health visits and eased requirements for provider participation in Medicare. The availability of third-party reimbursement for home health care services led to an increase in the types and numbers of agencies providing the services and, ultimately, to a change in the focus of those services.

Medicare regulations require home health agencies to obtain certification to participate as providers of services. In 1966, 85% of Medicare-certified agencies were visiting nurse associations and public health organizations (Knollmueller, 1985). Nursing provided general services, with emphasis on primary, secondary, and tertiary prevention. By 1987, there were 5,923 home health agencies. The number of visiting nurse associations and official agencies remained essentially the same, with hospital-based and proprietary agencies showing the largest rate of growth (National Association for Home Care, 1987). The number of agencies, of home health nurses, and of clients is expected to continue rising, with home health representing an ever increasing percentage of the total health care market (Selby, 1990).

The majority of home health agencies of the 1990s are specialized organizations. They employ nearly 54,000 nurses who provide services to clients with diagnosed illnesses; they focus on technical procedures and secondary prevention (Moses, 1990). The primary emphasis is on improvement or maintenance of clients' physiologic status. Efforts by primary payors to reduce costs have led agencies to decrease or eliminate consideration of environmental, economic, social, or psychological factors that may affect clients' health status. Home health care has grown from its modest, humanitarian beginnings to a multibillion dollar industry. (For a more complete discussion of the history of home health nursing, refer to Chapter 1.)

HOME HEALTH ISSUES

Home health practitioners of today are no less dedicated than were their predecessors. Unfortunately, nurses continue to face many practice and reimburse-

Use in Home Health Care Settings

ment crises. The issues confronting modern home health administrators and practitioners are different, and even more complex, than those faced by Lillian Wald and her contemporaries. The level of technology used in the home care setting has resulted in the need for practitioners with different skills. Home health agencies have begun to employ nurses who possess specific technical expertise from experience in acute care. These nurses may not be knowledgeable about community health nursing, however, and they may be uncomfortable in home settings, especially because the family controls a significant portion of the care process. Conversely, experienced community health nurses may be uncomfortable caring for clients who are acutely ill or who require technical procedures using equipment such as respirators or intravenous pumps. As stated by Cary (1988),

The home health care nurse of today and tomorrow not only must practice from the community health conceptual framework of prevention, health promotion, and risk reduction for clients, families, and groups, but must be technically skilled in direct care-giving activities and clinical judgment appropriate to the acuity levels of today's consumers. In addition, the home care professional must be confident in the autonomy of nursing practice, the interdisciplinary delivery mode, the client and community advocacy responsibilities, and the managed care activities required (pp. 342–343).

Other critical home health issues include: (1) a dramatic rise in the demand for home health services, (2) an increase in the acuity and service requirements of clients referred for home health care, and (3) restrictions on reimbursement for home health care.

HOME HEALTH CARE AND THE OMAHA SYSTEM

The Omaha System serves as a guide for home health care practice and documentation. It facilitates gathering data for integrated management information systems. As such, the Omaha System is a valuable tool for agency administrators and staff.

Harris (1988) noted that "an organized, legible clinical record is essential for home care services" (p. 191). The Omaha System provides an organizing framework for the client record. The System is congruent with the ANA *Standards of Home Health Nursing Practice* (1986) as well as the outcome effectiveness initiatives that are emerging in the 1990s (Lohn, 1990). Therefore, the Omaha System enhances professional documentation and accountability as it enables nurses to demonstrate application of the nursing process and the benefits of service. Simultaneously, the Omaha System enables nurses to expand the focus of client data to include increased visibility of negative client data. These data are essential to the reimbursement process because of ever changing regulations. Specific ways that home health practitioners and administrators can use the Omaha System include:

- To define agency expectations for practice and documentation during the orientation process
- To assist the practitioner in rapidly sorting more pertinent from less pertinent client data. Reimbursement for care provided by home health agencies has been increasingly tied to the ability of agency staff to document accurately and completely
- To guide the practitioner in the collection of relevant data in multiple categories, including Environmen-

169

tal and Psychosocial; these categories may be overlooked by home health practitioners who focus, often exclusively, on Physiologic and Health Related Behavior data

- To assist the practitioner in identifying and focusing on the client's primary health problems, and in identifying and documenting the client's knowledge, behavior, and status in relation to those problems
- To examine client progress during the period of home health service — a traditional concern for the practitioner and an increasing concern for the administrator
- To provide standard data for use in an integrated management information system
- To articulate the essence of home health nursing to other nurses, to third-party payors, and to society at large; the Omaha System assists administrators and staff to describe the agency, client, and nursing activities, as well as client change

The Visiting Nurse Services of Des Moines served as one of the three test agencies during the testing of the Problem Classification Scheme and development of the Expected Outcome – Outcome Criterion Schemes (see Chapter 4). In the following section, Rose Marie Serra describes the implementation and subsequent computer use with the Problem Classification Scheme. Referencing the problems from the Scheme to medical diagnoses has facilitated development of nursing care plans.

EXPERIENCES WITH THE OMAHA SYSTEM IN DES MOINES

by ROSE MARIE SERRA, RN, BSN, Assistant Director/Director of Clinical Services, Visiting Nurse Services, Des Moines, IA

Visiting Nurse Services of Des Moines, formerly known as the Public Health Nursing Association, became involved in the development of the Omaha System as one of three test agencies. In 1978, staff of each test agency were oriented to the concepts and use of the Problem Classification Scheme in the practice setting. The staff of Visiting Nurse Services were, for the most part, receptive and eager to participate in nursing research that had a potential impact on actual nursing practice. The staff were already adept at using the problem-oriented record system, a recommendation for implementing the Scheme. However, the adjustment to the process of writing problem-specific nursing care plans was another matter. Many staff were accustomed to using a medical diagnosis as the problem on the care plan and writing nursing interventions and goals for that diagnosis. For example, some staff were accustomed to identifying the medical diagnosis "diabetes mellitus" as the client's problem. They did not identify the nursing problems resulting from client's diabetes mellitus as 35. Nutrition: Impairment, 26. Integument: Impairment, 29. Circulation: Impairment, and 43. Technical Procedure: Impairment. The policy of allowing no medical diagnoses to be listed on the Problem List or Care Plan had to be strictly enforced.

As staff became more familiar with the Omaha System, they found themselves automatically thinking in terms of the Problem Classification Scheme when they completed the admission assessment of the client. They appreciated the sameness of terminology from nurse to nurse that resulted from using the Scheme; they felt it was helpful as they visited clients in other nurses' caseloads. They noted that use of the Scheme helped them direct their efforts toward identifying and handling those client problems that might be resolved with nursing intervention. In this way, they did not waste time and energy on problems that were clearly not appropriate for nursing involvement. After the initial testing period ended, the staff continued to use the Problem Classification Scheme. New nurses adjusted readily to the system.

Some modifications in the agency's documentation system were made as time went on. In order to decrease documentation time and eliminate redundancy, staff were allowed to group problems with similar interventions together instead of separately recording on each problem. Furthermore, the staff were allowed to discontinue the use of the Problem List because all identified problems for which nursing interventions were appropriate were listed on the Nursing Care Plan. This further decreased time spent on documentation.

The Visiting Nurse Services management decided to begin automation in 1983. The Problem Classification Scheme lent itself very easily to a computerized clinical record. Staff dictated their home visit documentation and transcriptionists entered the data into the record file. Many shortcuts were programmed into the automated record system, which saved both nursing and transcription time.

At the present time, agency staff are developing an automated system of nursing care plans. This system will identify the International Classification of Diseases (ICD9) codes listed on the physician's plan of treatment (HCFA 485) and display the client problems from the Problem Classification Scheme that may be associated with that medical diagnosis. In this way, the computer system prompts a nurse in terms of the fewest client problems that should be assessed for the usual manifestations of that disease. The system then displays the possible signs and symptoms, nursing interventions, and goals for those problems. The nurse selects only those problems, symptoms, interventions, and goals that are appropriate for that client. Additional problems, symptoms, interventions, and goals may be added to the plan as appropriate. Finally, the nurse is asked to enter an estimated number of visits necessary to accomplish the goals. The completed nursing care plan is printed and incorporated into the clinical record. To update the plan, the nurse simply looks at the screen for that client and adds or deletes data as appropriate. It is hoped that this new computer system will provide beginning statistical data linking client problems to medical diagnosis.

Application

Two case studies are presented; they describe visits with John Henry and Sarah Clark. These cases illustrate use of the Omaha System as a guide for practice and documentation of home health nursing at the Visiting Nurse Association of Omaha. The Problem Classification Scheme is the basis for data collection and identification of client problems or nursing diagnoses. The Intervention Scheme is used for planning and implementing services. Evaluation is facilitated through use of the Problem Rating Scale for Outcomes. Actual record forms used to document the delivery of home health care by the staff of the VNA of Omaha are included. Blank forms and instructions are included in the Appendix.

The John Henry case example (pp. 171–195) includes (1) a description of the referral process, (2) a dialogue between the nurse and the Henrys, and (3) the following VNA of Omaha forms:

Figure 10–1, Home Health Referral (p. 172)
Figure 10–2, Patient Information Record (p. 173)
Figure 10–3, Data Base/Problem List Worksheet (pp. 176–185)
Figure 10–4, Data Base (pp. 186–187)
Figure 10–5, Problem List (pp. 188–189)
Figure 10–6, Client Care Plan/Problem Rating Worksheet (pp. 190–191)
Figure 10–7, Problem Ratings/Plans (pp. 192–193)
Figure 10–8, Skilled Visit Report (pp. 194–195).

John Henry Case Example

REFERRAL PROCESS

John Henry is a fictional client whose problems typically warrant home health nursing services. He was seen in his private physician's office and subsequently referred to the VNA of Omaha. The verbal referral orders to initiate nursing service were taken by the intake nurse. She completed a Home Health Referral and initiated a Patient Information Record to be completed by the staff nurse/case manager during the admission home visit. The intake nurse phoned Mr. Henry to inform him of the referral and to ascertain his willingness to receive services. Information obtained during the phone contact was also entered onto the referral form and face-sheet. The forms were sent to a nursing supervisor, who assigned Mr. Henry to a case manager (Figs. 10–1 and 10–2).

USING THE PROBLEM CLASSIFICATION SCHEME

Cathi Alexander, the case manager, phoned the Henry home and scheduled a visit for the following morning. Based on physician orders and other referral information, Cathi planned the agenda for the first home visit. Medicare regulations designed to safeguard client rights require that the nurse discuss the proposed plan of care, payment for care, and client rights prior to provision of service. Therefore, Cathi would begin the visit to conform with these regulations. In addition to completion of Medicare and agency admission requirements, the agenda for the visit included the following:

■ Complete a physical assessment on Mr. Henry
■ Ascertain the Henrys' understanding of Mr. Henry's disease processes and the medical treatment regimen
■ Observe the physical environment
■ Observe the relationship between the Henrys and elicit verbal information regarding the Henrys' psychosocial status and needs
■ Explain the home care services prescribed by the physician
■ Initiate teaching
■ Develop a plan of care with the Henrys and schedule the next home visit

The following morning the nurse arrived at the Henry home and was met at the door by Mrs. Henry. After greeting the nurse warmly, Mrs. Henry introduced her to Mr. Henry, who was seated in the living room. They discussed Mr. Henry's signs and symptoms in relation to his diagnoses of Parkinson's disease and orthostatic hypotention. Also, they discussed his medication regime and their concerns about his medications. Cathi followed her planned agenda, modifying it to meet the Henrys' needs during the visit, which lasted almost 1 hour.

The visit dialogue is included here. Like the dialogue in Chapter 9, this visit can be incorporated into home health orientation.

The Henry Family Home Visit

CATHI: Good morning, Mrs. Henry, I'm Cathi Alexander from the Visiting Nurse Association. I spoke with you on the phone yesterday.

MRS. HENRY: Come in. John and I have been waiting for you.

(The nurse and Mrs. Henry walk into the living room where Mr. Henry is sitting. Mrs. Henry introduces the nurse to Mr. Henry.)

CATHI: Dr. Watson has requested that a visiting nurse see you two to three times a week to see how you're managing. Before I start, I have some forms here I'd like to review with you. There are also some papers for you to sign. We can never be 100% sure but Medicare should pay for my visits for now. If anything changes, I'll let you know before any services not covered by Medicare are provided.

(Cathi reviews admission forms required by the VNA and by Medicare and obtains Mr. Henry's signature on the applicable forms.)

```
For VNA Use Only        THE VISITING NURSE ASSOCIATION OF OMAHA        For VNA Use Only
```

Date: 08 / 14 / 89 H/Hold #: ___24___ CT: 70

Account #: 24

VNAM ✓ VNHR ____ VNCHS ____ Payment Discussed? Y ☒ N ☐ Fax Y ☐ N ☐

Source: (Name) MD

Relationship: _____ Phone: _____

Previous VNA Record?: N ☒ Y ☐ Date From ___/___/___ to ___/___/___

Rejected? ☐ on ___/___/___

SS #: 402-73-4554

Medicare #: 402-73-4554 A

Medicaid #: _____

Ins _____ # _____

Other # *doesn't want service if medicare won't pay*

Patient (Last Name First): Henry, John Birth Date: 5/26/ 1905 Sex: M ☒ F ☐ Marital Status: S ☐ M ☒ W ☐ D ☐ Sep ☐

Street Address: 4567 Main City: Omaha Zip: 68130 Phone: 544-1230

Spouse/Parent: Jane Birth Date: 12/6/11

Emergency Contact: Grace Jones Relationship: dgt. Phone: 543-2786

Hospital: NA from ___/___/___ to ___/___/___ SNF: from ___/___/___ to ___/___/___

Physician: Dr. Al Watson Address: 710 Drs. Bldg. Phone: 302-7913

Physician: Dr. John Abrams (cardiologist) Address: 602 Drs. Bldg Phone: 302-0345

Primary Diagnosis: (Dates) Orthostatic hypotension (8/14/89)

Secondary Diagnosis: (Dates) CHF (1/1/85) Parkinson's Disease (7/1/89)

Mental State:
Alert ☒   Depressed ☐
Forgetful ☐   Disoriented ☐
Other _____   Confused ☐

Functional Limits:
Mental ☐   Ambulation ☒
Speech ☐   Vision ☐
Other Cane   Respiratory ☐
   Hearing ☐

Range of Vital Signs and Lab:
BP 120/80 sit 100/76 stand P 42-100 R _____
Blood Sug. _____ Wt. _____

Lives Alone ☐ With Other ☒ Spouse H & P Req: Y ☒ N ☐ Pharmacy Skaggs

Significant Information: experiencing sl. ↓ in BP since init on Sinemet ↑, Dyazide dc'ed + Lanoxin dose ↓
Had Halter monitor x24° HR 42-100 c/o dizziness

Service: Nursing ☒ Physical Therapy ☐ Speech Therapy ☐ Occupational Therapy ☐ Home Health Aide ☐

Medical Orders/Plan of Treatment: F.W.B. ☐ N.W.B. ☐ P.W.B. ☐ _____ %

VO Dr. Watson

SNC 2-3x/wk x 9wks
Assess BP — more concerned re: diastolic ↓
Assess HR — report >120
Teach meds + assess compliance. (Refused Nitro-instruct not to take Lanoxin for chest pain)
Assess s/s vertigo
Safety teaching
Report progress/concerns to MD

Has app't c̄ cardiologist in 3 wks

Supplies: _____

Activity Tolerance: as tol

Diet: Lo salt

Allergies: NKA

Meds/Dosage: _____
Sinemet 25/100, tab ½ po BID
Lanoxin 0.125 mg, tab ½ po q̄ am
Mylanta 1-2 tbsp po @ HS PRN

D/C Dyazide

M.D. Signature _____

R.N. Signature *Patricia Whitted, RN*

Additional Information on Attached Sheet: Y ☐ N ☒

FIGURE 10–1 ■ The Home Health Referral is the initial document used to gather data before client service is initiated.

CATHI: Tell me how you're feeling, Mr. Henry.

MR. HENRY: I don't feel very good. I think that new medicine Dr. Watson ordered for my Parkinson's disease is making me sick. I feel like I'm going to throw up every time I take it and I'm dizzy every time I try to stand up.

CATHI: When do you take your medicine?

MRS. HENRY: I give it to him the first thing after he gets up in the morning. He's supposed to take it at night too, but I haven't been giving it to him because it makes him sick and he needs his rest.

```
-----------------------------------------------------------------------------
                    PATIENT   INFORMATION   RECORD                   PAGE    1
-----------------------------------------------------------------------------

Household #:       24
Address 1:    4567 MAIN ST., #4                Station: VNA MIDLANDS DIR SVC
Address 2:                                       Phone: 402 544-1234
City/St/Zip: OMAHA          NE 68130      Census Tract: 70.00
Directions:                              Monthly Income: 1,500
Case Manager:    CATHERINE ALEXANDER


                          ACCOUNTS IN HOUSEHOLD
Patient's Name:              Account #:     Birth Date:     Rel. to HH:
HENRY, JOHN                          24      5/26/1905      HEAD OF HOUSEHOLD
HENRY, JANE                       55512     12/06/1911 -NA  WIFE
-----------------------------------------------------------------------------

-----------------------------------------------------------------------------
Patient's Name:              Account #:
HENRY, JOHN                          24


** EMERGENCY INFORMATION       Relation:  Address:                Phone:
     JONES, GRACE              DAUGHTER                         402 543-2222

** ADMISSION INFORMATION
     Soc Sec #:    402-73-4554       Rel. to HH: HH- HEAD OF HOUSEHOLD
     Birth Date:     5/26/1905         Religion: 2- PROTESTANT
     Admit Date:     8/15/89      Referral Code: PRIVATE PHYSICIAN
     Refer Date:     8/14/89           Program: 201 - HOME HEALTH CARE
     1st Contact:    8/14/89              Race: 01- CAUCASIAN
     Care Started:   8/15/89               Sex: MALE
     Plan Establ.:   8/14/89       Marital Sts: MARRIED
     Discharged:     0/00/00     Discharge Reason:
     Special Instructions:
     ICDA Diagnosis:


** DIAGNOSIS INFORMATION
     61        CARDIAC
     50        NRV SYSTM/SNS ORGN DISORD

** FUNDING SOURCES            Billing #:     Comment:          Effect Date:
     01- MEDICARE             402734554A                          8/15/89
     11- PRIVATE PAY

** EMPLOYER - 33/ RETIRED

** OTHER AGENCIES             Contact:                      Phone:
     DR. AL WATSON                                       402 302-7913


** PHYSICIAN INFORMATION                      Orders Cover
                                        From Date:   To Date:
                                         8/15/89     10/13/89
```

FIGURE 10–2 ■ The Patient Information Record is a computer-generated facesheet that includes information obtained during the referral and admission process.

CATHI: Sometimes medications can make you feel nauseated when you take them on an empty stomach. Why don't you try taking the medicine just after breakfast and again just after dinner and see if that helps? The dizzy spells probably aren't caused by the medicines. Dr. Watson said your blood pressure is dropping when you stand up. That will make you dizzy. I'd like to check you over and see what I find.

(The nurse completes a brief physical assessment including sitting and standing blood pressure readings.)

CATHI: Your blood pressure is 104/64 when you're sitting and drops to 70/50 when you stand up. That fast drop will

make you feel lightheaded and dizzy for a few minutes until your body adjusts. Dr. Watson has changed your medication to try to get this under control. In the meantime, it's important that you go slowly when changing positions from lying to sitting and from sitting to standing. You should have something to hold onto when you stand so you don't fall if you become dizzy. And don't try to walk until the dizziness passes.

MR. HENRY: I guess I can do that. I just hope Dr. Watson figures this out fast. It's taking all my strength and it's hard on Jane, too. She has to do everything—I'm just no good.

MRS. HENRY: I really don't mind the extra work but it's hard on John. He used to be so active and now he can't even drive. I have to run all the errands and take him to the doctor.

CATHI: Do you have family or friends who can help?

MRS. HENRY: Our daughter, Grace, lives in town but she works and has a family of her own. She does help when she can. She took off work yesterday to help me take John to the doctor. I was afraid to try with just the two of us. He's so weak and dizzy.

CATHI: It's good that you have Grace to help. What about Mr. Henry's personal care? How are you managing that?

MR. HENRY: I'm afraid to get in the tub so Jane has been helping me with a sponge bath in the bathroom. We're managing.

CATHI: If it gets to be too much, we could send a home health aide to help you a couple of times a week. We could also have our occupational therapist visit to instruct you on energy conservation and to suggest equipment that might be helpful.

MR. HENRY: Well—maybe later.

CATHI: Okay, you keep it in mind. Dr. Watson said you have chest pain from time to time. When was the last time you had chest pain?

MR. HENRY: I had a little one this morning. Just a tight feeling in my chest. It didn't last very long. Sometimes they're worse and the pain starts in my chest and goes down my arm. I usually take one of these pills. They seem to help.

CATHI: This is your Lanoxin. It will help but only if you take it as prescribed once a day. Your heart beat is a little irregular and this medicine can help. If you're having chest pain we can ask Dr. Watson to prescribe nitroglycerin, that will help.

MR. HENRY: He wanted to give me some but I didn't want it. This works fine and I don't want any more pills than I already have.

CATHI: As I understand it, Dr. Watson is hoping to get you off the Lanoxin completely.

MRS. HENRY: Yes. Yesterday he did decrease the amount John takes.

CATHI: It's really important that you take it as prescribed once a day. If you take it every time you have chest pain, you will get too much and that's just as bad as not enough. Lanoxin is a very powerful drug and must be taken very carefully.

MR. HENRY: I never thought of that.

CATHI: I'll bring you more information about your pills on my next visit. I'll also call Dr. Watson to report on my visit today.

MRS. HENRY: Please be sure to tell him that the Parkinson's medicine is making John sick.

CATHI: I will. Maybe he will want to change something. Do remember to take it with food. I think that will help. I'd like to visit you again in 2 days to see how you're getting along.

MR. HENRY: I really appreciate your help. Thanks for coming.

CATHI: See you on Friday. Goodbye.

MR. & MRS. HENRY: Goodbye.

During the course of the visit, Cathi used a worksheet based on the Problem Classification Scheme as (1) a guide for obtaining information and (2) a form on which to record data. She also recorded on the Skilled Visit Report form. Following the visit, she returned to her office to complete admission paperwork and documentation of the visit. As an experienced nurse work-ing with a receptive family, Cathi was able to collect most of the data on the admission visit. Had the family been unreceptive, less data might have been obtained. Although the VNA policy allows three visits or 2 weeks for Data Base completion in order to provide flexibility, the staff are encouraged to complete the Data Base as quickly as possible. Cathi reviewed the worksheet and completed assessment statements for the Environmental, Psychosocial, and Physiological Domains. She made a mental note to discuss Mr. Henry's nutritional status and to obtain a health history during her next scheduled home visit. After the second visit, she completed the Data Base/Problem List Worksheet and turned it in for typing (Fig. 10–3).

The completed Data Base serves as a baseline against which future change can be measured (Fig. 10–4). The Data Base is updated annually and whenever significant changes occur. Such changes include hospitalization, birth or death of a family member, or a move to a new environment.

Analysis of data recorded on the worksheet facilitates identification of client and family problems on the Problem List (Fig. 10–5). Cathi identified one Family and four Individual problems. Of the five problems, one was a Potential problem and four were Actual problems with signs/symptoms. Cathi chose to identify Mr. Henry's anginal pain as a sign/symptom of the problem 29. Circulation: Impairment rather than identifying 24. Pain as a separate problem. Furthermore, Mr. Henry's nausea was viewed as a medication side effect rather than as a sign/symptom of the problem 30. Digestion-Hydration: Impairment. Cathi has learned through experience in using the Omaha System that identifying a limited and manageable number of problems or nursing diagnoses will enable her to focus planning, intervention, and documentation efforts on priority issues. More is not always better.

USING THE PROBLEM RATING SCALE FOR OUTCOMES

Just as use of the Problem Classification Scheme helps the nurse to focus data collection efforts, use of the Problem Rating Scale for Outcomes allows the nurse to identify areas and priorities for intervention (Figs. 10–6 and 10–7). Cathi completed Knowledge, Behavior, and Status ratings for five of the six problems. Ratings were not completed for the Potential problem of 38. Personal Hygiene because Mr. and Mrs. Henry had not expressed interest in working on this problem. During subsequent visits, Cathi would continue to collect data and complete ratings and a plan of intervention when the Henrys expressed readiness. Cathi was aware that problems and ratings are dynamic and can change during the course of service. The Problem List is subject to change in three ways:

- Addition of new problems
- Resolution of existing problems
- Change in the status of a problem based on the presence or absence of signs/symptoms, risk factors, or client interest

The Problem Rating Scale for Outcomes is used by the nurse to rerate priority problems at 2-month intervals in conjunction with recertifying the Physician Plan of Treatment. The Rating Scale is also used to rate each of the problems at the time Mr. Henry is dismissed from service. Comparison of the ratings over time allows the nurse to measure and document progress.

USING THE INTERVENTION SCHEME

Following completion of ratings, Cathi used the Intervention Scheme to develop and document an intervention plan. The Scheme provides cues and clues to the nurse during development of the plan. The ratings and plan were recorded by Cathi on a worksheet for entry into the clinical record. Cathi was especially concerned about Mr. Henry's circulatory status and chest pain, particularly in view of his failure to take his cardiac medications as prescribed. During the home visit, she had taken advantage of the opportunity to initiate teaching about Mr. Henry's medication regime. However, Cathi knew that insisting on too much change during the first home visit could interfere with the rapport she was attempting to establish with the Henrys. She also was aware that providing information in small amounts could facilitate learning.

A Skilled Visit Report form is used by all professionals to document each visit (Fig. 10–8). Home health care services provided by therapists, nurses, and social workers have different foci. However, the form is sufficiently generic to provide an acceptable documentation method for all. The front of the form incorporates portions of the Problem Classification Scheme and the entire Intervention Scheme, allowing the user to encode, rather than narrate, some of the data. The domains and problem areas of the Problem Classification Scheme, as well as the Medicare Treatment Codes, appear on the back of the form. This format serves as a reminder system for the staff. The form also includes information required by Medicare intermediaries, professional review organizations, and other reviewers; examples include spaces for documenting homebound status and time of visit. During the actual visit, Cathi recorded on the Skilled Visit Report form. This strategy serves two purposes. First, accuracy of data is improved when recording occurs immediately. Second, documentation time subsequent to the visit is decreased.

While in the office, Cathi contacted Mr. Henry's physician to report the results of the visit. She discussed with the physician her concern regarding Mr. Henry's misuse of Lanoxin for control of chest pain. She also mentioned that Mr. Henry did not want more pills. The physician agreed to prescribe a Transderm Nitro patch that can be effective for control of angina. This telephone communication was dictated and given to a secretary for transcription into the client record. Cathi also completed the medical orders (HCFA 485) and initiated a Medical Update and Patient Information form (HCFA 486) to be completed at the end of the billing cycle. On her next visit, Cathi implemented the revised treatment plan that she had discussed with Mr. Henry's

physician. She documented the visit on a Skilled Visit Report (Fig. 10–8B).

The Henry family example details use of the Omaha System as a guide for practice and documentation of home health nursing. The System was designed to be adaptable to a variety of formats and forms. This example used forms from the VNA of Omaha to illustrate the nurse's thinking as care was planned and provided.

1. The Problem Classification Scheme, the first component of the Omaha System, provided the basis for collection of baseline data and identification of client problems or nursing diagnoses. Data were collected on a Home Health Referral and Data Base/Problem List Worksheet and entered into the client record on a Patient Information Record, Data Base, and Problem List.
2. Initial ratings of client Knowledge, Behavior, and Status were identified for each priority problem using the Problem Rating Scale for Outcomes, the second component of the Omaha System. The ratings were recorded on a worksheet and entered in the client record on the Problem Ratings/Plans.
3. Standard language from the Intervention Scheme, the third component of the Omaha System, was used to provide clues and cues to the nurse in development of the nursing plan of care. The plan was recorded on a worksheet and entered in the client record on the Problem Ratings/Plans. A Skilled Visit Report, designed to incorporate portions of the Problem Classification Scheme as well as the Intervention Scheme, was used to record nurse-client interactions during the course of the home visit. This form is used by all agency professionals to record home visit data, actions, assessments, and short-term plans.

Using the Omaha System in Diabetic Care

Clients with the medical diagnosis "diabetes mellitus" are frequently the recipients of home health care. Omaha System users have struggled when applying the System to diabetic clients because a single nursing diagnosis is not equivalent to diabetes. This is especially true for those users who have based their practice on a medical model. It is important for users to remember that the Omaha System is based on a nursing model and includes only those client problems that nurses are licensed to diagnose and treat. The nurse does not deal directly with the diagnosis "diabetes." Nursing efforts are concentrated, instead, on identification and treatment of the constellation of problems that may arise for clients with this medical diagnosis.

Kathleen McLaughlin, a nurse specializing in diabetes education, has used the three components of the Omaha System to develop teaching tools for diabetes education. The 24 teaching plans address 10 client problems taken from the Problem Classification Scheme. The category Other has been used to identify two additional problems, Technical Information and Distress.

Text continued on page 196

DATA BASE/PROBLEM LIST WORKSHEET

Instructions: Circle **one** choice (Adequate, Not Assessed, Not Applicable, Health Promotion, Potential **or** Deficit/Impairment/ Actual). CIRCLE F (Family) **or** I (Individual) **only** when using Health Promotion, Potential, or Deficit/Impairment/Actual. If Potential is circled, Risk Factors must be listed. If Deficit/Impairment is circled, one or more Signs/Symptoms (S/S) must be circled. If S/S are circled, elaboration must be included in the comments section. Starred (*) items on the worksheet must be completed.

Date Admitted _____8/15/89_____
Date Completed _____8/17/89_____
Nurse Name _____Cathi Alexander_____
Family Name _____Henry_____
Household # _____24_____
Account # _____John - 24_____
Account # _____
Account # _____

DOMAIN I. ENVIRONMENTAL

01.   INCOME:
    (Adequate)   Not Assessed   Not Applicable   Health Promotion
*Source _pension, social security_
_____ Amount _adequate_
F   **Potential**, Risk Factors:_____
I   **Deficit,** S/S: 1) low/no income 2) uninsured medical expenses
3) inadequate money management 4) able to buy only
_____ necessities 5) difficulty buying necessities 6) other _____

02.   SANITATION:
    (Adequate)   Not Assessed   Not Applicable   Health Promotion
F   **Potential**, Risk Factors:_____
I   **Deficit,** S/S: 1) soiled living area 2) inadequate food storage/
disposal 3) insects/ rodents 4) foul odor 5) inadequate water
supply 6) inadequate sewage disposal 7) inadequate laundry
facilities 8) allergens 9) infectious/contaminating agents
_____ 10) other _____

03.   RESIDENCE:
    (Adequate)   Not Assessed   Not Applicable   Health Promotion
*Type _2 bedroom house, one floor_
                     (Own)   Rent
F   **Potential**, Risk Factors:_____
I   **Deficit,** S/S: 1) structurally unsound 2) inadequate heating/
cooling 3)steep stairs 4)inadequate/obstructed exits/entries
5) cluttered living space 6) unsafe storage of dangerous
objects/substances 7) unsafe mats/throw rugs 8) inadequate
safety devices 9) presence of lead-based paint 10) unsafe
gas/electrical appliances 11) inadequate/crowded living space
_____ 12) homeless 13) other _____

04.   NEIGHBORHOOD/WORKPLACE SAFETY:
    (Adequate)   Not Assessed   Not Applicable   Health Promotion
F   **Potential**, Risk Factors:_____
I   **Deficit,** S/S: 1) high crime rate 2) high pollution level
3) uncontrolled animals 4) physical hazards 5) unsafe play
_____ area 6) other _____

05.   OTHER: S/S: 1) other

*Environmental Assessment: _Adequate environment_

A

FIGURE 10-3 ■ (A–J) The Data Base/Problem List Worksheet is an assessment tool for obtaining family and individual information related to the entire Problem Classification Scheme; the tool was designed for use in the home health and public health settings.

DOMAIN II. PSYCHOSOCIAL

06. COMMUNICATION WITH COMMUNITY RESOURCES:

(Adequate) Not Assessed   Not Applicable   Health Promotion

*Transportation Resources _wife drives_

F
I   **Potential**, Risk Factors: _____
     Impairment, S/S: 1) unfamiliar with options/procedures for
obtaining services 2) difficulty understanding roles/regulations
of service providers 3) unable to communicate concerns to
service provider 4) dissatisfaction with services 5) language
——— barrier 6) inadequate/unavailable resources 7) other _____

07. SOCIAL CONTACT:

(Adequate) Not Assessed   Not Applicable   Health Promotion

*Support System _family & friends supportive_

F
I   **Potential**, Risk Factors: _____
Impairment, S/S: 1) limited social contact 2) uses health care
provider for social contact 3) minimal outside stimulation/
——— leisure time activities 4) other _____

08. ROLE CHANGE:

Adequate   Not Assessed   Not Applicable   Health Promotion
(F) **Potential**, Risk Factors: _____
I   (Impairment), S/S: (1) involuntary reversal of traditional male/
female roles 2) involuntary reversal of dependent/independent
——— roles 3) assumes new role 4) loses previous role 5) other

wife taking on more responsibilities

09. INTERPERSONAL RELATIONSHIP:

(Adequate) Not Assessed   Not Applicable   Health Promotion

F   **Potential**, Risk Factors: _____
I   **Impairment**, S/S: 1) difficulty establishing/maintaining
relationships 2) minimal shared activities 3) incongruent values/
goals 4) inadequate interpersonal communication skills
5) prolonged, unrelieved tension 6) inappropriate suspicion/
——— manipulation/compulsion/aggression 7) other _____

10. SPIRITUAL DISTRESS:

(Adequate) Not Assessed   Not Applicable   Health Promotion

F   **Potential**, Risk Factors: _____
I   **Actual**, S/S: 1) expresses spiritual concerns 2) disrupted
spiritual rituals 3) disrupted spiritual trust 4) conflicting
——— spiritual beliefs and medical regimen 5) other _____

11. GRIEF:

(Adequate) Not Assessed   Not Applicable   Health Promotion

F   **Potential**, Risk Factors: _____
I   **Impairment**, S/S: 1) fails to recognize normal grief responses
2) difficulty coping with grief responses 3) difficulty expressing
grief responses 4) conflicting stages of grief process among
——— family/individual 5) other _____

B

FIGURE 10-3 *Continued*

12. EMOTIONAL STABILITY:
(Adequate) Not Assessed   Not Applicable   Health Promotion
F   **Potential**, Risk Factors: _____
I   **Impairment**, S/S: 1) sadness/hopelessness/worthlessness
2) apprehension/undefined fear 3) loss of interest/involvement
in activities/self-care 4) narrowed perceptual focus 5) scattering
of attention 6) flat affect 7) irritable/agitated 8) purposeless
activity 9) difficulty managing stress 10) somatic complaints/
\#   chronic fatigue 11) expresses wish to die/attempts suicide
_____ 12) other _____

13. HUMAN SEXUALITY:
(Adequate) Not Assessed   Not Applicable   Health Promotion
F   **Potential**, Risk Factors: _____
I   **Impairment**, S/S: 1) difficulty recognizing consequences of
sexual behavior 2) difficulty expressing intimacy 3) sexual
\#   identity confusion 4) sexual value confusion 5) dissatisfied with
_____ sexual relationships 6) other _____
_____

14. CARETAKING/PARENTING:
(Adequate) Not Assessed   Not Applicable   Health Promotion
*Primary Caregiver: _self, wife_____
F   **Potential**, Risk Factors: _____
I   **Impairment**, S/S: 1) difficulty providing physical care/safety
2) difficulty providing emotional nurturance 3) difficulty providing
cognitive learning experiences and activities 4) difficulty
providing preventive and therapeutic health care 5) expectations
incongruent with stage of growth and development
\#   6) dissatisfaction/difficulty with responsibilities 7) neglectful
_____ 8) abusive 9) other _____
_____

15. NEGLECTED CHILD/ADULT:
Adequate (Not Assessed) Not Applicable   Health Promotion
F   **Potential**, Risk Factors: _____
I   **Actual**, S/S: 1) lacks adequate physical care 2) lacks emotional
nurturance/support 3) lacks appropriate stimulation/cognitive
\#   experiences 4) inappropriately left alone 5) lacks necessary
_____ supervision 6) inadequate/ delayed medical care 7) other _____
_____

16. ABUSED CHILD/ADULT:
Adequate (Not Assessed) Not Applicable   Health Promotion
F   **Potential**, Risk Factors: _____
I   **Actual**, S/S: 1) harsh/excessive discipline 2) welts/bruises/
burns 3) questionable explanation of injury 4) attacked
verbally 5) fearful/hypervigilant behavior 6) violent
\#   environment 7) consistently negative messages 8) assaulted
_____ sexually 9) Other _____
_____

C
FIGURE 10-3 *Continued*

17. **GROWTH AND DEVELOPMENT OF CHILD/ADULT:**   Household # ___24___
    Adequate (Not Assessed) Not Applicable Health Promotion
    Height_____ Weight_____ Head Circumference_____
    Feeding_____
    Newborn PA _____
F   **Potential,** Risk Factors: _____
I   **Impairment,** S/S: 1) abnormal results of development
    screening tests 2) abnormal weight/height/head circumference
    in relation to growth curve/age 3) age inappropriate behavior
4) inadequate achievement/maintenance of developmental
____ tasks 5) other _____

18. **OTHER:** S/S: 1) Other

Psychosocial Assessment: *Some family stress/disruption due to John's illness but many strengths evident*

DOMAIN III. PHYSIOLOGICAL

19. **HEARING:**
    (Adequate) Not Assessed Not Applicable Health Promotion
    Correction _____
F   **Potential,** Risk Factors: _____
I   **Impairment,** R _____ L _____ S/S: 1) difficulty hearing normal
speech tones 2) absent/abnormal response to sound
____ 3) abnormal results of hearing screening test 4) other _____

20. **VISION:**
    (Adequate) Not Assessed Not Applicable Health Promotion
    Correction _____
F   **Potential,** Risk Factors: _____
I   **Impairment,** R _____ L _____ S/S: 1) difficulty seeing small print/
    calibrations 2) difficulty seeing distant objects 3) difficulty
    seeing close objects 4) absent/abnormal response to visual
    stimuli 5) abnormal results of vision screening test
6) squinting/blinking/tearing/blurring 7) difficulty differentiating
____ colors 8) other _____

21. **SPEECH AND LANGUAGE:**
    (Adequate) Not Assessed Not Applicable Health Promotion
F   **Potential,** Risk Factors: _____
I   **Impairment,** S/S: 1) absent/abnormal ability to speak
    2) absent/abnormal ability to understand 3) lacks alternative
    communication skills 4) inappropriate sentence structure
5) limited enunciation/clarity 6) inappropriate word usage
____ 7) other _____

22. **DENTITION:**
    (Adequate) Not Assessed Not Applicable Health Promotion
    Correction _____
F   **Potential,** Risk Factors: _____
I   **Impairment,** S/S: 1) abnormalities of teeth 2) sore/swollen/
    bleeding gums 3) ill-fitting dentures 4) malocclusion 5) other
#
____

D

FIGURE 10-3 *Continued*

23. **COGNITION:**

(Adequate) Not Assessed   Not Applicable   Health Promotion

F   **Potential**, Risk Factors: _____

I   **Impairment**, S/S: 1) diminished judgment 2) disoriented to time/place/person 3) limited recall of recent events 4) limited recall of long past events 5) limited calculating/sequencing skills 6) limited concentration 7) limited reasoning/abstract

\#   thinking ability 8) impulsiveness 9) repetitious language/
_____ behavior 10) other _____

_____

24. **PAIN:**

(Adequate) Not Assessed   Not Applicable   Health Promotion

F   **Potential**, Risk Factors: _____

I   **Actual**, Description _____

Relieved by: _____
S/S: 1) expresses discomfort/pain 2) elevated pulse/respirations/blood pressure 3) compensated movement/

\#   guarding 4) restless behavior 5) facial grimaces 6) pallor/
_____ perspiration 7) other _____

_____

25. **CONSCIOUSNESS:**

(Adequate) Not Assessed   Not Applicable   Health Promotion

F   **Potential**, Risk Factors: _____

I   **Impairment**, S/S: 1) lethargic 2) stuporous 3) unresponsive
4) comatose 5) other _____

\#   _____
_____

26. **INTEGUMENT:**

(Adequate) Not Assessed   Not Applicable   Health Promotion

F   **Potential**, Risk Factors: _____

I   **Impairment**, S/S: 1) lesion 2) rash 3) excessively dry

\#   4) excessively oily 5) inflammation 6) pruritus 7) drainage
_____ 8) ecchymosis 9) hypertrophy of nails 10) other _____

_____

27. **NEURO-MUSCULO-SKELETAL FUNCTION:**

Adequate   Not Assessed   Not Applicable   Health Promotion
Assistive Devices _cane_ _____

_____

F   **Potential**, Risk Factors: _____
(I) (Impairment) S/S: 1) limited range of motion (2) decreased muscle strength 3) decreased coordination 4) decreased muscle tone 5) increased muscle tone 6) decreased sensation 7) increased sensation 8) decreased balance

\# (9) gait/ambulation disturbance (10) difficulty managing activities
_24_ of daily living (11) tremors/seizures 12) other _____

_____

unsteady, shuffling gait
vertigo c̄ position chg.
slight tremor of hands

E

FIGURE 10-3 *Continued*

28. **RESPIRATION:**
   (Adequate) Not Assessed   Not Applicable   Health Promotion
   Rate __18__ Assistive Devices _____

   F   **Potential**, Risk Factors:_____
   I   **Impairment**, S/S: 1) abnormal breathing patterns 2) unable to breathe independently 3) cough 4) unable to cough/expectorate independently 5) cyanosis 6) abnormal sputum
   #   7) noisy respirations 8) rhinorrhea 9) abnormal breath sounds
   _____ 10) other _____

29. **CIRCULATION:**
   Adequate   Not Assessed   Not Applicable   Health Promotion
   Temp _____ Assistive Devices _____

   BP: sitting R $^{104}/_{64}$ L _____ ; standing R $^{70}/_{50}$ L _____ ;
   lying R _____ L _____
   Pulses: apical _56 - 96_ radial_____ peripheral _____
   F   **Potential**, Risk Factors: _____
   (I)   (Impairment) S/S: 1) edema 2) cramping/pain of extremities
   3) decreased pulses 4) discoloration of skin/cyanosis
   5) temperature change in affected area 6) varicosities
   (7) syncopal episodes (8) abnormal blood pressure reading
   (9) pulse deficit (10) irregular heart rate 11) excessively rapid
   #   heart rate 12) excessively slow heart rate (13) anginal pain
   _24_ 14) abnormal heart sounds 15) other _____

   c/o vertigo c̄ position chg.
   HR irreg c̄ 2 skipped beats
   per min. Chest pain, occ.
   radiating down arm approx.
   once per day

30. **DIGESTION-HYDRATION:**
   (Adequate) Not Assessed   Not Applicable   Health Promotion
   Assistive Devices _____

   F   **Potential**, Risk Factors: _____
   I   **Impairment**, S/S: 1) nausea/vomiting 2) difficulty/inability to chew/swallow/digest 3) indigestion/reflux 4) anorexia
   5) anemia 6) ascites 7) jaundice/liver enlargement
   #   8) decreased skin turgor 9) cracked lips/dry mouth
   _____ 10) electrolyte imbalance 11) other _____

31. **BOWEL FUNCTION:**
   (Adequate) Not Assessed   Not Applicable   Health Promotion
   Assistive Devices _____

   F   **Potential**, Risk Factors: _____
   I   **Impairment**, S/S: 1) abnormal frequency/consistency of stool
   2) painful defecation 3) decreased bowel sounds 4) blood in
   #   stools 5) abnormal color 6) cramping/abdominal discomfort
   _____ 7) incontinent of stool 8) other _____

F

FIGURE 10-3 *Continued*

32. GENITO-URINARY FUNCTION:
(Adequate) Not Assessed   Not Applicable   Health Promotion
Assistive Devices _____

F   **Potential**, Risk Factors: _____
I   **Impairment**, S/S: 1) incontinent of urine 2) urgency/frequency
    3) burning/painful urination 4) difficulty emptying bladder
    5) abnormal urinary frequency/amount 6) hematuria
    7) abnormal discharge 8) abnormal menstrual pattern
\# 9) abnormal lumps/swelling/tenderness of male/female
____ reproductive organs 10) dyspareunia 11) other _____

33.   ANTEPARTUM/POSTPARTUM:
Adequate   Not Assessed (Not Applicable) Health Promotion
AP: *TPAL _____ EDC _____ Date OB Care _____
     Fetal Act/FHR _____
     L&D Prep _____ Abn Lab _____
     Danger Sig _____ Preterm Labor _____
PP: Del Date _____ Bonding _____
     8-point check _____
F   **Potential**, Risk Factors: _____
I   **Impairment**, S/S: 1) difficulty coping with pregnancy/body
     changes 2) inappropriate exercise/rest/diet/behaviors
\#   3) discomforts 4) complications 5) fears delivery procedure
____ 6) difficulty breast-feeding 7) other _____
*TPAL = Term (36–42 wk), Preterm (under 36 wk), Abortions, Living
Children

34.   OTHER: S/S: 1) other

*Physiological Assessment: _Poor NMS status c̄ general weakness & s/s of Parkinsons. Unable to be independent. Poor cardiac status c̄ evidence of orthostatic hypotension & irreg. heart rate_

DOMAIN IV. HEALTH RELATED BEHAVIORS
35.   NUTRITION:
(Adequate) Not Assessed   Not Applicable   Health Promotion
Height _5'10"_ Weight _190_ Diet _low salt_
F   **Potential**, Risk Factors: _____
I   **Impairment**, S/S: 1) weighs 10% more than average
     2) weighs 10% less than average 3) lacks established
     standards for daily caloric/fluid intake 4) exceeds established
     standards for daily caloric/fluid intake 5) unbalanced diet
     6) improper feeding schedule for age 7) nonadherence to
\#   prescribed diet 8) unexplained/progressive weight loss
____ 9) hypoglycemia 10) hyperglycemia 11) other _____

36.   SLEEP AND REST PATTERNS:
(Adequate) Not Assessed   Not Applicable   Health Promotion
F   **Potential**, Risk Factors: _____
I   **Impairment**, S/S: 1) sleep/rest pattern disrupts family
     2) frequently wakes during night 3) somnambulism
\#   4) insomnia 5) nightmares 6) insufficient sleep/rest for age/
____ physical condition 7) other _____

Household # _24_

G
FIGURE 10-3 *Continued*

37. PHYSICAL ACTIVITY:
(Adequate) Not Assessed   Not Applicable   Health Promotion
F   **Potential**, Risk Factors:_____
I   **Impairment**, S/S: 1) sedentary life style 2) inadequate/
\#   inconsistent exercise routine 3) inappropriate type/amount of
____ exercise for age/physical condition 4) other _____

walks within home; activity appropriate for physical status

38. PERSONAL HYGIENE:
Adequate   Not Assessed   Not Applicable   Health Promotion
F   (Potential) Risk Factors: _weakness_____
(I) **Impairment**, S/S: 1) inadequate laundering of clothing
    2) inadequate bathing 3) body odor 4) inadequate
\#   shampooing/combing of hair 5) inadequate brushing/flossing/
_24_ mouth care 6) other _____

wife assists

39. SUBSTANCE USE:
(Adequate) Not Assessed   Not Applicable   Health Promotion
F   **Potential**, Risk Factors:
I   **Impairment**, S/S: 1) abuses over-the-counter/street drugs
\#   2) abuses alcohol 3) smokes 4) difficulty performing normal
____ routines 5) reflex disturbances 6) behavior change 7) other

40. FAMILY PLANNING
Adequate   Not Assessed (Not Applicable) Health Promotion
Methods _____

F   **Potential**, Risk Factors: _____
I   **Impairment**, S/S: 1) inappropriate/insufficient knowledge of
    family planning methods 2) inaccurate/inconsistent use of
\#   family planning methods 3) dissatisfied with present family
____ planning method 4) other _____

41. HEALTH CARE SUPERVISION:
(Adequate) Not Assessed   Not Applicable   Health Promotion
*Routine care plans _Dr. Watson routinely once a_
month
*Emergency care plans _911_

f   **Potential**, Risk Factors: _____
I   **Impairment**, S/S: 1) fails to obtain routine medical/dental
    evaluation 2) fails to seek care for symptoms requiring
    medical/dental evaluation 3) fails to return as requested to
    physician/dentist 4) inability to coordinate multiple
    appointments/regimens 5) inconsistent source of medical/
\#   dental care 6) inadequate prescribed medical/dental regimen
____ 7) other _____

42. PRESCRIBED MEDICATION REGIMEN:
Adequate   Not Assessed   Not Applicable   Health Promotion
F   **Potential**, Risk Factors: _____
(I) (**Impairment**) S/S: (1) deviates from prescribed dosage/
    schedule (2) demonstrates side effects 3) inadequate system
    for taking medication 4) improper storage of medication 5)fails
\#   to obtain refills appropriately 6) fails to obtain immunizations
_24_ 7) other _____

taking Lanoxin PRN for chest pain. c̄/o nausea from Sinemet & not taking as prescribed

H
FIGURE 10-3 *Continued*

43. TECHNICAL PROCEDURE:

Adequate   Not Assessed   (Not Applicable)   Health Promotion

F   **Potential**, Risk Factors: _____

I   **Impairment**, S/S: 1) unable to demonstrate/relate procedure
accurately 2) does not follow/demonstrate principles of safe/
aseptic techniques 3) procedure requires nursing skill

\#   4) unable/unwilling to perform procedure without assistance

_____ 5) unable/unwilling to operate special equipment 6) other _____

Household # ___*24*___

44. OTHER: S/S: 1) Other

*Health Behavior
Assessment: *Deviation from medication regimen as prescribed; experiencing some side effects*

Significant Planning Factors: _____

*Homebound Status: *Weakness, unsteady, vertigo*

HEALTH HISTORY
Significant Medical History of Client(s)

Hospitalizations:

1/85 trt of CHF

Pregnancies:

NA

Surgeries:

Injuries:

FIGURE 10-3 *Continued*

MEDICAL HISTORY OF CLIENT AND FAMILY MEMBERS

Complete column(s) below indicating client's name(s) and relationship of other pertinent family members. Focus on specific family history as it contributes to client care.

Diagnosis   Name/Relationship

Diagnosis	John					
Diabetes						
Epilepsy						
Cardiac Disease	✓					
Hypertension						
CVA						
Arthritis/Gout						
Cancer						
Frequent Headaches/Migraines						
Asthma/Allergies						
Respiratory Disease						
SIDS						
GI Problems/Ulcers						
Kidney/Bladder Problems						
Phlebitis/Varicose Veins						
Drug/Alcohol Abuse						
Mental Retardation						
Mental Illness						
Other Parkinsons	✓					
Hypotension	✓					

ASSESSMENT/COMMENTS: _diagnosed c̄ CHF 4 yrs. ago — no medical problems prior to that. New diagnosis of Parkinson's Disease_

J

FIGURE 10-3 *Continued*

```
---------------------------------------------------------------------
                         * * * D A T A   B A S E * * *         PAGE   1
HOUSEHOLD #:     24     4567 MAIN ST., #4        STATION- VNA MIDLANDS DIR SVC
---------------------------------------------------------------------
                         ACCOUNTS IN HOUSEHOLD
Patient's Name:            Account #:        From Date:
HENRY, JOHN                     24           8/15/89
HENRY, JANE                   55512          9/14/89 - NOT ADMITTED
---------------------------------------------------------------------

DATE ADMITTED:   08/15/89

ENVIRONMENTAL DOMAIN:  All areas assessed with significant findings as
follows:  INCOME:  Source:  Pension, Social Security.  Amount:
Adequate.  RESIDENCE:  Type:  Two bedroom house, one floor, own.

A:  ADEQUATE ENVIRONMENT.

PSYCHOSOCIAL DOMAIN:  All areas assessed with significant findings as
follows:  COMMUNICATION WITH COMMUNITY RESOURCES:  Transportation
Resources:  Wife drives.  SOCIAL CONTACT:  Support System:  Family and
friends supportive.  ROLE CHANGE:  Wife taking on more
responsibilities.  Areas Not Assessed:  Neglected Child/Adult, Abused
Child/Adult, G&D of Child/Adult.

A:  SOME FAMILY STRESS/DISRUPTION DUE TO JOHN'S ILLNESS BUT MANY
STRENGTHS EVIDENT.

PHYSIOLOGICAL DOMAIN:  All areas assessed with significant findings as
follows:  NEURO-MUSCULO-SKELETAL FUNCTION:  Assistive Devices:  cane.
Unsteady, shuffling gait.  Vertigo with position changes.  Slight
tremor of hands.  RESPIRATION:  Rate 18.  CIRCULATION:  BP right
sitting 104/64, standing 70/50.  AP 56-96.  Complains of vertigo with
position change.  Heart rate irregular with 2 skipped beats per minute.
Chest pain, occasionally radiating down arm approximately once per day.
Areas Not Assessed:  Antepartum/Postpartum.

A:  POOR NMS STATUS WITH GENERALIZED WEAKNESS AND S/S OF PARKINSON'S.
UNABLE TO BE INDEPENDENT.  POOR CARDIAC STATUS WITH EVIDENCE OF
ORTHOSTATIC HYPOTENSION AND IRREGULAR HEART RATE.

HEALTH RELATED BEHAVIORS DOMAIN:  All areas assessed with significant
findings as follows:  NUTRITION:  Height 5 ft. 10 in., weight 190 lbs.
Low salt diet.  PHYSICAL ACTIVITY:  Walks within home, activity
appropriate for physical status.  PERSONAL HYGIENE:  Risk Factors:
Weakness.  Wife assists.  HEALTH CARE SUPERVISION:  Routine care plans:
Dr. Watson routinely once a month.  Emergency care plans:  911.
PRESCRIBED MEDICATION REGIMEN:  Taking LANOXIN p.r.n. for chest pain.
Complains of nausea from SINEMET, not taking as prescribed.

A:  DEVIATION FROM MEDICATION REGIMEN AS PRESCRIBED, EXPERIENCING SOME
SIDE EFFECTS.

SIGNIFICANT PLANNING FACTORS:  Homebound Status:  Weakness, unsteady,
vertigo.

HEALTH HISTORY:  Significant Medical History of Client:
                                                        ---------------
---------------------------------------------------------------------
```

A

FIGURE 10-4 ■ (*A and B*) The Data Base is a computer-generated form developed from the Data Base/Problem List Worksheet.

```
--------------------------------------------------------------------
                         * * * D A T A   B A S E * * *          PAGE    2
HOUSEHOLD #:     24      4567 MAIN ST., #4      STATION- VNA MIDLANDS DIR SVC
--------------------------------------------------------------------

Hospitalizations:
1/85 treatment of CHF

Medical History of Client and Family Members:

JOHN
Cardiac Disease
Hypotension
Parkinson's

ASSESSMENT/COMMENTS:  DIAGNOSED WITH CHF 4 YEARS AGO.   NO MEDICAL
PROBLEMS PRIOR TO THAT TIME.   NEW DIAGNOSIS OF PARKINSON'S DISEASE.
```
Cathi Alexander, PHN
```
                  Cathi Alexander, PHN/rip
```

```
--------------------------------------------------------------------
```
B

FIGURE 10-4 *Continued*

```
-----------------------------------------------------------------------
                   * * * P R O B L E M   L I S T * * *        PAGE   1
HOUSEHOLD #:     24    4567 MAIN ST., #4      STATION- VNA MIDLANDS DIR SVC
-----------------------------------------------------------------------
                      ACCOUNTS IN HOUSEHOLD
Patient's Name:              Account #:      From Date:
HENRY, JOHN                       24         8/15/89
HENRY, JANE                       55512      9/14/89 - NOT ADMITTED
-----------------------------------------------------------------------


* 08/15/89 FAMILY
              08C
           Role Change: Impairment

              0801
           Involuntary Reversal Of Traditional Male/Female
           Roles

* 08/15/89 HENRY, JOHN
              27C
           Neuro-Musculo-Skeletal Function: Impairment

              2702
           Decreased Muscle Strength

              2708
           Gait/Ambulation Disturbance

              2709
           Difficulty Managing Activities Of Daily Living

              2710
           Tremors/Seizures

* 08/15/89 HENRY, JOHN
              29C
           Circulation: Impairment

              2907
           Syncopal Episodes

              2908
           Abnormal Blood Pressure Reading

              2909
           Pulse Deficit

              2910
           Irregular Heart Rate

              2913
           Anginal Pain

* 08/15/89 HENRY, JOHN
              38B
           Personal Hygiene: Potential Impairment


-----------------------------------------------------------------------
           **
           **
           **
```

A

FIGURE 10−5 ■ (*A and B*) The Problem List is a computer-generated index of the client's health-related interests, concerns, and problems and is based on the Problem Classification Scheme.

```
-----------------------------------------------------------------------------
                        * * * P R O B L E M   L I S T * * *
HOUSEHOLD #:      24      4567 MAIN ST., #4                    PAGE    2
                                              STATION- VNA MIDLANDS DIR SVC
-----------------------------------------------------------------------------
* 08/15/89 HENRY, JOHN
              42C
         Prescribed Medication Regimen: Impairment

              4201
         Deviates From Prescribed Dosage/Schedule

              4202
         Demonstrates Side-Effects
                    Cathi Alexander, PHN
                 Cathi Alexander, PHN/rip
```

```
-----------------------------------------------------------------------------
         **
         **
         **
```

B

FIGURE 10-5 Continued

CLIENT CARE PLAN/PROBLEM RATING WORKSHEET

NAME: _Henry, John_   DATE: _8/15/89_

HH# _24_   ACCOUNT # _24_   ADMIT DATE: _8/15/89_

PROBLEM CLASSIFICATION SCHEME

DOMAIN I. ENVIRONMENTAL
01. Income
02. Sanitation
03. Residence
04. Neighborhood/workplace safety
05. Other

DOMAIN II. PSYCHOSOCIAL
06. Communication with community resources
07. Social contact
08. Role change
09. Interpersonal relationship
10. Spiritual distress
11. Grief
12. Emotional stability
13. Human sexuality
14. Caretaking/parenting
15. Neglected child/adult
16. Abused child/adult
17. Growth and development
18. Other

DOMAIN III. PHYSIOLOGICAL
19. Hearing
20. Vision
21. Speech and language
22. Dentition
23. Cognition
24. Pain
25. Consciousness
26. Integument
27. Neuro-musculo-skeletal function
28. Respiration
29. Circulation
30. Digestion-hydration
31. Bowel function
32. Genito-urinary function
33. Antepartum/postpartum
34. Other

DOMAIN IV. HEALTH RELATED BEHAVIORS
35. Nutrition
36. Sleep and rest patterns
37. Physical activity
38. Personal hygiene
39. Substance use
40. Family planning
41. Health care supervision
42. Prescribed medication regimen
43. Technical procedure
44. Other

Problem Rating Scale For Outcome

1	2	3	4	5
Poor	Fair	Average	Good	Excellent

INTERVENTION SCHEME CATEGORIES

I. Health Teaching, Guidance, and Counseling
II. Treatments and Procedures
III. Case Management
IV. Surveillance

TARGETS

01. Anatomy/physiology
02. Behavior modification
03. Bladder care
04. Bonding
05. Bowel care
06. Bronchial hygiene
07. Cardiac care
08. Caretaking/parenting skills
09. Cast care
10. Communication
11. Coping skills
12. Day care/respite
13. Discipline
14. Dressing change/wound care
15. Durable medical equipment
16. Education
17. Employment
18. Environment
19. Exercises
20. Family planning
21. Feeding procedures
22. Finances
23. Food
24. Gait training
25. Growth/development
26. Homemaking
27. Housing
28. Interaction
29. Lab findings
30. Legal system
31. Medical/dental care
32. Medication action/side effects
33. Medication administration
34. Medication setup
35. Mobility/transfers
36. Nursing care, supplementary
37. Nutrition
38. Nutritionist
39. Ostomy care
40. Other community resource
41. Personal care
42. Positioning
43. Rehabilitation
44. Relaxation/breathing techniques
45. Rest/sleep
46. Safety
47. Screening
48. Sickness/injury care
49. Signs/symptoms-mental, emotional
50. Signs/symptoms-physical
51. Skin care
52. Social work/counseling
53. Specimen collection
54. Spiritual care
55. Stimulation/nurturance
56. Stress management
57. Substance use
58. Supplies
59. Support group
60. Support system
61. Transportation
62. Wellness
63. Other (specify)

PROBLEM _08_

RATINGS
Knowledge _3_ Behavior _3_ Status _3_

PLANS

Category _I_ Target _11_ Specifics _Normal responses to role change_

Category _I_ Target _60_ Specifics _Active listening, offer emotional support_

Category _____ Target _____ Specifics _____

Category _____ Target _____ Specifics _____

Category _____ Target _____ Specifics _____

PROBLEM _27_

RATINGS
Knowledge _2_ Behavior _3_ Status _2_

PLANS

Category _I_ Target _46_ Specifics _slow position change, use cane or other support when standing or ambulating_

Category _IV_ Target _50_ Specifics _gait, strength, endurance_

Category _____ Target _____ Specifics _____

Category _____ Target _____ Specifics _____

Category _____ Target _____ Specifics _____

CASE MANAGER _Cathi Alexander, RN_

A

FIGURE 10-6 ■ (*A and B*) The Client Care Plan/Problem Rating Worksheet is a data-gathering guide to note both problem-specific client ratings and plans associated with the Problem Rating Scale for Outcomes and the Intervention Scheme.

CLIENT CARE PLAN/PROBLEM RATING WORKSHEET

NAME: _Henry, John_

HH# _24_ ACCOUNT # _24_

DATE: _8/15/89_

ADMIT DATE: _8/15/89_

PROBLEM CLASSIFICATION SCHEME

DOMAIN I. ENVIRONMENTAL
01. Income
02. Sanitation
03. Residence
04. Neighborhood/workplace safety
05. Other

DOMAIN II. PSYCHOSOCIAL
06. Communication with community resources
07. Social contact
08. Role change
09. Interpersonal relationship
10. Spiritual distress
11. Grief
12. Emotional stability
13. Human sexuality
14. Caretaking/parenting
15. Neglected child/adult
16. Abused child/adult
17. Growth and development
18. Other

DOMAIN III. PHYSIOLOGICAL
19. Hearing
20. Vision
21. Speech and language
22. Dentition
23. Cognition
24. Pain
25. Consciousness
26. Integument
27. Neuro-musculo-skeletal function
28. Respiration
29. Circulation
30. Digestion-hydration
31. Bowel function
32. Genito-urinary function
33. Antepartum/postpartum
34. Other

DOMAIN IV. HEALTH RELATED BEHAVIORS
35. Nutrition
36. Sleep and rest patterns
37. Physical activity
38. Personal hygiene
39. Substance use
40. Family planning
41. Health care supervision
42. Prescribed medication regimen
43. Technical procedure
44. Other

Problem Rating Scale For Outcome

1	2	3	4	5 /
Poor	Fair	Average	Good	Excellent

INTERVENTION SCHEME CATEGORIES

I. Health Teaching, Guidance, and Counseling
II. Treatments and Procedures
III. Case Management
IV. Surveillance

TARGETS

01. Anatomy/physiology
02. Behavior modification
03. Bladder care
04. Bonding
05. Bowel care
06. Bronchial hygiene
07. Cardiac care
08. Caretaking/parenting skills
09. Cast care
10. Communication
11. Coping skills
12. Day care/respite
13. Discipline
14. Dressing change/wound care
15. Durable medical equipment
16. Education
17. Employment
18. Environment
19. Exercises
20. Family planning
21. Feeding procedures
22. Finances
23. Food
24. Gait training
25. Growth/development
26. Homemaking
27. Housing
28. Interaction
29. Lab findings
30. Legal system
31. Medical/dental care
32. Medication action/side effects
33. Medication administration
34. Medication setup
35. Mobility/transfers
36. Nursing care, supplementary
37. Nutrition
38. Nutritionist
39. Ostomy care
40. Other community resource
41. Personal care
42. Positioning
43. Rehabilitation
44. Relaxation/breathing techniques
45. Rest/sleep
46. Safety
47. Screening
48. Sickness/injury care
49. Signs/symptoms-mental, emotional
50. Signs/symptoms-physical
51. Skin care
52. Social work/counseling
53. Specimen collection
54. Spiritual care
55. Stimulation/nurturance
56. Stress management
57. Substance use
58. Supplies
59. Support group
60. Support system
61. Transportation
62. Wellness
63. Other (specify)

PROBLEM _29_

RATINGS
Knowledge _2_ Behavior _2_ Status _2_

PLANS

Category _I_ Target _07_ Specifics _foods to avoid, relief of edema_

Category _I_ Target _35_ Specifics _balanced rest/activity_

Category _I_ Target _50_ Specifics _when to notify MD/RN (increased wt., edema, SOB, pain)_

Category _III_ Target _31_ Specifics _regular MD & cardiologist_

Category _IV_ Target _50_ Specifics _circ. status, chest pain, edema, SOB, orthostatic BP_

PROBLEM _42_

RATINGS
Knowledge _2_ Behavior _2_ Status _2_

PLANS

Category _I_ Target _32_ Specifics _Lanoxin, Sinemet, Mylanta_

Category _I_ Target _33_ Specifics _Lanoxin, Sinemet, Mylanta_

Category _III_ Target _31_ Specifics _coordinate c̄ MD_

Category _IV_ Target _32_ Specifics _prescribed meds_

Category _IV_ Target _33_ Specifics _compliance c̄ dose, frequency as prescribed_

CASE MANAGER _Cathi Alexander, RN_

B

FIGURE 10-6 _Continued_

```
--------------------------------------------------------------------------
            * * *  P R O B L E M   R A T I N G S/P L A N S  * * *      PAGE    1
HOUSEHOLD #:      24      4567 MAIN ST., #4        STATION- VNA MIDLANDS DIR SVC
--------------------------------------------------------------------------
                          ACCOUNTS IN HOUSEHOLD
Patient's Name:                  Account #:         From Date:
HENRY, JOHN                          24             8/15/89
HENRY, JANE                       55512             9/14/89 - NOT ADMITTED
--------------------------------------------------------------------------

* 08/15/89 HENRY, JOHN
            08
            ROLE CHANGE

            K3
            KNOWLEDGE - Basic knowledge

            B3
            BEHAVIOR - Inconsistently appropriate

            S3
            STATUS - Moderate signs/symptoms

            2
            Re-Evaluate Two Months
PLAN:
1. HTGC:  coping skills:  normal responses to role change.
2. HTGC:  support system:  active listening, offer emotional support.

* 08/15/89 HENRY, JOHN
            27
            NEURO-MUSCULO-SKELETAL FUNCTION

            K2
            KNOWLEDGE - Minimal knowledge

            B3
            BEHAVIOR - Inconsistently appropriate

            S2
            STATUS - Severe signs/symptoms

            2
            Re-Evaluate Two Months
PLAN:
1. HTGC:  safety:  slow position change, use cane or other support
when standing or ambulating.
2. S:  s/s - physical:  gait, strength, endurance.

* 08/15/89 HENRY, JOHN
            29
            CIRCULATION

            K2
            KNOWLEDGE - Minimal knowledge

            B2

--------------------------------------------------------------------------
HTGC = Health Teaching , Guidance , & Counseling
T & P = Treatments & Procedures
CM = Case Management       S = Surveillance
```

A

FIGURE 10–7 ■ (*A and B*) The Problem Ratings/Plans is a computer-generated form developed from the Client Care Plan/Problem Rating Worksheet.

```
------------------------------------------------------------------------
              * * *  P R O B L E M  R A T I N G S/P L A N S  * * *        PAGE   2
HOUSEHOLD #:     24    4567 MAIN ST., #4        STATION- VNA MIDLANDS DIR SVC
------------------------------------------------------------------------
              BEHAVIOR - Rarely appropriate

                  S2
              STATUS - Severe signs/symptoms

                  2
              Re-Evaluate Two Months
PLAN:
1. HTGC:  cardiac care:  foods to avoid, relief of edema.
2. HTGC:  mobility/exercise:  balanced rest/activity.
3. HTGC:  s/s - physical:  when to notify MD/RN (increased weight,
increased edema, SOB, pain).
4. CM:  medical/dental care:  regular MD and cardiologist.
5. S:  s/s - physical:  circulatory status, chest pain, edema, SOB,
orthostatic BP.

* 08/15/89 HENRY, JOHN
              42
              PRESCRIBED MEDICATION REGIMEN

                  K2
              KNOWLEDGE - Minimal knowledge

                  B2
              BEHAVIOR - Rarely appropriate

                  S2
              STATUS - Severe signs/symptoms

                  2
              Re-Evaluate Two Months
PLAN:
1. HTGC:  medication action side effects:  Lanoxin, Sinemet, Mylanta.
2. HTGC:  medication administration:  Lanoxin, Sinemet, Mylanta.
3. CM:  medical/dental care:  coordinate with MD.
4. S:  medication action side effects:  prescribed meds.
5. S:  medication administration:  compliance with dose, frequency
as prescribed.
```

Cathi Alexander, PHN
Cathi Alexander, PHN/rip

```
------------------------------------------------------------------------
HTGC = Health Teaching , Guidance , & Counseling
T & P = Treatments & Procedures
CM = Case Management      S = Surveillance
```

B

FIGURE 10-7 *Continued*

VISITING NURSE ASSOCIATION OF THE MIDLANDS SKILLED VISIT REPORT

H.H.# ___24___ Client Name _Nosby, John_ Date _8/15/89_ Time _10_ (a.m.) p.m. Unscheduled ( ) Explain

Homebound Due to _Generalized weakness, unsteady, shuffling gait w/cane + resting w/ position change_

CLIENT PROBLEMS (Circle #)

	SUBJECTIVE/OBJECTIVE	CAT	TARG	RX	INTERVENTIONS/COMMENTS
ENVIRONMENTAL:					
PSYCHOSOCIAL:					
(08) Role change	See data base	IV	49	A1	
PHYSIOLOGICAL:					
21. Speech and language:					
24. Pain:					
26. Integument: Lesion ___ Depth ___ Diameter ___ Drainage ___					
(27) Neuro-musculo-skeletal function:		I	46		Slow position change, use care, don't attempt to walk if dizzy
28. Respiration: Rate _18_ Resting ___ Activity ___ Lung Sounds _Clear_					
(29) Circulation: Pulse: Apical _R_ Radial _104/64_ Pedal _70/50_ Lying ___ Sitting ___ Standing ___	See data base. Chest pain this am-non-radiating. Relieved w/ Lanoxin	IV I	50 32 33	A1 A1 A1	Correct use of Lanoxin. Suggested Nitro for chest pain. Continued to refuse
Edema ___ Weight ___ Temp. ___					
30. Digestion-hydration:					
31. Bowel function:					
32. Genito-urinary function: Incontinent ( ) (Other) ___					
HEALTH RELATED BEHAVIORS:					
35. Nutrition: Intake ___					
(38) Personal hygiene: HHA SUPERVISORY VISIT POC ( ) Appropriate ( ) Inappropriate	See data base	III	41 43	A1	Offered HHA, OT consult. Want to manage on own for now
41. Health care supervision: MD Visit Date _8/14/89_					
42. Prescribed med(s): Know Comply _Lanoxin_ Yes/(No) Yes/No _Sinemet_ Yes/(No) Yes/No	Taking Lanoxin PRN Chest pain. Sinemet 1g am w/ % nausea	I	32 33	A1	Correct dose + frequency. Take Sinemet w/meals
43. Technical procedure:					
(Other) ___					

Assessment _Nausea possibly se of Sinemet, exhibiting s/s orthostatic hypotension, compliance w/meds poor_

Plan: Frequency and Reason _SNC 3x/wk to continued teaching + assessment of medically unstable client_

Signature _Cathi Alexander_ (RN) LPN RPT OTR SP MSS Employee # _504_

INTERVENTION SCHEME

CATEGORIES
I. Health Teaching, Guidance, and Counseling
II. Treatments and Procedures
III. Case Management
IV. Surveillance

TARGETS
01. Anatomy/physiology
02. Behavior modification
03. Bladder care
04. Bonding
05. Bowel care
06. Bronchial hygiene
07. Cardiac care
08. Caretaking/parenting skills
09. Cast care
10. Communication
11. Coping skills
12. Daycare/respite
13. Discipline
14. Dressing change/wound care
15. Durable medical equipment
16. Education
17. Employment
18. Environment
19. Exercises
20. Family planning
21. Feeding procedures
22. Finances
23. Food
24. Gait training
25. Growth/development
26. Homemaking
27. Housing
28. Interaction
29. Lab findings
30. Legal system
31. Medical/dental care
32. Medication action/side effects
33. Medication administration
34. Medication set-up
35. Mobility/transfers
36. Nursing care, supplementary
37. Nutrition
38. Nutritionst
39. Ostomy care
40. Other community resource
41. Personal care
42. Positioning
43. Rehabilitation
44. Relaxation/breathing techniques
45. Rest/sleep
46. Safety
47. Screening
48. Sickness/injury care
49. Signs/symptoms-mental/emotional
50. Signs/symptoms-physical
51. Skin care
52. Social work/counseling
53. Specimen collection
54. Spiritual care
55. Stimulation/nurturance
56. Stress management
57. Substance use
58. Supplies
59. Support group
60. Support system
61. Transportation
62. Wellness
63. Other (specify)

FIGURE 10–8 ■ (A and B) The Skilled Visit Report is a problem-specific guide that incorporates the Intervention Scheme; it is used to document home health services actually provided during one home visit.

A

VISITING NURSE ASSOCIATION OF THE MIDLANDS SKILLED VISIT REPORT

H.H.# _34_   Client Name _Army, John_   Date _8/17/89_   Time _10_ (a.m.) p.m.   Unscheduled ( ) Explain

Homebound Due to _unsteady, shuffling gait, unsteady ambulation, dizzy when stands_

CLIENT PROBLEMS (Circle #)

	SUBJECTIVE/OBJECTIVE	CAT	TARG	RX	INTERVENTIONS/COMMENTS
ENVIRONMENTAL:					
PSYCHOSOCIAL:					
PHYSIOLOGICAL:					
21. Speech and language:					
24. Pain:					
26. Integument:					
Lesion					
Depth					
Diameter					
Drainage					
(27) Neuro-musculo-skeletal function:	c/o vertigo when standing. Obs. ambulating - requires assist.	I / IV	46 / A17	A1	Use assistive devices at all times. Have wife or another person present for stand by assist.
28. Respiration: Rate _18_ Resting / Activity _Ø_ Lung Sounds _Ø_					
(29) Circulation: Pulse _60 irreg_ Apical _Radial_ _Pedal_ _R 108/62_ _100/60_ B/P _Lying Ø_ _Sitting Ø_ _Standing_	no c/o chest pain. Lightheaded w/position chg	III	50	A1	
Edema _Ø_ Weight _____ Temp. _____					
30. Digestion-hydration:					
31. Bowel function:					
32. Genito-urinary function: Incontinent ( ) _____ (Other)					
HEALTH RELATED BEHAVIORS:					
35. Nutrition: Intake					
38. Personal hygiene: HHA SUPERVISORY VISIT POC ( ) Appropriate ( ) Inappropriate					
41. Health care supervision					
MD Visit Date					
(42) Prescribed med(s): Know Comply _Lanoxin_ Yes/No Yes/No _Sinmet_ Yes/No Yes/No	Taking w/meals has decreased nausea	I / IV	31 / 32	A1 / A17	Dose, freq, action, s.e. of Sinmet. Agreed to try Transderm Nitro patch
43. Technical procedure: _____ (Other)					

Assessment _Minimal improvement of s/s orthostatic hypotension. Complient w/ Sinmet and receptive to teaching_

Plan: Frequency and Reason _3x/wk. Teach re: cardiac meds @ next HV. Continue assessment of medically unstable client_

Signature _Cathy Alexander_   (RN) LPN RPT OTR SP MSS   Employee # _504_

INTERVENTION SCHEME

CATEGORIES
I. Health Teaching, Guidance, and Counseling
II. Treatments and Procedures
III. Case Management
IV. Surveillance

TARGETS
01. Anatomy/physiology
02. Behavior modification
03. Bladder care
04. Bonding
05. Bowel care
06. Bronchial hygiene
07. Cardiac care
08. Caretaking/parenting skills
09. Cast care
10. Communication
11. Coping skills
12. Daycare/respite
13. Discipline
14. Dressing change/wound care
15. Durable medical equipment
16. Education
17. Employment
18. Environment
19. Exercises
20. Family planning
21. Feeding procedures
22. Finances
23. Food
24. Gait training
25. Growth/development
26. Homemaking
27. Housing
28. Interaction
29. Lab findings
30. Legal system
31. Medical/dental care
32. Medication action/side effects
33. Medication administration
34. Medication set-up
35. Mobility/transfers
36. Nursing care, supplementary
37. Nutrition
38. Nutritionist
39. Ostomy care
40. Other community resource
41. Personal care
42. Positioning
43. Rehabilitation
44. Relaxation/breathing techniques
45. Rest/sleep
46. Safety
47. Screening
48. Sickness/injury care
49. Signs/symptoms-mental/emotional
50. Signs/symptoms-physical
51. Skin care
52. Social work/counseling
53. Specimen collection
54. Spiritual care
55. Stimulation/nurturance
56. Stress management
57. Substance use
58. Supplies
59. Support group
60. Support system
61. Transportation
62. Wellness
63. Other (specify)

B

FIGURE 10-8 Continued

USING THE OMAHA SYSTEM FOR DIABETES EDUCATION
by KATHLEEN McLAUGHLIN, RN, MPH, CDE, Consultant, Health Education, Sparta, NJ

The importance of education in the treatment of diabetes has been emphasized by the American Diabetes Association (ADA). Former ADA president Harold Rifkin, MD, wrote in the introduction to *Goals for Diabetes Education*, "'treatment of diabetes' is largely an educational process" (Franz, Kronsick, Maschak-Carey, et al., 1986). Recognizing the importance of well planned patient teaching and cognizant of the limited time that nurses have to plan care, the New Jersey State Department of Health, Diabetes Control Program, initiated the development of a series of teaching plans incorporating concepts of the Omaha System (Table 10–1).

Each preprinted plan contains one or two nursing diagnoses from the Problem Classification Scheme. Although each plan includes all of the signs and symptoms of the nursing diagnosis, only those that are clearly relevant to diabetes education are addressed in the form of status or discharge goals. Because it is inappropriate for a client to be discharged without improvement in signs and symptoms, the status outcome goals are written for the client to exhibit no signs or symptoms at discharge (level 5).

Knowledge objectives are derived from *Goals for Diabetes Education* (Franz, et al., 1986) and cover areas for content/curriculum specified in National Standards for Diabetes patient education programs (American Diabetes Association, 1990). Behavior objectives have been developed by the author using behavior change theory. The acceptable levels of Knowledge and Behavior at discharge indicate the minimum acceptable level of movement along the Problem Rating Scale for Outcomes. For example, when the nurse indicates "minimal knowledge" on the admission assessment, the ap-

propriate discharge level for Knowledge may be "has basic knowledge." In a critical area, such as insulin administration, the appropriate discharge level would be "consistently appropriate behavior" (Martin, Scheet, Crews, et al., 1986, p. 72).

The teaching content segment contains an outline and cues for the nurse to specify factors that influence individual learning, teaching and evaluation methods, and materials to be used. The nurse, in consultation with the client, selects only those plans that are appropriate for the specific situation. Each teaching plan is devised individually for (1) the characteristics of the client and his/her environment that may influence learning, such as literary levels, disabilities, or barriers to change, (2) teaching methods and audiovisual materials to be used, (3) methods by which the Knowledge and Behavior objectives will be evaluated, and (4) the dates intervention begins and is accomplished.

The nursing diagnosis 35. Nutrition is used to illustrate application of a standard diabetic teaching plan for a client with type II diabetes who has been instructed to lose weight. The appropriate signs and symptoms are circled including (01) weighs 10% more than desirable, (04) exceeds established standards for caloric intake, and (07) nonadherence to prescribed diet.

The Status goals are selected by the client and nurse to identify a mutually acceptable short-term weight goal. The Knowledge and Behavior objectives that have been met on admission are dated and initialed; those yet to be met are discussed by the client and nurse. As each objective is met, it is dated and initialed on the teaching plan. Teaching-learning

TABLE 10–1 ■ Sample Diabetic Teaching Plan

Name: *Sarah M.*   Date of Birth *3-24-24*

INITIAL DIABETES EDUCATION STANDARD TEACHING PLAN #9 NUTRITION, TYPE II DIABETES

Nsg Dx: (35) Nutrition
Modifier: (circle one) health promotion, potential impairment, impairment
Signs and symptoms:
01. weighs 10% more than desirable
02. weighs 10% less than desirable
03. lacks established standards for daily caloric/fluid intake
04. exceeds established standards for daily caloric/fluid intake
05. unbalanced diet
06. improper eating schedule
07. nonadherence to prescribed diet
08. other: fails to incorporate Dietary Guidelines for Americans, American Heart Association and/or American Cancer Society recommendations
   into meal pattern

Special learner needs:
Reads at 10th grade level

Selected Audiovisual Materials
*Take Control of your Type II
   Diabetes Self-Care Diary,
   (Hoechst-Roussel, 1989)
Healthy Food Choices (ADA,
   1986)*

Prescribed diet: *1200 Calories, Low fat, No sugar*
Ht. *5'5"* Wt. *200#* DBW *125#* Excess pounds *75*
Actual WT, minus DBW = excess pounds
♂ DBW = 100 # plus 6 # for each inch over 5 feet
♀ DBW = 106 # plus 5 # for each inch over 5 feet

TABLE 10–1 ■ Sample Diabetic Teaching Plan *Continued*

DATE INTRODUCED	CONTENT OUTLINE	NURSE/CLIENT ACTIVITIES / AV AIDS	EVALUATION METHOD
	Knowledge Objectives:		
4-3-89	1. Treatment triad; meals, activity, hypoglycemic agents; and management elements; monitoring and continuing education	*Discussion*	*Verbal recall at one week*
	2. Role of food in nutrition, blood glucose and lipid control	*Use of AV materials*	
	3. Client's meal plan; types of foods, amounts, timing of meals and snacks, importance of consistency		
	4. Critical importance of meal plan		
	5. Reasons to attain and maintain desirable body weight		
	6. Need to learn more about sick day food intake		
	Behavioral Objectives:		
4-3-89	1. Accepts personal responsibility for own meal plan	*Use of daily log*	*Review log at each visit*
	2. Identifies elements in own eating pattern that need to change	*Paper & pencil activities* *Problem solving discussions*	
	3. Writes 7 day menu plan		
	4. Maintains food log for *3* days		*Review menu plans Review recipes for appropriate changes*
	5. Records problems, feelings about dietary changes in daily log		
	6. Modifies 3 favorite recipes		
	7. Determines role of own food intake on own blood glucose level		

STATUS GOALS

Within _2_ week(s), the client will:

	Date	Initials
35.01/2. identify a weight goal that is reasonable and directed toward desirable body weight: _25#_ by _July 4, 1989_.	_4-3-89_,	_KK_
35.03/4. know and accept established standards for daily calorie and fluid intake (prescribed meal plan)	_4-14-89_,	_KK_
35.05. eat a balanced diet	_PTA_,	—
35.06. eat on a consistent schedule	_PTA_,	—
35.07. adhere to prescribed diet	_4-14-89_,	_KK_
35.08. incorporate Dietary Guidelines for Americans, American Heart Association and/or American Cancer Society recommendations into meal plan.	_PTA -_,	—

KNOWLEDGE OBJECTIVES

Within _2_ week(s), the client will demonstrate basic knowledge of the role of nutrition in the management of diabetes by being able to:

1. State that appropriate food choices are important for good nutrition.	_4-3-89_,	_KK_
2. State how the balance of food intake and activity affects total body weight, blood glucose and lipid levels.	_4-4-89_,	_KK_
3. State that the treatment of choice for type II diabetes is adherence to a meal and activity plan that attains and maintains desired body weight.	_4-4-89_,	_KK_
4. State that the meal plan is a critical component in diabetes management.	_4-7-89_,	_KK_
5. List three personal reasons to attain/maintain normal body weight.	_4-10-89_,	_KK_
6. List the types and amounts of foods to be included in meals and snacks as indicated in his/her meal plan.	_4-10-89_,	_KK_

BEHAVIOR OBJECTIVES

Within _2_ week(s), the client will:

1. Identify and prioritize own eating patterns that need changing.	_4-10-89_,	_KK_
2. Write menu plans for seven days, including plans appropriate for weekdays and weekend days, that are relevant to personal lifestyle and within the guidelines of personal diet prescription.	_4-14-89_,	_KK_
3. Modify and prepare three personal favorite recipes to decrease sugar, salt, and fat content, and indicate satisfaction with the results.	_4-10-89_,	_KK_
4. Maintain a complete and accurate food diary which includes time of food intake, amount, method of preparation, and name of food (including brand names of processed foods) for at least _3_ days.	_4-7-89_,	_KK_
5. Determine how food intake may be influencing own blood glucose level when it is above _160_.	_4-12-89_,	_KK_
6. Note in the daily log, problems or feelings encountered in attaining prescribed meal plan goals, as this occurs.	_4-12-89_,	_KK_
7. Uses problem-solving techniques to increase dietary adherence.	_4-12-89_,	_KK_
Signature _Karen Kaiser, RN_	Initials	_KK_

Abbreviations: NA—Not applicable; PTA—Prior to admission

methods, audiovisual aids, and evaluation methods are selected by the nurse and client and documented prior to implementation.

Evaluation of client learning and behavior change is both ongoing and periodic. Therefore, alterations in the goals and objectives, teaching-learning strategies, audiovisual aids, and evaluation methods may be made as necessary. The diabetic teaching plans become part of the client's permanent record, thus they are available for review on subsequent admissions.

USING THE OMAHA SYSTEM IN INTERDISCIPLINARY PRACTICE

The John Henry case example and McLaughlin's teaching plan illustrate use of the Omaha System by home health nurses. Physical therapists, occupational therapists, speech pathologists, and social workers use the Omaha System in a similar manner as they provide and document home health service. In addition to serving as a tool for individual practitioners, the Omaha System is used at the VNA of Omaha and other locations to facilitate interdisciplinary collaboration. The VNA of the Midlands Hospice team uses the Omaha System as a tool for gathering, organizing, and interpreting data to plan and provide care. In a similar manner, the staff of Spaulding Rehabilitation Hospital Home Health Program are using the Problem Classification Scheme. Their implementation decisions and experiences are described by Joan Goldsberry.

Using the Omaha System in Hospice

The VNA of Omaha Hospice team consists of nurses, social workers, a pastoral counselor, and a physician. Services are provided to terminally ill clients of differing ages with a variety of medical diagnoses. Each newly referred client is visited by a nurse and a social worker. In addition to providing an explanation of the hospice program and ascertaining client and family readiness to participate, the nurse and social worker collect data using the VNA of Omaha Data Base as a guide. The client's attending physician is contacted to

ascertain that the client meets hospice admission criteria, to determine that the physician is in agreement with provision of hospice services to the client, and to obtain verbal medical orders for care. At the interdisciplinary group meeting, a primary nurse and a social worker report on the data gathered from the physician and from the client and family during their home visits. The group then uses the Problem Classification Scheme to identify problems. The members of the various disciplines tend to focus on different issues. For example, social workers are adept at identification of problem areas in the Psychosocial Domain such as 08. Role Change or 14. Caretaking/Parenting, whereas nurses and physicians identify physiologic and health-related behavior problem areas such as 24. Pain or 43. Technical Procedure. Use of the Problem Classification Scheme provides the group with a common ground and standard language for problem identification.

The team members collaborate to develop Knowledge, Behavior, and Status ratings for each problem using the Problem Rating Scale for Outcomes. The ratings are reviewed on a weekly basis. In this way, changes in a client's condition can be identified and the plan of care altered on a timely basis. The Intervention Scheme is used by the team to develop the plan of care for each problem. Use of the Scheme also assists in identifying the need to involve other disciplines, such as physical therapists, home health aides, or nutritionists, in provision of hospice services. The Problem Ratings and Plan in conjunction with the physician orders serve as the Interdisciplinary Plan of Care that is used by all disciplines, including on-call staff, providing service to hospice clients.

EXPERIENCES WITH THE OMAHA SYSTEM IN BOSTON

by JOAN GOLDSBERRY, RN, Director Home Health, Spaulding Rehabilitation Hospital, Boston, MA

Spaulding Rehabilitation Hospital in Boston (MA) specializes in rehabilitation care of patients with a wide variety of medical problems including arthritis, traumatic head injury, and spinal cord disease. The hospital is affiliated with The Massachusetts General Hospital, Harvard Medical School, and Tufts University School of Medicine. The home health agency, established in 1981, is certified as a Medicare provider and is accredited by the Joint Commission for Accreditation of Healthcare Organizations (JCAHO). Staff serve clients who reside in Boston and 27 towns within a 10- to 12-mile radius of the hospital. The agency employs 25 direct service professional staff as well as contract staff. Disciplines represented include nursing, physical therapy, occupational therapy, and speech language pathology. They make approximately 30,000 home visits per year.

When the home health agency was established, it was de-

cided that a problem-oriented record system would be appropriate for documenting services provided to clients. Many of the clients would receive service from multiple disciplines. It was determined that all disciplines providing service to a given client would document on a common record. The interdisciplinary team members would concurrently identify and address common problems from differing perspectives. Thus, a standard nomenclature for stating problems was important to assure coordination of approaches and to prevent duplication of effort. Management staff were aware of the Problem Classification Scheme (PCS) and felt that this tool offered the standard language they wanted for their clinical record. Therefore, the PCS was chosen for use in the record system.

Each health professional who provides care completes a discipline-specific assessment of client needs. Based on the assessment data obtained when the professional uses the Problem Classification Scheme as a guide, the problems are recorded on a Master Problem List. The caregiver also establishes goals and plans for each identified problem. Problems and plans are reviewed during weekly interdisciplinary team "patient care conferences." The purposes of the review are to facilitate common understanding and to coordinate efforts of all caregivers. The results of the conference are recorded in the clinical record in the form of problems, progress, and goals.

Staff response to use of the Problem Classification Scheme has been positive. Staff are introduced to the record during their orientation period. Members of all disciplines have expressed relief that the record contains a structured format and that the required terminology of the Problem Classification Scheme is not foreign to them. The standard nomenclature keeps all care providers focused on relevant patient problems while recognizing the unique contribution of each discipline to problem resolution.

USING THE OMAHA SYSTEM IN LONG-TERM CARE

Long-term care has been defined as assistance in the form of health care and supportive services for those in need of help with performance of activities of daily living (Halamandaris, 1987). Whereas long-term care used to be synonymous with care provided in a nursing home, today long-term care is increasingly being provided in the home and community settings. Approximately 5% of the over-65 population currently resides in nursing homes. It is estimated that another 10% of this age group who reside in their homes need the same level of care. Further, studies show that 80% of long-term care is performed by family caregivers (Eisenberg & Amerman, 1988).

It is predicted that the need for long-term care will increase in direct proportion to the increase in lifespan of the American population. The US General Accounting Office, in a 1987 report, indicated that 3.2 million elderly needed some degree of assistance to remain in their own homes. Long-term needs are not confined to the elderly. The Congressional Budget Office noted that by 1985, 7.4 to 12.5 million disabled adults would be in need of some degree of long-term care. These numbers do not include the estimated 10 million children who need long-term care assistance due to birth defects or accident-related disabilities (Halamandaris, 1987).

Access to and funding for long-term care is becoming an increasingly critical national issue. In response to this concern, a bipartisan congressional group, the Pepper Commission, was formed to prepare recommendations for a national program of comprehensive health care. Their recommendations included provisions for long-term home and community-based care for severely disabled people of all ages. These people were defined as those needing assistance with three out of five activities of daily living or those having a severe cognitive impairment. Case managers would determine the amount and type of services needed. Covered services would include:

- Home health care
- Physical, occupational, speech, and other appropriate therapy services
- Personal care services
- Homemaker chore services
- Grocery shopping and transportation
- Medication management
- Adult day care and social day care
- Respite care for caregivers
- Cost-effective training of family members for delivery of home-based family care, and support counseling for family caregivers (Pepper Commission, 1990)

The report included estimated costs for home care of $64.2 billion over the initial 5-year phase-in period. The commission report addresses revenue, but critics have indicated that the recommendations regarding funding are neither detailed nor specific.

There is little funding available at the present time to support long-term care. Medicare was designed to cover the costs for acute care, but it provides little coverage for the costs of chronic, maintenance level care. Private insurance typically does not cover these costs. Medicaid does pay for long-term care but only for those who meet restrictive income guidelines and, then, the care is frequently available only in nursing homes. Increasingly, state officials are initiating Medicaid waiver programs designed to provide long-term care to eligible people who continue to reside in their own homes. One of the first programs of this type, the Lombardi plan, or the Nursing Home Without Walls program, was initiated in the state of New York in an attempt to control nursing home costs. The program provides a broad range of services for clients who otherwise would require nursing home placement (Halamandaris, 1987). Many home health agencies, especially visiting nurse associations, provide long-term care to clients who can pay privately for the care. These programs are tailored to meet the needs of clients and their families. These agencies could provide more long-term care services if financing were more readily available (Halamandaris, 1987).

Community health personnel offer important benefits to children, adults, and elders who need long-term care services. The services can be "health promoting, responsive, and relevant to an extended number of people as well as cost-effective" (Ross, 1985, p. 338). "Community health nurses who work in a collaborative and ongoing way with their older client families are in a unique position to observe and document many phenomena associated with the process of healthy aging" (Ross, 1985, p. 346).

The long-term care program of the VNA of Omaha is typical of long-term home health care services offered by visiting nurse associations. The program is financed by a combination of sources, including fee-for-service payments, Medicaid, United Way, and private contributions. Designed for clients who are medically stable, the program offers home health aide care with limited nursing services. Clients who develop conditions requiring acute care are referred for Medicare-covered home health services until their conditions become stable.

Use of the Omaha System by staff of the VNA of Omaha in a long-term care program is illustrated by the Sarah Clark case example. Actual staff names are used, whereas the fictitious client represents a composite of the many people who receive care through this program. The Clark case study (pp. 200–225) includes (1) a description of the referral process and (2) the following VNA of Omaha forms:

Figure 10–9, Home Health Referral (p. 201)
Figure 10–10, Patient Information Record (p. 202)
Figure 10–11, Data Base/Problem List Worksheet (pp. 203–212)
Figure 10–12, Data Base (pp. 213–214)
Figures 10–13 and 10–19, Problem List (pp. 215 and 224)
Figure 10–14, Problem Ratings Scale Worksheet (pp. 216–217)
Figures 10–15 and 10–20, Problem Ratings/Plans (pp. 218–219 and 225)
Figure 10–16, Home Health Aide Care Plan (p. 220)
Figure 10–17, Long Term Care Visit Report (pp. 221–222)
Figure 10–18, Home Health Aide Progress Note (p. 223)

Sarah Clark Case Example

Sarah Clark is an 85-year-old widow who lives alone in a small, two bedroom home in a residential neighborhood. She referred herself to the VNA for assistance with bathing. She told the intake nurse that arthritis in her knees and hips had left her confined to a wheelchair and unable to get into the bathtub unassisted. The nurse contacted Mrs. Clark's physician who stated that, in addition to arthritis, Mrs. Clark had hypertension, congestive heart failure, and adult onset diabetes mellitus. All of her medical conditions were under good control with medication. Because Mrs. Clark was considered medically stable and primarily needed assistance with personal care, she was referred to the VNA Long-Term Care program (Figs. 10–9 and 10–10).

The referral was received by the supervisor and assigned to Joan Bellairs, who would be the nurse case manager for Mrs. Clark. Her duties included (1) conducting an initial assessment, (2) establishing the plan of care, (3) providing any nursing assistance needed by Mrs. Clark, (4) supervising the home health aide, and (5) conducting reassessments every 60 days.

Joan used the VNA of Omaha Data Base/Problem List Worksheet to guide her collection and assessment of data during her initial visit to Mrs. Clark (Fig. 10–11). When Joan returned to her office, she finished the Base/Problem List Worksheet by completing an assessment of each domain. Review of the completed data base also facilitated identification of Mrs. Clark's problems. Of the six problems, one was in the Environmental, three were in the Physiological, and two were in the Health Related Behaviors Domains. Signs and symptoms defined the Actual state of four problems, and risk factors led to the identification of two Potential problems. Clerical staff used the worksheet to develop a computer-generated Data Base and Problem List (Figs. 10–12 and 10–13).

Joan and Mrs. Clark identified two priority problem areas, 38. Personal Hygiene and 03. Residence during the admission visit. Together they agreed on a plan to address those problems. In addition, Joan developed plans for two physiologic problems that, although currently stable, represented areas requiring ongoing monitoring and health teaching. Joan used the Problem Rating Scale for Outcomes to develop Knowledge, Behavior, and Status ratings for each of the four priority problems; two problems were Actual and two were Potential. She recorded the plans and ratings on a worksheet that was used to develop a computer-generated form (Figs. 10–14 and 10–15). The categories and targets of the Intervention Scheme and client-specific comments also provided the basis for documentation of the Home Health Aide Care Plan (Fig. 10–16).

Joan completed the Physician's Orders; this form would be sent to the physician for signature. The Long-Term Care Visit Report, which was initiated during the home visit, was also completed and filed in Mrs. Clark's clinical record (Fig. 10–17A). Home health aide services were documented on special progress notes and filed in the clinical record (Fig. 10–18).

The second nursing visit to Mrs. Clark was scheduled in 14 days. This schedule represented Joan's assessment of Mrs. Clark's nursing needs as well as agency policy. In the interim, Joan implemented the plan to address the problem area 03. Residence and documented her interventions on an interim note. During the second home visit, Joan's activities were guided by the physician's orders and the nursing plan of care.

Joan's activities during the second home visit included surveillance and health teaching for the problem areas 27. Neuro-Musculo-Skeletal Function and 39. Circulation. The Home Health Aide Care Plan was reevaluated for appropriateness, and Mrs. Clark's satisfaction was ascertained. The nursing activities, Joan's assessment, and followup plans were recorded on a Long Term Care Visit Report and filed in the clinical record (Fig. 10–17B).

Joan determined that the plan for addressing the problem area, 03. Residence, had been successful in resolving the problem. Subsequent to the visit, she updated the Problem List and Problem Ratings/Plans to reflect that change (Figs. 10–19 and 10–20).

Mrs. Clark is both similar to and different from other

For VNA Use Only   **THE VISITING NURSE ASSOCIATION OF OMAHA**   **For VNA Use Only**

Date: _6_ / _19_ / _89_ H/Hold #: _55551_ _____ CT: _60_ _____

Account #: _____, _____, _____

SS #: _501-20-4126_ _____

VNAM _✓_ VNHR _____ VNCHS _____ Payment Discussed? Y ☐ N ☐ Fax Y ☐ N ☐

Medicare #: _501-20-4126 A_ _____

Source: (Name) _Self_ _____

Medicaid #: _____

Relationship: _____ Phone: _____

Ins _____ # _____

Previous VNA Record?: N ☒ Y ☐ Date From ___ / ___ / ___ to ___ / ___ / ___

Other # _____

Rejected? ☐ on ___ / ___ / ___

Patient (Last Name First): _Clark, Sarah_ _____ Birth Date: _5_ / _12_ / _1904_ Sex: M ☐ F ☒ Marital Status: S ☐ M ☐ W ☒ D ☐ Sep ☐

Street Address: _2342 So. 26th St_ _____ City: _Omaha_ _____ Zip: _68105_ Phone: _342-7123_

Spouse/Parent: _____ Birth Date: ___ / ___ / ___

Emergency Contact: _Judy Washington_ _____ Relationship: _niece_ _____ Phone: _734-8602_

Hospital: _na_ _____ from ___ / ___ / ___ to ___ / ___ / ___ SNF: from ___ / ___ / ___ to ___ / ___ / ___

Physician: _Dr. George Collins_ _____ Address: _127 So. 41st Ave_ _____ Phone: _559-1293_

Physician: _____ Address: _____ Phone: _____

Primary Diagnosis: (Dates) _Arthritis_

Secondary Diagnosis: (Dates) _QOOM, HTN, CHF_

Mental State:

Alert ☒   Depressed ☐
Forgetful ☐   Disoriented ☐
Other _____ Confused ☐

Functional Limits:

Mental ☐   Ambulation ☒
Speech ☐   Vision ☐
Other _____ Respiratory ☐
Hearing ☐

Range of Vital Signs and Lab:

BP _____ P _____ R _____
Blood Sug. _____ Wt. _____

Lives Alone ☒   With Other ☐ _____ H & P Req: Y ☐ N ☐ Pharmacy _____

Significant Information: _Needs help c̄ bath. Essentially confined to WC 2° severe arthritis_

Service: Nursing ☒   Physical Therapy ☐   Speech Therapy ☐   Occupational Therapy ☐   Home Health Aide ☒

Medical Orders/Plan of Treatment: F.W.B. ☐ N.W.B. ☐ P.W.B. ☐ _____ %

_V.O. 6/20/89_

RN to eval. general health status
Eval. compliance c̄ meds
RN determine frequency
HHA to assist c̄ tub bath –RN
determine frequency

Activity Tolerance: _____

Diet: _low salt, low carbohydrate_

Allergies: _NK_

Meds/Dosage: _____
Lanoxin 0.125 mg q̄ d
Micronase 5 mg q̄ d
Motrin 300 mg Q10
Dyazide 25 mg q̄ d
Micro-K 600 mg q̄ d
Darvocet N-100 T̄ q̄ 4-6° PRN

Supplies: _____

M.D. Signature _____

R.N. Signature _Carolyn Jorginson, RN_

Additional Information on Attached Sheet: Y ☐ N ☒

FIGURE 10–9 ■ The Home Health Referral is the initial document used to gather data before client service is initiated.

```
------------------------------------------------------------------------
                    PATIENT  INFORMATION  RECORD              PAGE   1
------------------------------------------------------------------------


Household #:   55551                    Station: VNCHS-HMS (LTC)
Address 1:   2342 SOUTH 26TH ST.          Phone: 402 342-7123
Address 2:                          Census Tract:  60.00
City/St/Zip: OMAHA        NE 68105  Monthly Income:   400
Directions:
Case Manager:   JOAN BELLAIRS

                        ACCOUNTS IN HOUSEHOLD
Patient's Name:              Account #:   Birth Date:   Rel. to HH:
CLARK, SARAH                   55551     5/12/1904     HEAD OF HOUSEHOLD
                                                      -------------------
------------------------------------------------------------------------
Patient's Name:              Account #:
CLARK, SARAH                   55551


**  EMERGENCY INFORMATION     Relation:  Address:            Phone:
    WASHINGTON, JUDY          NIECE                        402 734-8602

**  ADMISSION INFORMATION
    Soc Sec #:   501-20-4126        Rel. to HH: HH- HEAD OF HOUSEHOLD
    Birth Date:    5/12/1904          Religion: 2- PROTESTANT
    Admit Date:    6/20/89       Referral Code: PATIENT/FAMILY/FRIEND
    Refer Date:    6/19/89             Program: 270 - LTC - SNC D.C.
    1st Contact:   6/19/89                Race: 01- CAUCASIAN
    Care Started:  6/20/89               . Sex: FEMALE
    Plan Establ.:  6/20/89         Marital Sts: WIDOWED
    Discharged:    0/00/00      Discharge Reason:
    Special Instructions:
    ICDA Diagnosis:


**  DIAGNOSIS INFORMATION
    111       ARTHRITIS
    61        CARDIAC
    63        HYPERTENSION
    21        DIABETES

**  FUNDING SOURCES         Billing #:      Comment:        Effect Date:
    11- PRIVATE PAY                                           6/20/89

**  EMPLOYER - 33/ RETIRED

**  OTHER AGENCIES          Contact:               Phone:
    M.D.                    DR. GEORGE COLLINS     402 559-1293


                                            Orders Cover
**  PHYSICIAN INFORMATION             From Date:   To Date:




------------------------------------------------------------------------
```

FIGURE 10 – 10 ■ The Patient Information Record is a computer-generated facesheet that includes information obtained during the referral and admission process.

clients served by the Long-Term Care program. Like the majority of Long-Term Care clients, she has multiple, chronic conditions that require ongoing care. Unlike many other Long-Term Care clients, Mrs. Clark needs only assistance with personal care. Elderly clients frequently require a variety of community-based services, such as transportation, meals, and housekeeping. A home health nurse coordinates these services to prevent fragmentation of care.

Text continued on page 213

DATA BASE/PROBLEM LIST WORKSHEET

Instructions: Circle **one** choice (Adequate, Not Assessed, Not Applicable, Health Promotion, Potential **or** Deficit/Impairment/Actual).   CIRCLE F (Family) **or** I (Individual) **only** when using Health Promotion, Potential, or Deficit/Impairment/Actual. If Potential is circled, Risk Factors must be listed. If Deficit/Impairment is circled, one or more Signs/Symptoms (S/S) must be circled. If S/S are circled, elaboration must be included in the comments section. Starred (*) items on the worksheet must be completed.

Date Admitted _6-20-89_
Date Completed _6-20-89_
Nurse Name _Jean Bellairs, RN_
Family Name _Clark_
Household # _55551_
Account # _Sarah_
Account # _____
Account # _____

DOMAIN I. ENVIRONMENTAL

01.   INCOME:
(Adequate)   Not Assessed   Not Applicable   Health Promotion
*Source _social security, savings & interest_
_____ Amount $ _400/mo_

F   **Potential**, Risk Factors:_____
I   **Deficit**, S/S: 1) low/no income 2) uninsured medical expenses
3) inadequate money management 4) able to buy only
____ necessities 5) difficulty buying necessities 6) other _____

02.   SANITATION:
(Adequate)   Not Assessed   Not Applicable   Health Promotion
F   **Potential**, Risk Factors:_____
I   **Deficit**, S/S: 1) soiled living area 2) inadequate food storage/
disposal 3) insects/ rodents 4) foul odor 5) inadequate water
supply 6) inadequate sewage disposal 7) inadequate laundry
facilities 8) allergens 9) infectious/contaminating agents
____ 10) other _____

03.   RESIDENCE:
Adequate   Not Assessed   Not Applicable   Health Promotion
*Type _single family, 2 BR, 1 floor_
(Own)   Rent
F   **Potential**, Risk Factors:_____
I   (Deficit) S/S: (1) structurally unsound 2) inadequate heating/
cooling 3)steep stairs 4)inadequate/obstructed exits/entries
5) cluttered living space 6) unsafe storage of dangerous
objects/substances 7) unsafe mats/throw rugs (8) inadequate
safety devices 9) presence of lead-based paint 10) unsafe
gas/electrical appliances 11) inadequate/crowded living space
____ 12) homeless 13) other _____

1. _front porch wood rotting_

8. _no devices to facilitate safe bathing_

04.   NEIGHBORHOOD/WORKPLACE SAFETY:
Adequate   Not Assessed   Not Applicable   Health Promotion
F   **Potential**, Risk Factors:_____
I   **Deficit**, S/S: 1) high crime rate 2) high pollution level
3) uncontrolled animals 4) physical hazards 5) unsafe play
____ area 6) other _____

05.   OTHER: S/S: 1) other

*Environmental Assessment: _Env. essentially adequate posing no threats to health c̄ exception of residential deficits_

A

FIGURE 10–11 ■ (_A–J_) The Data Base/Problem List Worksheet is an assessment tool for obtaining family and individual information related to the entire Problem Classification Scheme; the tool was designed for use in home health and public health settings.

DOMAIN II. PSYCHOSOCIAL

Household # _55551_

06. COMMUNICATION WITH COMMUNITY RESOURCES:
(Adequate) Not Assessed   Not Applicable   Health Promotion
*Transportation Resources _niece assists, MOBY_

F
I
&
#

Potential, Risk Factors: _____
Impairment, S/S: 1) unfamiliar with options/procedures for obtaining services 2) difficulty understanding roles/regulations of service providers 3) unable to communicate concerns to service provider 4) dissatisfaction with services 5) language barrier 6) inadequate/unavailable resources 7) other _____

07. SOCIAL CONTACT:
(Adequate) Not Assessed   Not Applicable   Health Promotion
*Support System _niece visits weekly, church members visit weekly_

F
I
#

Potential, Risk Factors: _____
Impairment, S/S: 1) limited social contact 2) uses health care provider for social contact 3) minimal outside stimulation/ leisure time activities 4) other _____

08. ROLE CHANGE:
(Adequate) Not Assessed   Not Applicable   Health Promotion

F
I
#

Potential, Risk Factors: _____
Impairment, S/S: 1) involuntary reversal of traditional male/ female roles 2) involuntary reversal of dependent/independent roles 3) assumes new role 4) loses previous role 5) other

09. INTERPERSONAL RELATIONSHIP:
(Adequate) Not Assessed   Not Applicable   Health Promotion

F
I
#

Potential, Risk Factors: _____
Impairment, S/S: 1) difficulty establishing/maintaining relationships 2) minimal shared activities 3) incongruent values/ goals 4) inadequate interpersonal communication skills 5) prolonged, unrelieved tension 6) inappropriate suspicion/ manipulation/compulsion/aggression 7) other _____

10. SPIRITUAL DISTRESS:
(Adequate) Not Assessed   Not Applicable   Health Promotion

F
I
#

Potential, Risk Factors: _____
Actual, S/S: 1) expresses spiritual concerns 2) disrupted spiritual rituals 3) disrupted spiritual trust 4) conflicting spiritual beliefs and medical regimen 5) other _____

active in Baptist church

11. GRIEF:
Adequate   Not Assessed (Not Applicable) Health Promotion

F
I
#

Potential, Risk Factors: _____
Impairment, S/S: 1) fails to recognize normal grief responses 2) difficulty coping with grief responses 3) difficulty expressing grief responses 4) conflicting stages of grief process among family/individual 5) other _____

B

FIGURE 10–11 *Continued*

12. EMOTIONAL STABILITY:

(Adequate) Not Assessed   Not Applicable   Health Promotion

F   **Potential**, Risk Factors: _____

I   **Impairment**, S/S: 1) sadness/hopelessness/worthlessness
2) apprehension/undefined fear 3) loss of interest/involvement
in activities/self-care 4) narrowed perceptual focus 5) scattering
of attention 6) flat affect 7) irritable/agitated 8) purposeless
activity 9) difficulty managing stress 10) somatic complaints/
chronic fatigue 11) expresses wish to die/attempts suicide
_____ 12) other _____

13. HUMAN SEXUALITY:

Adequate (Not Assessed) Not Applicable   Health Promotion

F   **Potential**, Risk Factors: _____

I   **Impairment**, S/S: 1) difficulty recognizing consequences of
sexual behavior 2) difficulty expressing intimacy 3) sexual
identity confusion 4) sexual value confusion 5) dissatisfied with
sexual relationships 6) other_____
_____

14. CARETAKING/PARENTING:

(Adequate) Not Assessed   Not Applicable   Health Promotion

*Primary Caregiver: _self_

F   **Potential**, Risk Factors: _____

I   **Impairment**, S/S: 1) difficulty providing physical care/safety
2) difficulty providing emotional nurturance 3) difficulty providing
cognitive learning experiences and activities 4) difficulty
providing preventive and therapeutic health care 5) expectations
incongruent with stage of growth and development
6) dissatisfaction/difficulty with responsibilities 7) neglectful
_____ 8) abusive 9) other _____

15. NEGLECTED CHILD/ADULT:

Adequate   Not Assessed (Not Applicable) Health Promotion

F   **Potential**, Risk Factors: _____

I   **Actual**, S/S: 1) lacks adequate physical care 2) lacks emotional
nurturance/support 3) lacks appropriate stimulation/cognitive
experiences 4) inappropriately left alone 5) lacks necessary
_____ supervision 6) inadequate/ delayed medical care 7) other ____

16. ABUSED CHILD/ADULT:

Adequate   Not Assessed (Not Applicable) Health Promotion

F   **Potential**, Risk Factors: _____

I   **Actual**, S/S: 1) harsh/excessive discipline 2) welts/bruises/
burns 3) questionable explanation of injury 4) attacked
verbally 5) fearful/hypervigilant behavior 6) violent
environment 7) consistently negative messages 8) assaulted
_____ sexually 9) Other _____

C

FIGURE 10–11 *Continued*

17. **GROWTH AND DEVELOPMENT OF CHILD/ADULT:**
Household # __5555 1__

Adequate   Not Assessed   (Not Applicable)   Health Promotion
Height_____ Weight____ Head Circumference_____
Feeding_____
Newborn PA_____

F   **Potential**, Risk Factors: _____

I   **Impairment**, S/S: 1) abnormal results of development
screening tests 2) abnormal weight/height/head circumference
in relation to growth curve/age 3) age inappropriate behavior

\# 4) inadequate achievement/maintenance of developmental
_____ tasks 5) other _____

18. **OTHER:** S/S: 1) Other

Psychosocial Assessment: _Has adequate support system_ _____

DOMAIN III. PHYSIOLOGICAL

19. **HEARING:**
(Adequate)   Not Assessed   Not Applicable   Health Promotion
Correction _____

F   **Potential**, Risk Factors: _____

I   **Impairment**, R _____ L _____ S/S: 1) difficulty hearing normal

\# speech tones 2) absent/abnormal response to sound
_____ 3) abnormal results of hearing screening test 4) other _____

20. **VISION:**
(Adequate)   Not Assessed   Not Applicable   Health Promotion
Correction _glasses c̄ adequate correction_

F   **Potential**, Risk Factors: _____

I   **Impairment**, R _____ L _____ S/S: 1) difficulty seeing small print/
calibrations 2) difficulty seeing distant objects 3) difficulty
seeing close objects 4) absent/abnormal response to visual
stimuli 5) abnormal results of vision screening test

\# 6) squinting/blinking/tearing/blurring 7) difficulty differentiating
_____ colors 8) other _____

21. **SPEECH AND LANGUAGE:**
(Adequate)   Not Assessed   Not Applicable   Health Promotion

F   **Potential**, Risk Factors: _____

I   **Impairment**, S/S: 1) absent/abnormal ability to speak
2) absent/abnormal ability to understand 3) lacks alternative
communication skills 4) inappropriate sentence structure

\# 5) limited enunciation/clarity 6) inappropriate word usage
_____ 7) other _____

22. **DENTITION:**
(Adequate)   Not Assessed   Not Applicable   Health Promotion
Correction _____

F   **Potential**, Risk Factors: _____

I   **Impairment**, S/S: 1) abnormalities of teeth 2) sore/swollen/
bleeding gums 3) ill-fitting dentures 4) malocclusion 5) other

\#
_____

D

FIGURE 10-11 *Continued*

23. COGNITION:

F
I

(Adequate)   Not Assessed   Not Applicable   Health Promotion

Potential, Risk Factors: _____

Impairment, S/S: 1) diminished judgment 2) disoriented to time/place/person 3) limited recall of recent events 4) limited recall of long past events 5) limited calculating/sequencing skills 6) limited concentration 7) limited reasoning/abstract thinking ability 8) impulsiveness 9) repetitious language/ behavior 10) other _____

\#

Household # _55551_

24. PAIN:

F
(I)

Adequate   Not Assessed   Not Applicable   Health Promotion

Potential, Risk Factors: _____

(Actual) Description _arthritic pain LEs_

Relieved by: _medication_

S/S: (1) expresses discomfort/pain 2) elevated pulse/ respirations/blood pressure (3) compensated movement/ guarding 4) restless behavior 5) facial grimaces 6) pallor/ perspiration 7) other _____

\#

1. dull aching pain which worsens in cold or damp weather

25. CONSCIOUSNESS:

F
I

(Adequate)   Not Assessed   Not Applicable   Health Promotion

Potential, Risk Factors: _____

Impairment, S/S: 1) lethargic 2) stuporous 3) unresponsive 4) comatose 5) other _____

\#

26. INTEGUMENT:

F
I
\#

(Adequate)   Not Assessed   Not Applicable   Health Promotion

Potential, Risk Factors: _____

Impairment, S/S: 1) lesion 2) rash 3) excessively dry 4) excessively oily 5) inflammation 6) pruritus 7) drainage 8) ecchymosis 9) hypertrophy of nails 10) other _____

27. NEURO-MUSCULO-SKELETAL FUNCTION:

Adequate   Not Assessed   Not Applicable   Health Promotion

Assistive Devices _wheelchair, walker_

F
(I)

Potential, Risk Factors: _____

(Impairment) S/S: (1) limited range of motion 2) decreased muscle strength 3) decreased coordination 4) decreased muscle tone 5) increased muscle tone 6) decreased sensation 7) increased sensation 8) decreased balance (9) gait/ambulation disturbance (10) difficulty managing activities of daily living 11) tremors/seizures 12) other _____

\#

Spends most of time in wc using feet & arms to propel chair; is able to ambulate short distances c̄ walker & transfers unassisted

E

FIGURE 10-11 *Continued*

28. **RESPIRATION:**
(Adequate) Not Assessed   Not Applicable   Health Promotion
Rate _16_   Assistive Devices _____

F   **Potential**, Risk Factors: _____
I   **Impairment**, S/S: 1) abnormal breathing patterns 2) unable to
     breathe independently 3) cough 4) unable to cough/
     expectorate independently 5) cyanosis 6) abnormal sputum
7) noisy respirations 8) rhinorrhea 9) abnormal breath sounds
____ 10) other _____

29. **CIRCULATION:**
Adequate   Not Assessed   Not Applicable   Health Promotion
Temp _98.6_ Assistive Devices _____

     BP: sitting R $^{130}/_{70}$ L _____ ; standing R $^{124}/_{70}$ L _____ ;
     lying R _____ L _____
     Pulses: apical _76_ radial _76_ peripheral _____
F   (**Potential,**) Risk Factors: _hx of HTN & CHF_____
(I) **Impairment**, S/S: 1) edema 2) cramping/pain of extremities
     3) decreased pulses 4) discoloration of skin/cyanosis
     5) temperature change in affected area 6) varicosities
     7) syncopal episodes 8) abnormal blood pressure reading
     9) pulse deficit 10) irregular heart rate 11) excessively rapid
heart rate 12) excessively slow heart rate 13) anginal pain
____ 14) abnormal heart sounds 15) other _____

circulatory problems
controlled c̄ medication

30. **DIGESTION-HYDRATION:**
(Adequate) Not Assessed   Not Applicable   Health Promotion
Assistive Devices _____

F   **Potential**, Risk Factors: _____
I   **Impairment**, S/S: 1) nausea/vomiting 2) difficulty/inability to
     chew/swallow/digest 3) indigestion/reflux 4) anorexia
     5) anemia 6) ascites 7) jaundice/liver enlargement
8) decreased skin turgor 9) cracked lips/dry mouth
____ 10) electrolyte imbalance 11) other _____

A ODM controlled c̄ medication

31. **BOWEL FUNCTION:**
(Adequate) Not Assessed   Not Applicable   Health Promotion
Assistive Devices _takes MOM if no BM qod_____

F   **Potential**, Risk Factors: _____
I   **Impairment**, S/S: 1) abnormal frequency/consistency of stool
     2) painful defecation 3) decreased bowel sounds 4) blood in
     stools 5) abnormal color 6) cramping/abdominal discomfort
7) incontinent of stool 8) other _____

F

FIGURE 10-11 Continued

32. GENITO-URINARY FUNCTION:

(Adequate) Not Assessed   Not Applicable   Health Promotion

Assistive Devices _____

Household # _5555/_

F **Potential**, Risk Factors: _____

I **Impairment**, S/S: 1) incontinent of urine 2) urgency/frequency
3) burning/painful urination 4) difficulty emptying bladder
5) abnormal urinary frequency/amount 6) hematuria
7) abnormal discharge 8) abnormal menstrual pattern

\# 9) abnormal lumps/swelling/tenderness of male/female
_____ reproductive organs 10) dyspareunia 11) other _____

---

33. ANTEPARTUM/POSTPARTUM:

Adequate   Not Assessed (Not Applicable) Health Promotion

AP: *TPAL _____ EDC _____ Date OB Care _____
Fetal Act/FHR _____
L&D Prep _____ Abn Lab _____
Danger Sig _____ Preterm Labor _____

PP: Del Date _____ Bonding _____
8-point check _____

F **Potential**, Risk Factors: _____

I **Impairment**, S/S: 1) difficulty coping with pregnancy/body
changes 2) inappropriate exercise/rest/diet/behaviors

\# 3) discomforts 4) complications 5) fears delivery procedure
_____ 6) difficulty breast-feeding 7) other _____

*TPAL = Term (36–42 wk), Preterm (under 36 wk), Abortions, Living
Children

---

34. OTHER: S/S: 1) other

*Physiological Assessment: _Arthritis of LEs causing pain & interfering c̄ NMS function;_
HTN, CHF & AODM controlled c̄ medication

DOMAIN IV. HEALTH RELATED BEHAVIORS

35. NUTRITION:

(Adequate) Not Assessed   Not Applicable   Health Promotion

Height _5'3"_ Weight _130#_ Diet _low salt, low CHO_

F **Potential**, Risk Factors: _____

I **Impairment**, S/S: 1) weighs 10% more than average
2) weighs 10% less than average 3) lacks established
standards for daily caloric/fluid intake 4) exceeds established
standards for daily caloric/fluid intake 5) unbalanced diet
6) improper feeding schedule for age 7) nonadherence to

\# prescribed diet 8) unexplained/progressive weight loss
_____ 9) hypoglycemia 10) hyperglycemia 11) other _____

demonstrates good understanding
of modified diet & good
compliance

---

36. SLEEP AND REST PATTERNS:

(Adequate) Not Assessed   Not Applicable   Health Promotion

F **Potential**, Risk Factors: _____

I **Impairment**, S/S: 1) sleep/rest pattern disrupts family
2) frequently wakes during night 3) somnambulism

\# 4) insomnia 5) nightmares 6) insufficient sleep/rest for age/
_____ physical condition 7) other _____

G

FIGURE 10–11 *Continued*

37. PHYSICAL ACTIVITY:
    Adequate   Not Assessed   Not Applicable   Health Promotion

F   Potential, Risk Factors:_____
(I) (Impairment) S/S: (1) sedentary life style 2) inadequate/
\# inconsistent exercise routine 3) inappropriate type/amount of
_____ exercise for age/physical condition 4) other _____

essentially wc bound

38. PERSONAL HYGIENE:
    Adequate   Not Assessed   Not Applicable   Health Promotion

F   (Potential) Risk Factors: *requires assing 2° NMS impairment*
(I) Impairment, S/S: 1) inadequate laundering of clothing
    2) inadequate bathing 3) body odor 4) inadequate
\# shampooing/combing of hair 5) inadequate brushing/flossing/
_____ mouth care 6) other _____

39. SUBSTANCE USE:
    (Adequate) Not Assessed Not Applicable Health Promotion

F   Potential, Risk Factors:
I   Impairment, S/S: 1) abuses over-the-counter/street drugs
\# 2) abuses alcohol 3) smokes 4) difficulty performing normal
_____ routines 5) reflex disturbances 6) behavior change 7) other

40. FAMILY PLANNING
    Adequate   Not Assessed (Not Applicable) Health Promotion
Methods _____

F   Potential, Risk Factors: _____
I   Impairment, S/S: 1) inappropriate/insufficient knowledge of
    family planning methods 2) inaccurate/inconsistent use of
\# family planning methods 3) dissatisfied with present family
_____ planning method 4) other _____

41. HEALTH CARE SUPERVISION:
    (Adequate) Not Assessed Not Applicable Health Promotion
    *Routine care plans *sees MD at least annually, niece
or MOBY for transportation
    *Emergency care plans *Lifeline, 911*

f   Potential, Risk Factors: _____
I   Impairment, S/S: 1) fails to obtain routine medical/dental
    evaluation 2) fails to seek care for symptoms requiring
    medical/dental evaluation 3) fails to return as requested to
    physician/dentist 4) inability to coordinate multiple
    appointments/regimens 5) inconsistent source of medical/
\# dental care 6) inadequate prescribed medical/dental regimen
_____ 7) other _____

42. PRESCRIBED MEDICATION REGIMEN:
    (Adequate) Not Assessed Not Applicable Health Promotion
F   Potential, Risk Factors: _____
I   Impairment, S/S: 1) deviates from prescribed dosage/
    schedule 2) demonstrates side effects 3) inadequate system
    for taking medication 4) improper storage of medication 5)fails
\# to obtain refills appropriately 6) fails to obtain immunizations
_____ 7) other _____

*demonstrates adequate
understanding of meds
& takes as ordered*

H

FIGURE 10-11 *Continued*

43. TECHNICAL PROCEDURE:

Adequate   Not Assessed   (Not Applicable)   Health Promotion

F   **Potential**, Risk Factors: _____

I   **Impairment**, S/S: 1) unable to demonstrate/relate procedure
accurately 2) does not follow/demonstrate principles of safe/
aseptic techniques 3) procedure requires nursing skill

4) unable/unwilling to perform procedure without assistance

———5) unable/unwilling to operate special equipment 6) other ____

Household # _55551_

44.   OTHER: S/S: 1) Other

*Health Behavior
Assessment: _Requires assistance c̄ personal care; demonstrates good understanding of & compliance c̄ medical trt. plan_

Significant Planning Factors: _Highly motivated to remain in own home_

*Homebound Status: _Severe arthritis of LEs; essentially confined to wc & requires assistance to leave home_

HEALTH HISTORY
Significant Medical History of Client(s)

Hospitalizations:

1987 CHF

Pregnancies:

none

Surgeries:

none

Injuries:

none

FIGURE 10-11 *Continued*

MEDICAL HISTORY OF CLIENT AND FAMILY MEMBERS

Complete column(s) below indicating client's name(s) and relationship of other pertinent family members. Focus on specific family history as it contributes to client care.

Diagnosis	Name/Relationship Sarah					
Diabetes	1965					
Epilepsy						
Cardiac Disease	1987					
Hypertension	1987					
CVA						
Arthritis/Gout	1950					
Cancer						
Frequent Headaches/Migraines						
Asthma/Allergies						
Respiratory Disease						
SIDS						
GI Problems/Ulcers						
Kidney/Bladder Problems						
Phlebitis/Varicose Veins						
Drug/Alcohol Abuse						
Mental Retardation						
Mental Illness						
Other						

ASSESSMENT/COMMENTS: _Long term history of cardiac disease, HTN, arthritis & AODM_

J

FIGURE 10–11 *Continued*

```
-----------------------------------------------------------------------------
                          * * * D A T A   B A S E * * *                PAGE  1
HOUSEHOLD #:   55551      2342 SOUTH 26TH ST.     STATION- VNCHS-HMS (LTC)
-----------------------------------------------------------------------------
                          ACCOUNTS IN HOUSEHOLD
Patient's Name:              Account #:          From Date:
CLARK, SARAH                   55551             6/20/89
-----------------------------------------------------------------------------

DATE ADMITTED:  06/20/89

ENVIRONMENTAL DOMAIN:  All areas assessed with significant findings as
follows:  INCOME:  Source:  Social Security, savings and interest.
Amount:  $400/month.  $1,500 savings; $3,000 burial fund.  Helps
friends prepare income tax statements and taxes to supplement income.
RESIDENCE:  Type:  Single family, 2 bedroom, 1 floor/own.  Front porch
wood rotting.  No devices to facilitate safe bathing.
NEIGHBORHOOD/WORKPLACE SAFETY:  Stable, older homes, residential.

A:   ENVIRONMENT ESSENTIALLY ADEQUATE POSING NO THREATS TO HEALTH WITH
EXCEPTION OF RESIDENCE DEFICITS.

PSYCHOSOCIAL DOMAIN:  All areas assessed with significant findings as
follows:  COMMUNICATION WITH COMMUNITY RESOURCES:   Transportation
Resources:  Niece assists, MOBY.  SOCIAL CONTACT:  Support System:
Niece visits weekly, church members visit weekly.  SPIRITUAL DISTRESS:
Active in Baptist church.  CARETAKING/PARENTING:  Primary Caregiver:
Self.  Areas Not Assessed:  Human Sexuality.

A:   HAS ADEQUATE SUPPORT SYSTEMS.

PHYSIOLOGICAL DOMAIN:  All areas assessed with significant findings as
follows:  VISION:  Correction:  Glasses with adequate correction.
PAIN:  Description:  Arthritic pain left extremities.  Relieved by
medication.  Dull, aching pain which worsens in cold or damp weather.
NEURO-MUSCULO-SKELETAL FUNCTION:  Assistive Devices:  Wheelchair,
walker.  Spends most of time in wheelchair using feet and arms to
propel chair; is able to ambulate short distances with walker and
transfers unassisted.  RESPIRATION:  Rate 16.  CIRCULATION:  Temp 98.6,
BP sitting right 130/70, standing right 126/70, AP 76, PP 76.  Risk
Factors:  History of hypertension and CHF.  Circulatory problems
controlled with medication.  DIGESTION-HYDRATION:  AODM controlled with
medication.  BOWEL FUNCTION:  Assistive Devices:  Takes MOM if no BM
q.o. day.

A:   ARTHRITIS OF LEFT EXTREMITIES CAUSING PAIN AND INTERFERING WITH NMS
FUNCTION.  HTN, CHF, AND DM CONTROLLED WITH MEDICATIONS.

HEALTH RELATED BEHAVIORS DOMAIN:  All areas assessed with significant
findings as follows:  NUTRITION:  Height 5 ft. 3 in., weight 130 lbs.
Diet:  Low salt, low carbohydrate.  Demonstrates good understanding of
modified diet and good compliance.  PHYSICAL ACTIVITY:  Essentially
wheelchair bound.  PERSONAL HYGIENE:  Risk Factors:  Requires assist
secondary to NMS function impairment.  HEALTH CARE SUPERVISION:
Routine care plans:  Sees MD at least annually, niece or MOBY for
transportation.  Emergency care plans:  Lifeline, 911.  PRESCRIBED
MEDICATION REGIMEN:  Demonstrates adequate understanding of meds and

-----------------------------------------------------------------------------
```

A

FIGURE 10-12 ■ *(A and B)* The Data Base is a computer-generated form developed from the Data Base/Problem List Worksheet.

The Omaha System is well suited to the practice and documentation of Long-Term Care nurses. Use of the Problem Classification Scheme, the foundation of the Omaha System, facilitates collection of comprehensive data. A client with chronic health conditions may be adversely affected by environmental, social, mental, emotional, and mobility factors that must be considered in development of a plan of care (Korn, Iverson, & Pastor, 1989). Use of the Intervention Scheme provides cues and clues to the nurse in planning and implementing care. Rating the client's priority problems over time facilitates evaluation and enables the nurse to

```
-------------------------------------------------------------------
                    * * * D A T A   B A S E * * *           PAGE   2
  HOUSEHOLD #:   55551     2342 SOUTH 26TH ST.      STATION- VNCHS-HMS (LTC)
-------------------------------------------------------------------
takes as ordered.

A:  REQUIRES ASSISTANCE WITH PERSONAL CARE.  DEMONSTRATES GOOD
UNDERSTANDING OF AND COMPLIANCE WITH MEDICAL TREATMENT PLAN.

SIGNIFICANT PLANNING FACTORS:  Highly motivated to remain in own home.
Homebound Status:  Severe arthritis of lower extremities.  Essentially
confined to wheelchair and requires assistance to leave home.

HEALTH HISTORY:  Significant Medical History of Client

Hospitalizations:  1987 CHF

Medical History of Client and Family Members:

SARAH
Diabetes 1965
Cardiac Disease 1987
Hypertension 1987
Arthritis/Gout 1950

ASSESSMENT/COMMENTS:  LONG TERM HISTORY OF CARDIAC DISEASE, HTN,
ARTHRITIS, AND DIABETES.  Joan Bellairs, RN
                       Joan Bellairs, PHN/rip




-------------------------------------------------------------------
```

B

FIGURE 10-12 *Continued*

identify progress. The standard language of the Schemes helps the nurse to detail the scope of problems encountered in Long-Term Care clients, delineate the services provided by Long-Term Care staff, and describe the results of Long-Term Care services. Such information, whether relative to an individual client or to clients in the aggregate, is valuable in supporting the need for Long-Term Care to third-party payors, legislators, and the community in general.

Text continued on page 226

```
------------------------------------------------------------------
          * * *  P R O B L E M   L I S T  * * *          PAGE   1
HOUSEHOLD #:    55551    2342 SOUTH 26TH ST.    STATION- VNCHS-HMS (LTC)
------------------------------------------------------------------
                       ACCOUNTS IN HOUSEHOLD
Patient's Name:            Account #:        From Date:
CLARK, SARAH                 55551             6/20/89
------------------------------------------------------------------

 * 06/20/89 CLARK, SARAH
              03C
            Residence: Deficit

              0301
            Structurally Unsound

              0308
            Inadequate Safety Devices

 * 06/20/89 CLARK, SARAH
              24C
            Pain: Actual

              2401
            Expresses Discomfort/Pain

              2403
            Compensated Movement/Guarding

 * 06/20/89 CLARK, SARAH
              27C
            Neuro-Musculo-Skeletal Function: Impairment

              2701
            Limited Range Of Motion

              2708
            Gait/Ambulation Disturbance

              2709
            Difficulty Managing Activities Of Daily Living

 * 06/20/89 CLARK, SARAH
              29B
            Circulation: Potential Impairment

 * 06/20/89 CLARK, SARAH
              37C
            Physical Activity: Impairment

              3701
            Sedentary Life Style

 * 06/20/89 CLARK, SARAH
              38B
            Personal Hygiene: Potential Impairment

                    Joan Bellairs, PHN/rip
                    Joan Bellairs, PHN
------------------------------------------------------------------
         **
         **
         **
```

FIGURE 10–13 ■ The Problem List is a computer-generated index of the client's health-related interests, concerns, and problems and is based on the Problem Classification Scheme.

PHN *Joan Billows*

Problem Ratings Scale Worksheet

Date _6/20/89_   Household # _5555/_
Client # _5555/_

Problem # _03_

K _3_

B _3_

S _3_

MONTHS _6_

PLAN:

1. _CM: 15 – Abbey Foster for tub bars and chair_

2. _CM: 40 – AAA for Handyman Service_

3. _____

4. _____

Date _6/20/89_ Client # _5555/_

Problem # _27_

K _3_

B _3_

S _3_

MONTHS _6_

PLAN:

1. _HTGC: 35: ROM, balance rest/activity_

2. _HTGC: 46: transfers, obstacles to use of wc_

3. _T+P: 41: NHA to assist w/ tub bath_

4. _S: 50: increased swelling, decreased ROM_

01. Anatomy/physiology
02. Behavior modification
03. Bladder care
04. Bonding
05. Bowel care
06. Bronchial hygiene
07. Cardiac care
08. Caretaking/parenting skills
09. Cast care
10. Communication
11. Coping skills
12. Day care/respite
13. Discipline
14. Dressing change/wound care
15. Durable medical equipment
16. Education
17. Employment
18. Environment
19. Exercises
20. Family planning
21. Feeding procedures
22. Finances
23. Food
24. Gait training
25. Growth/development
26. Homemaking
27. Housing
28. Interaction
29. Lab findings
30. Legal system
31. Medical/dental care
32. Medication action/side
     effects
33. Medication administration
34. Medication set-up
35. Mobility/exercise
36. Nursing care, supplementary
37. Nutrition
38. Nutritionist
39. Ostomy care
40. Other community resource
41. Personal care
42. Positioning
43. Rehabilitation
44. Relaxation/breathing techniques
45. Rest/sleep
46. Safety
47. Screening
48. Sickness/injury care
49. Signs/symptoms – mental/emotional
50. Signs/symptoms – physical
51. Skin care
52. Social work/counseling
53. Specimen collection
54. Spiritual care
55. Stimulation/nurturance
56. Stress management
57. Substance use
58. Supplies
59. Support group
60. Support system
61. Transportation
62. Wellness
63. Other

I. HTCG:
II. T & P:
III. CM:
IV. S.

A

FIGURE 10-14 ■ (*A and B*) The Problem Ratings Scale Worksheet is a data-gathering guide to note both problem-specific client ratings and plans associated with the Problem Rating Scale for Outcomes and the Intervention Scheme.

PHN *Joan Bellaire*

Problem Ratings Scale Worksheet

Date 6/20/89   Household # 5555l
                Client # 5555l

Problem # 29

K 3

B 4

S 5

MONTHS 6

PLAN:

1. HTGC: 50 when to contact RN, MO

2. S: 50 vital signs, edema, report to MD PRN

3. _____

4. _____

Date 6/20/89 Client # 5555l

Problem # 38

K 4

B 3

S 5

MONTHS 6

PLAN:

1. see prob 27, # 3

2. _____

3. _____

4. _____

01. Anatomy/physiology
02. Behavior modification
03. Bladder care
04. Bonding
05. Bowel care
06. Bronchial hygiene
07. Cardiac care
08. Caretaking/parenting skills
09. Cast care
10. Communication
11. Coping skills
12. Day care/respite
13. Discipline
14. Dressing change/wound care
15. Durable medical equipment
16. Education
17. Employment
18. Environment
19. Exercises
20. Family planning
21. Feeding procedures
22. Finances
23. Food
24. Gait training
25. Growth/development
26. Homemaking
27. Housing
28. Interaction
29. Lab findings
30. Legal system
31. Medical/dental care
32. Medication action/side
    effects

33. Medication administration
34. Medication set-up
35. Mobility/exercise
36. Nursing care, supplementary
37. Nutrition
38. Nutritionist
39. Ostomy care
40. Other community resource
41. Personal care
42. Positioning
43. Rehabilitation
44. Relaxation/breathing techniques
45. Rest/sleep
46. Safety
47. Screening
48. Sickness/injury care
49. Signs/symptoms – mental/emotional
50. Signs/symptoms – physical
51. Skin care
52. Social work/counseling
53. Specimen collection
54. Spiritual care
55. Stimulation/nurturance
56. Stress management
57. Substance use
58. Supplies
59. Support group
60. Support system
61. Transportation
62. Wellness
63. Other

I. HTCG:
II. T & P:
III. CM:
IV. S.

B

FIGURE 10–14 *Continued*

```
------------------------------------------------------------------------
              * * *  P R O B L E M   R A T I N G S/P L A N S  * * *      PAGE   1
   HOUSEHOLD #:   55551     2342 SOUTH 26TH ST.      STATION- VNCHS-HMS (LTC)
------------------------------------------------------------------------
                          ACCOUNTS IN HOUSEHOLD
   Patient's Name:                  Account #:        From Date:
   CLARK, SARAH                       55551            6/20/89
------------------------------------------------------------------------

   * 06/20/89 CLARK, SARAH
                  03
                  RESIDENCE

                  K3
                  KNOWLEDGE - Basic knowledge

                  B3
                  BEHAVIOR - Inconsistently appropriate

                  S3
                  STATUS - Moderate signs/symptoms
   PLAN:
   1. CM:  durable medical equipment:  Abbey Foster for tub bars and
   chair.
   2. CM:  other community resource:  AAA for Handyman Service.

   * 06/20/89 CLARK, SARAH
                  27
                  NEURO-MUSCULO-SKELETAL FUNCTION

                  K3
                  KNOWLEDGE - Basic knowledge

                  B3
                  BEHAVIOR - Inconsistently appropriate

                  S3
                  STATUS - Moderate signs/symptoms

                  6
                  Re-Evaluate Six Months
   PLAN:
   1. HTGC:  mobility/exercise:  ROM, balance rest/activity.
   2. HTGC:  safety:  transfers, obstacles to use of wheelchair.
   3. T&P: personal care: HHA to assist with tub bath.
   4. S:  s/s - physical:  increased swelling, decreased ROM.

   * 06/20/89 CLARK, SARAH
                  29
                  CIRCULATION

                  K3
                  KNOWLEDGE - Basic knowledge

                  B4
                  BEHAVIOR - Usually appropriate


------------------------------------------------------------------------
   HTGC = Health Teaching , Guidance , & Counseling
   T & P = Treatments & Procedures
   CM = Case Management      S = Surveillance
```

A

FIGURE 10–15 ■ (*A and B*) The Problem Ratings/Plans is a computer-generated form developed from the Problem Ratings Scale Worksheet.

```
--------------------------------------------------------------------------------
              * * *   P R O B L E M   R A T I N G S/P L A N S   * * *        PAGE   2
HOUSEHOLD #:    55551      2342 SOUTH 26TH ST.         STATION- VNCHS-HMS (LTC)
--------------------------------------------------------------------------------
                S5
          STATUS - No signs/symptoms

                6
          Re-Evaluate Six Months
PLAN:
1. HTGC:  s/s - physical:  when to contact RN, MD
2. S:  s/s - physical:  vital signs, edema, and report to MD p.r.n.

 * 06/20/89 CLARK, SARAH
                38
          PERSONAL HYGIENE

                K4
          KNOWLEDGE - Adequate knowledge

                B3
          BEHAVIOR - Inconsistently appropriate

                S5
          STATUS - No signs/symptoms

                6
          Re-Evaluate Six Months
PLAN:
1. See Problem 27, #3.
                        Joan Bellairs, RN
                        Joan Bellairs, PHN/rip
```

```
--------------------------------------------------------------------------------
HTGC = Health Teaching , Guidance , & Counseling
T & P = Treatments & Procedures
CM = Case Management      S = Surveillance
```

B

FIGURE 10–15 *Continued*

THE VISITING NURSE ASSOCIATION OF OMAHA
Home Health Aide Care Plan–LTC

Funding Source _II_

Name of Patient _Clark, Sarah_   Account Number _55551_

Address _2342 So 26th St_   CT _60_   Phone Number _342-7123_

Directions to Home _____

Age _85_   Other family members in home _lives alone_   Activity Level _wheelchair_

Diagnosis(es) _degenerative arthritis LEs, AODM, HTN, CHF_   Mental status _alert_

In case of emergency contact: Name _Judy Washington (niece)_ Phone Number _734-8602_

Special Instructions/Precautions _assist with transfers._ _Diabetic - No nail care_

Frequency _1 x/wk_

Preferred Days & Times

Second Choice

	Monday	Tuesday	Wednesday	Thursday	Friday	Saturday	Sunday
					#1		
					#2		

BATH   Frequency

Bed _____
Sponge _____
Shower _____
_____
_____
Tub _use tub_   _1x/wk_
Chair _____
_____
_____

HAIR
✓ Comb c̄ HV
___ Set
✓ Shampoo PRN

NAILS
___ Trim toenails
___ Trim fingernails

OTHER CARE   Frequency

___ Weight
___ Shave
___ Oral care
___ Foot Soak
✓ Linen change
✓ Dress _assist_   _1x/wk_
✓ Other _lotion: esp. to_   _1x/wk_
legs & feet

VITAL SIGNS
✓ Blood pressure   c̄ HV
✓ Radial pulse
___ Apical pulse
___ Respirations

OTHER DUTIES

ANKLES   Frequency

___ Measure R
___ Measure L

RANGE OF MOTION/EXERCISE PROGRAM
(Specify)

Rom / LEs

SKIN
Check for redness/breakdown c̄ HV
✓ Hip
✓ Coccyx
✓ Heel
___ Elbow
___ Shoulder blades

REPORT TO NURSE IF: _BP over 90 diastolic, c/o ↑ pain_

Nurse's Signature _Joan Bellairs RN_

Date _6/20/89_

VNCHS–LTC   Sup. Review
Rev. 6/88   Schedule

FIGURE 10–16 ■ The Home Health Aide Care Plan is a tool for the nurse to communicate Intervention Scheme data to the home health aide who provides services.

VISITING NURSE COMMUNITY HEALTH SERVICES LONG TERM CARE VISIT REPORT

Pt. Act.# 55551 **Client Name** Sarah Clark **Date** 6/30/89

NC = No Change

CLIENT PROBLEMS	SUBJECTIVE/OBJECTIVE	CAT.	TARG.	INTERVENTIONS/COMMENTS
ENVIRONMENTAL/PSYCHOSOCIAL: Residence	See Data Base	III	15 40	Interested in referral for assistance in home repairs; willing to pay sliding fee
26. Integument: Lesion ___ Diameter ___ Drainage ___				
(27) Neuro-musculo-skeletal function: Ambulation Wheelchair	See Data Base	I	46	Slow position chg, positioning of wc & use of brakes
28. Respiration: Rate ___ Resting ___ Activity ___ Lung Sounds ___				
29. Circulation: Pulse ___ Apical ___ Radial ___ Pedal ___ B/P ___ Lying ___ Sitting ___ Standing ___ Edema ∅ Weight ___	See Data Base			
31. Bowel function: Continency ___				
32. Genito-urinary function: Continency ___				
35. Nutrition: Intake MOW				
36. Sleep/rest:				
38. Personal hygiene: HHA Sup. POC ( )Approp. ( )Inapp. Satisfied ___ Unsat. ___ Needs HHA due to: ___	"I can sponge myself but I'd like to get in the tub once a week"	II	41	Assisted into tub c̄ difficulty. Has tub chair. Lotion to body. NHA to assist weekly.
41. Medical/dental supervision: MD visit Date 4/__/89	"I see the Dr. about q̄ 6 mo"			
42. Prescribed med(s): Know ___ Comply ___ Yes/No Yes/No Yes/No Yes/No	Niece gets meds refilled. States purpose & freq. of each med correctly	IV	32 33	Reviewed all meds. Taking as prescribed
(Other Problems) ___				

Assessment: Has good understanding of health status & treatment. Requires assistance to safely manage tub bath.

Plan: Frequency and Reason NHA 1X/wk , RN for aide supervisor (q̄ 14d) + POC reassessment (q̄ 60d)

— Nurse Signature: Joan Bellaire RN ___ Employee #: 1071

INTERVENTION SCHEME

CATEGORIES
I. Health Teaching, Guidance, and Counseling
II. Treatments and Procedures
III. Case Management
IV. Surveillance

TARGETS
01. Anatomy/physiology
02. Behavior modification
03. Bladder care
04. Bonding
05. Bowel care
06. Bronchial hygiene
07. Cardiac care
08. Caretaking/parenting skills
09. Cast care
10. Communication
11. Coping skills
12. Day care/respite
13. Discipline
14. Dressing change/wound care
15. Durable medical equipment
16. Education
17. Employment
18. Environment
19. Exercises
20. Family planning
21. Feeding procedures
22. Finances
23. Food
24. Gait training
25. Growth/development
26. Homemaking
27. Housing
28. Interaction
29. Lab findings
30. Legal system
31. Medical/dental care
32. Medication action/side effects
33. Medication administration
34. Medication set-up
35. Mobility/exercise
36. Nursing care, supplementary
37. Nutrition
38. Nutritionist
39. Ostomy care
40. Other community resource
41. Personal care
42. Positioning
43. Rehabilitation
44. Relaxation/breathing techniques
45. Rest/sleep
46. Safety
47. Screening
48. Sickness/injury care
49. Signs/symptoms - mental/emotional
50. Signs/symptoms - physical
51. Skin care
52. Social work/counseling
53. Specimen collection
54. Spiritual care
55. Stimulation/nurturance
56. Stress management
57. Substance use
58. Supplies
59. Support group
60. Support system
61. Transportation
62. Wellness
63. Other (specify)

A

FIGURE 10–17 ■ (*A and B*) The Long Term Care Visit Report is a problem-specific guide that incorporates the Intervention Scheme; it is used to document long-term care services that are actually provided during each home visit.

VISITING NURSE COMMUNITY HEALTH SERVICES LONG TERM CARE VISIT REPORT

Pt. Act.# 55551 Client Name _Sarah Clark_ Date 7 / 3 / 89

NC = No Change

CLIENT PROBLEMS	SUBJECTIVE/OBJECTIVE	CAT.	TARG.	INTERVENTIONS/COMMENTS
ENVIRONMENTAL/PSYCHOSOCIAL: _Residence_	Handymen fixed porch and installed tub-bars. Work well	III	15 / 40	Problem-resolved
26: Integument: Lesion ___ Diameter ___ Drainage ___				
27: Neuro-musculo skeletal function: Ambulation ___ _NC_	Arthritis hurts when weather damp. Getting in tub seems to help.	I	35	Encouraged activity as tol.
28: Respiration: Rate ___ Resting ___ Activity ___ Lung Sounds ___				
29: Circulation: Pulse 72 / 72 Apical / Radial Pedal B/P 138/68 / 135/62 Lying / Sitting / Standing Edema ___ Weight ___	"I'm feeling fine." Denies NP, edema, palpitations.	I / IV	50 / 50	Reviewed Sx CHF NC - stable
31: Bowel function: Continency ___				
32: Genito-urinary function: Continency ___				
35: Nutrition: Intake ___ MOW				
36: Sleep/rest: ___				
38: Personal hygiene: HHA Sup. POC ✓ Approp. ( ) Inapp. Satisfied ___ Unsat. ___ Needs HHA due to.	"I really like my aide."			
41: Medical/dental supervision: MD visit Date ___				
42: Prescribed med(s): Know ___ Comply ___ Yes/No Yes/No ___ Yes/No Yes/No				
(Other Problems) ___				

Assessment: _Stable, no change in POC_

Plan: Frequency and Reason _RN q 14d for HHA supervision - reassess q 60 d.   HHA 1x/wk_

Nurse Signature: _Jean Bellairs RN_ Employee #: _1071_

INTERVENTION SCHEME

CATEGORIES
I. Health Teaching, Guidance, and Counseling
II. Treatments and Procedures
III. Case Management
IV. Surveillance

TARGETS
01. Anatomy/physiology
02. Behavior modification
03. Bladder care
04. Bonding
05. Bowel Care
06. Bronchial hygiene
07. Cardiac care
08. Caretaking/parenting skills
09. Cast care
10. Communication
11. Coping skills
12. Day care/respite
13. Discipline
14. Dressing change/wound care
15. Durable medical equipment
16. Education
17. Employment
18. Environment
19. Exercises
20. Family planning
21. Feeding procedures
22. Finances
23. Food
24. Gait training
25. Growth/development
26. Homemaking
27. Housing
28. Interaction
29. Lab findings
30. Legal system
31. Medical/dental care
32. Medication action/side effects
33. Medication administration
34. Medication set-up
35. Mobility/exercise
36. Nursing care, supplementary
37. Nutrition
38. Nutritionist
39. Ostomy care
40. Other community resource
41. Personal care
42. Positioning
43. Rehabilitation
44. Relaxation/breathing techniques
45. Rest/sleep
46. Safety
47. Screening
48. Sickness/injury care
49. Signs/symptoms - mental/emotional
50. Signs/symptoms - physical
51. Skin care
52. Social work/counseling
53. Specimen collection
54. Spiritual care
55. Stimulation/nurturance
56. Stress management
57. Substance use
58. Supplies
59. Support group
60. Support system
61. Transportation
62. Wellness
63. Other (specify)

FIGURE 10–17 *Continued*

B

VISITING NURSE ASSOCIATION OF THE MIDLANDS HOME HEALTH AIDE PROGRESS NOTE

Date 6/23/89   Patient Name Sarah Clark   Patient Number 55551

BATH*********************************OTHER CARE*********************************RANGE OF MOTION*********
                                                                              (SPECIFY)

✓	Tub
	Shower
	Sponge
	Bed
	Other

	Shave
	Oral Care
	Foot Care
✓	Linen Change
	Dress
✓	Skin Care (lotion)

LEs

CATHETER CARE***********
	Routine Pericare
	Urine Color
	Urine Amount
	Leakage

HAIR***********************
✓	Comb
	Set
	Shampoo

	Enema (type)
	Dressing Change
	Ambulate
	Other

NAILS******************
	Trim Fingernails
	Trim Toenails

VITAL SIGNS/WEIGHT***************
120/70	Blood Pressure
72	Radial Pulse
16	Respiration
	Weight
	Temperature

INCIDENTAL SERVICES****
	Prepare Lite Meal
	Take Out Trash
	One Load Laundry
	Wash Dishes
	Wet Mop Br Floor
	Vacuum Pt. Room

SKIN**************************
Check if redness/
Breakdown:
none   Hip
ANKLES******************
	Measurement Right
	Measurement Left

SUPPLIES***************

	Coccyx
	Heel
	Elbow
	Shoulder Blades
	Perineum
	HHA Eval Visit by
	Refused Service

COMMENTS: _____

_____   R. N. NE Visit
Report To R.N.
Hospitalized   RN Name _____

Arrived In Home 10:05am   5 Mileage   HOME HEALTH AIDE SIGNATURE Kathy Henry
Left Home 12:45am

VISITING NURSE ASSOCIATION OF THE MIDLANDS HOME HEALTH AIDE PROGRESS NOTE

Date 6/30/89   Patient Name Sarah Clark   Patient Number 55551

BATH*********************************OTHER CARE*********************************RANGE OF MOTION*********
                                                                              (SPECIFY)

✓	Tub
	Shower
	Sponge
	Bed
	Other

	Shave
	Oral Care
	Foot Care
✓	Linen Change
	Dress
✓	Skin Care (lotion)

LEs

CATHETER CARE***********
	Routine Pericare
	Urine Color
	Urine Amount
	Leakage

HAIR***********************
✓	Comb
	Set
✓	Shampoo

	Enema (type)
	Dressing Change
	Ambulate
	Other

NAILS******************
	Trim Fingernails
	Trim Toenails

VITAL SIGNS/WEIGHT***************
124/68	Blood Pressure
74	Radial Pulse
16	Respiration
	Weight
	Temperature

INCIDENTAL SERVICES****
	Prepare Lite Meal
	Take Out Trash
	One Load Laundry
	Wash Dishes
	Wet Mop Br Floor
	Vacuum Pt. Room

SKIN**************************
Check if redness/
Breakdown:
none   Hip
ANKLES******************
	Measurement Right
	Measurement Left

SUPPLIES***************

	Coccyx
	Heel
	Elbow
	Shoulder Blades
	Perineum
	HHA Eval Visit by
	Refused Service

COMMENTS: _____

_____   R. N. NE Visit
Report To R.N.
Hospitalized   RN Name _____

Arrived In Home 9:30am   5 Mileage   HOME HEALTH AIDE SIGNATURE Kathy Henry
Left Home 10:05am

FIGURE 10-18 ■ The Home Health Aide Progress Note is used to document the length of each visit and the services provided.

```
---------------------------------------------------------------
                    * * * PROBLEM LIST * * *           PAGE 1
HOUSEHOLD #: 55551      2342 SOUTH 26TH ST.  STN-VNCHS-HMS (LTC)
---------------------------------------------------------------
                    ACCOUNTS IN HOUSEHOLD
Patient's Name:              Account #:        From Date:
CLARK, SARAH                   55551            6/20/89
---------------------------------------------------------------
* 06/20/89 CLARK, SARAH
07/03/89   RESOLVED
              03C
           Residence Deficit

              0301
           Structurally Unsound

              0308
           Inadequate Safety Devices

* 06/20/89 CLARK, SARAH
              24C
           Pain:  Actual

              2401
           Expresses Discomfort/Pain

              2403
           Compensated Movement/Guarding

* 06/20/89 CLARK, SARAH
              27C
           Neuro-Musculo-Skeletal Function:   Impairment

              2701
           Limited Range of Motion

              2708
           Gait/Ambulation Disturbance

              2709
           Difficulty Managing Activities of Daily Living

* 06/20/90 CLARK, SARAH
              29B
           Circulation:  Potential Impairment

* 06/20/90 CLARK, SARAH
              37C
           Physical Activity:  Impairment

              3701
           Sedentary Life Style

* 06/20/89 CLARK, SARAH
              38B
           Personal Hygiene:   Potential Impairment
                              Joan Bellairs
                              Joan Bellairs, PHN/rip
---------------------------------------------------------------
```

FIGURE 10–19 ■ The Problem List is a computer-generated index of the client's health-related interests, concerns, and problems and is based on the Problem Classification Scheme; additional and resolved problem information is documented when appropriate.

```
------------------------------------------------------------
            * * * PROBLEM RATINGS/PLANS * * *        PAGE 1
HOUSEHOLD #:  55551      2342 SO. 26TH ST.  STN-VNCHS-HMS (LTC)
------------------------------------------------------------
                      ACCOUNTS IN HOUSEHOLD
Patient's Name:               Account #:         From Date:
CLARK, SARAH                     55551            06/20/89
------------------------------------------------------------
* 07/03/89 CLARK, SARAH
             03
             RESIDENCE

             K4
             KNOWLEDGE - Adequate Knowledge

             B5
             BEHAVIOR - Consistently Appropriate

             S5
             STATUS - No signs/symptoms
PROBLEM RESOLVED.
                                      Joan Bellairs
                              Joan Bellairs, PHN/rip
```

FIGURE 10–20 ■ The Problem Ratings/Plans is a computer-generated form developed from the Problem Ratings Scale Worksheet; pertinent changes in problem ratings and care plans are documented when appropriate.

SUMMARY

Documentation of home health services is becoming increasingly important as third-party payors and consumers are demanding that home health care providers be accountable for the services they provide. As the amount of time required for documentation escalates, home health agency administrators and staff are searching for methods to accurately and completely document their services in an efficient manner. The Omaha System is one such method. The John Henry and Sarah Clark case examples illustrated practice and documentation of home health nursing using the Omaha System. One client received acute care and the other received long-term care. In both cases, the staff nurse providing the care used the Omaha System to facilitate:

- Collection and assessment of baseline data and identification of client problems using the standard language and format of the Problem Classification Scheme
- Rating the client's Knowledge, Behavior, and Status for priority problems using the Problem Rating Scale for Outcomes
- Planning and implementing home health services using the Intervention Scheme to provide structure and standard language as well as cues and clues

The Omaha System offers a flexible tool for use in home health care. It is adaptable to a variety of forms and formats, as shown by the two case examples from the VNA of Omaha. Implementation of the System at Visiting Nurse Services of Des Moines and development of computerized care plans were described by Serra. The System is equally adaptable for use with a variety of medical diagnoses. Use of the System to plan and implement diabetic patient education was illustrated. In addition to serving as a tool for the practice of home health nurses, the Omaha System facilitates multidisciplinary practice. Examples of such practice at the VNA of Omaha and Spaulding Rehabilitation Hospital Home Health Programs were identified.

REFERENCES

American Diabetes Association (1990, January). National standards for diabetes patient education and American Diabetes Association review criteria. *Diabetes Care, 13*:60–65.

American Nurses' Association (1986). *Standards of Home Health Nursing Practice.* Kansas City, MO.

Cary, A. (1988, February). Preparation for professional practice: What do we need? *Nurs. Clin. North Am., 23*:341–352.

Eisenberg, D., & Amerman, E. (1988). Community-based long term care: Preparing for a new role. In Harris, M. (Ed.), *Home Health Administration* (pp. 263–270). Owings Mills, MD. Rynd Communications.

Franz, M., Kronsick, B., Maschak-Carey, T., et al. (1986). *Goals for Diabetes Education.* Alexandria, VA, American Diabetes Association, Clinical Education Program.

Halamandaris, V. (1987, October). Long-term care: Filling the gaps. *Caring, 6*:18–22.

Harris, M. (1988). *Home Health Administration.* Owings Mills, MD, Rynd Communications.

Knollmueller, R. (1985, January). The growth and development of homecare: From no-tech to high tech. *Caring, 4*:3–8.

Korn , K., Iverson, L., & Pastor, B. (1989). The need to reform the long-term care system. *Caring, 8*:42–51.

Lohn, K. (Ed.). (1990). *Medicare: A Strategy for Quality Assurance* Vol. I. Washington, DC, National Academy Press.

Martin, K., Scheet, N., Crews, C., et al. (1986). *Client Management Information System for Community Health Nursing Agencies: An Implementation Manual,* No. HRP-0907023. Rockville, MD, Division of Nursing, US DHHS, PHS, HRSA.

Morrissey-Ross, M. (1988, June). Documentation: If you haven't written it, you haven't done it. *Nurs. Clin. North Am., 23*: 363–371.

Moses, E. (1990, March). [Survey of RNs in US] Personal communication regarding unpublished data.

National Association for Home Care (1987, August 21). *NAHC Report,* No. 227. Washington, DC.

The Pepper Commission (1990, March 2). *Recommendations to the Congress.* Washington, DC, US Government Printing Office.

Ross, M. (1985). The elderly family. In Stewart, M., Innes, J., Searl, S., et al. (Eds.), *Community Health Nursing in Canada* (pp. 337–347). Toronto, Ontario, Gage.

Selby, T. (1990, February). Home health care finds new ways of caring. *Am. Nurse, 1*:12.

BIBLIOGRAPHY

Auerbach, M. (1985, November/December). Changes in home health care delivery. *Nurs. Outlook, 33*:290–291.

Belk, J. (1987, October). Long-term care: The time is now. *Caring, 6*:13–17.

Boesch, D. (Ed.) (1989, February). Prevent claims denials with effective documentation. *Hosp. Home Health, 6*:13–16.

Hackbarth, D., & Androwich, I. (1989, February). Graduate nursing education for leadership in home care. *Caring, 8*:6–11.

Halamandaris, V. (1988, February). Prospective payment: Blessing or curse. *Caring, 7*:10–11.

Hall, H. (1985, December). Home care and the values of public health. *Caring, 4*:38–39.

Humphrey, C. (1988, June). The home as a setting for care: Clarifying the boundaries of practice. *Nurs. Clin. North Am., 23*: 305–314.

Istre, S. (1988). The art and science of successful teaching. *Diabetes Educator, 15*(1):67–75.

Jewell, M., & Peters, D. (1989, September/October). An assessment guide for community health nurses. *Home Healthcare Nurse, 7*:32–36.

Keating, S., & Kelman, G. (1988). *Home Health Care Nursing: Concepts and Practice.* Philadelphia, J. B. Lippincott.

Kellogg, R. (1981). Home health nursing—it isn't just 8:00–4:00 anymore. In McCloskey, J., & Grace, H. (Eds.), *Current Issues in Nursing* (pp. 271–279). Boston, Blackwell.

Kilbane, K., & Blacksin, B. (1988, June). The demise of free care: The Visiting Nurse Association of Chicago. *Nurs. Clin. North Am., 23*:435–442.

Laxton, C. (Ed.) (1988, December). Home care services—Past, present, and future. *Caring, 7*:4–7.

Liszewski, D. (1987, June). Diversification and corporate restructuring revisited: Back to square one? *Nurs. Clin. North Am., 23*: 399–413.

Malloy, C., & Hartshorn, J. (1989). *Acute Care Nursing in the Home: A Holistic Approach.* Philadelphia, J. B. Lippincott.

Marter, L., Becker, H., Walker, L., et al. (1988, October). Home care nurses and quality care: Identifying the important skills. *Caring, 7*:38–40.

Martin, K., & Scheet, N. (1989). Nursing diagnosis in home health: The Omaha system. In Martinson, I., & Widmer, A. (Eds.), *Home Health Care Nursing* (pp. 67–72). Philadelphia, W. B. Saunders.

Miller, S. (1986). *Documentation for Home Health Care: A Record*

Management Handbook. Chicago, IL, Foundation of Record Education of the American Medical Record Association.

National Association for Home Care (1987, October). Long-term care: A women's issue. *Caring, 6:*67–74.

National Association for Home Care (1988, February). Alternative methods of reimbursement: A health and human services study. *Caring, 7:*32–35.

Powderly, K., & Smith, E. (1989, January/February). The impact of DRGs in health care workers and their clients. *Hastings Center Rep., 19:*16–18.

Seifer, S. (1987, April). The impact of PPS on home health care: A survey of 35 home health agencies. *Caring, 6:*11–12.

Shamansky, S. (1988, June). Providing home care services in a for-profit environment. *Nurs. Clin. North Am., 23:*387–398.

Stephany, T. (1990, April). A death in the family. *Am. J. Nurs., 90:*54–56.

CHAPTER ELEVEN

*T*he value of the cumulative school health record lies in the information it contains and the manner in which it is used. A record that is mandated by law to be kept, but which has little concrete data, is useless to the health professionals in the school setting. The impact of problem-oriented recording on nursing practice, delivery of health care, and revolutionizing of record keeping in all aspects of the health care industry is well documented (Yarnell & Atwood, 1974). In keeping with the trend in other health delivery sectors, school health is beginning to implement a problem-oriented approach to improve health care. (Christensen, 1981, p. 270)

School health nurses provide valuable, economical health and education services to individuals, families, groups, and communities throughout this country. Like community health nurses who practice in other settings, school nurses are facing increased pressures requiring their concern and involvement. These pressures relate to the changing student population and to professional, financial, and political issues. To contend with the current school health environment, to improve practice and documentation, and to facilitate communication, a school health nurse can use tools such as the Problem Classification Scheme, the Problem Rating Scale for Outcomes, and the Intervention Scheme.

SCHOOL HEALTH MILESTONES

School nursing programs were initiated in England late in the nineteenth century. In 1902, Lillian Wald established the first school health nursing service in this country. Wald designed a month-long demonstration project in which she assigned Lina Rogers Struthers, a Henry Street Settlement nurse, to four New York City schools. Rogers successfully cared for children with infectious diseases such as trachoma, pediculosis, ringworm, and scabies. Previously, these children were excluded from school for long periods. Because Rogers' efforts significantly reduced the absenteeism rate, 12 nurses began to work with individual children at schools. Further, they communicated with parents, doctors, and teachers about the children's health-related problems (Gardner, 1917). Their activities continued to focus on communicable diseases, especially smallpox, tuberculosis, and diphtheria.

The 1920s and 1930s were a time of phenomenal ex-

pansion of public health nursing, especially school health nursing. By the 1940s, approximately one-half of all public health nurses were employed in school health programs. However, the advent of antibiotics, establishment of sewage and water treatment programs, and a reduction in public health funding curtailed the expansion of school nursing programs. As a result, nursing positions were eliminated in some schools. (For a more complete discussion of the history of school health nursing, refer to Chapter 1.)

Although the goal of early school health programs was to reduce absenteeism, this focus soon expanded to include comprehensive and complex primary prevention services, health education, and environmental health measures.

Recently, "the purpose of school nursing is to enhance the educational process by the modification or removal of health-related barriers to learning and by promotion of an optimal level of wellness" (American Nurses' Associations, 1983, p. 1). Therefore, most school health programs involve extensive primary prevention and health education efforts. School nurses (1) monitor immunization status, (2) conduct screening programs for vision, hearing, and scoliosis, (3) initiate and coordinate referrals for diagnosis and treatment, (4) participate in classroom instruction, (5) provide medication and treatments under physicians' orders, (6) participate on interdisciplinary teams, and (7) screen the school setting for environmental problems and safety hazards.

CONTEMPORARY SCHOOL HEALTH

A contemporary school nurse provides services to healthy students, to those who are at high risk for devel-

Use in School Health Settings

oping health problems, and to those who have current, severe problems. For example, many children who attend rural and urban schools receive inadequate or marginal nutrition and health services. Some have survived low birth weight, birth trauma, and developmental delays as well as chronic and acute illnesses. Others exhibit learning disabilities or serious physical and emotional problems related to family instability, abuse, suicide, alcoholism, and drug use. Although the proportion of children residing in tenements has decreased since Wald's era, many of today's children are homeless, are living in shelters, or have resided in many foster care facilities. Children who experience an itinerant lifestyle are at risk for nutritional, physical, and emotional problems. In addition, their academic achievement is hampered by absences from and changes in schools.

Students frequently demonstrate the effects of diverse physical, emotional, social, or economic problems at school. Since Public Laws 94:142 and 99:457 were enacted, states are required to provide free and equal services and education opportunities for students with handicaps and developmental problems. In most instances, a contemporary school nurse has both the opportunity and the mandate to identify and address a variety of problems. A nurse, therefore, needs to practice sound principles of public health, especially epidemiology. To synthesize such practice, a school nurse must incorporate Leavell and Clark's (1965) three levels of prevention, encouraging the student and the student's family to accept the responsibility for health improvement (Perry, Luepker, Murray, et al., 1988). Primary prevention involves health promotion and specific protection; secondary prevention includes early diagnosis, prompt treatment, and disability limitation; tertiary prevention emphasizes rehabilitation.

The role of a school health nurse is complex. The nurse must balance professional obligations and expectations with demands of students, teachers, school principals, school board members, community health agency administrators, and the public. The nurse must be innovative as well as realistic.

The bright spot in school health is the school nurse. This individual, working in concert with the school and community health team, increases the potential for school health services to meet all expectations. The school nurse, in cost-effective fashion, not only provides services, but more importantly, also can serve as the focus and foundation of verifiable research in the future since standards for practice have been established. (Zanga & Oda, 1987, p. 416)

The school nurse's role has been characterized in various ways. Igoe (1980) described a school nurse's responsibilities regarding health service, health education, and a healthy environment. Wold (1981) described a school nurse as (1) deliverer of health services, (2) advocate for the health rights of children, (3) health counselor for individuals and groups, and (4) health educator in the school health program. Withrow (1988) identified five roles. The functional role includes on-call responsibilities to several schools. The primary role includes direct service and coordination. The team member role involves collaboration with many disciplines. The nurse practitioner role incorporates identification and management of specific health problems. The nurse teacher role focuses on dissemination of knowledge to support behavior change. Consultant and researcher were described by Withrow as additional, secondary roles. The role of the school nurse was summarized by the "Ten Commandments for the School Nurse."

1. Thou art the school nurse, responsible for promoting the health and well-being of all school children entrusted to thy care, thou shalt not be ignored nor allow others to be placed in thy role of primary health provider.

2. *Thou shalt not allow thy role to be taken in vain as to be considered as perhaps only the first-aid provider.*
3. *Thou shalt be included in those school functions relating to the child's health even if thou must invite thyself.*
4. *Thou shalt be honored and esteemed for thy abilities as a school nurse in the school, even if honored only by a few.*
5. *Thou shalt not allow others less knowledgeable than thee to kill thine enthusiasm for provision of an adequate school health program.*
6. *Thou shalt not tolerate the school's allegiance to others than thyself for provision of leadership of a good school health program even if thou must profoundly assert thyself.*
7. *Thou shalt not allow anyone to steal thy "prime time" at kindergarten registration or similar school program when thou canst publicly promote child health to the multitudes.*
8. *Thou shalt not state any falsehood regarding child health nor disregard primary parental responsibility, nor the school's responsibility regarding each child's health and safety.*
9. *Thou shalt cherish the belief that no one loves the child more or has their best interests more at heart than the child's Mom and Dad; however, in coveting this belief, thou art ever careful not to overlook the child not in possession of this type of parenting.*
10. *Thou shalt not covet the interests of thy school health program so exclusively as to overlook other aspects of the child's and teacher's school day. (Dworak, 1982, p. 314)*

SCHOOL HEALTH ISSUES

School health nurses face many professional and practice issues similar to those that concern other contemporary community health nurses. A decrease in the number of funded positions is a serious school nursing issue. This trend is occurring even though health-related student problems are increasing and many individuals and groups are encouraging an emphasis on prevention. "Despite wide acceptance and praise for the contributions of school nurses during the first half of the twentieth century, the number of nurses employed in schools has steadily declined in recent years, due in part to escalating costs and consequent budgeting cutbacks in school districts across the country" (Wold, 1981, p. ix). Approximately 48,000 registered nurses serve 48 million students in 17,000 largely independent school districts (Moses, 1990; Robert Wood Johnson Foundation, 1985; Zanga & Oda, 1987). Since 1972, the National Association of School Nurses has recommended that the maximal ratio in general student populations be one school nurse to 750 students (1989). At present, many nurses are required to serve a larger number of students.

Controversy surrounding the preparation of school nurses and scope of practice has increased even as the number of school health nurses has decreased. Nearly all school nurses were supervised by public health nursing directors prior to the 1950s. Recently, however, many nurses have become accountable to a school

nurse supervisor employed by the school district or to a school administrator. Although 28 states have school nursing consultants, ambiguity and conflict have increased, especially as attempts have been made to replace prepared school nurses with nonprofessional personnel. School nurses are struggling to define their domain (Withrow, 1988). "School health services are loved or hated, considered vital to the education process, or simply additional 'budget busters.' They work, or do not work, in meeting stated objectives, though professionals argue about what those objectives are and what they need to be for the future" (Zanga & Oda, 1987, p. 413). Additional issues confronting school health nurses relate to the changing student population. An increasing number of students (1) are members of vulnerable and dysfunctional families, (2) are involved in risk-taking behaviors, and (3) have severe physical, emotional, and mental handicaps as well as chronic illness. These changes in the student population have added to the school nurse's scope of practice dilemma. Should the nurse be a specialist for high-risk students, a generalist for all students, or both?

SCHOOL HEALTH AND THE OMAHA SYSTEM

School nurses need practical methods to assess students; they must document observations, conclusions, and interventions. The methods must allow them to demonstrate their professional expertise and emphasize the importance of nursing. Christensen (1981) noted that tools are needed for (1) communication, (2) planning nursing care, (3) client education, and (4) accountability, responsibility, and audit. For tools to be useful to a school nurse, they must be compatible with the nursing process as put forth in *Standards of School Nursing Practice* (American Nurses' Association, 1983) and *Evaluation Guide for School Nursing Practice* (National Association of School Nurses, 1985). In these publications, the nursing process is described as (1) data collection, (2) nursing diagnosis, (3) planning, (4) interventions, and (5) evaluation. School nurses have recently developed interest in incorporating nursing diagnosis into their professional practice.

Authors have described the value of the problem-oriented philosophy and format, as well as the nursing process, to school health records. Others have noted advances in automation and computer technology that have application to school health records. The Omaha System is a tool that can be beneficial to school health nurses and their students. The System is compatible with the nursing process, problem-oriented recording, and automation. Nurses can use the Omaha System in the school listing:

■ To clearly identify student health problems, provide appropriate services, and evaluate student progress during their school years, thus enhancing the potential for favorable outcomes

■ To provide the advantages of a problem-oriented

approach to practice documentation; the Omaha System can be used to create a school health record that is systematic, concrete, holistic, legally acceptable, and continuous, as well as adaptable and efficient

■ To explain clinical practice and documentation expectations during orientation of new school health nurses

■ To facilitate professional accountability regardless of the type, complexity, or intensity of the student's

health-related problem and the frequency of the student-to-nurse encounters throughout the kindergarten through twelfth grade years; such accountability is essential to developing quality assurance measures

■ To facilitate supervisor-staff conferences that involve review and evaluation

■ To explain student problems and nursing services in language that is understandable by and acceptable to other school personnel and parents

EXPERIENCES WITH THE OMAHA SYSTEM: A PROGRAM DIRECTOR'S PERSPECTIVE

by ESTHER DWORAK, RN, MSN, Director of School Health Program, Visiting Nurse Association of Omaha, Omaha, NE

The VNA of Omaha offers a comprehensive school health program to 23,000 kindergarten through twelfth grade students who attend 90 public and parochial schools. In addition to my position as director, staff include a supervisor, 12 staff nurses, a school health assistant, and a secretary. Funding for the program is provided through contracts with two countries.

At the annual fall school health conference in 1986, I was asked if the VNA's new publication, *Client Management Information System for Community Health Nursing Agencies: An Implementation Manual* (Martin, Scheet, Crews, et al., 1986), was available and how it was being implemented by our school nurses. The first query was simple to answer. How we, the VNA's school health program staff, were incorporating the Omaha System into the school health record was a different matter. The second question prompted me to recognize that we had yet to adapt and implement the Omaha System into our school health program.

Several of the school nurses had used the Omaha System during previous employment with the VNA home visit pro-

gram. The remainder of the staff had received no instruction and were not familiar with the Omaha System. After forming a three-member planning committee, we identified the need for all school nurses to become knowledgeable about a recording system that was becoming known nationally and internationally. Plans were made to provide inservice instruction for all school nurse staff.

In order to plan a relevant inservice program for school nurses it was important to clarify how the Omaha System could be used most effectively in the school nursing program. A year-long orientation plan was developed that included four phases (Table 11–1). The focal point became the application of problem-oriented recording and the three components of the Omaha System. The staff nurse member of the committee, a former home visit program nurse, furnished record examples from her school caseload. These records were easily adapted to the Problem Classification and Intervention Schemes.

The first inservice session lasted 1.5 hours. A synopsis of the entire research project was covered, along with details of

TABLE 11–1 ■ Orientation Plan

Phase 1. Inservice: included handouts and overheads

1. Introduction	5 minutes
2. Synopsis of VNA of Omaha research projects	5 minutes
3. Basic concepts (nursing process, Problem Classification Scheme, Problem Rating Scale for Outcomes, Intervention Scheme)	25 minutes
4. Large group work—example (Ima Breathless)	15 minutes
5. Small group work with five nurses/group—example (Willy Sweet)	15 minutes
6. Sharing of small group experiences	10 minutes
7. Plans for homework, next session, and future	10 minutes

Phase 2. Inservice: 1 month later

1. Group discussion—positives and negatives about homework	30 minutes
2. Report by two or three nurses—describe their selected student and their documentation	30 minutes
3. Future	15 minutes

Phase 3. Review all nurses' homework: 3 months later
1. Provide feedback on an individual basis.

Phase 4. Supervisory-staff shared visits to schools: during entire school year
1. Scheduled appointment with school nurse
2. Reviewed and discussed two to four representative records selected by school nurse

problem-oriented recording and the Omaha System. The group practiced applying the Problem Classification and Intervention Schemes using data from a hypothetical child who had allergic and asthmatic symptoms. Smaller groups then practiced using the Omaha System with a hypothetical example of a child with diabetes.

Next came the planning for future learning and meaningful use of the Omaha System. A self-adhering label with the 40 problems of the Problem Classification Scheme, as well as the categories and targets of the Intervention Scheme, was designed. School nurses attached the labels to the student health cards as they began to use the Omaha System.

School nurses were asked to (1) review their caseloads, (2) select one child with an existing health problem that had required a moderate amount of narrative health recording, and (3) apply the Omaha System to the existing record. In other words, nurses revised previous records or generated additional entries on a child's record using the new format. During a second inservice, 1 month later, each nurse brought one or more sample records to share with the other school nurses. This discussion was used for learning, not to judge recording.

The final phase in the orientation process involved a supervisory visit with each school nurse at an assigned school. Representative records were selected by the nurse, reviewed, and discussed. (More details about the shared visits are described later in this chapter.)

We have used a single card as a student health record for many years; this did not change with the introduction of the Omaha System. As the result of a recent revision, we are now using a folded, manila, 8.5 × 11″ file-type record with almost the entire inside reserved for narrative documentation of health data. Narrative documentation must remain brief, because the card may follow a child for 12 or more years.

Implementing the Problem Classification and Intervention Schemes provides a standard protocol for recording. From a director's perspective, I believe that using the Omaha System for documentation provides the school nurse with a professional method of recording that uses uniform and understandable terminology. Others who review the documentation can readily refer to the basic terminology of the Schemes at the bottom of the school card. The recording can and should remain relevant and significant to the child's health problems. The Schemes provide a focus for the student's specific needs and care. The Schemes limit the quantity of recording. Documentation becomes standard, orderly, and systematic.

The process of modifying the school health record and implementing the Omaha System caused us to consider and discuss general concerns about documentation in the school setting. As a result of the Family Education Rights and Privacy Act of 1974 (Public Law 93:380), school health records are accessible to parents as well as authorized school personnel. This law authorizes parents to see their child's school record and to request removal of information they consider inaccurate or an invasion of privacy. School nurses are advised to use a recording system that results in objective, accurate, and precise documentation. Recording should be directed toward relevant health problems. Superfluous data could place the nurse and school in jeopardy of parental criticism and even legal liability. Through use of the Problem Classification and Intervention Schemes, the school nurse is compelled to focus only on the child's health concerns and the actions required, provided, or recommended in order to relieve or alleviate the concerns.

So began the use of the Problem Classification Scheme and Intervention Scheme in the VNA of Omaha School Health Program. Can and does the Omaha System work? The answer is yes! Did we plan and schedule implementation in the most effective way possible? We are not certain. We have discussed the advantages and disadvantages of the gradual timetable that we used and the samples selected to introduce the Omaha System. Although gradual implementation produces less initial stress for school nurses, their proficiency increases slowly. Repetition and frequent practice are necessary to learn to use the Omaha System effectively. Scheduling adequate orientation and review is difficult because the school nurses' schedules are always busy and they have scattered work sites.

Are our school nurses enthusiastic about use of the Omaha System? As we concluded the four phases of the year-long orientation process, the answer remained open to speculation. Like all nurses, school nurses recognize that documentation is an important concern. The diverse demands on school nurses' time, the irregular recording required of them, and the lack of previous experience using the Omaha System make prompt, high quality documentation difficult. Our school nurses have modified and improved their recording practices, some easily and some through greater effort and more encouragement.

Those who understand the Omaha System the best are experienced VNA community health nurses who used the System in their home visit work. They were the least "flapped" when expected to use the Omaha System in school records.

Application

Application of the Omaha System in a school health program is illustrated through a case study involving a hypothetical school nurse, high school student, parent, vice principal, and physician. The narrative and record entries are intended to realistically represent current school nursing practice.

The data collection, data assessment, and problem identification steps of the diagnostic process are demonstrated as the school nurse applies the Problem Classification Scheme to client data. Steps in implementing interventions are described in relation to the Intervention Scheme. The nurse documents the process of evaluation even though she does not use the Problem Rating Scale for Outcomes. The case study depicts a method of applying the nursing process in a school setting. Because school nurses who use the Omaha System practice systematic problem-solving, they increase the potential for improving student outcomes.

Using the Omaha System with student data is illustrated on the narrative side of a student health record. A blank student health record and instructions appear in the Appendix. Substitution of codes for problems, intervention categories, and intervention targets eliminates the need for many words in the narrative. Nurses and others may refer to the lower left corner of the card for the coding dictionary.

Narrative documentation is not required on the records of many students, specifically not for those who have not evidenced health problems during their school years. School nurses document essential data on other portions of the student's health record. Sections were designed for (1) demographic, (2) emergency and special health information, (3) immunizations, (4) significant health history, (5) screening, (6) growth grid, and (7) audiometer threshold screening information. The entire card was developed by the VNA of Omaha school health staff. The VNA card is offered as an example, not a requirement. The Omaha System is compatible with a variety of forms used to record student services at a time when school nurses and administrators are becoming more sensitive to practice and documentation issues.

Sara Lynn Kent Case Example

REFERRAL PROCESS

Kathleen Steven, RN, is a school nurse assigned to several urban high schools. She regularly meets with school personnel to review possible student needs and concerns. During the second week of the fall semester, Ms. Green, Vice Principal, requested a meeting with the nurse. Ms. Green described reports she had received from several students that Sara Lynn Kent was eating little or nothing at lunch, had vomited in the restroom on more than one occasion, and was taking diet pills. The decision was made that the school nurse would confer with Sara about the reports.

USING THE PROBLEM CLASSIFICATION AND INTERVENTION SCHEMES

Sara was called to the nurse's office for a limited physical assessment. Sara's weight of 120 pounds was a 20-pound decrease from the previous year; her weight had dropped from 75% to 50% on the growth grid. Sara appeared pale and was defensive during the visit. She denied intentional vomiting and stated that, although she had taken diet pills a few times during the summer, she had taken none since. Sara denied mid-day hunger, stating she ate only a few crackers and sometimes fruit at lunch. During the visit, Kathleen discussed dietary needs and intake, dangers of diet pills, and long-term dangers of induced vomiting.

On Sara's return to the nurse's office a week later,

Kathleen checked her blood pressure, completed weight measurements, and obtained a menstrual history. Sara displayed more verbal cooperation and less defensiveness during the visit. The nurse explained to Sara that her stature, when compared to the national average, was at the 80th percentile on the growth grid, whereas her weight was on the 37.5th percentile. The nurse indicated that Sara had lost 14% of her body weight in 1 year. She again described Sara's nutrition needs and the dangers of eating disorders such as anorexia and bulimia.

The nurse planned and implemented a joint visit with Sara and her mother the following week. During the conference, Sara acknowledged that she had restricted her intake, taken some diet pills, and vomited several times at school. Although Sara's mother was pleased that her daughter had lost 20 pounds, she was concerned about Sara's behaviors. Kathleen described adolescent nutrition needs and the dangers of eating disorders; she recommended a nutrition evaluation and gave information about several resources.

The vice principal received a phone call from Sara's mother 1 week later. The mother reported that Sara had visited her family physician rather than seeking a nutrition evaluation. The physician expressed no concerns about Sara's weight or behaviors and did not recommend additional medical care. The vice principal called the nurse; they decided that the nurse would talk to Sara about regularly meeting with a school counselor. Sara was receptive to the recommendation.

The nurse conferred with the counselor 1 month later. Sara was becoming increasingly verbal and positive in small group sessions. The counselor saw no further indications of damaging behaviors or negative physical symptoms.

Sara Lynn stopped at the school nurse's office just before school closed in June. Sara Lynn was cheerful as she talked to Kathleen; she was looking forward to summer vacation. Her height was unchanged; her weight was 122 pounds.

Kathleen based her practice and documentation on the family nursing process (see Chapter 3) as she interacted with Sara Lynn and other students. School nurses need tools to structure and improve documentation because they see many students briefly or sporadically and have little time available for recording. Due to limited space on the health card, school nurses must identify pertinent nursing diagnoses and interventions and record that data logically and concisely. All required documentation can be included on the health card, thus eliminating the need for other forms and duplication of effort. The data of each encounter are recorded, followed by the (1) appropriate nursing problem number, (2) pertinent objective and subjective data, (3) intervention category, (4) targets, and (5) pertinent details. In this way, school health nurses and other readers are able to quickly scan a health record, examining the card for ongoing concerns and interventions (Fig. 11–1).

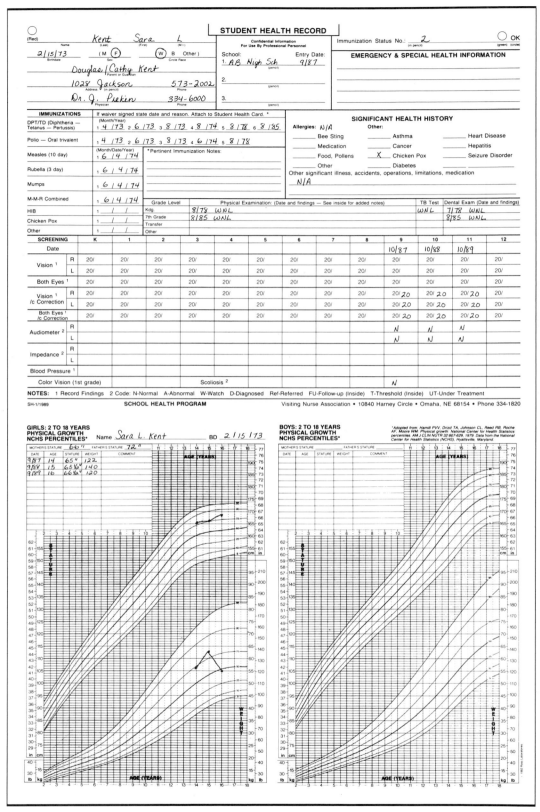

FIGURE 11–1 ■ (*A–D*) The Student Health Record depicts health-related data on one side (*A and B*) and student-nurse interactions on the other (*C and D*); narrative documentation is designed to use the Problem Classification Scheme and Intervention Scheme. (Fig. 11–1*B* used and reprinted with permission of Ross Laboratories, Columbus, OH 43216, from NCHS Charts, © 1976, Ross Laboratories.)

Name _Sara L. Kent_   BD _2 / 15 / 73_   Confidential Information For Use By Professional Personnel

DATE	ADDITIONAL INFORMATION REGARDING HEALTH PROBLEMS AND FOLLOW-UP (See problem classification and intervention schemes below. Also audio thresholds.)	Sign name/title directly after recording. (no initials)

9/2/89 — #35; III, 50. Conf. with vice principal, Ms. Green. Other students report minimal lunch intake; vomiting in rest room several times, and use of diet pills. Follow-up planned.   K. Stevens, RN

9/9/89 — #35 Conf. with student. Pale, defensive. Denies intentional vomiting. States took OTC diet pills a few times last summer, none since. Lunch usually 2-3 crackers, maybe fruit. Denies hunger.   IV, 37, 50: general health and nutritional assessment completed. Wt 120#, 20# wt loss since 9/88.   Changed from 75% to 50% on growth grid.   I, 25, 37: nutritional needs, dangers of diet pills and induced vomiting.   K. Stevens, RN

9/16/89 — #35 BP 102/82, LMP 8/9/89. Verbally responsive, less defensive. Body posture tense, anger observed in face.   IV, 50, 47: wt 120# Reviewed growth grid and 14% body wt loss in yr.   I, 25: dangers of anorexia and bulemia and nutritional needs.   K. Stevens, RN

9/23/89 — #35, I, 35; III, 50, 47. Conf. with student and mother. Sara described hx of restricted intake, some diet pills, vomited several times at school.   Mother — pleased about wt loss; concerned about Sara's behaviors.   III, 38: several resources.   K. Stevens, RN

9/30/89 — #35; III, 31 Vice principal received TC from mother. She reports appt. with Dr. Pichen who indicated no concerns with wt. or behaviors.   III, 11, 59: RN initiated referral to small discussion group led by school counselor. Sara — receptive to recommendation.   K. Stevens, RN

10/29/89 — #35; III 50, 49 Conf. with counselor. More verbal and positive in small group sessions. No further indications of negative behaviors.   K. Stevens, RN

6/4/90 — #35 Student in office. Cheerful. Wt 122# Healthy appearance   IV, 49, 50: student reports maintaining healthful diet, activity levels, and stabilizing wt.   K. Stevens, RN

PROBLEM CLASSIFICATION SCHEME

Environmental
01 Income
02 Sanitation
03 Residence
04 Neighborhood/workplace safety
05 Other

Psychosocial
06 Communication with community resources
07 Social contact
08 Role change
09 Interpersonal relationship
10 Spiritual distress
11 Grief
12 Emotional stability
13 Human sexuality
14 Caretaking/parenting
15 Neglected child/adult
16 Abused child/adult
17 Growth and development
18 Other

Physiological
19 Hearing
20 Vision
21 Speech and language
22 Dentition
23 Cognition
24 Pain
25 Consciousness
26 Integument
27 Neuro-musculo-skeletal function
28 Respiration
29 Circulation
30 Digestion-hydration
31 Bowel function
32 Genito-urinary function
33 Antepartum/postpartum
34 Other

Health Related Behaviors
35 Nutrition
36 Sleep and rest patterns
37 Physical activity
38 Personal hygiene
39 Substance misuse
40 Family planning
41 Medical/dental supervision
42 Prescribed medication regimen
43 Technical procedure
44 Other

INTERVENTION SCHEME

Categories
I   Health Teaching, Guidance, and Counseling
II   Treatments and Procedures
III Case Management
IV   Surveillance

Targets
01 Anatomy/physiology
02 Behavior modification
03 Bladder care
04 Bonding
05 Bowel care
06 Bronchial hygiene
07 Cardiac care
08 Caretaking/parenting skills
09 Cast care
10 Communication
11 Coping skills
12 Day care/respite
13 Discipline
14 Dressing change/wound care
15 Durable medical equipment
16 Education
17 Employment
18 Environment
19 Exercises
20 Family planning
21 Feeding procedures
22 Finances
23 Food
24 Gait training
25 Growth/development
26 Homemaking
27 Housing
28 Interaction
29 Lab findings
30 Legal system
31 Medical/dental care
32 Medication action/side effects
33 Medication administration
34 Medication set up
35 Mobility/exercise
36 Nursing care, supplementary
37 Nutrition
38 Nutritionist
39 Ostomy care
40 Other community resource
41 Personal care
42 Positioning
43 Rehabilitation
44 Relaxation/breathing techniques
45 Rest/sleep
46 Safety
47 Screening
48 Sickness/injury care
49 Signs/symptoms - mental/emotional
50 Signs/symptoms - physical
51 Skin care
52 Social work/counseling
53 Specimen collection
54 Spiritual care
55 Stimulation/nurturance
56 Stress management
57 Substance use
58 Supplies
59 Support group
60 Support system
61 Transportation
62 Wellness
63 Other

AUDIOMETER THRESHOLD SCREENINGS
(Frequencies Recorded in Decibel Intensity)

		500	1000	2000	3000	4000	6000	8000
DT	R							
GR	L							
DT	R							
GR	L							
DT	R							
GR	L							
DT	R							
GR	L							
DT	R							
GR	L							
DT	R							
GR	L							
DT	R							
GR	L							
DT	R							
GR	L							
DT	R							
GR	L							
DT	R							
GR	L							
DT	R							
GR	L							

C, D

FIGURE 11–1 (Continued)

EXPERIENCES WITH THE OMAHA SYSTEM: A SUPERVISOR'S PERSPECTIVE

by ELIZABETH CERNECH, RN, BA, Supervisor of School Health Program, Visiting Nurse Association of Omaha, Omaha, NE

The Omaha System and problem-oriented recording were introduced to the school nurses initially through two examples of documentation and a plan that was described by Esther Dworak. As the final phase of that plan, shared staff-supervisory school visits were conducted to review documentation skills and use of the Omaha System. Nurses who had hospital experience or who recently had attended schools of nursing or assessment courses were more familiar with the problem-oriented method of recording. For them, using the Omaha System was a simple adjustment or transition. As their records were evaluated, only minor suggestions and positive reinforcement were required.

During the staff-supervisory visits, it became apparent that some nurses were experiencing difficulty with recording in general. These nurses needed continuing, individual assistance. An approach was developed to augment the initial orientation plan. On an individual basis, the supervisors assisted those nurses who needed more guidance to:

- Compile previous narrative documentation about a student's health problems
- Use the Problem Classification Scheme to identify problems from student data and list those problems on a worksheet
- Record pertinent objective and subjective information
- Analyze what interventions had been used; identify the corresponding categories, targets, and student-specific information from the Intervention Scheme
- Compare the narrative documentation to the new entries that were based on the Omaha System

When the nurse could see an entire page of narrative documentation condensed to one-third page or less, the concept of the Omaha System became a practical reality. In some instances, the quantity of recording was not significantly decreased, but the quality was significantly improved.

In August, 1988, the school nurse staff participated in the Physical Assessment Skills Seminar (PASS Project), which consisted of several modules. The first module, an introduction to nursing assessment, was presented in two sessions. The first session included nursing process, nursing diagnosis, and techniques of assessment as well as a reintroduction of the Omaha System. A second session included a brief synopsis of the research project, basic concepts of the Omaha System, large group work based on previous recording, small group work, and discussion. Experienced staff were able to describe their feelings, ideas, and adaptations to the System and its relationship to school nursing. During this session, examples of simple, singular student health problems were recorded and discussed. It was determined that such examples would be more helpful in an orientation session and would give confidence to staff who expect to document more complicated health concerns in the future. The group sessions resulted in common expectations for both new and experienced staff.

At the conclusion of the second session, the staff were instructed to record according to the Omaha System whenever the revised individual health record was used. The purpose was to integrate both the new health record and the Omaha System into the school nurses' practice in a gradual, manageable fashion.

Shared staff-supervisory school visits were scheduled for new nurses. During the visit, a supervisor guided each nurse through the Omaha System process step by step, using an actual record. The staff nurse's documentation was evaluated by the supervisor. Staff were always encouraged to consult with each other if questions or concerns arose. Later, on-site visits were scheduled only as deemed necessary by the supervisors. Records were monitored periodically and at the end of the school year.

All staff were given the opportunity to present a sample of their documentation for peer review and discussion during the regularly scheduled staff meetings throughout the rest of the school year (Fig. 11 – 2). The primary purpose of the presentations involved the Omaha System, but the staff also needed a general review of documentation. Each nurse met with the supervisor before such a presentation for consultation and assistance as needed. The staff were asked to provide a variety of student problems to prevent repetition. Since staff presentations were given approximately every 2 weeks, the schedule helped keep the subject current and prevented "out of sight, out of mind" attitudes. Regular inclusion on the staff meeting agenda suggested a priority status for documentation issues. These group sessions provided an opportunity to practice the Omaha System and to share knowledge and abilities. The sessions required staff to critically examine their own documentation as well as that of other school nurses. The group sessions provided a positive exercise and were integrated into the staff meetings for the following school year.

At the conclusion of the second school year, supervisors assumed that the nurses were using the Omaha System on all new student records. When the supervisors realized that use was not consistent, a committee of supervisors and staff nurses was convened. The committee identified several areas of concern: (1) confusion between the problems, targets, and their respective definitions; (2) difficulty remembering the steps for using the Omaha System; and (3) lingering resistance to change.

The committee developed a plan of action for assisting school nurses to become proficient with the Omaha System and to improve the quality of their documentation. First, ex-

DATE	ADDITIONAL INFORMATION REGARDING HEALTH PROBLEMS AND FOLLOW-UP (See problem classification and intervention schemes below. Also audio thresholds.)	Sign name/title directly after recording. (no initials)
	Example 1	
12/04/89	#20. Teacher reports student having difficulty seeing chalkboard from classroom seat. II, 42, 47: Goodlite results (R) 20/50, (L) 20/50, both 20/40. Hyperopia WNL. Enc. preferential classroom seating. III, 31: vision referral sent home. B. Cernech, RN	
12/20/89	#19. Failed audio screening. IV, 47: rescreen in approx. 2 wks. B. Cernech, RN	
1/10/90	#19, 24. C/o (L) earache since a.m. Teacher reports freq. ear infecs. with slight hearing loss. II, 47, 50: otoscopic exam reveals (L) TM pink with good light reflex. Audio threshold results abnormal. III, 31: results of threshold and otoscopic exam sent home. Enc. to seek medical eval. B. Cernech, RN	
1/15/90	#19, 24. Seen by Dr. Stanley 1/11/90 regarding earache and audio results. Dx acute otitis media with antibiotic regime. III, 31: Dr. to rck in 1 wk. Dr. requests school nurse to repeat audio in 1 wk. To repeat audio and otoscopic exam 1/19/90 and report findings to parent. B. Cernech, RN	
	Example 2	
1/03/90	#26. Eruptions (R) corner of mouth: erythematous area 2.5cm. diameter, scattered pustules. Clear, nonodorous exudate with dark yellow crust. Student c/o area "itches". Scratching same. Student does not know cause. I, 51: handwashing. II, 14, 50: cleaned site with soap. Patted dry. Placed 2x2 dressing over site. III, 31: TC to father, prepared written referral. To see Dr. today. D. Gustafson, RN	
1/05/90	#26. Referral complete. Has Neosporin to apply t.i.d. after skin care. IV, 50: decreased crust, no pustules. I, 51: handwashing, skin care, and medication regime. D. Gustafson, RN	
	Example 3	
10/14/89	#33. Conf. with student upon counselor request. Ultrasound reveals EDC 2/01/90. Medical care initiated. Will live with parents and raise baby. I, 25, 49, 50: initiated anticip. guidance. I & III, 40, 16: enc. prenatal/Lamaze class. Gave info. re: comm. resources for same. TC to mom to review student visit and reinforce need for prenatal/Lamaze class and counseling. J. Stanton, RN	
11/08/89	Absent. J. Stanton, RN	
12/13/89	Absent. #33. III, 11, 59: TC with mom. Student home with viral illness. Currently attending prenatal classes. J. Stanton, RN	
1/25/90	#33. IV, 50: feeling well. Due to deliver. J. Stanton, RN	
4/04/90	#33. Delivered 7 lb. 12 oz. male approx. 6 wks. ago. C/o fatigue from late nights. III, 31: RTC for 6 wk. check-up next wk. VNA HV nurse seeing student and babe. I, 49, 50: postpartal changes. J. Stanton, RN	
	#14. Baby has URI with congestion. Using cool mist vaporizer. I, 48: care of ill infant. III, 22, 37: info. re: WIC qualifications relayed to student per request. J. Stanton, RN	

FIGURE 11-2 ■ Examples of problem-oriented documentation using the Omaha System and the Student Health Record.

pectations were clarified. More examples of appropriate record entries were generated to demonstrate these expectations. Second, a reference guide was developed. The guide was designed for use by experienced staff as well as for new staff at the time of orientation. The guide contained (1) the definitions and codes for the Problem Classification Scheme and Intervention Scheme and (2) the new examples.

Examples of Documentation

VNA of Omaha school nurses selected excerpts from actual student records that portrayed use of the Omaha System. During the months after orientation, nurses discussed these excerpts during staff meetings. The plan served to promote (1) correct use of the Omaha System by all school nurses, (2) understanding of application with diverse students, and (3) continuing emphasis on documentation as an essential component of school nursing practice. The three examples in Figure 11-2 illustrate adequate, concise, and understandable documentation for three encounters that involve actual nurses and fictitious students. Relatively simple student-nurse interactions that focus on screening and a skin rash are included, as well as a more complex situation involving teenage pregnancy.

EXPERIENCES WITH THE OMAHA SYSTEM: A SCHOOL NURSE'S PERSPECTIVE

by CATHY ADEN, RN, MSN, (formerly) School Nurse, Visiting Nurse Association of Omaha, Omaha, NE

Using the Omaha System has allowed me to document student services in a realistic, yet comprehensive manner. The System provides a method for tracking a student's health and health care needs throughout the school years.

The school nurses at the VNA of Omaha implemented the Omaha System on a gradual basis. We first began documentation in the Omaha System format on all new kindergarten and transfer students' records. We then used the Omaha System format on the records of the students who had special problems or physiologic needs. These problems ranged from a slight hearing loss to the need for four-time-a-day catheterization or tracheal suctioning.

At the group orientation to the documentation system, each nurse was responsible for selecting a few school records and applying the format of the Omaha System. The group met at a later date to follow up on recording needs and concerns. As a school nurse with experience using the Omaha System, I assisted other school nurses on an individual basis. Even with such a homogeneous group as 12 school nurses who had worked together for a number of years, it was evident that we all had varying personalities, skills, concerns, and expectations about documentation (Aden & Warren, 1991). By working together as a group and combining our experience and skills, we were able to solve problems and move forward with implementation.

One important issue that we addressed during implementation was the requirement that school personnel as well as school nurses be able to read and understand the documentation. For example, teachers, counselors, and secretaries need access to students' health records at various times and for various reasons. We chose to print the complete list of problems, interventions, and targets on a self-adhesive label for the school nurse to attach to the bottom of the narrative section of the school card. This self-adhesive label addressed both concerns. Two years after the System was in place, the school card itself was changed. When the new card was printed, the words and coding of the Omaha System were incorporated onto the record.

School nurses address acute care as well as chronic health care needs and consciously attempt to promote health and wellness. They provide holistic care that encompasses all four domains of the Omaha System. The increasing complexity of meeting the health care needs of today's students calls for a well defined documentation system. We as school nurses need to be able to track continuity of care from problem identification through resolution.

I worked with one student who had severe cardiac problems. Daily, for a period, I used the Omaha System to record assessments, planning, and activities associated with the student's changing needs. Using the Omaha System produced a series of entries that demonstrated a clear pattern of care that could be understood by anyone. The increased specificity of recording and decreased unnecessary commentary were remarkable (Fig. 11–3).

For students with multiple handicaps, I found that the use of the Omaha System assisted me in formulating the nursing/health care section of the yearly Individual Educational Plans (IEPs). Federal law requires an annual IEP for every child in a special education program. By definition, a child with multiple handicaps has a complex health status that requires a nurse to conduct a thorough and systematic assessment. After assessment, the nurse identifies problems and determines their priorities before planning and implementing interventions. Using the Omaha System can facilitate documentation of complex assessments and interventions, as illustrated in Figure 11–3.

Our group of school nurses had been accustomed to documenting in an unfocused, narrative style. To change to the Omaha System format, we needed to deliberately incorporate the nursing process. We began to consider, identify, plan, intervene, evaluate, and record to specific concerns. As we became comfortable with the changed thought and recording process, we integrated it into all progress notes. School nurses now record in the Omaha System format on all new students every year. In time, all students served by the VNA of Omaha school nurses will have a clear, problem-focused, and holistic record that reflects the philosophy of the family nursing process.

SUMMARY

A school health nurse needs tools to facilitate clinical practice and documentation in the rapidly changing school setting. School nurses share many concerns with their community health nurse peers, but they also face unique issues and demands.

Experiences with the Omaha System have been delineated in this chapter by a school health director, a supervisor, and a staff nurse. Application of the Omaha System was illustrated through health records from five diverse students. The severity of the students' health-related problems varied markedly as did the frequency of student-nurse interaction. In each example, the Omaha System provided a tool for the school nurse to use as a framework for practice and documentation — a framework that was consistent with the nursing process and principles of sound school nursing practice.

Name _____ BD __/__/__	Confidential Information For Use By Professional Personnel	
DATE	**ADDITIONAL INFORMATION REGARDING HEALTH PROBLEMS AND FOLLOW-UP** (See problem classification and intervention schemes below. Also audio thresholds.)	**Sign name/title directly after recording. (no initials)**

Example

Date	Entry
9/14/86	#27 IV, 25: ht. 43½" with L knee bent. C Aden, RN
1/26/87	#27 IV, 25: legs extended ht. 47" Hip to heel R 25", L 26" C Aden, RN
8/29/87	#41 IV, 31, 50: yearly update. Dental exam, hosp. EEG, CT scan, LP, pneumonia. On Phenobarb and Tridone for seizures. C Aden, RN
2/27/88	#26 Hosp. for pneumonia. Back to school today. 3# wt. loss in 10 days. 4 spots reddened skin lower spinal column. Reddened areas on buttocks. Red area 2.5cm diameter R hip. Skin breakdown 2cm diameter on coccyx, not yet open wound. I, 51: Cloth diapers, keep open to air, positions change q 30 min. See flow sheet. C Aden, RN
3/13/88	#28. II, 50: Crackling lung sounds bilat. heard on auscultation, worse in RLL. IV, 50: eyes drawn, weak, decreased appetite. I, 50: increase fluids during school day to 3 oz. q 2 hr. III, 31: report possible relapse to mother. C Aden, RN
3/20/88	#28. IV: physical condition improved. C Aden, RN
8/30/88	#28, 30 IV, 39, 50: yearly update. Pneumonia, gastrostomy now in place. C Aden, RN
9/11/88	#27, 28, 29, 30. II, 50: see flow sheet for results of physical assessment. III, 50: conf with school staff. Rec. mother request physical exam. ASAP. C Aden, RN
9/25/88	#41 IV, 32, 21: drs. exam resulted in decreased formula and increased Phenobarb. C Aden, RN #32 IV, 50: brownish stain in diaper noticed 9/22 by school staff and foster mother. Stain plus changes in seizure cycle (see flow sheet) suggest menstrual flow C Aden, RN
12/18/88	#32 III, 50: see prev. entry. Letters to neurologist re: continuation of 9/88 concerns. C Aden RN
1/22/89	#28. Noticeable increase in clear to white mucus coughed up < 1 wk. Lung auscultation reveals bilat. fine inspiratory/expiratory crackles and wheezes. R eye swelled, decreased appetite, wt. loss. I, 48: increased fluids. Take temp (ax) 3x/day. III, 31: recommend phys. exam by dr. C Aden, RN
2/26/89	#28 IV, 50: dx pneumonia. Out of school at this time. C Aden, RN
4/2/89	#30 G-tube spillage. III, 50: spillage and G-tube care reviewed with mother. C Aden, RN
4/30/89	#30 Possible dehydration secondary to sweating in warm weather. III, 48: teacher-nurse conf. TC to mother who gives water po. School staff give nothing po per direction of foster mother. Order from Dr. Picken to give 2-4 oz. water per G-tube am + pm at school. C Aden, RN

FIGURE 11–3 ■ Example of problem-oriented documentation for a student with multiple handicaps using the Omaha System and the Student Health Record.

REFERENCES

Aden, C., & Warren, J. (1991). A validation study of NANDA's taxonomy I. In Carroll-Johnson, R. (Ed.), *Classification of Nursing Diagnosis: Proceedings of Ninth National Conference.* Philadelphia, J. B. Lippincott.

American Nurses' Association (1983). *Standards of School Nursing Practice.* Kansas City, MO.

Christensen, M. (1981). Systematic assessment. In Wold, S. (Ed.), *School Nursing: A Framework for Practice* (pp. 245–280). St. Louis, C. V. Mosby.

Dworak, E. (1982, May). Ten commandments for the school nurse. *J. School Health,* 52:314.

Gardner, M. (1917). *Public Health Nursing.* New York, Macmillan.

Igoe, J. (1980, August). Changing patterns in school health and school nursing. *Nurs. Outlook,* 28:486–492.

Leavell, H. & Clark, E. (1965). *Preventive Medicine for the Doctor in His Community* (3rd ed.). New York, McGraw-Hill.

Martin, K., Scheet, N., Crews, C., et al. (1986). *Client Management Information System for Community Health Nursing Agencies: An Implementation Manual* (No. HRP-0907023). Rockville, MD, Division of Nursing, US DHHS, Public Health Service (PHS), Health Resources and Services Administration (HRSA).

Moses, E. (1990, March). [Survey of RNs in US] Personal communication regarding unpublished data.

National Association of School Nurses (1985). *Evaluation Guide for School Nursing Practice.* Scarborough, ME.

National Association of School Nurses (1989). *Resolutions and Policy Statements of the National Association of School Nurses.* Scarborough, ME.

Perry, C., Luepker, R., Murray, D., et al. (1988, September). Parent involvement with children's health promotion: The Minnesota home team. *Am. J. Public Health,* 78:1156–1160.

Robert Wood Johnson Foundation (1985). *Special Report,* No. 1. Princeton, NJ, Robert Wood Johnson Foundation Communications Office.

Withrow, C. (1988). The community health nursing in the schools. In Stanhope, M., & Lancaster, J. (Eds.), *Community Health Nursing: Process and Practice for Promoting Health* (pp. 779–790). St. Louis, C. V. Mosby.

Wold, S. (1981). *School Nursing: A Framework for Practice.* St. Louis, C. V. Mosby.

Zanga, J., & Oda, D. (1987, December). School health services. *J. School Health,* 57:413–416.

BIBLIOGRAPHY

Allensworth, D., & Kolbe, L. (1987, December). The comprehensive school health program: Exploring an expanded concept. *J. School Health*, 57:409–412.

Carvey, A., Kittell, S., & Hadeka, M. (1987, November). A method for documentation in school health services. *J. School Health*, 57:390–391.

Crosby, F., & Dunn, J. (1988, September/October). Teaching nursing diagnoses to school nurses: A standardized measure of the cognitive effect. *J. Contin. Educ. Nurs.*, 19:211–215.

Disparti, J. (1988). School health. In Caliandro, G., & Judkins, B. (Eds.), *Primary Nursing Practice* (pp. 151–167). Glenview, IL, Scott, Foresman/Little, Brown.

Dolan, J., Fitzpatrick, M., & Herrmann, E. (1983). *Nursing in Society: A Historical Perspective* (15th ed.). Philadelphia, W. B. Saunders.

Donahue, M. (1985). *Nursing, the Finest Art: An Illustrated History.* St. Louis, C. V. Mosby.

Dunn, J., & Crosby, F. (1988, September/October). Teaching nursing diagnoses to school nurses: A curriculum plan. *J. Contin. Educ. Nurs.*, 19:205–215.

Freeman, R., & Heinrich, J. (1981). *Community Health Nursing Practice* (2nd ed.). Philadelphia, W. B. Saunders.

Gibbons, L. (1990, February). Health records simplified by computer. *School Nurse*, 6:7–8.

Goodwin, L., Igoe, J., & Smith, A. (1984, October). Evaluation of the school nurse achievement program: A follow-up survey of school nurses. *J. School Health*, 54:335–338.

Kalisch, P., & Kalisch, B. (1986). *The Advance of American Nursing* (2nd ed.). Boston, Little, Brown.

MacDonough, G. (1979). School nursing. In Fromer, M. (Ed.), *Community Health Care and the Nursing Process* (pp. 396–412). St. Louis, C. V. Mosby.

Mayo, R. (1976, August). A nurse can be a man or a woman. *Am. J. Nurs.*, 76:1318–1319.

Mayshark, C., Shaw, D., & Best, W. (1977). *Administration of School Health Programs* (2nd ed.). St. Louis, C. V. Mosby.

Meeker, R., DeAngelis, C., Berman, B., et al. (1986, Fall). A comprehensive school health initiative. *Image*, 18:86–91.

Miller, E., & Hopp, J. (1988, May). Perceptions of school nursing by school districts. *J. School Health*, 58:197–199.

Newton, J. (Ed.) (1987). *School Health: A Guide for Health Professionals.* Elk Grove Village, IL, Committee on School Health, American Academy of Pediatrics.

Oda, D. (1981, September). A viewpoint on school nursing. *Am. J. Nurs.*, 81:1677–1678.

Oda, D. (1982). School health services: Growth potential for nursing. In Aiken, L. (Ed.), *Nursing in the 1980s: Crises, Opportunities, Challenges* (pp. 359–379). Philadelphia, J. B. Lippincott.

Pigg, Jr., R. (1989, January). The contribution of school health programs to the broader goals of public health: The American experience. *J. School Health*, 59:25–30.

Shiao, P., & McKaig, C. (1989, October). Categorizing school health office visits by nursing diagnoses. *School Nurse*, 5:18–20.

Simmons, D. (1985). Recent innovations and installations of nursing information systems. In Hannah, K., Guillemin, E., & Conklin, D. (Eds.), *Nursing Uses of Computers and Information Science* (pp. 31–35). New York, North-Holland.

Stember, M. (1985). Nursing role in school health. In Jarvis, L. (Ed.), *Community Health Nursing: Keeping the Public Healthy* (2nd ed.) (pp. 295–309). Philadelphia, F. A. Davis.

Wald, L. (1934). *Windows on Henry Street.* Boston, Little, Brown.

Will, G. (1990, April 23). Mothers who don't know how. *Newsweek*, 80.

Williams, C. (1977, April). Community health nursing—what is it? *Nurs. Outlook*, 25:250–254.

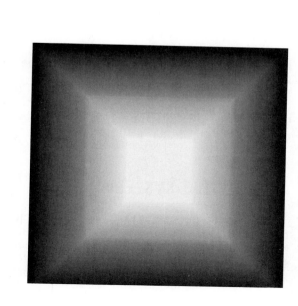

CHAPTER TWELVE

*T*he need, the relevance—indeed, the potential—in personal health service programs for obtaining group-level data—by conducting a community diagnosis, for instance, or monitoring the health status over time of those receiving care in a particular program—appear to be less obvious. Yet, if the concept of public health practice is to have meaning in the area of personal health care services, it must be operationalized in relevant and viable practice terms which are clear to all. (Williams, 1977, p. 252)

Excellent nursing practice and documentation skills are required of staff nurses and supervisors employed in voluntary, official, proprietary, school-based, and hospital-based community health programs. All of these community health nurses provide services to individuals, families, groups, and communities. Their work is highly autonomous, although they often function within organized agencies or programs that have established policies, procedures, and systems. Other agency employees, supervisors, and peers are available as sources of information and support regarding professional practice and documentation issues.

In contrast, a small but growing number of community health nurses are practicing in less traditional and less structured settings. The findings of a 1988 survey indicate that approximately 46,000 nurses are employed in untraditional settings (Moses, 1990). Some nurses have direct links to established community health agencies, health-care providers, and social service agencies; other nurses develop solo practices or organize new provider groups independent of traditional provider groups. For nurses working in alternative health care settings, the use of realistic, flexible tools that increase the structure of their practice, documentation, and data management is critical. The Problem Classification Scheme, the Problem Rating Scale for Outcomes, and the Intervention Scheme are tools that can be of benefit in new settings.

ALTERNATIVE SYSTEMS

Alternative community health delivery systems tend to evolve in response to nurses' search for autonomous practice and public pressure. Usually the systems are structured for population-focused care, thus attracting and serving target population groups or aggregates. The target groups are designated populations within specific social systems rather than particular individuals or families. Often those who comprise a target group share personal or environmental characteristics; in other instances, group members share potential and actual risks for illness, premature death, or disability. The client groups vary from affluent to homeless, educated to illiterate, employed to unemployed, and from healthy to terminally ill. The behavior of some aggregates is considered deviant by the public. Group members may feel disengaged, disenfranchised, defeated, helpless, inert, and despairing (Freeman & Heinrich, 1981).

Examples of alternative delivery systems include:

Urban Ghetto Systems. Family practice clinics, free clinics, neighborhood health centers
Rural Systems. Migrant health programs, mobile clinics, health screening and referral projects
Aged, Disabled, and Related Systems. Adult day care centers, group homes for disabled, health maintenance centers, hospice programs, retirement homes
Women/Children Systems. Birthing and midwifery centers, day care centers for preschoolers, maternal-child nursing clinics, shelters for abused women
Occupational Health Systems. Mental health programs, wellness programs
Health Maintenance/Preferred Payment Organizations. Preventive and therapeutic health programs, physician-nurse caseload system
Other Delivery and Related Systems. Discharge planning systems, prison and related health systems (Corrigan, 1986)

Nurses employed in these alternative programs refer to themselves as community health nurses, public health nurses, home health nurses, primary care nurses, clinical nurse specialists, nurse practitioners, or

Use in Alternative Community Health Delivery Systems

private practitioners. Such nurses use interpersonal, diagnostic, problem-solving, technical, and management skills with individuals, aggregates, and communities, just like nurses employed by organized community health agencies. Nurses in alternative programs, however, need special knowledge and the ability to apply that knowledge to the (1) population-focused care required by clients, (2) nontraditional setting, and (3) high proportion of non-nursing personnel who are employed or volunteer within that setting. As community health nurses work with target populations or special communities, they are concerned about the following:

1. Analyzing the population, based on statistical information as well as on comments from members and group leaders.
2. Defining special health problems or hazards arising from or associated with the environment and/or living habits, as well as identifying resources.
3. Setting goals and priorities with leaders of the group and other concerned citizens, based on needs of the community.
4. Providing services in ways sensitive to the different cultural values and attitudes of the special community and appreciating the value differences between [themselves] and these special groups.
5. Evaluating the impact of nursing services on the special community. (Freeman & Heinrich, 1981, p. 481)

Community health nurses in nontraditional settings may be very independent as they pioneer new roles and create their own positions and job descriptions. There may be few or no other nurses employed in a particular setting. Often, immediate supervisors or boards to whom these nurses report do not include nurses or other health care professionals.

ALTERNATIVE HEALTH DELIVERY ISSUES

Community health nurses who practice in alternative delivery systems are confronted by the same issues as other public health, home health, and school nurses. Decreases in reimbursement for community health services and changes in consumer expectations run counter to the increasing demand for services, the rise in number of dysfunctional families, and the complexity of professional nursing practice. (These issues are described in Chapters 9, 10, and 11.)

Community health nurses who practice in alternate delivery systems need general and special skills. Nurses benefit from educational preparation at the baccalaureate or graduate level that includes epidemiology, biostatistics, community development, policy formation, and administration (Williams, 1988). This preparation helps nurses develop competence in the areas of social policy, group dynamics, leadership, decision-making, communication, and management (Campbell, 1988). Attributes such as clinical and consulting expertise, business and marketing skills, political savvy, self-confidence, flexibility, and energy, as well as the development of a professional network, increase the nurse's chances for success (Muff, 1982). When the target population consists of a specific ethnic, religious, cultural, or social group, a community health nurse needs extensive knowledge and sensitivity regarding that group. In addition, a nurse needs extensive technical skills to meet the care requirements of certain population subgroups. Nurses who practice within untraditional settings are likely to face additional issues, however, some of which are emotionally charged and personally distressing. Such issues include: (1) high-risk client populations such as troubled children, prisoners, migrant workers, and the homeless; (2) inadequate facilities, equipment, organizational systems, and job security; (3) little professional support within the setting and even within nursing itself.

ALTERNATIVE HEALTH DELIVERY AND THE OMAHA SYSTEM

The Omaha System offers a flexible tool to community health nurses and others practicing within new delivery systems. The Problem Classification Scheme, the Problem Rating Scale for Outcomes, and the Intervention Scheme serve as a framework for implementing nursing diagnoses, nursing interventions, and client outcomes. The Omaha System can be used when the client is defined as an individual, a family, or a group. Based on the nursing process, the Omaha System is compatible with the American Nurses' Association Standards (1986a, 1986b) and can serve as a guide to professionals in alternative settings. Community health agency staff can use the Omaha System in the following ways:

- To provide a practice and documentation framework that enables a nurse and administrator to organize, prioritize, and analyze client data; this data management can occur at the individual, aggregate, and community levels
- To select and adapt the portions of the Omaha System that are most relevant to the target population, the setting, and the staff as well as to the type and length of encounters between clients and staff
- To develop a quality assurance program that involves the client record and relates to effectiveness of care and client outcomes
- To communicate a community health nurse's and administrator's client-specific concerns to other nurses, health care professionals, paraprofessionals, and lay persons who are part of the delivery system
- To generate data that explain and justify the role of a nurse and other practitioners to persons outside the delivery system

In order to demonstrate application of the Omaha System in a variety of nurse-managed community health programs, nine examples have been selected for inclusion in this chapter. The structure, administration, staff, target population, and systems described with each of these programs differ markedly from one another and from traditional home health or public health home visit programs. Some programs in this chapter involve clients and community health nurses who are closely associated with other established health care agencies and institutions; in contrast, programs are described in which community health nurses practice independently or even in isolation. Many of the nurses have an opportunity to develop a community-oriented nursing practice and the potential for conducting quantitative and qualitative research (Goeppinger, 1988). Diversity exists among the nine examples, but so do similarities. In each program:

- Nurses are leaders and exhibit innovation, humanism, flexibility, determination, independent practice, and a high degree of professional competence
- The programs are designed to meet the health-related needs of target populations
- Nurses, other employees, and clients have benefited from the use of the Omaha System

CASE MANAGEMENT AND COMMUNITY COLLABORATION

Case management is one of the community health nurse's most important skills. The term has become popular in conversation and publications, but it is anything but novel. Community health nursing history is filled with leaders like Phoebe, Madame d'Youville, Nightingale, Wald, Dock, and Freeman who wrote about and, more importantly, practiced case management successfully at multiple levels.

Lillian Wald and Lavinia Dock seemed to fear no person or organization as they practiced case management at the beginning of the twentieth century. At the individual or family level, they did not hesitate to ask friends, relatives, and socialites to provide services and goods for needy families. At the community and national level, they were equally energetic and brash. Through coordination with other nurses, with politicians and businessmen, they established nursing services that were reimbursed by private insurance companies, public schools, and the American Red Cross.

In the tradition of community health nursing leaders, Adrienne Massel exemplifies commitment to general systems theory, the concept of community as client, and the nursing process. In a community of 34,000, Massel has identified powerful subsystems and has expanded her professional skills and enthusiasm far beyond the circle of public health nurses, programs, and clients in her Beloit, Wisconsin, agency. She has established community-based working relationships with local citizens and leaders in order to improve the continuity and quality of client services. She has articulated the benefits of community health nursing services and convinced non-nurses of the value of using a nursing model, the Omaha System.

THE BELOIT INITIATIVE AND THE OMAHA SYSTEM
by ADRIENNE MASSEL, RN, MSN, Public Health Nurse, Beloit Health Department, Beloit, WI

The police chief in our community approached city officials with a plan for an alternative human service delivery system in June, 1988. The chief developed the plan in response to long-standing frustration expressed by police officers who recognized that they continue to treat the symptoms of community problems rather than the underlying social causes. City officials encouraged him to develop the plan further. As a public health nurse from the Beloit Health Department, I worked with the police chief to develop the health aspects of the service delivery proposal and to incorporate the Omaha System into that proposal by assembling a team of various community representatives.

The Service Delivery System is comprised of four concepts or strategies. They are as follows:

Colocation of services: Community agency personnel who provide services for high-risk populations would locate offices in two centers, both established in high-risk neighborhoods. Included would be public health nurses and police officers as well as other health and human service providers. The staff at the centers would offer recreational as well as professional services to citizens of all ages.

Community involvement: Professionals would use a variety of strategies to elicit community participation, including the establishment of a citizen advisory board. The board members would serve as a link between professionals and neighborhood residents. Another strategy would involve a door-to-door canvas, encouraging residents to use the services at the two centers.

Team approach: A team approach would be used to organize and integrate services. For a given client, the team composition would vary according to that client's needs. Many individuals and families, especially those who have serious social, economic, educational, and health-related problems, are involved with multiple community agencies. The cooperative efforts of personnel from more than one human service agency are usually necessary to resolve these problems.

Problem-oriented communication: To facilitate effective, co-ordinated client care, human service team members would use the Problem Classification Scheme, the Problem Rating Scale for Outcomes, and the Intervention Scheme. The standard terminology of the Omaha System would enhance communication within the team, especially since members represent various disciplines and various agencies. In addition, the System would provide a tool for developing client-specific care plans.

I was familiar with the Omaha System, having introduced it to our staff nurses in 1982. Our nurses use the Problem Classification Scheme to identify client problems in the care plans of agency records. After acquainting the police chief with the Scheme, the chief determined that the Omaha System was an excellent communication tool for the Service Delivery System. The Omaha System (1) is client-centered, (2) consists of terminology that personnel from a variety of disciplines can understand, (3) is computer-compatible, and (4) furnishes a logical, progressive method for addressing the diagnosis and treatment of client problems. Thus, the Omaha System was incorporated into the problem-oriented communication strategy.

The proposal for an Initiative in Alternative Human Service Delivery System was submitted for funding to a national foundation by the City of Beloit in December, 1988. Because the proposal was rejected, the system has not been fully implemented; however, interest remains among community agencies, and progress continues.

Beloit city officials recognized that the proposed Beloit Initiative in Alternative Human Service Delivery had merit for effectively addressing community problems. Subsequently, they established a new city position, that of Director of Community Resources. The director will manage a revised Beloit Initiative Program. Members of a committee headed by the Beloit Health Officer, Donald Burandt, MD, are reviewing the concepts of the program and rewriting the grant proposal with a holistic health focus. Committee members, city officials, and human service personnel are optimistic about the future of the Service Delivery program and its value to the community.

AMBULATORY CARE CENTERS

The concept of ambulatory care is neither new nor original. Four programs that originated during the eighteenth and nineteenth centuries provided the historic roots for the current ambulatory care movement. First, Quakers and Joseph Warrington, a physician, organized ambulatory care services beginning in 1786. The staff of the Philadelphia Dispensary were not affiliated with any hospital; they provided medical, surgical, and obstetric services. Second, during 1889, Jane Adams and Ellen Gates Starr opened Hull House in a Chicago neighborhood to provide educational, philan-thropic, civic, and social activities for families. Health-related problems such as inadequate nutrition were among their concerns. Third, Lillian Wald and Mary Brewster established the Henry Street Settlement in New York City in 1893 as an experiment in public health nursing. They saw families at the House and at first-aid sites. They established a milk station and distributed milk, just one of their preventive strategies to decrease infant mortality. Finally, Ada Mayo Stewart began an occupational health nursing program for employees and families of Vermont Marble Company in 1895.

Closely associated with the development of ambulatory care services is the nurse practitioner movement. The term was introduced with a graduate program established by Ford and Silver at the University of Colorado in 1965. The demand for more cost-effective care by consumers and third-party payors has encouraged tremendous growth in ambulatory care; the trend away from acute care toward ambulatory care is pervasive.

An ambulatory care nurse functions as a "specialized generalist" in collaboration with other health care professionals and paraprofessionals. The nurse serves as a health educator, administrator, consultant, and researcher. Specific functions include eliciting histories and performing physical examinations; assessing health and illness status; providing health screening, education, and counseling; assisting with health maintenance and prevention activities; and initiating appropriate diagnostic and therapeutic procedures with physician consultation (Selleck, Sirles, & Sloan, 1988).

An ambulatory care client receives care from staff in a structured system while remaining outside the hospital. Recipients of care may occupy any point of the health-illness spectrum and are members of all socioeconomic groups; age and ethnicity also are diverse. Zielstorff describes below a satellite health center, but similar settings include (1) free-standing or hospital-based emergency clinics, (2) surgery centers, (3) disease-specific clinics and offices, (4) residential centers for senior citizens, (5) community health centers, and (6) occupational health centers. The staff in these settings provide services that address acute, episodic client needs or long-term, chronic client needs. The services provided, the nature of client problems, and client progress all require documentation in a comprehensive, yet concise, manner. Zielstorff describes the process at Massachusetts General Hospital as she and a multidisciplinary staff implemented the Omaha System in their ambulatory care program.

COORDINATED LONG-TERM CARE AND THE OMAHA SYSTEM*

by RITA ZIELSTORFF, RN, MS, Assistant Director, Laboratory of Computer Science, Massachusetts General Hospital, Boston, MA

In 1984, the Massachusetts General Hospital (MGH) founded the MGH Coordinated Care Program for the elderly. The demonstration project was intended to show that improved coordination of care of high-risk elders after discharge from the hospital can reduce unnecessary utilization of hospitals, nursing homes, and emergency rooms. Selected patients were followed by multidisciplinary teams consisting of a nurse, social worker, and a geriatrician consultant. During hospitalization, each team assessed the patient for post-discharge needs, then followed the patient after discharge to make sure that the designated package of services was delivered. In addition, each patient in need of a primary physician was linked to an MGH satellite health center. Home visits were carried out as needed by the teams and full functional reassessments were done every 6 months. Close communications with all of the community agencies involved in the patient's care was a high priority.

The Coordinated Care Teams at MGH and the physicians, nurse practitioners, and nutritionists at the health centers used a common automated record system, COSTAR, for this project (Zielstorff, Jette, Barnett, et al., 1985; Zielstorff, et al., 1986a; Zielstorff, et al., 1990; Zielstorff, Jette, Gillick, et al., 1986b). The MGH Coordinated Care Plan was developed and divided into three major sections: Problems, Health Appraisal, and Management. The admission information and problems sections are illustrated in Figure 12–1; the solid lines are for recording the data from the current visit that is then transcribed into the system by a clerk. The care plan was produced before every visit and incorporated all the most recent notes about every active problem.

The MGH record system requires that all providers use a common vocabulary to record their observations and findings, as described by Zielstorff in Chapter 8. The COSTAR lexicon of medical diagnoses, laboratory tests, procedures, and physical examination was incorporated into the system, but nurses and social workers found this vocabulary to be inadequate for their purposes. The Problem Classification Scheme was added to the system, along with terms to record assessments and interventions. We made some adjustments to the vocabulary because of the special nature of this population. For example, problem terms relating to child and maternal development were deleted. We added the following eight problem terms to the vocabulary to reflect the special problems addressed by the teams in this project.

Environmental	Problems with coordination of care
	Physical layout inadequate
Psychosocial	Denial
	Living arrangement problem
	Problems with formal care
	Problems with informal caregivers
Physiological	Endocrine/metabolic function impairment
Health Related Behaviors	Inadequate understanding of disease

At the end of the 3-year project, we evaluated the usefulness of the Problem Classification Scheme for multidisciplinary coordination of long-term care in the elderly. All disciplines had equal access to all of the vocabulary terms and could choose whatever term seemed most appropriate for

*The MGH Coordinated Care Program was supported by Grant 9991, Robert Wood Johnson Program for Hospital Initiatives in Long-Term Care. The implementation and evaluation of the enhanced COSTAR system was supported by Grant 1 R18 HS05261, National Center for Health Services Research, Office of the Assistant Secretary for Health (OASH).

```
                        MGH COORDINATED CARE PLAN

PRIMARY MD: DR. ALAN MICHAELS
PRIMARY NURSE PRACT: SHEEHY,MARGARET                 UNIT:# DEMO-014
1ST COORDINATOR: BARKER,ANN B,RN                         DEMO, TEST
DATE OF ADM TO MGH: 1/2/85                       (M) 85 YRS   (4/6/01)
DATE OF DISCH FROM MGH: 5/21/85                     123 ANY ST   2ND FL
LAST DATA ENTRY: 1/15/86                               REVERE, MA 02151
PRINTED: 10/22/86                                HOME PHONE: 234-4346


DATE:_____ PROVIDER:_____ SITE:_____
TYPE: ___INIT ___FU ___DISH ___CONF ___UPDATE  PRINT AT:_____
MODE: ___TELE ___PERSONAL ___OTH WITH: ___PT ___FAM/FRNDS ___LMD ___OTH

   HEALTH HX                                                  1/3/85
        HAS HAD DIABETES FOR 10 YRS, CONTROLLED ON TOLAZAMIDE.
        SAYS LMD IN CHELSEA DIED 6 MOS AGO, HAS NOT SEEN AN MD
        SINCE THEN.

                            [ANN BARKER,RN]


   REASON FOR ADMISSION                                       1/3/85
        DIABETES MELLITUS, UNCONTROLLED HYPERGLYCEMIA
                            [ANN BARKER, RN]


   HOSPITAL SUMMARY                                           1/10/85
        ADMITTED 1/2/85 W/ ACUTE ALCOHOLIC EPISODE &
        UNCONTROLLED HYPERGLYCEMIA, CONDITION STABILIZED ON 1200
        CAL DIAB DIET & DAILY TOLAZAMIDE.   PROBLEMS OF
        ALCOHOLISM AND DEPRESSION WILL NEED FOLLOW UP.  INTIALLY
        CONFUSED IN HOSPITAL, BUT MENTATION IS ADEQUATE ON
        DISCHARGE

                            [MARK A RANDALL,MD]

   PATIENT PROFILE
        84-YEAR OLD FRAIL MAN WHO LIVES ALONE.  WIFE DIED 14 MOS
        AGO.   TWO DAUGHTERS LIVE IN OHIO, COMMUNICATE
        INFREQUENTLY.  LANDLADY "CHECKS UP ON HIM" EVERY DAY,
        OCCASIONALLY SHOPS FOR FOOD FOR HIM.
                            [ANN B BARKER,RN]
 _____
 _____
 _____
 _____
 _____

 *********************************************************************
                              PROBLEMS
 *********************************************************************

 ALLERGIES/SENSITIVITIES

     * DRUG REACTION
           REPORTS RASH AFTER SULFA FOR UTI 5 YRS AGO
```

A

FIGURE 12–1 ■ (*A and B*) The header information and problem sections of the Massachusetts General Hospital Coordinated Care Plan incorporate terminology from the Problem Classification Scheme. (From Coordinated Care Program, Massachusetts General Hospital, Boston, MA.)

describing a particular patient problem. Although medical diagnosis vocabulary was used to describe 54% of the problems in this acutely ill population, Omaha terms were used to describe 38% of the problems. The remaining 8% of the problems was defined using the MGH-added terms. The terms from the Environmental, Health Related Behaviors, and Psychosocial Domains were particularly valuable because the COSTAR lexicon did not include many terms for problems from these domains.

The Problem Classification Scheme proved highly useful for this project, for several reasons:

■ We found it to be an easily understandable vocabulary for multiple disciplines, easy to teach and to use.
■ From a clinical point of view, consistent use of terms that were clear and simple facilitated interdisciplinary communication in this fully integrated automated record system. In addition, physicians became much more aware of so-

```
MAJOR DIAGNOSES/PROBLEMS

    DIABETES MELLITUS                                         1/10/85
         S: FEELING "OK" AT HOME, NO DIZZINESS OR SWEATS.  O: VS
         AS NOTED, PULSES OK, SEE LAB TESTS.  A: IMPROVING  P:
         CONTINUE PRESENT REGIMEN
                               [ALAN MICHAELS,MD] [1/30/85]

    SUBSTANCE MISUSE                                           1/5/85
       ALCOHOL ABUSE
           GOAL: IMPROVEMENT  [1/4/85]
           REPORTED BY LANDLADY.  PT. ADMITS TO GIN IN BEER "MOST
           DAYS"
                               [ANN B BARKER,RN]

    DEPRESSION                                                1/24/85
         APPEARS  UNKEMPT,  FLAT  AFFECT,  LITTLE  INTEREST  IN
         SURROUNDINGS.  HAS NO SOCIAL CONTACTS BESIDES LANDLADY.
    ─────────────────────────────────────────────────────────
    ═════════════════════════════════════════════════════════
    ─────────────────────────────────────────────────────────
    ─────────────────────────────────────────────────────────


OTHER DIAGNOSES/PROBLEMS

    SOCIAL ISOLATION                                           2/5/85
         GOAL: IMPROVEMENT   [1/5/85]
         HAS REFUSED TO GO BACK TO GOLDEN AGE CLUB.   SAYS IT
         REMINDS HIM TOO MUCH OF WHEN HIS WIFE WAS ALIVE.  MIGHT
         CONSIDER OTHER ACTIVITIES.
                               [RUTH M SHERIDAN,MSW]

    NONCOMPLIANCE, PRESCRIBED DIET                            1/26/85
         GOAL: IMPROVEMENT   [1/4/85]
         DOING  BETTER  AT  HOME  WITH  HOME  DELIVERED  MEALS,  AND
         AIDE.  CHO STILL TO HIGH.  DENIES ALCOHOL.
    ─────────────────────────────────────────────────────────
    ─────────────────────────────────────────────────────────
    ─────────────────────────────────────────────────────────
    ─────────────────────────────────────────────────────────
```

B

FIGURE 12–1 *Continued*

cial, psychological, and environmental problems in these patients, because these problems were given names of equal rank with medical diagnoses, and they were integrated into the patient's problem list along with medical diagnoses.

■ Because the clinical records were also intended to be used as a data base for research, we were concerned with the validity and reliability of the vocabulary. The published data about development of the vocabulary satisfied that concern.

NURSE-MANAGED CLINICS

Nurse-managed clinics are similar to, yet different from, ambulatory care centers. Similarities are historic development, physical setting, diversity of clients served, and the need for clients to come to the site. Differences are staffing and services. Ambulatory care centers have been described in relation to Zielstorff's experiences. In contrast, a community health nurse, alone or with peers, provides services independently at nursing centers or nurse-managed clinics. Thus, the services available to a client are nursing-focused, with the services of other health care providers available through consultation or referral. "A hallmark of a nursing center is its flexibility and willingness to provide services in non-traditional ways" (Fenton, Rounds, & Iha, 1988).

Prevention and health maintenance are the foci of most nurse-managed clinics that have been described in nursing literature. The clinics, depicted in this chapter by Bataillon, were established by the VNA of Omaha in 1974. In 1975, community health nurses in a rural area of Pennsylvania established a multiphasic health screening program for elders. Working from a central office, two satellite offices, and a mobile unit, nurses provide services to clients who have not been seeing a physician. Program objectives involve health education, referral and followup, and coordination (Young & Gottke, 1985). In 1977, the University of Connecticut School of Nursing faculty established a nursing center for older adults with the following goals: (1) preventive health maintenance—precrisis interventions, (2) early detection of health problems—precrisis interventions, (3) health maintenance for chronic problems—postcrisis interventions, and (4) coordination of care—crisis continuum (Thibodeau & Hawkins, 1987). Since then, community health agency staff and nursing faculty have established nurse-managed health centers for older adults in many states. Like Bataillon's example, nurses at other sites use a problem-oriented approach for documentation and program evaluation.

The establishment of so many nurse-managed centers for older adults reflects several trends. This is the age group experiencing the greatest growth, the highest prevalence of chronic illness, sometimes the most precipitous decrease in income, and often the strongest desire to maintain independence. Because of nursing centers, the elderly may receive primary care services that would not be available otherwise. Many nurse-managed centers have been established in inner cities and rural areas for the same reasons. Services offered by the staff of a nursing center were identified by Wilson, Patterson, and Alford (1989):

- Health assessment
- Health problem detection
- Direct care including injections and nail care
- Laboratory tests
- Monitoring health problems
- Individual and group health teaching involving how to stay well and live with chronic health problems
- Individual teaching of self-care for minor problems
- Medication review and teaching
- Assistance in coping with physical and mental health problems
- Referrals to other health professionals, including physicians
- Teaching how to use the health care system and community resources

Not all nursing centers or clinics are designed for older adults. Many local and county health departments have pediatric, antepartum/postpartum, and sexually transmitted disease clinic programs as well as services for clients across the age span. Community health nurses employed in all centers need methods for documenting services. The Omaha System allows a nurse to structure documentation in a way that increases the potential to retrieve and aggregate data. Data are especially meaningful if client problems are defined as Actual, Potential, or Health Promotion (Hays, 1990; Mundt, 1988) and if interactions emphasize health teaching, guidance, and counseling (Fenton, et al., 1988). As indicated by Bataillon, the brevity and sporadic nature of nurse-client encounters require particular skill as a documentation system is being developed and used to record nursing diagnoses, nursing interventions, and client progress.

HEALTH MAINTENANCE CENTERS AND THE OMAHA SYSTEM

by PAMELA BATAILLON, RN, MSN, Director of Clinical Services, Visiting Nurse Association of Omaha, Omaha, NE

Nurse-managed Health Maintenance Centers were initiated in 1974 by the Visiting Nurse Association of Omaha. Located in highrise apartment buildings for the elderly, senior centers, and churches, these nursing centers were found to be an acceptable, accessible, and cost-efficient method of delivery of community health nursing services to ambulatory elders. Twenty-eight such nursing centers are currently operational under VNA of Omaha auspices.

The purpose of the Health Maintenance Center is to provide individual health promotion and maintenance services to the ambulatory older adult population. An experienced community health nurse is assigned to each site, providing approximately 15 to 30 minutes of services to those clients who have scheduled appointments. Goals of the program include (1) assisting persons to develop and maintain resources that enhance their well-being, (2) identifying persons at risk for disease, (3) promoting knowledge of self-care techniques for health promotion and disease prevention, and (4) assessing client needs for other health services and providing advocacy, liaison, and referral.

Individual assessment, according to a defined data base, is initiated on the first visit and continues throughout the nurse-client contacts. Emphasis is placed on (1) determining the level of self-care abilities and limitations of each client and (2) assisting the client in developing the necessary health promotion and self-care activities.

The client record in the Health Maintenance Center is based on the Problem Classification Scheme and the Problem Rating Scale for Outcomes of the Omaha System (see the Appendix for record forms and instructions). The record was designed to provide documentation that reflects and enhances the professional practice of the clinic nurses. The design facilitates documentation during a client visit, a necessity due to the time constraints upon the nurse.

The client record consists of a folder, the Data Base, and the Problems/Plans/Ratings/Progress forms. The use of the client folder as part of the record has eliminated the need for additional paper to record frequently used information. The Data Base and Problems/Plans/Ratings/Progress forms were designed to promote quick, concise, and clear documentation. The record provides the following benefits:

Folder
  Facilitates easy retrieval of pertinent information
  Provides space for (1) client's name, age, and address/phone; (2) physician's name and phone number; (3) medical diagnoses; and (4) current medications
  Serves as a quick reference to a nurse other than the primary nurse
Data Base
  Follows the course of most client interviews
  Provides space for subjective and objective data
  Facilitates a client profile or assessment statement
  Encourages documentation of regularly scheduled reappraisals
Problems/Plans/Ratings/Progress
  Facilitates easy access to a problem list and associated plans
  Encourages rating the client's Knowledge, Behavior, and Status for each problem at the time of identification and at regular internals
  Provides space for documentation of activities at each visit

Clients who visit the Health Maintenance Centers vary markedly in terms of their health and illness knowledge as well as in type and severity of medical diagnoses. Clients who use the Centers live independently and manage their own self-care with varying degrees of proficiency. They do require professionals, however, to evaluate the presence or absence of signs and symptoms. Professional evaluation is viewed as a universal need of this population. To date, the problem areas identified most frequently by the Health Maintenance Center staff nurses are 41. Medical/Dental Supervision, 42. Prescribed Medication Regimen, and 43. Technical Procedure.

The client record has been modified for use at two of the newest Health Maintenance Centers. At the first site, the new client completes a Health History/Modified Data Base form. This practice allows nurses to spend less time collecting data so they can focus on problem areas sooner. At the second site, all clients receive foot care. The record has been modified to reflect greater emphasis on assessment of the feet; a separate section emphasizes cardiovascular status.

The Health Maintenance Center client record will be refined by the involved nurses to reflect future site or target population needs. Since the Problem Classification Scheme and the Problem Rating Scale for Outcomes provide the basic framework for the client record, such modifications do not hinder nurses who are transferred between sites or impede compilation of data from multiple sites.

Future plans for use of documented data involve (1) identifying trends in outcomes for the health maintenance clinic population, and (2) correlating the rating scale with tools measuring functional abilities and independent activities of daily living (IADLs). These data are being collected as part of the VNA research grant activities. The results of this research will be valuable to actual and potential funding sources, as well as to the knowledge base relative to this growing population of American society.

THE HOMELESS

Street dweller, bag lady, box tenant, grate man, car resident, transient, telephone booth occupant, and *homeless* are all terms used to describe the men, women, and children who have no acceptable shelter. The homeless population of the US is increasing; it is currently estimated at 2 to 3 million (Berne, Dato, Mason, et al., 1990; Lindsey, 1989). "The new generation of homeless is younger and more heterogeneous, and includes more women than the former population" (Francis, 1987, p. 230). Many women bring one or more children to the shelters including children who are as young as newborns (Bern, et al., 1990; Rafferty, 1989).

The recent growth in this target population has occurred for many reasons. The first factor is the deinstitutionalization of psychiatric residents. Often former residents do not receive coordinated mental health services or do not have adequate living arrangements following discharge from state and county hospitals. It has been estimated that one-third to two-thirds of the homeless are former residents of inpatient mental health facilities (Ferguson, 1989; Francis, 1987). Homelessness is also a consequence of layoffs, an absence of job skills, abuse, divorce, family violence, urban renewal with low-income housing shortages, alcoholism, drug abuse, physical illness and disability, antisocial behavior, and old age.

The homeless as a target population have a history of physical as well as mental morbidity and mortality. They are vulnerable to accidental injury and assault—the leading causes of death and disability. They are also vulnerable to hypothermia, malnutrition, peripheral vascular disease, and communicable disease such as tuberculosis, skin infestations, and respiratory infections. The homeless have limited access to health care services. The clinics established in many cities are among their few options. Frequently, clinics are established in conjunction with shelters and soup kitchens organized by volunteers and employees from the Salvation Army or local churches. Such clinics are funded by private donations as well as foundation, federal, and state grants.

Community health nurses who work with homeless clients are faced with unique problems—problems that involve practice and documentation. Edie Iwan, VNA of Omaha community health nurse, has been providing health-related services to the homeless for 4 years through a Nebraska State Health Department Maternal Child Health Block Grant (90M-16/C). The seven shelters where she works vary as to organization, staffing, services offered, policies, and resources. At each shelter, however, Iwan addresses persistent dilemmas. First, homeless clients need bedrest for illnesses and injuries on occasion; injuries of the feet occur frequently. However, most shelter policies require that clients leave during the day. Therefore, the community health nurse must work with shelter staff to allow for exceptions. Second, when medications, especially antibiotics, are prescribed, the staff need to be creative and resolute. If the client is scheduled to come to the shelter for medications and does not appear, a staff member may need to search that person's usual haunts. Third, infections and infestations such as lice require nursing intervention for the shelter staff as well as the client.

The Omaha System can provide the framework for the client record and for obtaining aggregate client data at homeless centers. This approach was chosen by staff at the VNA of Omaha and the University of Kentucky.

Both records incorporate the Problem Classification Scheme and the Intervention Scheme. A community health nurse who works with a homeless population needs a simple, clear record system to track intermittent, unpredictable client contacts. It is not unusual for nursing services to be provided to a homeless client over an extended period of time at more than one shelter. At the aggregate level, health-related data based on the Omaha System can produce valuable information. As described by Stanhope and Blomquist, this information has been useful to demonstrate client trends as well as changes in the needs of the homeless. These data substantiate the importance of nursing services and provide the basis for obtaining further funding; they offer the potential to communicate health-related problems of the homeless to the public.

A HOMELESS CLINIC AND THE OMAHA SYSTEM*

by MARCIA STANHOPE, RN, DSN, FAAN, Professor and Principal Investigator, University of Kentucky College of Nursing, Lexington, KY; and KATHLEEN BLOMQUIST, RN, PhD, Assistant Professor and Contract Researcher/Evaluator, University of Kentucky College of Nursing, Lexington, KY

The nurse-managed clinic operated by the University of Kentucky College of Nursing in conjunction with the Community Kitchen, Inc., a nonprofit, multiservice organization, has offered primary health care services to the homeless and very poor of Lexington since 1981. In October, 1986, the College of Nursing was awarded a contract from the Division of Nursing to expand and evaluate existing clinic services. Documentation of the health problems of the population, the impact of nursing care on the health status of the population, and the evaluation of the cost-effectiveness of the nurse-managed clinic were but a few of the contract activities.

The clinic population, staff, and services have grown significantly since 1986. Nurse clinicians and nurse practitioners cared for about 900 clients who made over 5,000 visits to the clinic in 1989. To describe the activities in the clinic, nursing faculty, who comprise the majority of the clinic staff, wanted a computer-applicable system of codes for client problems, nursing interventions, and client outcomes suitable for use in an ambulatory care setting. The Omaha System was selected over other nursing diagnosis systems because it enabled the staff to describe and encode problems of the client population and nursing interventions. The domains, problems, and modifiers of the Problem Classification Scheme, the numeric ratings of the Problem Rating Scale for Outcomes, and the general categories and specific targets of the Intervention Scheme allowed a variety of useful analyses.

A computerized client form was developed for use in the clinic. It was designed to include demographic, housing status, alcohol and drug use, mental health problem, and medical problem data as well as acuity/chronicity and severity information. In addition, the form allowed the staff to use the Omaha System and to document client problems, problem ratings, and nursing interventions.

Client data based on the Problem Classification Scheme were analyzed for the contract years 1986 to 1989 (see Table 12–1). It was found that 75% of all client problems was coded with the Actual modifier by the nursing staff. The probability of encountering a client with problems in the Physiological Domain was greater than for the three other domains combined. However, client problems were identified in all domains. Of the 44 nursing problems listed in the Scheme, 16 accounted for 86% to 91% of all client problems encountered. Twenty-eight problems occurred in less than 2% of all encounters.

Records were also examined in relation to the Intervention Scheme and the frequency of occurrence of the 60 targets of nursing action. Seventeen of the 60 targets of nursing intervention accounted for 88% of all nursing actions. Forty-two targets accounted for less than 1% of the total objects of encounters. When the four intervention categories and the 1986 client data were reviewed, Surveillance followed by Treatments and Procedures accounted for the majority of nursing actions. However, by 1989, the trend had changed; Health Teaching, Guidance, and Counseling as well as Treatments and Procedures were the most frequently used intervention categories.

The Omaha System has been useful to the clinic staff in describing trends in client problems and nursing interven-

*Funded by contract 240-86-0082 US Department of Health and Human Services, Health Resources and Services Administration, Division of Nursing.

TABLE 12-1 ■ Aggregate Data Trends Noted in the Homeless Population: 1986-1989*

PROBLEMS: ACCOUNTED FOR 86-91% OF ALL IDENTIFIED PRIMARY PROBLEMS	
1. Integument	9. Prescribed Medication Regime
2. Circulation	10. Substance Misuse
3. Pain	11. Health Care Supervision
4. Respiration	12. Nutrition
5. Neuro-Musculo-Skeletal Function	13. Income
6. Vision	14. Emotional Stability
7. Genito-Urinary Function	15. Digestion-Hydration
8. Other (Physiological Domain)	16. Hearing

CATEGORIES	
1986	
1. Surveillance (31%)	3. Health Teaching, Guidance, and Counseling (26%)
2. Treatments and Procedures (30%)	4. Case Management (14%)
1989	
1. Health Teaching, Guidance, and Counseling (36%)	3. Surveillance (26%)
2. Treatments and Procedures (32%)	4. Case Management (6%)

TARGETS: ACCOUNTED FOR 88% OF ALL RECORDED	
1. Signs/symptoms — physical	10. Durable medical equipment
2. Medical/dental care	11. Medication administration
3. Stimulation/nurturance	12. Skin care
4. Sickness/injury care	13. Signs/symptoms — mental/emotional
5. Support system	14. Substance use
6. Dressing change/wound care	15. Medication set-up
7. Supplies	16. Communication
8. Nutrition	17. Medication action/side effects
9. Transportation	

*In rank order.

tions. Health promotion class topics have been based on the problems of the clients. Audits of records have been done using the Omaha System to compare data over several years in a consistent manner. Data about numbers of problems and interventions per contact have been used in cost and efficiency analyses. Preliminary analyses indicate that a modified Omaha System is a useful method of coding client problems in an ambulatory/primary care setting.

NEIGHBORHOOD COLLABORATION

The elderly have been described as a primary, at-risk target population for the community health nurse. This population group is experiencing a critical lack of preventive and health maintenance services, especially since the onset of Medicare (Bremer, 1987). Comprehensive services must be made available to the elderly so that the World Health Organization goal of access to basic health care for all is met (Ulin, 1989).

Ambulatory care or nurse-managed centers have been described by Zielstorff and Bataillon as one means of offering preventive, health maintenance, and curative services to the elderly at a minimal fee. Additional programs are needed for the elderly, especially for the frail elderly who are unable to travel conveniently to the centers.

The goal of the Block Nurse Program, begun in St. Paul, MN, by Martinson and others, is to deliver needed, comprehensive, and economical services in clients' homes. Without this alternative of nursing services, personal care services, and companionship provided by neighborhood employees and volunteers, evaluators estimated that 85% of the clients would require nursing home admission; this finding was included in a 1985 Block Nurse Program external evaluation. Often, the lack of services leads to a "revolving door syndrome" and frequent expensive readmissions to the hospital (Bremer, 1987). Therefore, "the client, family, and block nurse together develop a plan of care that works for them. The nurse can take time to build trust, explore alternatives, reconsider objectives, and encourage growth and independence" (Jamieson, 1989, p. 1291). The Block Nurse Program addresses the goal of basic health care for all as well as a second World Health Organization goal, that of community involvement.

The community health nurses of the Block Nurse Program and the Ramsey County Public Health Nursing Service have been closely associated since the Block Nurse Program was instituted. Marjorie Jamieson and the Ramsey County administrators, Barbara O'Grady and Mary Lou Christensen, have practiced as expert, community-focused nurses for many years. After thoughtful consideration, they determined that the Omaha System offered a practice and documentation tool that was applicable to sound public health nursing practice and to the Block Nurse Program.

THE BLOCK NURSE PROGRAM AND THE OMAHA SYSTEM

by MARJORIE JAMIESON, RN, MS, Executive Director, The Block Nurse Program, Inc., St. Paul, MN; and SUZANNE CLARKE, RN, BSN, Assistant Director, The Block Nurse Program, Inc., St. Paul, MN

St. Anthony Park, a neighborhood in St. Paul, is a community of about 7,000 residents. Almost 13% of the residents are over age 65, a statistic that is similar to the national average. In 1981, the Block Nurse Program was started in St. Anthony Park by a group of nurses and other concerned citizens. The purpose was to provide an alternative way of delivering and financing care needed by the elderly residents of this neighborhood.

The Block Nurse Program represents a unique, collaborative effort. Professional nurses, paraprofessionals, and trained volunteers provide services to their elderly neighbors in St. Anthony Park. Services include (1) nursing, (2) personal care, (3) housekeeping, (4) companionship, and (5) other in-home services. Both staff and clients live in the community; a sense of ownership has developed as St. Anthony Park residents have come to view the program as their own. A local board of directors plans and directs the program. The staff of Ramsey County Public Health Nursing Service hires the nurses and home health aides who live in the community and provides quality assurance and administrative services for the program.

The goal of the Block Nurse Program is to allow elderly people to remain in their own homes. Without the program, many elders would be forced to enter nursing homes. Residents of the St. Anthony Park neighborhood 65 years and older are eligible for services, based upon need and regardless of ability to pay. Some services are covered by Medicare, Medicaid, private insurance, and other sources. Services not covered by third-party payors are billed to the client based upon ability to pay. Community fundraising efforts and grants provide money for nonreimbursable services.

The Omaha System was chosen as an assessment, care planning, and evaluation tool. Two characteristics of the Omaha System made it particularly useful for this project.

■ A computer-ready system meant that nursing diagnosis and client outcome information could become part of the project's data base, available for future reports.
■ The assessment process would be simplified for the

nurse, who could circle and check appropriate data on a preprinted form instead of writing volumes of narrative notes.

Primary block nurses, who are public health nurses, use the Problem Classification Scheme during their assessment visit. As case managers, they develop a care plan for nursing practice that is based on the categories and targets of the Intervention Scheme. To evaluate client status and measure goal attainment, the nurse uses the Problem Rating Scale for Outcomes every 6 months.

At the request of the primary nurses, the care plan form was organized so that the Physiological Domain appears first on the form. This request occurred because many nurses are accustomed to doing a head-to-toe physical assessment before moving to the other domains. Following the Physiological Domain are the Health Related Behaviors, the Psychosocial and the Environmental Domains. The nurses have found that the opening interview and assessment flow smoothly since the care plan was organized in this way. The first page of the Family Nursing Diagnosis and Care Plan is included as Figure 12–2.

Based on the success of the St. Anthony Park program, it was decided to seek funding for replication and evaluation. A 3-year project was recently funded by the US Department of Health and Human Services (DHHS), Division of Nursing, and the W. K. Kellogg Foundation. The goals of the project are to test the replicability of the model in three socioeconomically diverse communities and to collect data on a projected 1,000 clients. Project sites are two other neighborhoods in St. Paul and the rural community of Atwater, MN. A Block Nurse Program has also been established in the Prospect Park neighborhood of Minneapolis and a sixth program is being developed in Birmingham, AL. Aggregate client data will be available to educators, researchers, public policy makers, legislators, insurance companies, community organizers, and others interested in community-based health and long-term care.

RESIDENTIAL CENTERS

Most clients who use community health nurse services at ambulatory care or health maintenance centers are living independently and are capable of controlling many aspects of their lives. Although several of the health maintenance sites described by Bataillon in this chapter are located at congregate living facilities, residents must elect to seek service from the health maintenance program. Furthermore, when ambulatory care and health maintenance clients make a conscious deci-

sion to seek care from the community health nurse, they must go to that nurse.

In contrast, the children who are described by Warner in the following section are a special population with special needs. They do not make decisions about health care services or many other aspects of their lives. The personnel of the Child Milieu Enhancement Project have control over access, content, organization, and staffing of health-related services available to the residents. Thus, children in the residential home are a captive audience for nurses and other health care

FAMILY NURSING DIAGNOSIS AND CARE PLAN

Source: Omaha VNA

Family Number: _____
Client(s) Name(s): _____
Member(s) Number: _____

Date of Assessment: _____
Nurse Signature _____

CLIENT PROBLEM/NURSING DIAGNOSIS
DIRECTIONS:
CIRCLE one choice (Adequate, Not Assessed, Not Applicable, Health Promotion, Potential or Deficit/Impairment/Actual).
If Potential is circled, risk factors must be listed.
If Deficit/Impairment is circled, one or more Signs/Symptoms (S/S) must be listed.
Date and sign subsequent information.
Date deficit if identified after initial assessment.

CARE PLAN AND OUTCOME
DIRECTIONS:
Vulnerable client problems/nursing diagnoses are numbers 14, 15, 16, 23. These identified problems must have a plan to reduce vulnerability.
Vulnerability Assessed　　　Date _____
Highly Vulnerable?　　　Yes _____　No _____
Homebound due to: _____

DOMAIN III: PHYSIOLOGICAL

19. HEARING:
ADEQUATE　　NOT ASSESSED　　NOT APPLICABLE　　HEALTH PROMOTION
CORRECTION
POTENTIAL, RISK FACTORS: _____
IMPAIRMENT, R _____ L _____　　S/S:1) difficulty hearing normal speech tones
2) absent/abnormal response to sound
3) abnormal results of hearing screening test
4) other _____

20. VISION:
ADEQUATE　　NOT ASSESSED　　NOT APPLICABLE　　HEALTH PROMOTION
CORRECTION
POTENTIAL, RISK FACTORS: _____
IMPAIRMENT, R _____ L _____　　S/S: 1) difficulty seeing small print/calibrations 2) difficulty seeing distant objects
3) difficulty seeing close objects 4) absent/abnormal reponse to visual stimuli
5) abnormal results of vision screening test 6) squinting/blinking/tearing/blurring
7) difficulty differentiating colors
8) other _____

21. SPEECH AND LANGUAGE:
ADEQUATE　　NOT ASSESSED　　NOT APPLICABLE　　HEALTH PROMOTION
POTENTIAL, RISK FACTORS: _____
IMPAIRMENT, S/S:1) absent/abnormal ability to speak 2) absent/abnormal ability to understand 3) lacks alternative communication skills
4) inappropriate sentence structure
5) limited enunciation/clarity
6) inappropriate word usage
7) other _____

DATE　　ADDITIONAL INFORMATION

	Rating Scale	Date
Knowledge		
Behavior		
Status		

SERVICE PLAN
GOAL:
DATE MET: _____　CAT　TARGET
INTERVENTIONS:

DATE　　ADDITIONAL INFORMATION

	Rating Scale	Date
Knowledge		
Behavior		
Status		

SERVICE PLAN
GOAL:
DATE MET: _____　CAT　TARGET
INTERVENTIONS:

DATE　　ADDITIONAL INFORMATION

	Rating Scale	Date
Knowledge		
Behavior		
Status		

SERVICE PLAN
GOAL:
DATE MET: _____　CAT　TARGET
INTERVENTIONS:

21

FIGURE 12–2 ■ A portion of the Ramsey County (MN) Block Nurse Program Family Nursing Diagnosis and Care Plan that is based on the Omaha System. (From Block Nurse Program, Inc., St. Paul, MN.)

providers. These children, however, may have little interest in preventive or therapeutic health practices; they represent a real challenge to community health nurses. Most of these children have a history of serious problems prior to admission, problems that may interfere with their adjustment to a home as well as to their physical, emotional, social, and educational development. They have been removed from their family of origin or foster family(ies); their sense of security and self-worth may be diminished.

The community health nurses and other staff described by Warner are child-oriented, caring people. Because of these characteristics, they are interested in completing a thorough assessment of each child from a psychosocial, physiologic, and health-related behavior perspective. They want to provide appropriate interventions and monitor the child's progress during the time of residency. By adapting the Omaha System, they have developed such a framework for their practice and documentation.

THE CHILD MILIEU ENHANCEMENT PROJECT AND THE OMAHA SYSTEM*

by SANDRA WARNER, RN, PhD, Associate Professor, University of Texas Health Science Center at San Antonio, San Antonio, TX

The Child Milieu Enhancement Project was designed as an innovative undertaking that allowed nurses to (1) enhance the care available for disadvantaged, orphaned, and abused children, (2) test the heuristic and problem-solving value of a nursing practice model, (3) analyze the cost benefits and effectiveness of nursing care, (4) computerize the recordkeeping system, and (5) practice autonomously in a nontraditional setting. The project generated needed data by translating the quality and cost-effectiveness of nursing interventions into measurable outcomes through a documentation and reporting process. Data generated by the Enhancement Project have the potential to justify this Project as a legitimate alternative to traditional health care.

The project was implemented in a Children's Home that provides intake and residential care for 48 dependent, neglected, abused, and predelinquent children. The ages of the children range from 4 to 18 years. Administered by a religious organization, the Home receives funds from United Way, private donors, and Medicaid. A nurse, four social workers, 12 houseparents, and nine support staff comprise the staff of the Children's Home. The Home's professional staff members were involved in the project, as were four faculty members from the University of Texas Health Science Center at San Antonio and eight consultants. The faculty members included the project director, a clinical specialist in psychiatric nursing, a pediatric nurse practitioner, and an evaluator. The consultants included a programmer, an economist, a social worker, a psychiatric nurse, two psychologists, a psychiatrist/pediatrician, and an information systems manager.

The time and energy spent by community health nurses in developing the Omaha System was greatly appreciated, for it served as a prototype for materials developed for the Child Milieu Enhancement Project. For example, the Problem Classification Scheme and the Problem Rating Scale for Outcomes, two components of the Omaha System, were adapted or "pediatricized" to become the Child Clinical Assessment Tool (CCAT) and the Child Problem Rating Scale.

These two forms, adapted for a younger population who lived in a residential care facility, were used to assess children's problems and quantify their severity. Portions of the CCAT and the Child Problem Rating Scale are included as Figure 12-3.

The CCAT was tailored to meet the needs of the children within the framework of the Child Milieu Enhancement Model. For example, elements from each of the model's three components are represented in the CCAT. These components include Dimensions of Practice, Environmental Modes, and Recipients of Care. The Child Problem Rating Scale allowed staff to rate the severity of the child's problem on a Likert-type scale. Whether a problem related to knowledge deficits, behaviors, and/or physical status, change over time was documented by rating the same problem at a later date. These two forms represent a large part of the Home's computerized recordkeeping system and reflect the child care provided from admission to discharge.

All child care record data were programmed onto an IBM PC computer. The comprehensive list of the child's problems within the CCAT was indexed by Environmental Mode elements and further sorted by pagination and subgroupings as Education, General Health, and Systems. Such sorting allowed staff to quickly locate and code by number and/or letter any child-specific condition for entry into the computer. The programmers also devised a way to track and code model usage by default, once the problem was identified and given its corresponding ratings.

Once data were entered into the computer, files became available for browsing, editing, printing, and generating reports. Multiple reports were generated from the data base by combining different variables. For example, a yearly summary of the percentage of population by ethnicity, insurance coverage, and average length of stay has value for reports to the US DHHS and the United Way. Reports from the Nurse's Log were generated by combining up to three variables. For example, the ethnicity of the children seen by physicians for respiratory ailments was indexed with the current calendar year.

While attempting to create the necessary forms to implement and test a practice model, project personnel needed a

*Funded for 3 years by the Division of Nursing, US DHHS 1 D10 NU 600013.

38. Sexuality:

ASSESSMENT

A. Risk Factors

   a. The observable responses, actions or activities of the child which may stem from the child's family of origin.

   b. The observable responses, action or activities which stem from the child's current living conditions inclusive of dorm living, school, off-campus activities, parental visits and therapy visits.

B. Impairment

   00. no impairment
   01. difficulty recognizing consequences of sexual behavior
   02. difficulty expressing appropriate intimacy
   03. sexual identity confusion (reversal of traditional male/female roles)
   04. sexual value confusion in child
   05. dissatisfied with sexual relationships
   06. misunderstanding information related to sexual activity
   07. inappropriate sex play

   Rating Scales   K   B   S   (1-4)

   1
   2
   3
   4
   5
   6
   7

(ACTION PLAN WITH ANY RATING -- EVALUATION THEREIN)

B

PERSONAL INTERNAL: Psychological Processes

	PAGE
*EMOTIONS	
Dominate Coping Patterns	36
Eating Disorders	37
Emotional Stability*	38
Grief/Loss	39
Spirituality	40
Substance Misuse	41
PERSONAL EXTERNAL: (interrelatedness from person outward)	
Individuation/Separation	42
Interpersonal Relationships	43
Sexuality	44
*DORM ENVIRONMENT	
Adjustment to Institutional Living	45
*PLACEMENT	
Role change	46
*VISITATION	
Coping Patterns related to Dysfunctional Family	47

*Categories most frequently used in Plan of Service

A

Name _____   Social Security# _____

Date _____   Problem _____

Child Problem Rating Scale

		1	2	3	4

A. Knowledge:
   the ability of the
   child to remember
   and interpret
   information.

B. Behavior:
   the observable re-
   sponses, actions or
   activities of the
   child fitting the
   occasion or purpose.

C. Status:
   the condition of the
   child in relation to
   objective and subjec-
   tive defining charact-
   eristics.

KNOWLEDGE	BEHAVIOR	STATUS
1 no knowledge	1 not appropriate	1 extreme signs/symptoms
2 minimal knowledge	2 rarely appropriate	2 moderate signs/symptoms
3 basic knowledge	3 frequently appropriate	3 minimal signs/symptoms
4 superior knowledge	4 consistently appropriate	4 no signs/symptoms

This instrument will be used to rate any identified impairment
and document change over time.

C

FIGURE 12–3 ■ (A–C) Selected portions of the Child Clinical Assessment Tool and Child Problem Rating Scale developed for the University of Texas Health Science Center Child Milieu Enhancement Project that incorporates the Problem Classification Scheme and Problem Rating Scale for Outcomes. (From Child Milieu Enhancement Project, University of Texas Health Science Center, San Antonio, TX.)

firm foundation and springboard upon which to base their work. In the Omaha System, they found a parent for their fledgling project. Although major portions of the CCAT were derived from the Omaha System, differences in focus, content, and usage do exist. The Omaha System was developed for use with clients who span the health-illness and age continua. In contrast, the CCAT was devised for a relatively healthy, young population, although an effort was made to include an exhaustive list of all possible problems. In addition, the CCAT was conceived within the framework of the Child Milieu Enhancement model, whereas the Omaha System is defined by the nursing process. The content of the CCAT has an interdisciplinary focus, including concerns about Education, Dorm Environment, Placement, and Visita-tion, which are unique to staff employed in residential care settings.

The CCAT is used not only for assessments but also for interdisciplinary care planning and evaluation. When staff experience inculcation or repetition in relation to an acceptable model, they are likely to use that model. During a staffing session, social workers, child care workers, and nurses report their areas of responsibility and expertise in terms of subgroupings of the CCAT. This exercise provides a comprehensive review of a child and results in feelings of appreciation for each person's role in caring for a particular child. Although differences in form, content, and usage exist, the relationship between the Omaha System and the CCAT remains obvious.

PARISH NURSING PROGRAMS

Phoebe of Cenchrea (60 AD) has been identified as an expert case manager and community coordinator from a nursing heritage. Phoebe, the first visiting nurse identified by name, was a friend of St. Paul and an ordained deaconess in the early Christian church. As such, she was a parish worker, friendly visitor, and district nurse. Phoebe was one of many women and men who joined religious orders that were being organized in Europe to address human concerns.

Jean Denton indicates that the field of parish nursing is new and yet still related to history. Although 20 centuries have passed, many similarities exist between the community health nursing experiences of Phoebe of Cenchrea and Jean Denton. The focus of both is community-oriented health care, which is not simply practice outside institutional settings. Parish nursing practice involves clients of all ages across the health-illness continuum. Denton identifies several target population groups for the parish nurse; these groups vary in their severity of risk.

The diversity of a parish nurse's client population as well as the variety of interventions used require a flexible method of documentation. Like many other community health nurses described in this chapter, the parish nurse's client contacts vary markedly in frequency, length, and intensity. Little time is available for documentation, so Denton wanted a system that was based on a nursing model and provided the structure for recording pertinent information. Thus, she has adapted the Problem Classification Scheme and the Intervention Scheme of the Omaha System to accommodate the needs of her setting.

PARISH NURSING AND THE OMAHA SYSTEM

by JEAN DENTON, RN, MA, Director of Health Ministries, St. Paul's Episcopal Church, Indianapolis, IN

The field of parish nursing represents an evaluation of both nursing practice and church ministry. A nurse in a church draws on clinical experience both from ministry and from nursing to work with the church community to address health needs throughout a local congregation. Responsibilities are broad and vary from congregation to congregation. The potential for the role is enormous, because the roots of health and the roots of faith share common soil.

A parish nurse as health minister works at all three levels of prevention. Primary prevention activities are aimed at wellness promotion, a natural focus for a church community where wellness is built into the nature of relationships. Health risk appraisal, classes to teach safe babysitting, exercise classes, an educational series on mind-body-spirit con-nectedness, and meditation groups are a few examples of primary prevention opportunities. Through these programs, a parish nurse can assist people to remain well. Secondary prevention is addressed by the parish nurse as hidden risk factors are identified. Examples of such activities include blood pressure screening and offering support to high-risk groups such as children of divorced parents or people who are grieving. The nurse and parishioners are involved in tertiary prevention as the nurse (1) supports the lay pastoral visitation teams who care for shut-ins, (2) advocates for parishioners' rights in the health care system, and (3) counsels individuals and families about personal health and sickness-related issues.

Whenever a parish nurse has a one-to-one contact with a

parishioner, it behooves that nurse to record the interaction. Subsequent interactions with the parishioner are more meaningful when seen in connection with former interactions. A simple recordkeeping system is necessary, given the diverse nature of the work.

When a parish nursing program was initiated at St. Paul's Episcopal Church in 1989, several documentation options were considered. The Omaha Problem Classification Scheme (PCS) was chosen since it offered a quick and useful method to record initial and subsequent client contacts. The PCS applies to all ages and is comprehensive in scope, being born from more traditional fields within community health nursing. Using a data base that circumscribes the four domains provides basic information that can be shared as appropriate with clergy and lay pastoral visitors. It also simplifies problem identification by offering comprehensive categories, including 10. Spiritual Distress. The freedom to select Health Promotion, Potential, or Actual modifiers to delineate problems encourages the parish nurse to generate a comprehensive list of parishioner concerns. The problem categories can be fit onto a concise, preprinted record that encourages recordkeeping because it is user friendly.

The Intervention Scheme has been adapted for our parish nursing program at St. Paul's. The categories describe the general scope of a nurse's practice, and the targets provide more details. The four basic intervention categories are appropriate for all kinds of nursing activities, whether they involve office-based or home-based interactions. The opportunity to develop additional targets in conjunction with the four categories helps describe nursing practice with increasing specificity. In parish nursing, additional targets such as empathic listening, prayer, reminiscing, massage, and visualization are used frequently (Fig. 12–4).

The simplicity of the Omaha System promotes the collection and analysis of statistical data as well as recordkeeping for me as a parish nurse. As any field grows, more questions will be asked to help define it. Questions important to defining the scope of clinical practice for parish nursing include:

1. What kinds of problems do parish nurses deal with?
2. What kinds of interventions are most successful when addressing problems through the faith community?
3. How many and what kind of referrals were made to community agencies?

Using a flexible and well developed framework like the Omaha System has facilitated answering such questions and defining the practice of parish nursing.

HEALTH MINISTRIES PROJECT
ST. PAUL'S EPISCOPAL CHURCH
CLINICAL RECORD

DATA BASE

Name   Date

Address   Phone

Directions   Emergency contact

                                    Emergency phone #

Referral source

Primary Clergy

Physician   Phone

ENVIRONMENTAL

Housing

Income

Medical insurance

Transportation

Impressions:

PSYCHOSOCIAL/SPIRITUAL

Sex   Birthday   Marital status   Education   Mental Status

Experience with church

Impact of religious beliefs

Experience with grief

Family support system/Role

Lay Pastoral Care

Other health providers

Attorney   Living Will?   Durable power of attorney?

Impressions:

A

PHYSIOLOGICAL

Height   Weight   Ideal weight   B/P   P   R   Blood Type

Medical history

Chief complaint

Skin   Infections

Ears and eyes   Neoplasms

Dental   Mental/neurological

Cardiovascular   Accidents

Respiratory   Surgeries

Endocrine   Last physical exam/pap

Musculoskeletal   Significant family history

Gastrointestinal

Genito-urinary   Pain

Impressions:

HEALTH BEHAVIORS

Nutrition/diet

Habits

Functional limitations/ADLs

Sleep

Medical supervision

Medications

Impressions:

B

INTERVENTIONS

T for teaching, counseling, guidance
P for procedures, technical activities
C for case management, advocacy, referral
S for surveillance, detection, monitoring

DATE

TPCS	01.	Anatomy/physiology
TPCS	02.	Behavior modification
TPCS	03.	Bladder care
TPCS	04.	Bonding
TPCS	05.	Bowel care
TPCS	06.	Bronchial hygiene
TPCS	07.	Cardiac care
TPCS	08.	Caretaking/parenting skills
TPCS	09.	Cast care
TPCS	10.	Communication
TPCS	11.	Coping skills
TPCS	12.	Day care/respite
TPCS	13.	Discipline
TPCS	14.	Dressing change/wound care
TPCS	15.	Durable medical equipment
TPCS	16.	Education
TPCS	17.	Employment
TPCS	18.	Environment
TPCS	19.	Exercises
TPCS	20.	Family planning
TPCS	21.	Feeding procedures
TPCS	22.	Finances
TPCS	23.	Food
TPCS	24.	Gait training
TPCS	25.	Growth/development
TPCS	26.	Homemaking
TPCS	27.	Housing
TPCS	28.	Interaction
TPCS	29.	Lab finding
TPCS	30.	Legal system
TPCS	31.	Medical/dental care
TPCS	32.	Medication action/side effects
TPCS	33.	Medication administration

DATE

TPCS	34.	Medication set-up
TPCS	35.	Mobility/exercise
TPCS	36.	Nursing care, supplementary
TPCS	37.	Nutrition
TPCS	38.	Nutritionist
TPCS	39.	Ostomy care
TPCS	40.	Other community resource
TPCS	41.	Personal care
TPCS	42.	Positioning
TPCS	43.	Rehabilitation
TPCS	44.	Relaxation/breathing techniques
TPCS	45.	Rest/sleep
TPCS	46.	Safety
TPCS	47.	Screening
TPCS	48.	Sickness/injury care
TPCS	49.	Signs/Symptoms -mental/emotional
TPCS	50.	Signs/symptoms - physical
TPCS	51.	Skin care
TPCS	52.	Social work/counseling
TPCS	53.	Specimen collection
TPCS	54.	Spiritual care
TPCS	55.	Stimulation/nurturance
TPCS	56.	Stress management
TPCS	57.	Substance use
TPCS	58.	Supplies
TPCS	59.	Support group
TPCS	60.	Support system
TPCS	61.	Transportation
TPCS	62.	Wellness
TPCS	63.	Other - Reminiscing
TPRS	64.	Other - Visualization
TPRS	65.	Other - Massage

PROGRESS NOTES

D

PROBLEM LIST

H for Health promotion
P for Potential deficit
A for Actual problem

DATE

Environmental

DATE

HPA	01	Income
HPA	02	Sanitation
HPA	03	Residence
HPA	04	Neighborhood/ workplace safety
HPA	05	Other environmental

Psychosocial

HPA	06	Communication with community
HPA	07	Social contact
HPA	08	Role change
HPA	09	Interpersonal relationship
HPA	10	Spiritual distress
HPA	11	Grief
HPA	12	Emotional stability
HPA	13	Human sexuality
HPA	14	Caretaking/parenting
HPA	15	Neglected child/adult
HPA	16	Abused child/adult
HPA	17	Growth and development
HPA	18	Other psychosocial

Physiological

HPA	19	Hearing
HPA	20	Vision
HPA	21	Speech and Language
HPA	22	Dentition
HPA	23	Cognition
HPA	24	Pain
HPA	25	Consciousness
HPA	26	Integument
HPA	27	Neuro-musculo-skeletal function
HPA	28	Respiration
HPA	29	Circulation
HPA	30	Digestion-hydration
HPA	31	Bowel function
HPA	32	Genito-urinary function
HPA	33	Antepartum/postpartum
HPA	34	Other physiological

Health Related Behaviors

HPA	35	Nutrition
HPA	36	Sleep and rest
HPA	37	Physical activity
HPA	38	Personal hygiene
HPA	39	Substance misuse
HPA	40	Family planning
HPA	41	Health care supervision
HPA	42	Prescribed medication regimen
HPA	43	Technical procedure
HPA	44	Other health related behavior

PLANS

C

FIGURE 12–4 ■ (*A–D*) The Health Ministries Project, St. Paul's Episcopal Church (IN) Clinical Record incorporates the Problem Classification Scheme and the Intervention Scheme. (Courtesy of St. Paul's Episcopal Church, Indianapolis, IN.)

CORRECTIONAL INSTITUTIONS

There is no more captive population for the community health nurse than the men, women, and youth who are inmates of correctional institutions. Furthermore, this target group is at high risk for serious health problems involving (1) physical violence and suicides, (2) drug and alcohol abuse, (3) psychiatric illness, (4) communicable disease, (5) unhealthy living conditions, (6) overcrowding, (7) chronic illness, and (8) impaired parenting and child care. Inmates and their families experience profound stressors specific to detention, including:

■ Losses, such as loss of job, freedom, family contacts, dignity, food choices, privacy, and sexual activity
■ Threats such as those of physical violence or homosexual advances
■ Physical discomfort related to sleeping, eating, and other personal functions
■ Drug and/or alcohol withdrawal
■ Fears such as fear of impending trial or infidelity of a spouse or other companion (Freeman & Heinrich, 1981, p. 535)

The serious health-related problems of inmates, professional isolation, and the emotional overtones of correctional settings make the role difficult for the community health nurse. "Nurses as employees of a correctional system experience conflicting expectations. On one hand, they are employees of an institution whose mission is security and public safety. On the other hand, they are health care providers who are responsible for delivery of safe and ethical nursing care" (Gulotta, 1986–87, p. 5).

Margie Knappenberger describes the characteristics of a community health nurse's role and a jail setting, which justify the need for objective, precise, concise, and complete documentation. During incarceration, inmates may experience problems outlined in the Psychosocial, Physiological, and Health Related Behaviors Domains of the Problem Classification Scheme; using these domains provides the nurse with an assessment tool. In addition, many inmates experience problems in the Environmental Domain after release; these problems include access to health care, income, and housing. In the following description and on the forms developed for a correctional institution, Knappenberger delineates adaptation of the Problem Classification Scheme and the Intervention Scheme to her target population and setting.

A JAIL HEALTH PROGRAM AND THE OMAHA SYSTEM

by MARGIE KNAPPENBERGER, RN, MSN, Clinical Nurse Specialist, Corrections, Visiting Nurse Association of Omaha, Omaha, NE

Nursing service in the Sarpy County jail began in 1982 with the provision of care to a diabetic client. Prior to that, health-related services were provided by the jail deputy. Inmates had access to health care professionals in the emergency room of a local hospital or in doctors' offices. Since 1982, service delivery has expanded to provide a wide range of care for an inmate population that has risen from 44 to 136; the average daily population is 90 inmates.

The jail is located inside the Sarpy County Law Enforcement Center, which also houses the Sheriff's Department. It is located next to the county courthouse. Viewed as a community, the population groups served by the nurse include (1) inmates, (2) deputies (jail and road), (3) courthouse and sheriff office personnel, and (4) civilians in emergency situations. The group served primarily is the inmate population. Inmate subgroups include men, women, and juveniles who have committed adult crimes. Young adult males comprise the largest subgroup, although inmates range in age from 15 to 77.

Nursing responsibilities include developing the health care program and coordinating the health care of the inmate population. Advocacy and role development of the nurse are major activities. Service delivery is provided in a clinic, a classroom, and an inmate living area.

Positive health-related behaviors that include seeking preventive care have not been a priority of the inmate population at the Sarpy County Jail. Therefore, when incarcerated, some inmates have had many health problems. Sick-call priorities include (1) risk for suicide, (2) drug and alcohol abuse, (3) use of medications, (4) injuries and accidents in jail, (5) infectious diseases, (6) mental impairments, and (7) chronic health problems. In addition, priority is given to juveniles and US Immigration violators.

The majority of nursing activities are based on results of the inmate health assessment. Contact with a nurse begins when an inmate fills out a Health Questionnaire (Fig. 12–5). The form focuses primarily on the Physiological Domain of the Problem Classification Scheme. The purpose of the Health Questionnaire is twofold. One, its use allows a nurse more time during the interview to focus on priority health problems such as 39. Substance Misuse and 12. Emotional Stability. Usually, young adult males do not have many physiologic problems. Second, it provides a nonthreatening approach for questions about mental health (see Question 22:

Emotional). It has generated more revealing data than direct questioning had before.

The nurse reviews the Health Questionnaire with the inmate. The nurse then interviews the inmate using the Adult Data Base (Fig. 12–6). It is designed to identify (1) use of health care services prior to incarceration, (2) use of medications, (3) health behaviors and coping strategies, and (4) past health history. When a physical examination is completed, it is recorded on the Adult Data Base (see forms).

Client problems are determined from responses to the Health Questionnaire and entries in the Adult Data Base. Both forms are available in Spanish; they were translated by a VNA public health nurse, Rachel Dowd. The problems are recorded on the Inmate Profile. This document is kept in a notebook separate from the health record so that the Problem List is easily accessible. Problems identified by nursing not only drive the health care services for the inmate, but are also used in developing health classes, expanding service delivery, and obtaining health equipment.

A Progress Notes form provides a means for using a problem-oriented format (Fig. 12–7). A coding system at the bottom of the page is used to decrease recording time. It allows the nurse to refer to other forms or parts of forms without rewriting the same information. A category from the Intervention Scheme is used frequently on the Progress Notes; that category is HTGC—Health Teaching, Guidance, and Counseling.

The Omaha System has been adapted for documentation in a jail setting. The process of adapting the Omaha System and designing forms was accomplished despite time constraints and the quick turnover of the inmate population. After use in the jail health program, the problem Gambling Addiction was added. The purpose of using the two data base forms and the Problem Classification Scheme is to provide a systematic, concise, and easy method for identifying the inmate's priority problems, especially those that require nursing intervention.

The goal of the Jail Health Program is to improve or maintain optimal health. It is hoped that the promotion of health during incarceration will enhance an inmate's physical, mental, and social well-being and, possibly, prevent future incarceration.

Text continued on page 271

VISITING NURSE COMMUNITY HEALTH SERVICES

SARPY COUNTY LAW ENFORCEMENT CENTER
HEALTH SERVICES UNIT

HEALTH QUESTIONNAIRE

The Health Services Unit of the Sarpy County Law Enforcement Center wants to help you maintain or improve your health. Please complete this form about your health. Please print.

Name _____
      LAST   **FIRST**   **MIDDLE**

1. Do you have allergies (sensitivity) to any of the following? If so, please list.

                                      List   Kind of Reaction

Medicines   No _____ Yes _____ _____

Foods   No _____ Yes _____ _____

Clothing   No _____ Yes _____ _____

Pollens   No _____ Yes _____ _____

Other   No _____ Yes _____ _____

3. Are you on a special diet? No _____ Yes _____ If so, what type? _____

What do you eat in a normal day (outside of jail)?

Breakfast _____

Lunch _____

Dinner _____

Snacks _____

4. I use the following items: I have these items with me:

_____ None   _____ Glasses   _____

                                   _____ Contact Lenses _____

                                   _____ Dentures   _____

                                   _____ Artificial Limb _____

                                   _____ Brace   _____

                                   _____ Ostomy Equipment _____

                                   _____ Wheelchair   _____

                                   _____ Walker/Cane   _____

                                   _____ _____ _____

Explain _____

A

FIGURE 12–5 ■ (*A–D*) The Health Questionnaire was developed by the VNA of Omaha for the Sarpy County (NE) Law Enforcement Center.

5. Are you employed?   No _____ Yes _____

6. What is your job/occupation? _____

7. Marital Status?   Single _____ Married _____ Separated _____ Divorced _____ Widowed _____
   Other _____

8. What is the highest level of education you have completed? _____

9. Do you have health insurance?   No _____ Yes _____

   List _____

10. Do you have dental insurance?   No _____ Yes _____

   List _____

11. Are you active duty/retired/dependent military?   No _____ Yes _____
    If yes, please circle correct category.

12. Are you eligible for VA benefits?   No _____ Yes _____

Please place a check mark in the box next to each symptom or problem you are having. If you are having no problems, check no difficulty.

13. Breathing

_____ NO DIFFICULTY

_____ fever   _____ stuffy nose
_____ coughing   _____ difficulty breathing when lying down
_____ earache   _____ pain
_____ wheezing   _____ recent infection
_____ shortness of breath   _____ past infections
_____ sore throat

   Explain: _____
   _____
   Medications: _____

14. Circulation and Heart:

_____ NO DIFFICULTY

_____ palpitations   _____ swelling
_____ dizziness   _____ headache
_____ bruising   _____ fainting
_____ chest pain   _____ calf pain
_____ increased sweating

   Explain: _____
   _____
   Medications: _____

15. Stomach/bowels:

_____ NO DIFFICULTY

_____ nausea/vomiting   _____ constipation
_____ difficulty swallowing   _____ diarrhea
_____ indigestion   _____ pain
_____ bleeding   _____ change in habits
_____ heartburn   _____ hemorrhoids

   Explain: _____
   _____
   Medications: _____

B

FIGURE 12–5 *Continued*

16. Bladder/kidney

_____ NO DIFFICULTY

_____ trouble holding urine   _____ color change
_____ burning   _____ difficulty starting stream
_____ bloody urine   _____ pain/pressure
_____ frequent urination   _____ increased/decreased urination
_____ discharge

Explain: _____
_____

Medications: _____

17. Muscles/bones:

_____ NO DIFFICULTY

_____ cramping   _____ trouble moving
_____ aches/pains   _____ weakness
_____ swelling   _____ stiff/sore joints

Explain: _____
_____

Medications: _____

18. Reproductive: Female only

_____ NO DIFFICULTY

_____ bleeding   _____ change of life problem
_____ discharges   _____ pain
_____ blister/sores   _____ itching
_____ history of infections   _____ burning

At what age did you start menstruating? _____

Date of last menstrual period _____ (first day)   Menopause _____

Regular menstruations? _____ Irregular menstruations? _____ Any spotting? _____

How many pregnancies have you had? _____ Births _____ Stillborns _____ Abortions _____ Miscarriages _____

Are you pregnant now?   no _____ yes _____   Was it planned?   no _____ yes _____

Which birth control method do you use? _____

Explain: _____
_____

Medications: _____

19. Skin:

_____ NO DIFFICULTY

_____ sores   _____ temperature/color change
_____ dryness/cracking   _____ lumps
_____ excessive moisture   _____ changes in moles
_____ rash   _____ history of infections
_____ itching   (scabies, lice, ringworm)

Explain: _____
_____

Medications: _____

20. Nerves:

_____ NO DIFFICULTY

_____ numbness   _____ paralysis
_____ tingling   _____ poor coordination
_____ tremors   _____ forgetfulness
_____ seizures/convulsions

Explain: _____
_____

Medications: _____

C

FIGURE 12–5 *Continued*

21. Vision/Hearing/Speech:

_____ NO DIFFICULTY

_____ blurred/double vision
_____ light sensitivity
_____ difficulty seeing
_____ ringing in ears

_____ difficulty hearing
_____ difficulty speaking
_____ voice changes
_____ pain/pressure

Explain: _____

Medications: _____

22. Emotional:

_____ NO DIFFICULTY

_____ nervousness
_____ tension
_____ anxiety
_____ history of mental health hospitalizations

_____ depression
_____ irritability
_____ history of mental health problems

Many people experience abuse/violence in their relationships. Is anything like this happening in your life? no____ yes____

Do you use discipline in your home? no_____ yes _____

Explain: _____
_____
_____

Medications: _____

23. Anything else you want to add? _____
_____
_____
_____
_____
_____
_____

_____   _____
Date   Inmate Signature

                                    _____
                                    Community Health Nurse Signature

D

FIGURE 12–5 _Continued_

```
          VISITING NURSE COMMUNITY HEALTH SERVICES

          SARPY COUNTY LAW ENFORCEMENT CENTER
                 HEALTH SERVICES UNIT

                   ADULT DATA BASE

Name_____

Date Incarcerated _____    Birthdate _____ Age _____

Date of Release _____    First Incarceration:

Date of Initial Assessment _____      No _____   Yes _____

Dr. or Health Care Provider:                  Dentist:

     Name_____        Name_____

     Location/Phone_____        Location/Phone_____

     Last Contact_____        Last appointment_____

     Why_____        Condition_____
==================================================================================
Height    _____                                    Medications

Weight    _____         Kind              Amt/Frequency          How Long

Temp (F) _____         _____

Pulse     _____        _____

Resp.     _____        _____

B.P.      _____        _____

_____  _____         _____

_____  _____         _____
==================================================================================
Health Behaviors

Smoking:     No _____  _____pk/yr  Pipe - yes_____  Chew - yes_____  Cigar - yes_____

Coffee/Tea:  No _____     Cups _____/day     Soft Drink:  No _____   Glasses _____/day

Alcohol:     No _____     Drinks _____/day/wk/mo   Type _____

             Last Drink _____   History of DTs  No ___  Yes ___  _____

             _____

Drugs:       No _____   _____/day/wk/mo   Type _____

             Last Use _____   History of Withdrawal  No ___  Yes ___  _____

             _____

Sleep:       Hours/night _____    Naps _____   Problems getting to sleep _____

             Problems awakening at noc _____

Exercise:    _____/wk/mo x _____ min _____

Family History

HD_____       DM_____       Hypertension_____

CA_____       CVA_____       TB_____

Psychosocial

Coping Patterns_____

_____

Support Systems_____
```

A

FIGURE 12–6 ■ (*A and B*) The Adult Data Base developed by the VNA of Omaha for the Sarpy County Law Enforcement Center incorporates the Problem Classification Scheme.

Name_____   Page 2

ADULT DATA BASE

Chief Complaint:_____

_____

History of Present Illness:_____

_____

_____

_____

Past Health History:

Surgeries_____

_____

Hospitalizations_____

_____

Illnesses_____

_____

Injuries_____

_____

Physical Examination:

General Appearance_____

Skin_____

Ears_____

_____

Nose_____

Mouth/Throat_____

_____

Neck_____

Chest_____

Heart_____

Abodomen_____

_____

Back_____

_____

_____

Extremities/Functional Ability_____

_____

Genito-urinary_____

Neurological/Mental Status_____

_____

_____

_____
Community Health Nurse

B

FIGURE 12-6 *Continued*

VISITING NURSE COMMUNITY HEALTH SERVICES

SARPY COUNTY LAW ENFORCEMENT CENTER
HEALTH SERVICES UNIT

Progress Notes

Date   Progress Notes

8/89

KEY

1. See "Nurse Request Form"
2. See "Medical History"
3. See "Health Questionnaire"
4. See "Adult Data Base"
5. See "Injuries and Identification Marks"
6. See "Flow Sheet"
7. See "Inmate Profile: Medications/Treatments"
8. See "Inmate Profile: Nursing Care"
9. See "Inmate Profile: Lab/Diag Test/Surgery/Consultation"
10. See "Inmate Profile: Nursing Problems/Medical Problems"
11. Oriented to jail environment
12. Oriented to jail services
13. Return to clinic PRN
14. HTGC: Health Teaching, Guidance, and Counseling

FIGURE 12-7 ■ The Progress Notes developed by the VNA of Omaha for the Sarpy County Law Enforcement Center incorporate the Intervention Scheme.

THE MIGRANTS

As a target population, migrant and other seasonal farmworkers have limited access to organized health care, social services, and education programs. "The lives of migrant workers are difficult and dehumanizing. They have little or nothing to call their own, are uneducated, and are virtually powerless to make it otherwise, because most of their energies are directed toward the act of simply maintaining life, such as it is" (Geary & Crane, 1985, p. 506).

Migrant workers share many similarities to people who are homeless. Both aggregates face many of the same episodic and chronic health problems as well as barriers to care, often in relation to their poverty and powerlessness. Migrant workers, in addition, face grave risks and unique barriers. By definition, migrants are a mobile group. Even if they obtain adequate health services at one location, they will follow the stream or route soon, moving on to a new location. The vast majority of migrants are hispanic, usually of Mexican descent, and have limited English language skills. Thus, they must deal with language and cultural barriers. Living conditions at migrant worker camps increase their health risks. Often they have substandard facilities for shelter and sanitation. Migrant camps are usually geographically distant from a local community; rarely do migrants own any means of transportation. These fac-

tors increase a sense of isolation and the chance of violence among the migrant workers.

A migrant worker's health status is further comprised by a disproportionate number of occupational hazards. Frequent, serious injuries occur from (1) falls, (2) machinery accidents, (3) weightbearing and posture stresses, and (4) exposure to weather, pesticides, dust, pollen, insects, and animals (Freeman & Heinrich, 1981; Geary & Crane, 1985).

The migrant population presents serious challenges to community health nurses, challenges that involve practice as well as documentation. In the following section, Mary Jule Kulka describes community health nurses who are pioneering new roles in an Illinois migrant program. Such programs are possible because of nurses' innovation and dedication and the help of federal and state funding. Kulka and her staff have thoughtfully organized and scheduled their services to meet the health needs of the migrant workers. To help address the grave issue of continuity of care, they have developed both an English and a Spanish version of a client record system to fit their clients and setting. Furthermore, they share the record with the migrants during the period of service. When a migrant worker is ready to move on, nurses duplicate the client record, asking the worker to show the record to health care providers at the next site.

MIGRANT NURSING AND THE OMAHA SYSTEM*

by MARY JULE KULKA, RN, MS, Clinical Services Director, Nursing Assessment Referral Network, Illinois Migrant Council, Aurora, IL

The Illinois Migrant Health Project is a program of nurse-managed primary care services available to the migrant and seasonal farmworkers in Illinois. Our service population has changed very little over the last 18 years. Most farmworkers come to the state in family groups that include an average of four to five children. However, our outreach efforts over the last 2 years have identified an increasing number of single men who leave their families behind in Texas or Mexico. These farmworkers are the poorest members of the nation's workforce. In surveys conducted during 1986 and 1988, we found that over 94% of our population earned incomes below federal poverty guidelines. Virtually 100% of the population we serve is uninsured.

Limited resources force migrants to choose between economic necessity and their personal health needs.

Rather than jeopardize their job security by seeking early intervention, migrant workers often defer treatment until health problems have become critical. For many migrant

workers, our program offers their initial, and only, opportunity to obtain basic health services.

The Nursing Assessment and Referral Network (NARN), the core of the Illinois Migrant Health Project, involves the extensive use of registered nurses who provide direct care and case management services. Each of our six NARN sites is staffed on a seasonal schedule by a team comprised of a professional nurse or Regional Nursing Coordinator and a bilingual community health worker. Once the migrant or seasonal farmworkers are enrolled in our health project, the nurse begins to work with the clients through outreach visits to the camps or drop-in office visits. Services are available during daytime and evening hours. The nurse:

- Assesses episodic and chronic health problems
- Refers clients to local contracted physicians for medical care followup
- Conducts patient education
- Provides overall case management to assure quality and continuity of health care and linkages with needed social services

To facilitate these interventions and avoid duplicating efforts, our health care teams coordinate efforts and interact closely

*The Project is funded primarily by US DHHS Section 329, with additional funds received from other private and community sources.

with local health departments, community health centers, hospitals, and other migrant programs.

Continuity and quality of client care were of utmost priority in the process of developing the NARN system for primary care. We use a manual that includes all relevant clinical and administrative policies and procedures; our practice is guided by nursing care protocols and nonphysician supervision protocols that are revised on an annual basis. Since the health care team members function according to a "clinic without walls" outreach approach, it became necessary to develop a care plan that meets many different needs. Some of these needs are: (1) effective, culture-sensitive communication between a client and the health care team; (2) simplified documentation through use of an acceptable standard system; (3) an efficient and effective means of recording because of the large number of clients served; (4) clues for the nurse through a standard system of assessments and interventions; and (5) all essential information needed by various team members to provide health promotion and prevention services for the individual client.

Continuity of care is facilitated by giving each client a copy of the Individual Care Plan when they leave our geographic area (Fig. 12–8). The original remains in the client's chart. When the client returns at the start of the work season, a new Individual Care Plan is initiated. Furthermore, the care plan is translated into Spanish. Most clients speak and read only Spanish, so an English version does not promote healthy attitudes and self-care practices.

The Individual Health Care Plan has been revised three times since its conception and use at the beginning of the 1989 season. All of the health care teams have participated in these changes. Therefore, they feel a sense of ownership in its adoption. Our current Plan includes assessment areas, critical for adequate communication between clients and team members. Such areas are (1) language and literary skills, (2) family risk data, (3) client strengths and weak-

nesses, and (4) chronic disease data, especially concerning diabetes and hypertension. A client with chronic disease is one of the most difficult to track, so this last area is of particular concern.

The Individual Health Care Plan provides the baseline data to develop nursing diagnoses. The Omaha Problem Classification Scheme, developed by community health nurses, is used for this purpose. When reviewing nursing diagnostic systems, the Omaha System was the only one that matched the needs of our professional nurses to those of our migrant clients. Since, again, efficiency was needed, each professional nurse reviewed all of the 40 problems and identified those that were most relevant before we developed a master list used in the Care Plan.

A list of interventions was developed from the suggestions of each nurse. Another grid format was designed to facilitate charting. The targets of the Omaha Intervention Scheme are listed at the end of the Care Plan, helping health team members to document their services. Because the Intervention Scheme is new and unfamiliar, nurses have had some difficulty adjusting to it. They are not used to recording interventions in this manner; they are used to extensive narrative documentation. Before the influx of migrant workers began during the spring of 1990, inservices were scheduled to enhance the documentation of interventions to the best advantage. Thus, staff had the opportunity to practice their documentation skills and receive encouragement for their efforts.

Evaluation of the Individual Health Care Plan was completed during the fall of 1989. All of the health care team members, the professional nurses in particular, felt that the Plan was a great asset to both the clients and staff. They recognized that it enhances continuity and is very efficient. Precious nursing time is saved because we do not chart with narrative notes. Needless to say, it has been a successful implementation. Without the availability of the Omaha System, it would not have been possible. It has been important to have this standard system to promote quality and efficient client care.

Illinois Migrant Health Project
Individual Health Care Plan   19_____

ILLINOIS

Name _____ Area_____ Type of Work _____

Birth date _____ Current Medications:_____

Chronic Condition(s):_____   _____

MIGRANT HEALTH PROJECT

_____   _____
Language: English / Spanish
Literate: English / Spanish ___ non literate
Family: At risk members _____
        Family strengths _____
        Family weakness _____
        Others _____

Assessments: Dates											
Pulse											
Blood pressure											
Urine test											
Blood glucose											
Fasting/post-prandial											
Weight											
Thirst A or N											
Appetite											
Urination											
Visual changes											
Pain, headaches											
Other											
Initial											

A = abnormal
N = normal
↑ = increased
↓ = decreased

Nursing Diagnosis:

Environmental:	Resolved Date
Income – Deficit	
_____ uninsured health expense	
_____ inadequate money management	
_____ other	
Sanitation – Deficit	
_____ inadequate food storage	
_____ insects/rodents	
_____ inadequate laundry facilities	
_____ other –	
Residence Deficit	
_____ inadequate/crowded living space	
_____ other –	
Workplace Safety	
_____ pesticide hazard	
_____ fertilizer hazard	
_____ physical hazard	
_____ other –	

Physiological	Resolved Date
Deficit	
_____ Vision	
_____ Integument	
_____ Neuro-musculo-skeletal	
_____ Circulation BP	
_____ Genito-urinary function	
_____ other	
Health Related	
Nutrition	
_____ non-adherence to prescribed diet	
_____ weight is 10% more/less than average	
_____ other –	
Prescribed mediation regimen	
_____ deviates from prescribed dosage.	
_____ fails to obtain refills appropriately	
_____ other –	
Other	

See other side for interventions

Approved: 1989 Nurse Signature _____ Date_____
Revised: 1989

A

FIGURE 12–8 ■ (*A and B*) The Illinois Migrant Health Project Individual Health Care Plan incorporates the Problem Classification Scheme and the Intervention Scheme. (Courtesy of Illinois Migrant Council, Aurora, IL.)

Interventions:

Dates													
Diet teaching													
Medication compliances													
Obtains refills appropriately													
Proper dosage													
System for taking meds.													
Side effects of medications													
Exercise													
Future check-ups													
Risk factors													
Meal scheduling													
Weight													
Proper skin care													
Allay concerns of client/family													
Other													
Other													
Initial													

Goals: (As contracted with Client that includes by date _____)

Nurse Signature _____ Date_____

Client Signature _____ Date_____

Targets for Intervention Schemes

01.	Anatomy/physiology	33.	Medication administration
02.	Behavior modification	34.	Medication set-up
03.	Bladder care	35.	Mobility/exercise
04.	Bonding	36.	Nursing care, supplementary
05.	Bowel care	37.	Nutrition
06.	Bronchial hygiene	38.	Nutritionist
07.	Cardiac care	39.	Ostomy care
08.	Caretaking/parenting skills	40.	Other community resource
09.	Cast care	41.	Personal care
10.	Communication	42.	Positioning
11.	Coping skills	43.	Rehabilitation
12.	Day care/respite	44.	Relaxation/breathing techniques
13.	Discipline	45.	Rest/sleep
14.	Dressing change/wound care	46.	Safety
15.	Durable medical equipment	47.	Screening
16.	Education	48.	Sickness/injury care
17.	Employment	49.	Signs/symptoms - mental/emotional
18.	Environment	50.	Signs/symptoms - physical
19.	Exercises	51.	Skin care
20.	Family planning	52.	Social work/counseling
21.	Feeding procedures	53.	Specimen collection
22.	Finances	54.	Spiritual care
23.	Food	55.	Stimulation/nurturance
24.	Gait training	56.	Stress management
25.	Growth/development	57.	Substance use
26.	Homemaking	58.	Supplies
27.	Housing	59.	Support group
28.	Interaction	60.	Support system
29.	Lab findings	61.	Transportation
30.	Legal system	62.	Wellness
31.	Medical/dental care	63.	Other
32.	Medication action/side effects		

Revised 6/15/88

B

FIGURE 12-8 *Continued*

SUMMARY

Documentation is an important aspect of nursing practice in alternative delivery systems. In this chapter, community health nurses described their practice settings, target populations, nursing responsibilities, and use of the Omaha System. Some nurses used the entire Problem Classification Scheme, the Problem Rating Scale for Outcomes, and the Intervention Scheme. Others adapted portions of the Omaha System to fit their needs. The flexibility inherent in the Omaha System allowed nurses working in widely diverse alternative settings to develop useful client record systems.

Nurses in the nine settings indicated that they practiced with a holistic approach, expressing concern for the client as a individual, family, group, and community. Because of their comprehensive approach to clients, they developed documentation materials that reflected their practice. They wanted effective yet efficient methods of communicating the use of the nursing process. Thus, they each selected the Omaha System as a tool to help describe their practice to peers, other health care professionals, other human service providers, and the public.

REFERENCES

American Nurses' Association (1986a). *Standards of Community Health Nursing Practice.* Kansas City, MO.

American Nurses' Association (1986b). *Standards of Home Health Nursing Practice.* Kansas City, MO.

Berne, A., Dato, C., Mason, D., et al. (1990, Spring). A nursing model for addressing the health needs of homeless families. *Image*, 22:8–13.

Bremer, A. (1987, August). Revitalizing the district model for the delivery of prevention-focused community health nursing services. *Family Community Health*, 10:1–10.

Campbell, B. (1988, January). Program attunes students to population-focused care. *Nurs. Health Care*, 9:43–45.

Corrigan, M. (1986). [Evolving community health delivery systems with implications for community health nursing.] Unpublished data compiled from multiple sources.

Fenton, M., Rounds, L., & Iha, S. (1988, August). The nursing center in a rural community: The promotion of family and community health. *Family Community Health*, 11:14–24.

Ferguson, M. (1989, August). Psych nursing in a shelter for the homeless. *Am. J. Nurs.*, 89:1060–1062.

Francis, M. (1987, December). Long-term approaches to end homelessness. *Public Health Nurs.*, 4:230–235.

Freeman, R., & Heinrich, J. (1981). *Community Health Nursing Practice* (2nd ed.). Philadelphia, W. B. Saunders.

Geary, J., & Crane, J. (1985). Following the migrant stream. In Hall, J., & Weaver, B. (Eds.), *Distributive Nursing Practice: A Systems Approach to Community Health* (2nd ed.) (pp. 506–517). Philadelphia, J. B. Lippincott.

Goeppinger, J. (1988, December). Challenges in assessing the impact of nursing service: A community perspective. *Public Health Nurs.*, 5:241–245.

Gulotta, K. (1986–87, Spring/Summer). Factors affecting nursing practice in a correctional health care setting. *J. Prison & Jail Health*, 6(1):3–22.

Hays, B. (1990). *Relationships Among Nursing Care Requirements, Selected Patient Factors, Selected Nurse Factors, and Nursing Resource Consumption in Home Health Care.* Unpublished doctoral dissertation, Case Western Reserve University, Cleveland, OH.

Jamieson, M. (1989, October). Nursing our neighbors. *Am. J. Nurs.*, 89:1290–1291.

Lindsey, A. (1989, March/April). Health care for the homeless. *Nurs. Outlook*, 37:78–81.

Moses, E. (1990, March). [Survey of RN in U.S.] Personal communication regarding unpublished data.

Muff, J. (Ed.) (1982). *Socialization, Sexism, Stereotyping: Women's Issues in Nursing.* St. Louis, C. V. Mosby.

Mundt, M. (1988). An analysis of nurse recording in family health clinics of a county health department. *J. Community Health Nurs.*, 5(1):3–10.

Rafferty, M. (1989, December). Standing up for America's homeless. *Am. J. Nurs.*, 89:1614–1617.

Selleck, C., Sirles, A., & Sloan, R. (1988). The community health nurse as family nurse practitioner in primary/ambulatory care. In Stanhope, M., & Lancaster, J. (Eds.), *Community Health Nursing: Process and Practice for Promoting Health* (pp. 760–778). St. Louis, C. V. Mosby.

Thibodeau, J., & Hawkins, J. (1987, August). Evolution of a nursing center. *J. Ambulatory Care Manag.*, 10:30–39.

Ulin, P. (1989, May/June). Global collaboration in primary health care. *Nurs. Outlook*, 37:134–137.

Williams, C. (1977, April). Community health nursing: What is it? *Nurs. Outlook*, 25:250–254.

Williams, C. (1988). Population-focused practice: The basis of specialization in public health nursing. In Stanhope, M., & Lancaster, J. (Eds.), *Community Health Nursing: Process and Practice for Promoting Health* (pp. 292–303). St. Louis, C. V. Mosby.

Wilson, R., Patterson, M., & Alford, D. (1989, June). Services for maintaining independence. *J. Gerontol. Nurs.*, 15:31–37.

Young, C., & Gottke, S. (1985, May/June). Multiphasic health screening for the rural elderly. *Home Healthcare Nurse*, 3:41–46.

Zielstorff, R., Jette, A., & Barnett, G. (1990, December). Issues in designing an automated record system for clinical care and research. *Adv. Nurs. Sci.*, 13:75–88.

Zielstorff, R., Jette, A., Barnett G., et al. (1985). A COSTAR system for hospital-based coordination of long-term care for the elderly. In Ackerman, M. (Ed) *Proceeding Ninth Annual Symposium on Computer Applications in Medical Care* (pp. 17–21). New York: IEEE Press.

Zielstorff, R., Jette, A., Barnett G., et al. (1986a). A COSTAR-based multidisciplinary record system for long-term care practice and research. In Salamon, R., Blum, P., & Jorgensen, M. (Eds.), *Medinfo '86* (pp. 844–848). North Holland, Elsevier.

Zielstorff, R., Jette, A., Gillick, M., et al. (1986b). Functional assessment in an automated medical record system for coordination of long-term care. *Geriatr Rehab*, 1:43–57.

BIBLIOGRAPHY

Andersen, E., & McFarlane, J. (1988). *Community as Client: Application of the Nursing Process.* Philadelphia, J. B. Lippincott.

Archer, S., & Fleshman, R. (1978, November). Doing our own thing: Community health nurses in independent practice. *J. Nurs. Admin.*, 8:44–51.

Arlton, D., & Miercort, O. (1980, January). A nursing clinic: The challenge for student learning opportunities. *J. Nurs. Educ.*, 19:53–58.

Barger, S. (1985). Nursing centers: Here today, gone tomorrow? In McCloskey, J., & Grace, H. (Eds.), *Current Issues in Nursing* (2nd ed.) (pp. 752–760). Boston, Blackwell.

Bowdler, J. (1989, July). Health problems of the homeless in America. *Nurse Pract.*, 14:44–51.

Brickner, P., Scharer, L., Conanan, B., et al. (1985). *Health Care of Homeless People.* New York, Springer.

Buhler-Wilkerson, K. (1987, January/February). Left carrying the bag: Experiments in visiting nursing, 1877–1909. *Nurs. Res.*, 36:42–47.

Carr, E. (1982). A model for private practice: Requirements for success. In Muff, J. (Ed.), *Socialization, Sexism, Stereotyping: Women's Issues in Nursing* (pp. 413–423). St. Louis, C. V. Mosby.

Christy, T. (1970, March). Portrait of a leader: Lillian D. Wald. *Nurs. Outlook, 18:*50–54.

Crane, J. (1985). Springfield, Massachusetts: The sisters of providence health care for the homeless program. In Brickner, P., Scharer, L., Conanan, B., et al. (Eds.), *Health Care of Homeless People* (pp. 311–321). New York, Springer.

Damrosch, S., & Strasser, J. (1988). The homeless elderly in America. *J. Gerontol. Nurs., 14*(10):26–29.

Daugherty, L., & Buchanan, G. (1985). Nursing role in ambulatory care. In Jarvis, L. (Ed.), *Community Health Nursing: Keeping the Public Healthy* (2nd ed.) (pp. 263–275). Philadelphia, F. A. Davis.

del Bueno, D. (1985, May/June). Bandwagons, parades, and panaceas. *Nurs. Outlook, 33:*136–138.

DeMuth J. (1989, September). Patient teaching in the ambulatory setting. *Nurs. Clin. North Am., 24:*645–654.

Dolan, J., Fitzpatrick, M., & Herrmann, E. (1983). *Nursing in Society: A Historical Perspective* (15th ed.). Philadelphia, W. B. Saunders.

Donahue, M. (1985). *Nursing the Finest Art: An Illustrated History.* St. Louis, C. V. Mosby.

Felton, G., Kelly, H. Renehan, K., et al. (1985, November/December). Nursing entrepreneurs: A success story. *Nurs. Outlook, 33:*276–280.

Ford, L. (1982). Nurse practitioners: History of a new idea and predictions for the future. In Aiken, L., & Gortner, S. (Eds.), *Nursing in the 1980s: Crises, Opportunities, Challenges* (pp. 231–247). Philadelphia, J. B. Lippincott.

Freeman, R. (1974, November/December). Nurse practitioners in the community health agency. *J. Nurs. Admin., 4:*21–24.

Glascock, J., Webster-Stratton, C., & McCarthy, A. (1985, January/February). Infant and preschool well-child care: Master's- and nonmaster's-prepared pediatric nurse practitioners. *Nurs. Res., 34:*39–43.

Glassman, J., & DeVincenzo, D. (1984, Summer). Primary care nursing in a prison setting. *J. Prison & Jail Health, 1:*52–56.

Gresham-Kenton, L., & Wisby, M. (1987, August). Development and implementation of nurse-managed health programs: A problem-oriented approach. *J. Ambulatory Care Manag., 10:*20–29.

Hall, J., & Weaver, B. (1985). *Distributive Nursing Practice: A Systems Approach to Community Health* (2nd ed.). Philadelphia, J. B. Lippincott.

Hastings, C., & Muir-Nash, J. (1989, May/June). Validation of a taxonomy of ambulatory nursing practice. *Nurs. Econom., 7:*142–149.

Hastings, G., Vick, L., Lee, G., et al. (1980, July). Nurse practitioners in a jailhouse clinic. *Med. Care, 18:*731–744.

Hazard, M., & Kemp, R. (1983, April). Keeping the well-elderly well. *Am J. Nurs., 83:*567–570.

Jamieson, M. (1987, September). The St. Anthony Park block nurse program. *Am. J. Public Health, 77:*1227–1228.

Jamieson, M., Campbell, J., & Clarke, S. (1989). The block nurse program. *Gerontologist, 29*(1):124–127.

Jarvis, L. (Ed.) (1985). *Community Health Nursing: Keeping the Public Healthy* (2nd ed.). Philadelphia, F. A. Davis.

Kalisch, P., & Kalisch, B. (1986). *The Advance of American Nursing* (2nd ed.). Boston, Little, Brown.

Kark, S. (1981). *Community-oriented Primary Care.* New York, Appleton-Century-Crofts.

Kee, C. (1984, June). A case for health promotion with the elderly. *Nurs. Clin. North Am., 19:*251–262.

Kick, E. (1989, September). Patient teaching for elders. *Nurs. Clin. North Am., 24:*681–686.

Kinlein, M. (1977). *Independent Nursing Practice With Clients.* Philadelphia, J. B. Lippincott.

Knollmueller, R. (1989, October). Case management: What's in a name? *Nurs. Manag., 20:*38–42.

Kus, R. (1990). Nurses and unpopular clients. In McCloskey, J., & Grace, H. (Eds.), *Current Issues in Nursing* (3rd ed.) (pp. 554–558). St. Louis, C. V. Mosby.

Lenehan, G., McInnis, B., O'Donnell, D., et al. (1985, November). A nurses' clinic for the homeless. *Am. J. Nurs., 85:*1237–1240.

Lundeen, S. (1990). Nursing centers: Models for autonomous practice. In McCloskey, J., & Grace, H. (Eds.), *Current Issues in Nursing* (3rd ed.) (pp. 304–309). St. Louis, C. V. Mosby.

McDonald, D. (1986, June). Health care and cost containment for the homeless: Curricular implications. *J. Nurs. Educ., 25:*261–264.

McNeil, J., & Bergner, L. (1975, July/August). Use of mobile unit to provide health care for preschoolers in rural King county, Washington. *Public Health Rep., 90:*344–348.

Milio, N. (1970). *9226 Kercheval: The Storefront That Did Not Burn.* Ann Arbor, MI, University of Michigan Press.

Moccia, P. (1988). Occupational health. In Caliandro, G., & Judkins, B. (Eds.), *Primary Nursing Practice* (pp. 168–182). Glenview, IL, Scott, Foresman.

Pearson, L. (1988, April). Providing health care to the homeless— another important role for NPs. *Nurse Pract., 13:*38–48.

Rafferty, M. (1989, December). How nurses are helping the homeless. *Am. J. Nurs., 89:*1618–1619.

Rauschenbach, B., Frongillo, E., Thompson, F., et al. (1990, January). Dependency on soup kitchens in urban areas of New York state. *Am. J. Public Health, 80:*57–60.

Reilly, E., & McInnis, B. (1985). Boston, Massachusetts: The Pine Street Inn Nurses' Clinic and tuberculosis program. In Brickner, P., Scharer, L., Conanan, B., et al. (Eds.), *Health Care of Homeless People* (pp. 291–299). New York, Springer.

Reuler, J. (1989, August). Health care for the homeless in a national health program. *Am. J. Public Health, 78:*1033–1035.

Roberts, D., & Heinrich, J. (1985, October). Public health nursing comes of age. *Am J. Public Health, 75:*1162–1172.

Roemer, M. (1988, September). Resistance to innovation: The case of the community health center. *Am. J. Public Health, 78:*1234–1239.

Shapiro, S., & Shapiro, M. (1987, Spring). Identification of health care problems in a county jail. *J. Community Health, 12:*23–30.

Sheps, S., Schechter, M., & Prefontaine, R. (1987, Spring). Prison health services: A utilization study. *J. Community Health, 12:*4–22.

Silberstein, C. (1985). Nursing role in occupational health. In Jarvis, L. (Ed.), *Community Health Nursing: Keeping the Public Healthy* (2nd ed.) (pp. 263–275). Philadelphia, F. A. Davis.

Silberstein, C. (1988). The community health nurse in occupational health. In Stanhope, M., & Lancaster, J. (Eds.), *Community Health Nursing: Process and Practice for Promoting Health* (pp. 791–804). St. Louis, C. V. Mosby.

Slavinsky, A., & Cousins, A. (1982, June). Homeless women. *Nurs. Outlook, 30:*358–362.

Smith, G. (1989, March/April). Using the public agenda to shape PHN practice. *Nurs. Outlook, 37:*72–75.

Stewart, M., Innes, J., Searl, S., et al. (Eds.) (1985). *Community Health Nursing in Canada.* Toronto, Ontario, Gage.

Strasser, J. (1978, December). Urban transient women. *Am. J. Nurs., 78:*2076–2079.

Verran, J. (1981, May). Delineation of ambulatory care nursing practice. *J. Ambulatory Care Manag., 4:*1–13.

Walsh, L. (1988, April). Alternative health care delivery systems— nursing opportunity or threat? *Nurse Pract., 13:*56–64.

Widmer, A., & Martinson, I. (1989). Alternative systems and models of care. In Martinson, I., & Widmer, A. (Eds.), *Home Health Care Nursing* (pp. 25–34). Philadelphia, W. B. Saunders.

Wold, S. (Ed.) (1990). *Community Health Nursing: Issues and Topics.* Norwalk, CT, Appleton & Lange.

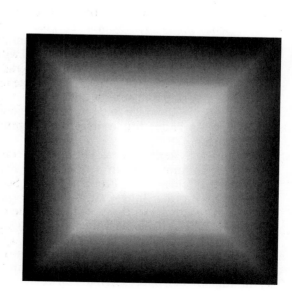

CHAPTER THIRTEEN

*I*t appears that the home health care nurse [community health nurse] of today and tomorrow not only must practice from the community health conceptual framework of prevention, health promotion, and risk reduction for clients, families, and groups, but must be technically skilled in direct care-giving activities and clinical judgment appropriate to the acuity levels of today's consumers. . . While the concepts can be taught in the classroom, the integration of these concepts in the graduates' practice functions and role can only be initiated through multiple, progressive practicum experiences throughout a program of study. This is imperative in both undergraduate and graduate level programs. (Cary, 1988, pp. 342–343)

The sense of change, growth, frustration, and excitement that community health nurses are experiencing is not limited to those employed in a practice setting. Undergraduate and graduate students and their faculty members are also encountering the evolution in community health nursing practice. Exposure to this evolution is inevitable whether students are (1) making home visits in a home health, public health, or combination agency; (2) providing services in an alternative delivery system; or (3) participating in a school nurse program (see Chapters 9 to 12).

Students begin a community health nursing course with a variety of biases and expectations. Frequently, their sentiments range from moderate intrigue, to discomfort, to fear (Cary, 1988; Lentz & Meyer, 1979; Magnan, 1989). Faculty members and agency staff hear or sense many of the students' preconceptions when they encounter statements like, "Community health nursing is a waste of time. I want to deal with sick people. I plan to work in a hospital when I graduate" (Tansey & Lentz, 1988, p. 174). The challenge for faculty and agency staff is to provide enthusiasm, support, and structure to encourage students to reconsider their preconceptions and attitudes regarding community health nursing.

The Omaha System serves as a bridge between acute care and community health settings. The Problem Classification Scheme, the Problem Rating Scale for Outcomes, and the Intervention Scheme provide structure for students as they begin a unique experience. Use of the Omaha System encourages clear and practical communication. Thus, it promotes unity between service and education, not separatism. As students develop confidence and skill with a community health nursing role, many learn to appreciate the chal-

lenges, independence, and leadership the role allows. Gaining competence using the Omaha System in documentation improves a student's transition to an employee role. That is especially true if a new graduate is employed in community health and confronts agency requirements for recording reimbursement-driven documentation.

NURSING EDUCATION ISSUES

The presence of students at the VNA of Omaha and other community health agencies has long been debated. "The placement of students in a home health care agency has the potential to both help and hinder the work of the agency" (Androwich & Andresen, 1988, p. 715). Likewise, students and faculty members who are associated with a community health agency will have both positive and negative experiences.

It is not expected that dilemmas associated with student affiliation will be resolved soon. Most public health and home health agencies, however, are facing financial constraints and diminishing flexibility in relation to referrals, numbers of visits, and length of involvement with individual clients, families, and groups. Simultaneously, nursing faculty members are recognizing the critical need to assign students to clients of varied educational, economic, social, and ethnic backgrounds and to introduce the concept of the client as an individual, family, group, or community. The merging of nursing practice and education is contingent upon positive clinical experiences for students (Stewart, Innes, Searl, et al., 1985). Only with adequate

Use in Nursing Education

exposure can students develop the skills they need for entry level practice in acute care, long-term care, or community health settings. These service and education dilemmas promote interest in collaboration; the exposure mutually benefits students, agencies, and the families of the community.

Specific issues pertinent to students and a community health service setting include:

- Grounding of practice skills—nursing students need to be involved with clients and professionals in order to develop competence, self-confidence, and independence. Progress along the novice-expert continuum requires experience in the service setting.
- Gap between theory and practice—students, faculty, and practitioners must recognize and increase their interdependence in order to benefit clients and enhance the emerging profession of nursing. Students and faculty bring new perspectives, knowledge, and enthusiasm to the agency. Staff nurses and supervisors functioning as expert community health nursing practitioners serve as important role models.
- Continuity of care—the needs of public health or home health clients are rarely identical to students' schedules. Faculty members and agency staff must work collaboratively to be responsive to clients and to ensure adequate communication among those involved in a specific client's care.
- Costs—students increase the pool of staff able to conduct home visits. Simultaneously, they consume agency resources in relation to staff time, space, and materials.

STUDENTS AND THE OMAHA SYSTEM

The VNA of Omaha has provided a clinical site for students for over 25 years. During those years, students were introduced to the practice of community health nursing in a traditional manner. They communicated with staff nurses about specific families, particularly at the beginning and end of their affiliation. Faculty members were responsible for supervising students as they planned, conducted, documented, and evaluated home visits. Students were expected to record visit data on progress notes and to update other areas of the record occasionally, but they were not responsible for the entire record. Students and their faculty advisors did not develop competence with the Problem Classification Scheme, the Problem Rating Scale for Outcomes, the Intervention Scheme, or the client record. One VNA staff member served as a liaison to the faculty and students, but specific questions about service or documentation were usually directed to any of the VNA supervisors.

VNA of Omaha administrators decided to modify and centralize the student program in 1988. The new program became known as the Student Learning Center. Within the Center, communication and supervision were simplified. Multiple contacts among students, faculty, staff, and supervisors were replaced by student, faculty, and coordinator contacts. Simultaneously, students became accountable for the entire client record that incorporated the three components of the Omaha System.

The amount of documentation for which a student is responsible does vary by agency and student program. As indicated above, students at the VNA of Omaha have been responsible for part or all of the client record.

A clinical record based on the Omaha System is beneficial for students regardless of their degree of responsibility. Students gain more understanding and skill, however, when they are given more responsibility. Ways in which the Omaha System can be used with students include:

- To introduce a method compatible with the conceptual framework that guides the college's program
- To demonstrate that the concepts of the nursing process have relevance and value for a service setting and that they do serve as a guide to clinical practice and documentation, thus decreasing the gap between theory and practice
- To introduce the world of community health nursing through a standard, easily understood system of client problems, nursing interventions, and client outcomes
- To demonstrate the community health nurse's autonomy in clinical practice and documentation
- To provide a framework for identifying pertinent nursing diagnoses in a community health setting
- To offer a method for evaluating client progress at a time when the health care system is becoming outcome-oriented
- To provide an efficient method of organizing the activities and services provided to clients
- To enhance student efficiency and productivity, thus increasing the cost benefits of students to the agency
- To enhance verbal and written communication among students, faculty, and agency staff, thus facilitating continuity of care
- To facilitate the transition from student to practitioner through exposure to clinical and documentation expectations similar to those of a staff nurse, thus facilitating progress along the novice-to-expert continuum described by Benner in 1984.

The descriptions written by Kay Bennett, Christine Merritt, and Virginia Aita focus on use of the Omaha System at the VNA of Omaha. Bennett, the VNA Student Coordinator, provides an overview of the student program, the schedule, and the client record orientation process. In collaboration with faculty, Bennett is responsible for (1) conducting orientation; (2) scheduling student-staff shared visits; (3) obtaining public health and home health client referrals; (4) supervising service and documentation; (5) providing advice about families, community resources, and other concerns; (6) conducting home visits when students are not available; (7) scheduling consultants and guest speakers to meet with students; and (8) serving as a liaison for group work sessions that focus on the community as the client.

Merritt and Aita write about their experiences as faculty members at University of Nebraska Medical Center and Bishop Clarkson College. Merritt describes her own orientation to the Omaha System and that of her students. She has identified strategies to assist students through the orientation process. Aita and her colleagues Mary Margaret Schaffner and Marlene Mahoney were among the first faculty members involved when the Student Learning Center was established. Aita outlines the schedule and steps they have developed to introduce the students to the interrelated principles of the nursing process, documentation, and the Omaha System.

VNA OF OMAHA STUDENT PROGRAM

by KAY BENNETT, RN, BSN, Student Learning Center Coordinator, Visiting Nurse Association of Omaha, Omaha, NE

The Student Learning Center Program is designed to introduce baccalaureate students who are associated with various colleges of nursing to the world of community health nursing. Using the Omaha System as a framework for practice and documentation has provided a means to implement the two purposes of the student program: (1) to establish and maintain a structure and support system within the VNA for clinical teaching of community health nursing at the baccalaureate level and (2) to provide community health nursing services for those individuals and families in the community for whom there is a need that can be met by a student. These clients otherwise do not meet the criteria for service from available funding sources (Visiting Nurse Association, 1989). I begin the students' orientation program with a brief overview of the organizational structure and various services of the VNA. The students view a videotape designed to describe the purpose and value of the VNA's client record as well as the components of the Omaha System. The videotape depicts the "why" of documentation. Each student receives a booklet that contains (1) introductory information on the Omaha System, (2) examples of each record form, and (3) directions for completing the record. Although the Omaha System may be new to students, faculty have introduced the nursing process and the concepts of nursing diagnosis, nursing interventions, and outcomes of care during previous classes.

The world of community health nursing is strange and even frightening to students whose experiences have been limited to acute care settings. Each student is assigned to accompany a staff nurse on one home visit in order to decrease student stress and anxiety. During the semester, the faculty members and I make additional shared visits as appropriate. I encourage students to read the client records before or after shared home visits. Students also talk to staff nurses about documentation. This plan helps students develop skills in identifying essential data and understanding the agency's documentation procedures. After one shared visit, students have a better grasp of agency practice and documentation expectations.

Another orientation session, scheduled at the end of the first week, focuses on the "how" of documentation. Students view a videotape of a simulated home visit and review a sample record and their instruction booklet. Discussion includes clinical practice and documentation expectations.

A large posterboard is kept in the student room throughout the semester. Each record form or section is mounted on the board, clearly labeled, and accompanied by instructions. This board provides a visual method of introducing each part of the record as well as the record as a whole. Some students prefer to learn about the client record as a total unit. Others feel overwhelmed by that approach, preferring to focus on only one section at a time.

Each student is expected to read a client record and discuss the family situation, visit plan, and anticipated documentation with a faculty member before making the first solo home visit. After the visit, the faculty member and I assist the student to document that visit. We repeat the process as needed. Being able to document nursing practice on unfamiliar client record forms is a challenge for students. When students develop skill and comfort in the community health setting, they gain a deep sense of achievement, satisfaction, and belonging.

Students have a caseload of three clients whose needs vary from preventive to therapeutic health care. Each student manages the caseload, a responsibility that includes (1) scheduling, planning, and conducting visits; (2) communicating with physicians and other community personnel; and (3) documenting family and service data. Due to the variety of clients, students are introduced to a wide range of community health nursing practices, community resources, and documentation requirements encountered by VNA staff nurses.

Faculty members and I review every client record at least three times during the semester. We evaluate the students' documentation skills, looking for evidence of clear, concise, and accurate entries on each record form. Through record review and discussion, we also determine if students understand the three components of the Omaha System and the nursing process. We give students encouragement and guidance concerning any deficits in specific areas of client records. For the most part, students view the VNA of Omaha record and the Omaha System as "necessary hazards" of their community health clinical experience. Toward the end of the semester, they become more comfortable about documentation; they are pleased with their own abilities to learn new skills, and they understand the benefits of the Omaha System.

Faculty members have met several times during the semester to review and revise the procedures for the student program. Record review, faculty evaluations, and student evaluations were valuable in revising record orientation plans, the record itself, and recording instructions. Subsequent revisions resulted in improvements for students as well as better understanding of the Omaha System by faculty. We are beginning to work on a utilization review plan that will include a schedule and procedures for conducting audits of all client records. The unique spirit of collaboration that exists within the student program promotes creativity, productivity, and high quality client services.

FACULTY AND THE COMMUNITY HEALTH NURSING EXPERIENCE

by CHRISTINE MERRITT, RN, MS, MPH, (formerly) Assistant Professor, University of Nebraska Medical Center College of Nursing, Omaha, NE

Faculty who use the Omaha System in conjunction with a student clinical practicum at the VNA of Omaha attend orientation sessions with new VNA staff nurses. The experience is both beneficial and humbling. Faculty gain a true appreciation of what students will experience as they repeat the same process, that of learning a new approach to the basic and familiar task of recording. Feeling disorganized, mentally "all thumbs," and somewhat overwhelmed is common for faculty and all students of the System. Such feelings should be expected. Faculty, staff, and students need to be encouraged at this point, to be told that what they feel is part of the process. In time, with practice using the Omaha System and through consultation with experienced staff, the System will become familiar and seem simple and logical. I, like other faculty members who initiated the new Student Learning Center, needed one semester to adjust to the VNA of Omaha student program, the client record, and the Omaha System. By the second semester, we felt very comfortable with our skills. In their evaluations, students reacted intuitively to our increasing sense of adequacy. The percentage of students who selected the most positive response to the evaluation statement "I understand the VNA clinical record" increased from 5% at the end of the first semester to 55% at the end of the second semester!

The Omaha System uses a problem-oriented format that is familiar to students. Any student, however, must restructure existing cognitive patterns relative to the component parts of both the Omaha System, a new concept, and their familiar recording style, a known concept. Whether the student is a professional nurse with many years of experience or a generic baccalaureate student, the issues are essentially the same. The papers look different and are labeled with unfamiliar headings, but the terminology is familiar. *Learning* each part of the System as an individual document is essential, but *thinking* of each part as a component piece of an integrated whole helps to minimize confusion and ease understanding and acceptance of why each one is necessary. The recurring complaint is that learning the System is "too much" but, viewed as a whole, it is easier to see that each piece has a separate and important function.

The data base comes first. It is a straightforward family systems assessment tool. All other parts of the record flow from this document. Priority problems identified in each of the four domains of the Problem Classification Scheme are transferred to the Problem Rating Scale for Outcomes form. Problems are rated and rerated periodically, usually two or even three times during the semester. Any changes or additions to the initial information gathered on the data base are reflected on the Data Base Update. The Family Visit Record or the Skilled Visit Report is the working document for recording. Both forms follow the "SOAP" format, with space allowed for subjective, objective, assessment, and plan data. On these forms, "S" and "O" data are recorded to specific client problems in the left-hand column. Nursing care is codified by category and target number in the center columns and may be elaborated upon in the right-hand intervention column. Overall assessment ("A") and specifics of the plan for the next visit ("P") are documented across the bottom of the page.

Specific sections of the VNA client record are directly related to the Problem Classification Scheme, the Problem Rating Scale for Outcomes, and the Intervention Scheme of the Omaha System. It is important that students understand the distinct purposes and organization of each section of the record and component of the Omaha System. It is equally important that they understand the relationships among all sections of the record and all components of the Omaha System. Each component of the Omaha System includes a numeric coding system. Some numbers are the same, but they must *not* be interchanged. For example, "3" could refer to a domain, problem, sign/symptom, problem rating, category, *or* target. It is necessary, therefore, to clarify the point of reference by using the correct words with their corresponding numbers in oral and written communication.

The Omaha System facilitates brevity and efficient use of nursing time on the task of documentation. It provides a structure for identifying essential information in relation to legal requirements, reimbursement, and quality assurance. No additional words, sentences, or paragraphs are required or necessary—a standard that is often difficult for students to accept. On inpatient units, many students are taught to record everything that takes place while the patient is in their care, including every item consumed from a meal tray. The faculty member needs to challenge students to make decisions about what is essential client record information in light of identified problems and established goals for each client. The development of documentation skills benefits students after graduation.

Faculty members can expect students to be confused at first. Feeling overwhelmed follows closely behind, and it is easy for students to become discouraged and even angry at this time. One-to-one faculty and student consultation is most helpful even though it is labor-intensive and exhausting for faculty. As students develop comfort and skill with community health nursing practice and documentation, they increase their competence in making independent nursing judgments. Faculty members need to remind students that the nurse who provides direct care is best prepared to make sound judgments, and the student is that nurse. Senior students have acquired the skills to make these judgments capably, but they may lack confidence in their own abilities. The community health nurse practicum is the time for students to blossom; many do so during the semester. Students mature quickly if faculty members ask for data, assessments, and rationale, following up with validation for correct decisions. Usually, two positive tutorial sessions give most students the knowledge and confidence to proceed on their own. By mid-term, students are sailing along and, from this point forward, faculty need only review and fine-tune completed documentation.

STUDENTS AND THE COMMUNITY HEALTH NURSING EXPERIENCE

by VIRGINIA AITA, RN, MSN, Instructor, Bishop Clarkson College of Nursing, Omaha, NE

Community health nursing students who participate in the Student Learning Center learn the process of documentation by using the VNA Omaha System. The key lies in matching the students' developing understanding of clinical experience to the format and content of the record. The advantage of this approach is that the students' experiences of working through the nursing process will be enhanced as each unit of the client record is completed. Because students are responsible for the entire VNA record, they actually apply the nursing process in a practice setting.

A standard orientation timetable emerged as Bishop Clarkson College faculty and students gained experience in establishing and maintaining client records. This three-step timetable became our guide to introducing the five units of the record (Table 13–1). It is important to remember that each student's response to clients and clinical practice varies. Therefore, the introduction of each unit of the record needs to be synchronized with a student's unique understanding of a client's situation.

Our students and those from other colleges of nursing begin the community health rotation with a 2-week theoretical orientation held at their college base. The VNA of Omaha orientation program begins the third week of the semester; this orientation was previously described by Bennett. With the first solo home visit, the student begins to use the home visit report form and document client services. Faculty mem-

TABLE 13–1 ■ Weeks of a Clinical Semester for Introducing Client Record Sections

WEEK 3 to 4
Referral form and client data/face sheet completed by the VNA intake staff
Home visit report form and interim notes

WEEK 5 to 6
Data Base/Problem List Worksheet or Data Base Update and Problem List Continuation
Initial Problem/Ratings/Plans

WEEK 15 to 16
Dismissal Problem Ratings/Plans and Transfer/Discharge Summary

bers and a Student Coordinator need to be available when students return from their home visits. They must guide students as they begin to synthesize their understanding of those visits with the nursing process, the Omaha System, and the client record instructions.

Students begin using an initial data base and problem list or a Data Base Update and Problem List Continuation about the fifth or sixth week of the semester. Students are encouraged to review the instruction booklet as they begin this portion of the client record. Usually, they spend 2 to 3 weeks collecting health status data and identifying problems concerning their client families. The Data Base/Problem List Worksheet is used to complete the initial data base and problem list. If a student is caring for a family with a data base initiated in the past, the student completes a Data Base Update, re-evaluates the problems, and completes the Prob-

lem List Continuation form. Concurrently, each Clarkson student prepares a family care plan; this course requirement is separate from the VNA record. The experience of identifying family problems for the VNA data base helps students complete the Clarkson care plan.

The second stage of documentation involves care planning in addition to problem identification. Each student is asked to review the entire client record and the Clarkson College care plan. Based on this review, students complete the Problem Rating/Plan unit. This unit of recording usually is accomplished easily. Students have already experienced the initial assessment, planning, and intervention stages of the nursing process and have made many visits to their clients' homes. Students are expected to refine their plans and interventions during the remaining weeks of the semester. They re-evaluate data specific to the Knowledge, Behavior, and Status ratings and modify ratings as appropriate. Students identify intervention strategies with clients to accomplish the goals identified on the Problem Rating/Plan form and the Clarkson care plan. By this time, faculty members usually observe that students have developed confidence with documentation.

Students complete the final stage of recording, the Transfer/Discharge Summary, about week 15 or 16. Simultaneously, students are expected to re-evaluate the Problem Ratings/Plans and the Clarkson College care plan goals. This terminal evaluation allows students to complete the nursing process, the three components of the Omaha System, and the record itself. Use of the client record system has enabled students to implement the nursing process. This is an important objective of the community health nursing course.

STUDENTS AND THE CLIENT RECORD

The Omaha System provides a tool to introduce undergraduate and graduate students to clinical practice and documentation in a community health setting. The format and instructions for the client record used in the Student Learning Center are patterned from those developed for the public health and home health programs (see Chapters 9 and 10). Such similarity is not required.

Many students do not view documentation as an essential component of nursing practice in any setting. An occasional faculty member will share this opinion. Community health nursing staff may need to remind students and faculty about agency policies and the critical nature of accurate, timely, and appropriate documentation. Students and faculty need to understand the ramifications of documentation for agency survival, whether students are participating in programs of public health, home health, long-term care, or alternative delivery systems. For example, the way a student documents services can produce financial or legal difficulties for agency personnel, whether the services are reimbursed by Medicare, Medicaid, a health department, private pay, *or* other sources. "At the student

level, a faculty member may request that students chart in depth on a family's psychosocial status. This may lead Medicare reviewers to believe that the patient is being primarily followed for nonreimbursable psychological problems versus an unstable physical condition. . . If visits are not documented correctly, however, denials for Medicare reimbursement may follow" (Androwich & Andresen, 1988, p. 716).

Students and faculty must become familiar with the client record and the complexities involving documentation at a specific clinical site. Records, policies, and expectations vary among community health agencies, but many similarities exist. "While nurses in other health care systems document because of legal and professional accountability, the home health care [*and* public health] nurse must also document in accordance with financial accountability consideration — that clients can continue to get needed services and that the agency will receive reimbursement for the service rendered to the client" (Cary, 1988, p. 343).

The establishment of a Student Learning Center with a coordinator, a standard client record, and documentation consultants has improved the quality of record-keeping by students at the VNA of Omaha. Faculty members from each college maintain autonomy and independence concerning other student assignments. For example, all faculty groups represented in this chapter require students to produce additional paperwork to fulfill course requirements. Creighton University faculty members Beth Furlong and Patricia Ehrhart made a conscious decision to eliminate care plans that were previously required of all community health nursing students, whether they were affiliated with the VNA of Omaha or other community agencies. They encourage students to demonstrate their knowledge of the nursing process by applying it directly to the client record. Forms completed by a Creighton University student depict a fictitious client and record. The name used for the client is Esther Earl, and the forms used are as follows:

A Student Learning Center record and instructions are included in the Appendix.

DIVERSE STUDENTS AND THE OMAHA SYSTEM

Faculty members of various schools and colleges have introduced associate degree, diploma, baccalaureate, and graduate students to the Omaha System.

Often, the introduction was incorporated into a traditional one-semester community health nursing course during which the student makes home visits to clients.

The Omaha System has been successfully introduced to students in other ways. Faculty members whose specialty is not community health nursing have presented the System during a unit involving the nursing process or nursing diagnosis. Community health faculty have introduced the Omaha System to individual students who are participating in an independent practicum or project. Some projects involve student-family encounters. Others include neighborhood or community assessment projects with the client defined as a group (Chambers, 1990).

Community health faculty work with many students who do not enter nursing education programs when they are 17 or 18 years of age. Often, the introduction of the Omaha System must be tailored to meet the needs of older students. For example, college graduates ranging from 22 to 50 years of age are students in an accelerated nursing program (Furlong & Ehrhart, 1990). The entire 8-week course is brief and intense. All concepts, including the Omaha System, must be introduced efficiently and effectively. The faculty maintains close, individual contact with students to determine their level of understanding and skill.

Mary Dooling describes the introduction of the Omaha System to baccalaureate completion students in a small collegiate program. Dooling outlines personality, age, and experience characteristics typical for her students. She incorporates those characteristics into methods she uses to present community health nursing and the Omaha System. She, too, has tailored her methods to complement her students' learning needs.

Text continued on page 297

For VNA Use Only	THE VISITING NURSE ASSOCIATION OF OMAHA	For VNA Use Only

Date: _10_ / _30_ / _89_ H/Hold #: _VNCHS 59241_ CT: _63_

Account #: _____ , _____

SS #: _485-50-0421_

VNAM _____ VNHR _____ VNCHS _✓_ Payment Discussed? Y ☐ N ☐ _Na_ Fax Y ☐ N ☒

Medicare #: _____

Source: (Name) _Dora Mueller, RN   VNAM_

Medicaid #: _____

Relationship: _____   Phone: _____

Ins _____ # _____

Previous VNA Record?: N ☐ Y ☒ _VNAM_ Date From _7_ / _24_ / _89_ to _10_ / _30_ / _89_

Other # _____

Rejected? ☐ on ___ / ___ / ___

Patient (Last Name First): _Earl, Esther_   Birth Date: _8_ / _14_ / _43_   Sex: M ☐ F ☒   Marital Status: S ☐ M ☐ W ☐ D ☒ Sep ☐

Street Address: _3221 North 52nd St_   City: _Omaha_   Zip: _68104_   Phone: _475-7749_

Spouse/Parent: _____   Birth Date: ___ / ___ / ___

Emergency Contact _Ann Johnson_   Relationship: _friend_   Phone: _432-9043_

Hospital: _____ from ___ / ___ / ___ to ___ / ___ / ___   SNF: from ___ / ___ / ___ to ___ / ___ / ___

Physician: _Brian Allen_   Address: _621 So 40th St._   Phone: _334-7220_

Physician: _____   Address: _____   Phone: _____

Primary Diagnosis: (Dates) _Pulmonary hypertension_

Secondary Diagnosis: (Dates) _Diabetes, COPD, Seizures, Ascites, Obesity_

Mental State:
Alert ☒   Depressed ☐
Forgetful ☐   Disoriented ☐
Other _____   Confused ☐

Functional Limits:
Mental ☐   Ambulation ☒
Speech ☐   Vision ☐
Other _____   Respiratory ☐
Hearing ☐

Range of Vital Signs and Lab:
BP _144/80_   P _88_   R _20_
Blood Sug. _____   Wt. _____

Lives Alone ☒   With Other ☐ _____   H & P Req: Y ☐ N ☐   Pharmacy _____

Significant Information: _SOB č exertion O₂ @ 2L cont. during day, 4L at HS per NC. Dismissed by VNAM as medically stable. Needs cont. assess. + monitoring. Tends to be non-compliant_

Service: Nursing ☒   Physical Therapy ☐   Speech Therapy ☐   Occupational Therapy ☐   Home Health Aide ☐

Medical Orders/Plan of Treatment: F.W.B. ☒   N.W.B. ☐   P.W.B. ☐ _____ %

Students to start NV this wk.
Frequency 1x/wk
to assess CVP, edema, med use;
health + safety teaching.

Activity Tolerance: _limited_
Diet: _low Na +_
Allergies: _NKA_
Meds/Dosage: _Dilantin 400mg po BID_
K-dur 20 meq ii po BID
Aldactone 25mg 4 tabs po tid
Diabeta 2.5mg ī po q̄ am
Theodur 200mg ii po BID
Lasix 80mg 4 tabs po q̄ am, 2 tabs q̄ noon
Lanoxin 0.25 ī po q̄ am
Medroxy progesterone ii tabs po tid
Ventolin 2-3 puffs q̄ 6 hr

Supplies: _____

M.D. Signature _____

R.N. Signature _Jean Lemphe, RN_

Additional Information on Attached Sheet: Y ☐ N ☒

FIGURE 13-1 ■ The Home Health Referral is the initial document used to gather data before client service is initiated.

```
--------------------------------------------------------------------------
                  PATIENT   INFORMATION   RECORD                    PAGE   1
--------------------------------------------------------------------------

Household #:   59241                        Station: VHCHS-NORTH
Address 1:   3221 NORTH 52ND STREET           Phone: 402 475-7749
Address 2:                              Census Tract:  63.00
City/St/Zip: OMAHA          NE 68104    Monthly Income:    360
Directions:  * STUDENT LEARNING CENTER.
Case Manager:

                      ACCOUNTS IN HOUSEHOLD
Patient's Name:             Account #:   Birth Date:    Rel. to HH:
EARL  *, ESTHER               59241     8/14/1943      HEAD OF HOUSEHOLD
--------------------------------------------------------------------------
--------------------------------------------------------------------------
Patient's Name:             Account #:
EARL  *, ESTHER               59241


** EMERGENCY INFORMATION      Relation:  Address:              Phone:
   JOHNSON, ANN               FRIEND                        402 432-9043

** ADMISSION INFORMATION
   Soc Sec #:    485-50-0421      Rel. to HH: HH- HEAD OF HOUSEHOLD
   Birth Date:    8/14/1943          Religion:  -
   Admit Date:    11/10/89      Referral Code: VNA
   Refer Date:    10/30/89          Program: 701 - STUDENT CENTER
   1st Contact:   11/10/89             Race:  -
   Care Started:  0/00/00              Sex: FEMALE
   Plan Establ.:  0/00/00      Marital Sts: DIVORCED
   Discharged:    0/00/00      Discharge Reason:
   Special Instructions:
   ICDA Diagnosis:


** DIAGNOSIS INFORMATION

** FUNDING SOURCES          Billing #:      Comment:          Effect Date:

** EMPLOYER -   /

** OTHER AGENCIES           Contact:              Phone:
   MD                       DR BRIAN ALLEN     402 334-7220


                                         Orders Cover
** PHYSICIAN INFORMATION                 From Date:  To Date:




--------------------------------------------------------------------------
```

FIGURE 13-2 ■ The Patient Information Record is a computer-generated facesheet that includes information obtained during the referral and admission process.

```
------------------------------------------------------------------------
              * * * D A T A   B A S E * * *                   PAGE    1
HOUSEHOLD #:    59241    3221 NORTH 52ND STREET    STATION- VHCHS-NORTH
------------------------------------------------------------------------
                        ACCOUNTS IN HOUSEHOLD
Patient's Name:            Account #:        From Date:
EARL  *, ESTHER              59241            7/24/89
------------------------------------------------------------------------

DATE ADMITTED:  07/24/89

ENVIRONMENTAL DOMAIN:  All areas assessed with significant findings as
follows:  INCOME:  Source:  Reluctant to disclose exact source.  States
doesn't have steady income, in appeal process for Medicaid.  Amount:
$360.  RESIDENCE:  Type:  Single level/own.

A:  MAIN DEFICIT REGARDING INCOME, OTHERWISE, NO OTHER EVIDENT
ENVIRONMENTAL DEFICITS AT THIS TIME.

PSYCHOSOCIAL DOMAIN:  All areas assessed with significant findings as
follows:  COMMUNICATION WITH COMMUNITY RESOURCES:  Transportation
Resources:  Waiting for son to get car; son's car being repaired.
SOCIAL CONTACT:  Support System:  Lady friends; close friend, Ann
Johnson.  EMOTIONAL STABILITY:  Death of mother and a friend during
past year.  Also financial problems.

A:  POTENTIAL PROBLEM IN REGARD TO EMOTIONAL STABILITY SECONDARY TO
RECENT DEATHS OF MOM AND A FRIEND, ALSO DUE TO FINANCIAL SITUATION.

PHYSIOLOGICAL DOMAIN:  All areas assessed with significant findings as
follows:  VISION:  Correction.  Glasses for distance.  DENTITION:
Correction:  Full set dentures.  CONSCIOUSNESS:  Alteration in oxygen
secondary to COPD, seizures.  NEURO-MUSCULO-SKELETAL FUNCTION:
Assistive Devices:  Walker, wheelchair.  History of seizure disorder.
Due to massive obesity, client most of day utilizes wheelchair.
RESPIRATION:  Rate 20.  Assistive Devices:  Home oxygen 2 liters per
nasal prongs.  COPD.  Dyspnea with activity.  CIRCULATION:  Temp 99.6.
BP sitting left 154/60, AP 86 and regular.  Hypertension.  Extreme
ascites secondary to corpulmonale.

A:  ALTERATION IN RESPIRATORY STATUS SECONDARY TO COPD.  ALTERATION IN
CIRCULATORY STATUS SECONDARY TO CORPULMONALE, MASSIVE OBESITY,
HYPERTENSION, LEADING TO DECREASED ENDURANCE.

HEALTH RELATED BEHAVIORS DOMAIN:  All areas assessed with significant
findings as follows:  NUTRITION:  Height 5 ft. 2 in., weight 230 lbs.
Diet:  2gm. sodium, restricted fluids 1500cc.  Diabetes mellitus.
HEALTH CARE SUPERVISION:  Emergency care plans:  911 or call friend.
PRESCRIBED MEDICATION REGIMEN:  Varies time of taking meds.  States
takes an extra "DILANTIN pill to keep from having seizures".

A:  RECEPTIVE TO TEACHING REGARDING HEALTH CARE AND SAFETY.  COMPLIANCE
WITH MED REGIME MAY BE QUESTIONABLE AND WITH DIET.

SIGNIFICANT PLANNING FACTORS:  Assessment of CVP, NMS, nutritional
status, med regime, and compliance.  Teaching regarding med actions and
side effects.  Monitor vital signs, s/s of exacerbation COPD,

------------------------------------------------------------------------
```

A

FIGURE 13-3 ■ (*A and B*) The Data Base is a computer-generated form developed from the Data Base/Problem List Worksheet.

```
---------------------------------------------------------------------
                    * * *  D A T A   B A S E  * * *           PAGE   2
HOUSEHOLD #:    59241     3221 NORTH 52ND STREET    STATION- VHCHS-NORTH
---------------------------------------------------------------------
```

management of ADL in home environment. Homebound Status: Decreased
endurance secondary to COPD, massive obesity.

HEALTH HISTORY: Significant Medical History of Client:

```
HOSPITALIZATIONS:                    PREGNANCIES:
Hospitalized approximately 5X        2 children (sons) 19 y/o & 20 y/o
 during past year, most recent
 7/19-7/23/89
```

Medical History of Client and Family Members:

ESTHER
Diabetes, Type II
Epilepsy
Hypertension
Respiratory Disease
Massive obesity

ASSESSMENT/COMMENTS: 44 Y/O WHITE FEMALE POST-HOSPITALIZATION 7/19/89
TO 7/23/89 FOR COPD, MASSIVE ASCITES, NON-INSULIN DEPENDENT DIABETIC,
SEIZURE DISORDER, EPISODES OCCURRING OF "PETITE MAL".

Iva Mueller, RN
                    Iva Mueller, RN/rip

B

FIGURE 13-3 *Continued*

```
          Visiting Nurse Community Health Services
                    Student Learning Center
---------------------------------------------------------
            D A T A   B A S E   U P D A T E
---------------------------------------------------------
```

Client Name _Carl, Esther_   Account # _59241_

Date	Initials	Domain	Data Base
11/17/91	SS	I	Income: now receiving medicaid.
		II	Emotional stability: depressed affect, talks alot
			about mother - deceased 1 yr ago.
		III	NMS function: seldom uses wc or walker, steadies
			self on furniture. No seizures for 4 mos.
			Circulation: 2+ pedal pitting edema bilat which
			slowly developed since 11/10. Ascites ↑ greatly since
			11/10 c̄ 12 # wt gain
		IV	Nutrition: poor compliance c̄ ↓ Na+ diet and
			fluid restrictions. Substance misuse: smokes
			apx 2 pks/day cigarettes. Turns off O₂ when
			smoking. ? safety. Prescribed med regimen:
			not taking diuretics as ordered, doesn't take at
			same time q day.

FIGURE 13–4 ■ The Data Base Update is used to document pertinent data obtained after the initial Data Base is completed.

```
                    Visiting Nurse Community Health Services
                          Student Learning Center
---------------------------------------------------------------------
* * * P R O B L E M   L I S T  (Actual, Potential, and Health Promotion) * * *
---------------------------------------------------------------------

Client Name  Earl, Esther                              Account #  59241
```

Date Identi-fied	Signa-ture	Problem (Name, Number, Modifier, and S/S[1])	Problem Change and Date[2]
11/17/89	Susan Stevens	12 Emotional stability: impairment	
		01 sadness 06 flat affect	
07/24/89	S Stevens	27 Neuro-musculo-skeletal function: impairment	
		03 decreased coordination/balance	
		08 gait/ambulation disturbance	
		09 difficulty managing ADLs	
07/24/89	S Stevens	28 Respiration: impairment	
		01 abnormal breath patterns	
		07 abnormal breath sounds	
07/24/89	S Stevens	29 Circulation	
		01 edema	
07/24/89	S Stevens	35 Nutrition: impairment	
		01 wt 10% more than average	
		04 exceeds established stand. for daily caloric intake	
		05 unbalanced diet	
11/17/89	S Stevens	39 Substance misuse: impairment	
		03 smokes	
7/24/89	S Stevens	42 Prescribed medication regimen: impairment	
		01 deviates from prescribed dosage/schedule	

---
[1] Copy problem information from Data Base/Problem List Worksheet. Name and number = write those of 40 problems which were identified. Modifier = write A (Actual), P (Potential), or HP (Health Promotion) as was identified for each problem. S/S = one or more must be recorded for an actual problem.

[2] To describe change, use Resolved for actual problems, Prevented for Health Promotion or Potential, or leave blank if record closed and problem still exists.

FIGURE 13–5 ■ The Problem List is an index of the client's health-related interests, concerns, and problems and is based on the Problem Classification Scheme.

```
                    Visiting Nurse Community Health Services
                             Student Learning Center
    ------------------------------------------------------------------
                  * * * P R O B L E M   R A T I N G S / P L A N S * * *
    ------------------------------------------------------------------

    Client Name  Earl, Esther                              Account #  59241

    Problem 29 Circ: imp.
    Date 11/17/89  Date          Date          Date          Date          Date
    (Initial      (Interim/      (Interim/     (Interim/     (Interim/     (Interim/
    Rating)       Dismissal)     Dismissal)    Dismissal)    Dismissal)    Dismissal)
    K  3          K  _____       K  _____      K  _____      K  _____      K  _____
    B  2          B  _____       B  _____      B  _____      B  _____      B  _____
    S  2          S  _____       S  _____      S  _____      S  _____      S  _____
    *  8 (wks)    ____ wks/      ____ wks/     ____ wks/     ____ wks/     ____ wks/
    months        months         months        months        months        months
    Susan Stevens
    Signature     Signature      Signature     Signature     Signature     Signature
    Plan & Date:
```

11/17/89 I HTGC: on cardiac care: elev. legs when sitting, avoid constricting
clothing 50: S/S physical: what/when to report to MO. III Cm: 31 med/dent
care: report to MO PRN IV Surv: 50 S/S physical: BP, VS, measure abd
+ ankles

```
    Problem 35 Nutrition: imp
    Date 11/17/89  Date          Date          Date          Date          Date
    (Initial      (Interim/      (Interim/     (Interim/     (Interim/     (Interim/
    Rating)       Dismissal)     Dismissal)    Dismissal)    Dismissal)    Dismissal)
    K  3          K  _____       K  _____      K  _____      K  _____      K  _____
    B  2          B  _____       B  _____      B  _____      B  _____      B  _____
    S  2          S  _____       S  _____      S  _____      S  _____      S  _____
    *  8 (wks)    ____ wks/      ____ wks/     ____ wks/     ____ wks/     ____ wks/
    months        months         months        months        months        months
    Susan Stevens
    Signature     Signature      Signature     Signature     Signature     Signature
    Plan & Date:
```

11/17/89 I HTGC: 37 nutrition: 2 Gm Na+ diet, restrict fluid oi anat/
physiol: rel of nut. pattern to S/S III Cm: 31 med/dent care: report to
MO PRN IV Surv: 37 nutrition: compliance c̄ prescribed diet

```
    ------------------------------------------------------------------
    KBS Numerical rating codes:   1=Poor  2=Fair  3=Average  4=Good  5=Excellent
    * Rerate scheduled
    Plan:  Use format from Intervention Scheme (i.e., 1 category:  1 or more
    targets:  client specific comments).
```

A

FIGURE 13–6 ■ (*A and B*) The Problem Ratings/Plans serves as a tool to develop and document problem-specific client ratings and plans associated with the Problem Rating Scale for Outcomes and the Intervention Scheme.

```
                    Visiting Nurse Community Health Services
                             Student Learning Center

         -----------------------------------------------------------------
                  * * * P R O B L E M   R A T I N G S / P L A N S * * *
         -----------------------------------------------------------------

         Client Name  Earl, Esther                        Account #  59241
         ================================================================
         Problem 39 Subst. misuse: imp
         Date 11/17/89  Date_____  Date_____  Date_____  Date_____  Date_____
         (Initial     (Interim/   (Interim/   (Interim/   (Interim/   (Interim/
         Rating)      Dismissal)  Dismissal)  Dismissal)  Dismissal)  Dismissal)
         K 3          K _____     K _____     K _____     K _____     K _____
         B 2          B _____     B _____     B _____     B _____     B _____
         S 3          S _____     S _____     S _____     S _____     S _____
         * 8 (wks)/       wks/        wks/        wks/        wks/        wks/
         months       months      months      months      months      months
         Susan Stevens
         Signature    Signature   Signature   Signature   Signature   Signature
         Plan & Date:
         11/17/89 I HTGC 01 anat/physiol.: s/s-physical-rel. between smoking/
         resp./cardiac status 02 behavior mod: techn. to ↓/stop smoking
         46 safety: O₂ precautions
```

```
         Problem 42 Pres med reg: imp
         Date 11/17/89  Date_____  Date_____  Date_____  Date_____  Date_____
         (Initial     (Interim/   (Interim/   (Interim/   (Interim/   (Interim/
         Rating)      Dismissal)  Dismissal)  Dismissal)  Dismissal)  Dismissal)
         K 2          K _____     K _____     K _____     K _____     K _____
         B 2          B _____     B _____     B _____     B _____     B _____
         S 2          S _____     S _____     S _____     S _____     S _____
         * 8 (wks)/       wks/        wks/        wks/        wks/        wks/
         months       months      months      months      months      months
         Susan Stevens
         Signature    Signature   Signature   Signature   Signature   Signature
         Plan & Date:
         11/17/89 I HTGC 32 med act ISE; 33 med adm: as pres. by MD
         III. CM 31 med/dent care report to MD PRN  IV Sur 33 med adm:
         compliance 50 s/s-phys: adverse rx
```

```
         KBS Numerical rating codes:  1=Poor  2=Fair  3=Average  4=Good  5=Excellent
         * Rerate scheduled
         Plan:  Use format from Intervention Scheme (i.e., 1 category:  1 or more
         targets:  client specific comments).
```

B

FIGURE 13–6 *Continued*

VISITING NURSE ASSOCIATION OF THE MIDLANDS SKILLED VISIT REPORT

H.H.# _59244_   Client Name _Earl, Esther_   Date _11/10/89_   Time _15_   a.m. (p.m.)   Unscheduled ( ) Explain

Homebound Due to _Obesity, SOB c̄ min exertion, requires O₂ cont._

CLIENT PROBLEMS (Circle #)

ENVIRONMENTAL: _Home uncluttered_

PSYCHOSOCIAL:

PHYSIOLOGICAL:

	SUBJECTIVE/OBJECTIVE	CAT	TARG	RX	INTERVENTIONS/COMMENTS
	See data base				
21. Speech and language:					
24. Pain:					
26. Integument:					
Lesion					
Depth					
Diameter					
Drainage					
27. Neuro-musculo-skeletal function:					
28. Respiration:	denies prod cough. Using	IV	50		
Rate _22_ Dyspnea	O₂ @ 2L per n/c				
Resting Activity					
Lung Sounds					
29. Circulation:	Abd. ascites - pt. states	IV	50		
Pulse _86_ _2t_	normal				
Apical Radial Pedal					
B/P _R 140/70_					
Lying _↓_ Sitting Standing					
Edema _↓ bilat pedal_					
Weight _231#_ Temp.					
30. Digestion-hydration:					
31. Bowel function:					
32. Genito-urinary function:					
Incontinent ( )					
(Other)					
HEALTH RELATED BEHAVIORS:					
35. Nutrition:	Drinking pepsi during HV	IV	37		Will keep food diary for 1 wk.
Intake _fruit - apple for lunch_					
38. Personal hygiene: HHA SUPERVISORY VISIT					
POC ( ) Appropriate ( ) Inappropriate					
41. Health care supervision					
MD Visit Date					
42. Prescribed med(s): Know Comply	States confused by meds. Doesn't	IV	33		
Yes/No Yes/No	always take @ same time. See				
Yes/No Yes/No	data base. Smoked 2 cig during				
43. Technical procedure:	HV. Turned off O₂ see data base	IV	57		Will approach issue of smoking when
(Other) _Substance abuse_					rapport estab.

Assessment _Needs health teaching re: meds, diet, safety issues of smoking ī O₂ use_

Plan: Frequency and Reason _RN 1 wk., complete assessment, initiate teaching_

Signature _Susan Stevens, CSRN_   RN   LPN   RPT   OTR   SP   MSS   Employee #

INTERVENTION SCHEME

CATEGORIES

I. Health Teaching, Guidance, and Counseling
II. Treatments and Procedures
III. Case Management
IV. Surveillance

TARGETS

01	Anatomy/physiology
02	Behavior modification
03	Bladder care
04	Bonding
05	Bowel Care
06	Bronchial hygiene
07	Cardiac care
08	Caretaking/parenting skills
09	Cast care
10	Communication
11	Coping skills
12	Daycare/respite
13	Discipline
14	Dressing change/wound care
15	Durable medical equipment
16	Education
17	Employment
18	Environment
19	Exercises
20	Family planning
21	Feeding procedures
22	Finances
23	Food
24	Gait training
25	Growth/development
26	Homemaking
27	Housing
28	Interaction
29	Lab findings
30	Legal system
31	Medical/dental care
32	Medication action/side effects
33	Medication administration
34	Medication set-up
35	Mobility/transfers
36	Nursing care, supplementary
37	Nutrition
38	Nutritionist
39	Ostomy care
40	Other community resource
41	Personal care
42	Positioning
43	Rehabilitation
44	Relaxation/breathing techniques
45	Rest/sleep
46	Safety
47	Screening
48	Sickness/injury care
49	Signs/symptoms-mental/emotional
50	Signs/symptoms-physical
51	Skin care
52	Social work/counseling
53	Specimen collection
54	Spiritual care
55	Stimulation/nurturance
56	Stress management
57	Substance use
58	Supplies
59	Support group
60	Support system
61	Transportation
62	Wellness
63	Other (specify)

FIGURE 13-7 ■ (A and B) The Skilled Visit Report is a problem-specific guide that incorporates the Intervention Scheme; it is used to document community health services that are actually provided during each home visit.

A

VISITING NURSE ASSOCIATION OF THE MIDLANDS SKILLED VISIT REPORT

H.H.# 59241   Client Name Earl, Esther   Date 4/17/89   Time 2:00   a.m. / p.m.   Unscheduled ( ) Explain

Homebound Due to Dyspnea w/ amb., on O₂ Cont.   Compromised CV status

CLIENT PROBLEMS (Circle #)

INTERVENTION SCHEME CATEGORIES

I. Health Teaching, Guidance, and Counseling
II. Treatments and Procedures
III. Case Management
IV. Surveillance

TARGETS

01 Anatomy/physiology
02 Behavior modification
03 Bladder care
04 Bonding
05 Bowel care
06 Bronchial hygiene
07 Cardiac care
08 Caretaking/parenting skills
09 Cast care
10 Communication
11 Coping skills
12 Daycare/respite
13 Discipline
14 Dressing change/wound care
15 Durable medical equipment
16 Education
17 Employment
18 Environment
19 Exercises
20 Family planning
21 Feeding procedures
22 Finances
23 Food
24 Gait training
25 Growth/development
26 Homemaking
27 Housing
28 Interaction
29 Lab findings
30 Legal system
31 Medical/dental care
32 Medication action/side effects
33 Medication administration
34 Medication set-up
35 Mobility/transfers
36 Nursing care, supplementary
37 Nutrition
38 Nutritionist
39 Ostomy care
40 Other community resource
41 Personal care
42 Positioning
43 Rehabilitation
44 Relaxation/breathing techniques
45 Rest/sleep
46 Safety
47 Screening
48 Sickness/injury care
49 Signs/symptoms-mental/emotional
50 Signs/symptoms-physical
51 Skin care
52 Social work/counseling
53 Specimen collection
54 Spiritual care
55 Stimulation/nurturance
56 Stress management
57 Substance use
58 Supplies
59 Support group
60 Support system
61 Transportation
62 Wellness
63 Other (specify)

CLIENT PROBLEMS	SUBJECTIVE/OBJECTIVE	CAT	TARG	RX	INTERVENTIONS/COMMENTS
ENVIRONMENTAL:					
PSYCHOSOCIAL: (12) Emotional stability	Bland affect. Talked about rel. c̄ mother—deceased 1 yr ago. (post that 20 yo son planning marriage—thinks he is too young	I	44		Allowed to vent feelings, active listening.
PHYSIOLOGICAL:					
21. Speech and language:					
24. Pain:					
26. Integument: Lesion Depth Diameter Drainage					
27. Neuro-musculo-skeletal function:	SOB c̄ walking. Doesn't like to walk. Use W.C. See data base				
28. Respiration: O₂ 0.24 p/m NC cont. Rate 22 Resting / Activity Lung Sounds clear					
(29) Circulation: Pulse 78 Apical / Radial R 163/70 Pedal B/P Lying 24 ankles Sitting / Standing Edema 2+ ankles Weight 243# Temp.	↑ edema in ankles ↑ ascites 2# wt↑. States has ↓ activity which has occurred ↑ in s/s ↓ wt	IV III	50 31		Will report s/s to md for fu
30. Digestion-hydration:					
31. Bowel function:					
32. Genito-urinary function: Incontinent ( ) ___ (Other) ___					
HEALTH RELATED BEHAVIORS:					
35. Nutrition: Intake	↓ appetite. Diff. c̄ fluid restriction	I	37		Reviewed food diary, disc. ↓ Na+ foods
38. Personal hygiene: HHA SUPERVISORY VISIT POC ( ) Appropriate ( ) Inappropriate					
41. Health care supervision MD Visit Date					
(42) Prescribed med(s): Know Comply Lasix Yes/No Yes/No Lanoxin Yes/No Yes/No	See data base	I	32 33		
43. Technical procedure: ___ (Other) ___					

Assessment ↑ s/s requiring medical fu. Interested in learning about diet, meds. S/s depression evident.

Plan: Frequency and Reason RV 1 wk to cont. assess + teaching. Report to md + od up appt.

Signature Susan Stevens, CSN7   RN   LPN   RPT   OTR   SP   MSS   Employee # ___

FIGURE 13-7 Continued

B

CLIENT FAMILY NAME *Earl, Esther*

HOUSEHOLD NUMBER *59241*

INTERIM NOTES

DATE

| 11/17/89 | TC to Dr. Brian Allen. Reported ↑ edema, ascites + wt. Made appt to see her in his office 11/19/89 at 10:30am   Susan Stevens CSN4 |
| 11/17/89 | tc to pt. to inform of MD appt. Says she will be able to go - will have friend Ann take her.   Susan Stevens CSN4 |

FIGURE 13–8 ■ The Interim Notes are used to document information generated through methods other than the home visit, such as (1) phone calls, (2) not home, not found visits, and (3) visits to hospitals and clinics.

Visiting Nurse Community Health Services
Student Learning Center

* * * D I S M I S S A L / T R A N S F E R   S U M M A R Y * * *

Client _Earl, Esther_   Date _12/7/89_

Nurse _Susan Stevens_   HH # _59241_

Date service began: _11/10/89_

Number of visits: _4_

Status of client/family when care began and at discharge:
11/10 Wt. 231# , BP 140/70 , RP 86, R 22. LS diminished, dyspnea c̄ activity. On O₂
@ 2L   1+ pedal edema LEs bilat. Noncompliant c̄ diet, meds, smoking.
12/7 Wt 252# , BP 150/70 , RP 84, R 22 Cont. O₂ 2+ pedal edema bilat. More
compliant c̄ diet, meds

Type of services provided:
Surveillance s/s
Referral to md for fu due to wt gain & increased pedal edema. Appt 11/19.
Teaching re: diet, meds, cardiac precautions, O₂ safety

Other agencies/resources contacted:
1. MD
2. Mobile Meals

Disposition/Transfer Plan:
Receptive to cont'd NVs. Because of poor follow through
c̄ diet, highly suggest client continue to be followed.

FIGURE 13–9 ■ The Dismissal/Transfer Summary reflects the number of home visits and types of community health services provided to a client; a copy of the form is mailed to the source of referral as a method of communicating appreciation and indicating client progress.

EXPERIENCES WITH BACCALAUREATE COMPLETION STUDENTS

by MARY DOOLING, RN, MSN, Instructor, University of Missouri–St. Louis School of Nursing, St. Louis, MO

I teach Community Health Nursing in a baccalaureate completion program at the University of Missouri – St. Louis. Community health nursing is a required course offered during the senior year. My students are a varied group and are graduates of 2-year associate degree and 3-year diploma programs. Their nursing experience ranges from a few to 25 years. Their current practice specialties include psychiatric, geriatric, pediatric, obstetric, medical-surgical, critical care, and, occasionally, home health nursing.

During the course, each student cares for one family in the community. Families are referred by a variety of agencies, which include (1) day care for the elderly, (2) church groups, (3) referrals by other faculty members, (4) hospitalized patients the students have cared for while at work, and (5) various community agencies such as the Multiple Sclerosis or Arthritis Societies. One faculty member coordinates a grant to provide services to pregnant teens and refers a large number of eligible families.

The majority of our students work full-time as RNs while carrying full academic loads. The philosophy, goals, and mission statements of the program support adult learners. Our philosophy emphasizes immediate application of classroom learning and recognizes that students fulfill many roles, the student role being only one.

Students usually have had no prior experience in community health nursing and no theory related to it, because most perform clinical practice in acute care settings. Not surprisingly, they appear anxious and uncomfortable during the first several weeks of the course. Most students have never considered community health nursing as an employment option.

Students follow one family from the eighth week to the sixteenth week of a 16-week semester. Because students accept referrals from a variety of agencies, they need an extensive orientation before caring for their families. They also take a course in family nursing care while enrolled in the community health nursing course. This course is another valuable component of the orientation process.

During orientation, students perform role play to rehearse the differences between a helping and a social relationship.

Contracting with families is also demonstrated. As community health nursing faculty, we participate with students in an exercise designed to show them how subtly a negative, judgmental attitude can convey a sense of hopelessness to clients.

Students are introduced to one component of the Omaha System, the Problem Classification Scheme, during this portion of the course. I emphasize the Environmental, Psychosocial, and Health Related Behaviors Domains. Students are less familiar with these three domains when they start their community practice. However, they begin to gain self-confidence quickly as they come to recognize the conceptual simplicity and concreteness of the Problem Classification Scheme.

Students are given a sample record and then asked to document services they provided and their families' responses after each home visit. Our emphasis is on patient teaching and preventive health measures, because many students need to develop skills in these areas. Their initial reaction is often, "But I'm not doing anything for the family." This reaction disappears, however, as they learn to focus on relationship-building, teaching, guidance, and helping families to help themselves. One of our primary goals is to help students develop expertise as advocates for families in need of resources. In addition, we want students to help families identify and focus on health-related concerns. Frequently, students are amazed at how much they can accomplish in these two areas.

As I have worked with students who are registered nurses, especially those who have years of experience in acute care settings, I have found that they need very concrete orientation to community health nursing practice. Introducing the students to the Problem Classification Scheme, giving them a chance to apply it, and providing for faculty feedback are three essential parts of their orientation process. Students are not used to considering lifestyle and environment as factors that might affect health care for a family. The Problem Classification Scheme has become an important part of my community health nursing course.

STUDENTS, A CLINIC, AND THE OMAHA SYSTEM

Community health nursing practice has been highly valued and visible in Canada probably more than in the US (Stewart, Innes, Searl, et al., 1985). Because of this tradition, community health is a very important focus of the nursing program at the University of New Brunswick, Canada. Faculty and students established a nurse-managed screening clinic as a community service as well as a setting in which senior nursing students learn the expanded role of a nurse. The clinic is similar to those described by Bataillon in Chapter 12.

Faculty members recognized the need for a structured documentation system when they established the clinic. They wanted to use a nursing model as the basis for the client record. In 1983, the faculty members selected the Problem Classification Scheme as the framework for recording client services in the clinic and for home visits. At present, the value of implementing the total Omaha System is being evaluated by the faculty.

NURSING STUDENT–MANAGED SCREENING CLINIC

by VALERIE GILBEY, BN, RN, BEd, MSc, Associate Professor, Faculty of Nursing, University
of New Brunswick, Fredericton, New Brunswick, Canada; and SHIRLEY ALCOE, BA, RN, BEd,
MA, MEd, EdD, Professor, Faculty of Nursing, University of New Brunswick, Fredericton,
New Brunswick, Canada

The curriculum developed by the faculty of nursing at The University of New Brunswick has a major community health emphasis. One goal is to prepare graduates to function in a primary health care setting. Since 1980, senior students in the basic program have been acquiring experience in an adult screening clinic conducted under the auspices of the faculty.

To prepare for the actual experience, nursing students are divided into pairs and are given the opportunity to develop their skills through simulating the entire assessment process. The assessment measures include a health history, Health Hazard Appraisal (HHA), height and weight, blood pressure, Fit Kit (fitness/exercise test), hemoglobin, urinalysis, and vision and hearing tests. Each student works with a peer as a client to complete an assessment and identify areas of concern based on the Omaha Problem Classification Scheme. If the peer-client wishes to undertake changes, an attempt is made to set realistic goals. The student (1) discusses all test results with the peer-client, (2) considers the implications of the identified health risks, and (3) suggests strategies for change. Relevant health information is provided, along with counseling regarding health problems and risks. At the conclusion of this experience, the student presents a record to the instructor that contains a completed health history and assessment. Most students identify problems with the modifier Health Promotion or Potential Impairment, although the modifier Actual Impairment is used occasionally. Short- and long-term goals and nursing approaches are established and progress notes recorded. Written feedback is given by the instructor, but no grade is given. In addition, students may choose to discuss concerns with their instructors.

The nursing student's next assignment is to work with an adult from the community who has responded to an invitation to visit the screening clinic. Initial attendance at the clinic takes place through three scheduled visits over a 6-week period. Clients frequently return for reassessment visits in the following year. The assessment measures and the actions taken at subsequent reassessment visits focus on the basis of the initial assessment and the client's presenting need at the time of followup. The nursing student who has a returning client uses the Problem Classification Scheme as a means of standardizing the language in the client's record. The nurse is able to reassess previously identified concerns, determine the client's present status, and assess any new problems. This standard language facilitates understanding for all students and faculty who use the record.

The Problem Classification Scheme is used by students in family home visit experiences as well as in the Screening Clinic. Several nursing students may be involved with a multiproblem family over a period of years. The students and faculty members find that the Problem Classification Scheme facilitates understanding of clients' nursing needs and ensures continuity.

Furthermore, the Problem Classification Scheme lends itself to research in that presenting problems can be sorted and classified easily. Currently, a study is underway to determine the nature of problems identified in well adults attending the Screening Clinic and the impact of the experience on health behaviors.

SUMMARY

The Omaha System offers a variety of benefits for students as they are introduced to community health clinical practice and documentation. A community health setting is a particular challenge to faculty because it differs markedly from the more individually focused, procedure-oriented, structured environment of acute care settings. In contrast, a community health nursing student is expected to develop a holistic approach to clients, whether they are individuals or a family, group, or community. In addition, a student is expected to synthesize data from environmental, psychosocial, physiological, and health-related behaviors information.

The Omaha System provides a student with a systematic way to record client data. Several approaches
to assist students in developing and refining documentation skills were described in this chapter. The Student Learning Center at the VNA of Omaha was described by Bennett, Aita, and Merritt. Their students represent several baccalaureate programs. Dooling outlined her program with baccalaureate completion students in another community. In contrast to the student-client encounters in home visit programs, Gilbey and Alcoe describe their experience with a nursing student-managed screening clinic. Their students use the Omaha System to collect and document client data obtained during clinic visits.

Faculty members in diverse settings have identified benefits of the Omaha System. Typically, they cite favorable results when the System is used for orientation, data collection, and documentation. One additional benefit of the Omaha System involves data management and research. Gilbey and Alcoe are collecting data on the client population served by their nursing student-managed clinic, and they plan to analyze those data. Just as aggregate data can be valuable to staff and administrators employed in community health agencies or schools, aggregate data collected by students can be useful to students and faculty. Such data, used in relation to quality assurance issues, can be used to examine the effectiveness of nursing care provided by students. Furthermore, financial issues such as cost benefits and productivity of students who use the Omaha System can be explored.

REFERENCES

Androwich, I. & Andresen, P. (1988). Student programs. In Harris, M. (Ed.), *Home Health Administration* (pp. 715–736). Owings Mills, MD, Rynd Communications.

Cary, A. (1988, June). Preparation for professional practice: What do we need? *Nurs. Clin. North Am., 23*:341–351.

Chambers, B. (1990, May). [Graduate student experiences with the Omaha system.] Personal communication regarding unpublished data.

Furlong, E., & Ehrhart, P. (1990, April). [Accelerated student experiences with the Omaha system.] Personal communication regarding unpublished data.

Lentz, J., & Meyer, E. (1979, September). The dirty house. *Nurs. Outlook, 27*:590–593.

Magnan, M. (1989, February). Listening with care. *Am. J. Nurs., 89*:219–221.

Stewart, M., Innes, J., Searl, S., et al. (Eds.) (1985). *Community Health Nursing in Canada.* Toronto, Ontario, Gage.

Tansey, E., & Lentz, J. (1988, July/August). Generalists in a specialized profession. *Nurs. Outlook, 36*:174–178.

Visiting Nurse Association (VNA) (1989, Fall). [*Policies Related to Student Learning Center.*] Unpublished report.

BIBLIOGRAPHY

Aydelotte, M. (1985). Approaches to conjoining nursing education and practice. In McCloskey J., & Grace, H. (Eds.), *Current Issues in Nursing* (2nd ed.) (pp. 288–313). Boston, Blackwell.

Benner, P. (1984). *From Novice to Expert.* Menlo Park, CA, Addison-Wesley.

Blakney, J., & Chandler, V. (1988, May). Expanded student participation: A response to tighter regulations. *Caring, 7*:36–37.

Blank, J., & McElmurry, B. (1988). A paradigm for baccalaureate public health nursing education. *Public Health Nurs., 5*(3): 153–159.

Deiman, P., Jones, D., & Davis, J. (1988, September/October). BSN education and PHN practice: Good fit or mismatch? *Nurs. Outlook, 36*:231–233.

Figge, E., & Parker-Etter, S. (1985). The home health agency: A case management approach to client care. In Hall, J., & Weaver, B. (Eds.), *Distributive Nursing Practice: A Systems Approach to Community Health* (2nd ed.) (pp. 464–472). Philadelphia, J. B. Lippincott.

Firlit, S. (1985). Nursing theory and nursing practice: Separate or linked? In McCloskey, J., & Grace, H. (Eds.), *Current Issues in Nursing* (2nd ed.) (pp. 6–19). Boston, Blackwell.

Flynn, B., Ray, D., & Selmanoff, E. (1987). Preparation of community health nursing leaders for social action. *Int. J. Nurs. Stud., 24*(3):239–248.

Foyt, M. (1989, June). Dear graduate nurse. *Am. J. Nurs., 89*:816–817.

Harris, M. (1984, November/December). Student programs benefit nursing service agencies. *Home Healthcare Nurse, 2*:34–35.

Lewis, J., & Glover, L. (1987, January). Joint efforts between education and the community. *J. Gerontol. Nurs., 13*:23–26.

Lundeen, S. (1990). Nursing centers: Models for autonomous practice. In McCloskey, J., & Grace, H. (Eds.), *Current Issues in Nursing* (3rd ed.) (pp. 304–309). St. Louis, C. V. Mosby.

MacAvoy, S. (1989). Continuing education in nursing diagnosis: Issues, strategies, and trends. In Carroll-Johnson, R. (Ed.), *Classification of Nursing Diagnoses: Proceedings of the Eighth Conference* (pp. 67–72). St. Louis, C. V. Mosby.

Mallison, M. (Ed.) (1989, September). Case Western leads revival of onsite clinical training. *Am. J. Nurs., 89*:1224, 1231.

Morrissey-Ross, M. (1988, June). Documentation: If you haven't written it, you haven't done it. *Nurs. Clin. North Am., 23*: 363–371.

Rajek, N. (1987, May). Developing an evening clinical experience for baccalaureate community health nursing students. *J. Nurs. Educ., 26*:197–200.

Rossi, L. (1989). Nursing diagnosis education in practice settings. In Carroll–Johnson, R. (Ed.), *Classification of Nursing Diagnoses: Proceedings of the Eighth Conference* (pp. 63–66). St. Louis, C. V. Mosby.

Secretary's Commission on Nursing (1988a, December). *Secretary's Commission on Nursing: Final Report,* Vol. I. Washington, DC, DHHS.

Secretary's Commission on Nursing (1988b, December). *Secretary's Commission on Nursing: Support Studies & Background Information,* Vol. II. Washington, DC, DHHS.

Smith, S. (1981, October). Sound off!: 'Oremization,' the curse of nursing. *RN, 44*:83.

Stein, K., Friedman, M., Eigisti, D., et al. (1987, April). Evaluating the use of a data base system with community health nursing students. *J. Nurs. Educ., 26*:162–163.

Thobaben, M., & Bohannan, J. (1990, March/April). Home health nursing: The relationship between education and practice. *Home Healthcare Nurse, 8*:49–52.

Wilson, J., & Brown, S. (1986, November/December). Nurse-owned agency offers management training for nursing students. *Home Healthcare Nurse, 4*:23–35.

CHAPTER FOURTEEN

*A*s we review the history of the attempts to assess the quality of health care, there seems to be a very clear message for nursing. The public is demanding accountability with documented evidence that the health care to which they are entitled is available, accessible, and cost-effective and that it produces the desired outcomes. The structures in which the care is delivered, the practitioners by whom it is delivered, and the process by which it is delivered will all be parts of the outcome evaluation by the consumer. (Walton, 1975, p. 31)

Increasing attention is being directed toward evaluating the quality of care provided in home and community settings. This attention is related to a variety of factors. First, the acuity level of client illness outside the hospital is escalating, making high quality care crucial. The rising acuity is related to efforts by the private business community and by the federal and state governments to control the rising costs of hospital-based health care. These efforts have had a major effect on hospital admission rates as well as lengths of stay. Increasingly, hospitals are used only when care cannot be provided in other settings, resulting in the development of the "sicker and quicker" phenomenon. Patients are more acutely ill when they enter hospitals and are dismissed sooner, returning home with care and treatment requirements that were considered highly technical, at the cutting edge of hospital treatment, just a few years ago (Sovie, 1987). The technologic advances in care available to clients in some hospitals and community settings have precipitated new, complex ethical issues. Further, state and local governments have begun to focus attention on preventive services. But despite these efforts, the AIDS epidemic, the increase in the homeless population, and the escalating use of illegal drugs are precluding easy solutions. These public health problems are straining monetary and human resources.

A second factor fostering quality assurance scrutiny involves negative publicity about community health care. Such publicity was generated by testimony during hearings of the House Select Committee on Aging. Quality of care in the home was compared by the American Bar Association (1986) to a black box, an unknown entity. Although there has been negative publicity about care provided by home care paraprofessionals, monitoring all home health care personnel and services is difficult. The Committee report identified four variables that limit standardization of quality assurance measures for home health care. These include the rapid growth and change of the industry, the diversity of agency types, lack of standard service definitions, and fragmented funding leading to fragmented services.

The third concern relates to greater reimbursement restrictions being imposed on community health nursing agencies by Medicare, other third-party payors, and state and local governments. These restrictions were described in Chapters 2 and 10. Between 1983 and 1985 there was a 38% increase in the number of patients discharged from hospitals into home care services. During the same period, the number of Medicare home health claims that were denied increased from 1.5% to 10%, and the average number of visits per patient decreased from 26 to 12 (Halamandaris, 1988). Concurrently, state and local elected officials have begun to ask public health agencies to justify the costs of service provided by their staffs. There is an increasing focus on the outcomes of care. In some cases, budget cuts have led to decreases in number of staff positions and clients served. There is a danger that the health care system is increasingly being driven by reimbursement regulations, creating a danger that clients may go without necessary community health care. Current regulations dictate that an agency must prove not only that the staff are providing high quality care, but that the care provided is worth the cost (Buck, 1988). Just as concern about cost was the dominant health care industry theme in the 1970s and 1980s, concern over quality is expected to dominate the 1990s. Surveillance and control strategies will become increasingly important.

Use in Quality Assurance Programs

QUALITY ASSURANCE DEFINED

Quality, an elusive concept, is synonymous with degree of excellence. *Quality assurance, quality improvement, quality control,* and *circles of quality* are terms used with increasing frequency throughout business and industry. In relation to health care, quality is the degree to which health services for individuals and populations increase the likelihood of desired health outcomes and are consistent with current professional knowledge (Lohn, 1990).

Many definitions of quality assurance related to health care have been developed. Various definitions emphasize a systematic evaluation method; they focus on determining excellence and imply that care can be improved as a result of these quality assurance activities. The American Nurses' Association (1986) definition of quality assurance is "activities to estimate and increase the level of excellence in the alteration of the health status of consumers, attained through review of providers' performance of diagnostic, therapeutic, prognostic, and other health care activities" (p. 18).

The purposes of a quality assurance program are to (1) measure how well the agency services meet specific expectations and standards and (2) identify ways in which the quality of care can be improved. A major objective of a quality assurance program is to mold the attributes and characteristics of the community health agency into a whole that is perceived as high quality by both consumers and providers of the agency services.

Utilization management, risk management, and quality assurance activities are frequently integrated within community health nursing agencies. Quality assurance programs are designed to examine the quality of services and the effects on the client; risk management programs are intended to identify and control areas of risk that could result in financial loss to the agency; and utilization review activities involve monitoring the appropriateness of services in relation to established utilization criteria (Barlow, 1989). This chapter incorporates utilization management and risk management under the label of quality assurance.

HISTORIC PERSPECTIVE

Although increasing emphasis is being placed on quality of health care, this is not a new concern. Florence Nightingale was one of the first to advocate the establishment of standards for provision of care and to suggest how data could be collected to evaluate attainment of those standards. An 1858 publication compared mortality rates of soldiers and those of civilians to illustrate the low standards for care of military personnel. The comparison was used by Nightingale to advocate for improvement of military care.

Quality of nursing care in the US was affected by two major movements that originated in the early 1900s. The first movement addressed licensure of nurses. State nursing associations led the way in seeking legislation mandating registration of nurses. North Carolina became the first state to pass such legislation in 1903. State licensure regulations addressed the general areas of preliminary education, professional training, licensing tests, and registry. By 1923, all the states had some type of legislation relating to licensure of nurses.

The second quality assurance movement grew from an interest in regulating education of health care providers. This trend was evident first in medicine. The Flexner Report, funded by the Carnegie Foundation, was published in 1910. It detailed the results of a study of medical schools and recommended initiation of standards for the training of physicians. As these recommendations were instituted, many medical schools were forced to close. The Flexner Report also stimulated interest in standards for training nurses. Between 1912 and 1939, three organizations concerned with regulation of nursing education were formed. The National Organization for Public Health Nursing examined nursing programs in colleges and universities that prepared public health nurses. The Association of Collegiate Schools of Nursing established education standards for its members. The accreditation of basic nursing education programs was initiated by the National League for Nursing Education; this program continues at present under the auspices of the National League for Nursing. During the 1950s and 1960s, nurses began to focus on the process of delivering nursing care. Research was directed toward the development of tools that could be used to measure nursing performance. Three tools developed during this era were the Slater Nursing Competencies Rating Scale, the Quality Patient Care Scale (QualPaCS), and the Phaneuf Nursing Audit (Wandelt & Phaneuf, 1972). The Slater Nursing Competencies Rating Scale and the QualPaCS measure competency of the nurse as care is being provided. The Phaneuf Nursing Audit, designed to measure quality of care received by a patient during an episode of care, is applied to the record following completion of care.

ROLE OF THE FEDERAL GOVERNMENT

The federal government began to widen its role in payment for health services with the enactment of Medicare and Medicaid in 1965. As health care costs rose, so did concern regarding the quality of care being purchased. Medicare conditions of participation provide structural standards that must be maintained in order for community health agencies to participate in the Medicare program. The conditions mandate that agencies monitor the extent to which their services are appropriate, adequate, effective, and efficient. Specifically, agencies are required to (1) review the appropriateness of continued care for each patient at 60-day intervals; (2) conduct a clinical record review of open and closed cases on a quarterly basis; (3) establish a professional advisory group that reviews policies, procedures, and clinical care; and (4) produce an annual evaluation of the total program of services provided (Wagner, 1988).

Professional review organizations (PROs), established by the 1983 Social Security Amendments, stress quality of care and cost containment. PROs' criteria for care are based on local patterns of practice. Their activities include medical care evaluation, continued stay review, and admissions certification. In addition, PRO staff monitor access to care and cost of care.

PROs focused their initial review efforts on federally funded care provided in hospitals. The Medicare Quality Assurance Act of 1985 expanded PRO authority to include review of services offered by health maintenance organizations (HMOs) and competitive medical plans (CMPs). Further, the Act strengthened quality assurance programs and improved access to post-hospital care by requiring hospitals to provide discharge planning to Medicare beneficiaries.

The authority of PROs was expanded again in 1986 to allow for investigation of consumer complaints and review of care provided at skilled nursing facilities and home health agencies participating in the Medicare program. PRO staff review a sample of clients readmitted to a hospital within 31 days of discharge. Any care provided during the period between hospitalizations is subject to review through examination of the agency's clinical record. A professional review organization has the authority to initiate sanctions against individuals and agencies found to be providing substandard care.

The federal government is continuing to emphasize quality of care. Members of Congress addressed this issue as part of the Omnibus Budget Reconciliation Act of 1987 (OBRA). The Act contained provisions designed to safeguard the rights of Medicare beneficiaries and guarantee quality of home health services. Recently, Congress passed an OBRA of 1989 that further focuses federal attention on outcome. The Health Care Financing Administration (HCFA) has revised procedures for survey of home health agencies participating in the Medicare program. The revisions increase the emphasis on client outcome in the evaluation of health services. Lang and Marek describe current federal initiatives related to quality of care.

CONTEMPORARY FEDERAL INITIATIVES

by NORMA LANG, RN, PhD, FAAN, Dean and Professor, University of Wisconsin-Milwaukee, School of Nursing, Milwaukee, WI; and KAREN MAREK, RN, MSN, Project Assistant/Doctoral Candidate, University of Wisconsin-Milwaukee, School of Nursing, Milwaukee, WI

There currently is a national emphasis on methods of collecting and synthesizing health care outcome data to determine effectiveness and quality of care delivered. The need for nursing data and the standardization of these data have never been more critical.

The Department of Health and Human Services (DHHS), through the Health Care Financing Administration (HCFA) and Public Health Services (PHS), has launched the Medical Treatment Effectiveness Program (MEDTEP). This program has the long-term goal of shifting the focus in assessment of health care services, research, and financing from processes to outcomes. The purpose of MEDTEP is to improve the effectiveness and appropriateness of health care services by enhancing our understanding of which health care practices are most effective (American Medical Peer Review Association, 1989). The three program components are (1) research on patient outcomes and clinical effectiveness, (2) collection and analysis of data, and (3) dissemination and assimilation of findings.

In addition, the Omnibus Budget Reconciliation Act (OBRA) of 1989 included a provision to establish an Agency for Health Care Policy and Research within the Public Health Service. The purpose of this agency is "to enhance the quality and appropriateness and effectiveness of health care services, and access to such services, through the establishment of a broad base of scientific research and through the promotion of improvements in clinical practice and in the organization, financing, and delivery of health care services" (Congressional Record—House, 1989). The newly established agency will include the Office of the Forum for Quality and Effectiveness in Health Care. This office will be responsible for development, periodic review, and refinement of clinical guidelines and standards of quality performance measures.

One aspect of MEDTEP is the development of a uniform clinical data set (UCDS). The purpose is to standardize the collection of health care clinical information as well as create a large epidemiologic data base for use in MEDTEP. Quality assessments by the professional review organizations will be based on the information generated by the UCDS.

The current UCDS is based primarily on medical information. The evaluation and measurement of health care, especially long-term and community-based care, under medical diagnosis or technical procedures provides an inadequate data base (Lang, 1988). It is essential that nursing information be included. Nursing information provides the most descriptive and valid indicators of the quantity and quality of health care. This is an ideal opportunity for community health nurses to demonstrate the effectiveness of their services.

The Omaha System has made a major contribution to the standardization of nursing information. With standardization there is the ability to build an epidemiologic base for nursing data. These data, however, must be included in the national health care data base if nursing care is to be considered in the national health care system.

ROLE OF NURSING AND OTHER ORGANIZATIONS

Accreditation of community health nursing agencies is another method of examining quality of nursing care. Two organizations presently offer accreditation programs: the Community Health Accreditation Program (CHAP), a subsidiary of the National League for Nursing (NLN), and the Joint Commission for Accreditation of Healthcare Organizations (JCAHO). Both programs provide an opportunity for participating agencies to engage in self-review as well as peer review. The evaluation process emphasizes physical and organization structures and personnel qualifications. Both accrediting organizations require that agencies maintain active programs of quality assurance.

The American Nurses' Association (ANA) has been active in promotion of quality nursing care in relation to an individual practitioner rather than an agency. ANA efforts have had three foci. The first effort, initiated in 1958, addressed certification of nurses. Specialties in which certification is available include community health and school nursing. The second effort involves establishment of standards for nursing practice in a variety of practice areas. The standards incorporate structure, process, and outcome criteria and are intended to form the basis for quality assurance programs. The third effort addresses quality assurance programs. A model for quality assurance, developed by Lang, was adopted by the ANA in 1976. This model is closely related to a problem-solving process and the nursing process. The model can be used to evaluate an individual nurse's performance, client care, or a total agency. The circular model consists of components that are described as follows:

- Identify values
- Identify standards and criteria
- Secure measurements
- Make interpretations
- Identify and choose courses of action
- Take action (American Nurses' Association, 1976)

QUALITY ASSURANCE PROGRAMS IN COMMUNITY HEALTH

All programs of quality assurance measure care against predetermined standards or broad statements of acceptable levels of achievement. In order to be used in evaluation, the standards must be further delineated through the use of criteria. Evaluation criteria are statements describing specific, measurable qualities of a standard. Evaluation standards and criteria have been classified by Donabedian (1966) as relating to structure, process, or outcome. This classification has become widely accepted by the health care industry.

Quality assurance efforts by the staff of community health nursing agencies have incorporated standards and criteria primarily related to examination of structure and process. Increasing attention is being directed toward development of outcome standards, however, HCFA officials have indicated that outcomes of care will be the future format for determining the quality of home care provided to Medicare beneficiaries. The Community Health Accreditation Program of the NLN has integrated measurable patient outcomes into its Standards for Agency Accreditation. JCAHO is currently undertaking a similar revision of its accreditation standards. The new emphasis on evaluation of outcomes is desirable, but it is essential that evaluation of structure and process not be discarded (Donabedian, 1966; Lieske, 1985).

Assessment of community health services is difficult for various reasons. Many assessment tools require lengthy and repeated observations of health care professionals. The presence of an observer in a client's home is impractical and alters the client-practitioner interaction. Therefore, quality assurance activities in community health agencies traditionally emphasize review of clinical records. Community health record systems, however, are frequently "not well developed and do not necessarily include the relevant clinical or functional measures along which it is desirable to document change" (Kane & Kane, 1988, p. 141).

The Omaha System offers a framework that has value for quality assurance activities. The framework has the capability of providing a single, unified structure for the clinical practice, documentation system, and data management plans throughout the agency. Furthermore, the System is comprehensive and relevant to community health settings.

The Omaha System delineates agency expectations and standards for practice as a necessary precursor to quality assurance programs. The four domains of the Problem Classification Scheme provide a comprehensive structure for collecting and assessing client data. The Intervention Scheme suggests activities and actions for addressing identified client problems. Evaluation of problem-specific client outcomes is facilitated through use of the Problem Rating Scale for Outcomes.

The Omaha System provides clear, standard language for documentation. The clinical record is logical and concise; extraneous information is avoided. A reviewer can easily follow the thoughts of a care provider, thus facilitating assessment of expertise and quality of practice.

The Omaha System is compatible with a variety of approaches used by the VNA of Omaha quality assurance program. Such approaches include utilization review, peer review, patient satisfaction surveys, incident reports, supervisory shared visits, and staff development. The Omaha System is integrated throughout the quality assurance program.

QUALITY ASSURANCE AT THE VNA OF OMAHA

The goals of the VNA of Omaha quality assurance program are to (1) validate that quality care is being provided by staff who are qualified and who comply with value-based predetermined standards set by the agency; (2) confirm that all input from clients and other consumers is reviewed and used to ensure quality care for the future; (3) determine that all available resources are used appropriately to ensure high quality, comprehensive care; and (4) identify problem areas, recommend and implement action plans, and evaluate the impact of changes on the overall quality of the care delivered. A Quality Assurance Committee composed of management and supervisory staff is responsible for directing quality assurance activities. The program is a circular process that includes:

- Ongoing collection and monitoring of information about all aspects of service delivery that have an impact on client care
- Evaluating the information collected in order to identify problems or opportunities to improve service delivery; evaluation may be done simply as a matter of observation of trends, or by comparing information against predetermined standards
- Communicating recommendations and implementing action where appropriate to improve service delivery or resolve problem areas
- Reassessing problem areas to determine if there was resolution and improvement in service delivery

Utilization Review

Utilization review is directed toward assuring that services provided are needed and that the level of care is both appropriate and cost effective. A utilization review program is mandated for all home health care provider agencies by the Medicare conditions of participation. Services are measured against standards that include: (1) criteria for admission to and dismissal from agency services; (2) eligibility for services by various care providers such as physical therapists, social workers, and home health aides; (3) number and frequency of services provided; and (4) referral to other community resources.

VNA of Omaha utilization reviews are conducted quarterly by a committee composed of health care professionals from the community at large and the management staff of the agency. Members include nurses, physical therapists, speech therapists, occupational therapists, and social workers. Data examined include actual client records and statistical reports. The standards related to utilization review are (1) 90% of reviewed cases must show that appropriate resources are used and agency services are appropriate, and (2) 100% of recommendations are implemented and followed up for re-evaluation. Committee members receive an orientation to the agency that includes a review of the agency's clinical record and the Omaha System. Use of the Omaha System to document client care has enabled reviewers to identify the complexity of client problems addressed by care providers, the numbers and types of interventions planned and provided, and the response of the client to care. Further, use of standard language to document client care has made comparisons easier.

Peer Review

Peer review is defined by the American Nurses' Association (1976) as the process by which registered nurses actively engaged in the practice of nursing appraise the quality of nursing care in a given situation in accordance with established standards of practice. Peer review is implemented to assure and improve quality, encourage professional growth, restructure inadequate evaluation, and support primary nursing. Difficulties associated with peer review include legal issues, difficulty placing blame and praise for outcomes, absence of an evaluation tool, costs and risks, and staff resistance (Jackson, 1989). Some community health agencies have established peer review programs, but these programs are not federally mandated. Their results vary greatly. Effective, formal peer review programs require effort and commitment on the part of the staff and management.

Peer review may include process standards, outcome standards, or a combination of process and outcome standards. The record audit has been the primary method used in the peer review process. An instrument as the Phaneuf Nursing Audit may be used or agency staff may develop their own instrument with accompanying standards and criteria. Gail Scoates describes the VNA of Omaha home health care peer review process and review tools that were developed by agency staff.

PEER REVIEW AT THE VNA OF OMAHA

by GAIL SCOATES, RN, MS, Director of Professional Practice, Visiting Nurse Association of Omaha, Omaha, NE

The staff of the VNA of Omaha home health care program participate in a peer review process that incorporates the Omaha System. Over a 2.5-year period, a staff committee was responsible for developing documentation standards and tools for record review. Currently, all home health nursing and rehabilitation staff serve as reviewers and provide records for evaluation by others. The peer review process has three major components that will be explained in the following paragraphs.

The first component involves examination of records for completeness and adherence to agency documentation policies. Attention is given to consistent use of the Omaha System as a framework that reflects sound and logical practice. A checklist tool is used by reviewers to delineate the presence of each record form and its required data elements in a client record. After a review is completed, results are compiled and evaluated by the Peer Review Committee. Recommendations are made to agency management staff and may include clarification of policies and suggestions for educational programs or changes in protocols. Since the peer review process was initiated, management staff have been receptive to and acted on peer review committee suggestions. That responsiveness of management staff has continued as additional components have been added. Examples of specific recommendations made by the Committee include changes in methods of data collection on admission visits and an inservice program on hypothermia. Evaluation of subsequent review findings have clearly indicated improvement in compliance with agency and regulatory documentation standards.

The second component entails examination of records in accordance with guidelines for home care established by the peer review organization (PRO). In 1986, PROs were given authority to review home health records of clients readmitted to a hospital within 31 days of discharge. The peer review committee identified a need to evaluate records according to the guidelines used by the PRO and to educate staff about the guidelines. Findings have (1) confirmed delivery of high quality care, (2) led to clarification of documentation requirements, and (3) indicated the need for selected staff inservice programs.

Finally, the peer review committee initiated development of a series of Intervention Guidelines as the third component of the peer review process. The Guidelines have two purposes. First, they serve as a tool to assist in planning and delivering problem-specific nursing care. Second, they are used as a record review tool to evaluate quality of care delivery. The goals of this component of peer review are to determine whether care provided meets acceptable standards and to provide clear direction for education and orientation within a clinical arena in an effort to improve the quality of care delivery.

Guideline development began with selection of commonly identified client problems from the Problem Classification Scheme (PCS). The Intervention Scheme provided an organized format for delineating specific nursing actions or activities. Problem-specific activities were identified for each intervention category of the Scheme. The nurse uses the Guidelines to assist in care planning by selecting the activities appropriate for a specific client, an approach that provides a general guideline for nursing intervention yet allows for attention to specific client needs. An example of the care planning/intervention guides, those that were developed for the problem Circulation, is included in Table 14–1. Care planning/intervention guides for all 40 problems of the Problem Classification Scheme appear in the pocket guide published as a companion to this text.

The first step in the peer review process involves determining which problems have been identified and are accompanied by nursing care plans. A master list is available, correlating medical diagnostic categories with possible client problems from the PCS. As an example, Table 14–2 illustrates the master list for the category of cardiovascular diseases.

TABLE 14–1 ■ Intervention Guide

29. Circulation
 I. Health Teaching, Guidance, and Counseling
  01. anatomy/physiology:
   a) circulatory system
   b) other
  07. cardiac care:
   a) prescribed diet
   b) foods to avoid
   c) fluid restriction
   d) relief of edema
   e) medical alert bracelet
   f) factors contributing to risk of increased cardiac impairment (smoking, clothing, weight, exercise, and stress)
   g) sexual activity
   h) avoidance of Valsalva maneuver
   i) other
  11. coping skills:
   a) dealing with disease process
   b) other
  15. durable medical equipment:
   a) oxygen
   b) support hose
   c) monitor
   d) other
  35. mobility/transfers:
   a) prescribed activity
   b) balanced rest/activity
   c) pacing
   d) energy conservation
   e) other
  41. personal care:
   a) foot care
   b) nail care
   c) hygiene
   d) other
  46. safety:
   a) infection control
   b) other
  50. signs/symptoms—physical:
   a) s/s CHF
   b) vital signs (temperature, pulse, respiration, and BP)
   c) signs/symptoms of deep vein thrombosis
   d) pain
   e) when to notify physician/nurse
   f) other
  56. stress management:
   a) relaxation techniques
   b) other
  63. other:
 II. Treatments and Procedures
  07. cardiac care:
   a) pacemaker check
   b) apply support hose
   c) no code
   d) other
  15. durable medical equipment:
   a) cardiac equipment
   b) other
  41. personal care:
   a) nail care
   b) other
  63. other:
 III. Case Management
  15. durable medical equipment:
   a) cardiac equipment
   b) other
  23. food:
   a) home delivered meals
   b) other
  31. medical/dental care:
   a) coordination with physician

TABLE 14–1 ■ Intervention Guide *Continued*

   b) other
  40. other community resource:
   a) Heart Association
   b) other
  43. rehabilitation:
   a) occupational therapy
   b) cardiac rehabilitation
   c) other
  61. transportation:
   a) resource
   b) other
  63. other:
 IV. Surveillance
  31. medical/dental care:
   a) compliance with scheduled appointments
   b) other
  35. mobility/transfers:
   a) prescribed activity
   b) balance rest/exercise
   c) pacing
   d) energy conservation
   e) other
  37. nutrition:
   a) compliance with prescribed diet
   b) hydration
   c) other
  49. signs/symptoms—mental/emotional:
   a) coping mechanisms
   b) other
  50. signs/symptoms—physical:
   a) circulatory status
   b) weight
   c) edema
   d) orthostatic BP
   e) signs/symptoms of deep vein thrombosis
   f) chest pain
   g) condition of feet/integument
   h) shortness of breath
   i) other
  63. other:

TABLE 14–2 ■ Problems Frequently Associated With Cardiovascular Diseases

(Myocardial infarction, congestive heart failure, hypertension, angina, peripheral vascular disease)

Possible Problems

29	Circulation
35	Nutrition
24	Pain
28	Respiration
37	Physical Activity
42	Medications
26	Integument
44	Other: Technical Information

The next step of the peer review process requires sophisticated nursing judgment. Reviewers determine if actions and activities have been implemented appropriately, are overlooked, or are inappropriate. Reviewers are encouraged to make positive comments as well as suggestions for improvement in documentation or care delivery. A compilation of results from this component of peer review is used to make recommendations similar to those that arise from the other peer review components.

The concept of peer review with evaluation of documentation and care delivery can be very stressful when initially introduced. By using a gradual process of moving from record audit to a comprehensive evaluation of care delivery, peer review and evaluation have been well accepted by VNA of Omaha personnel. The implementation process has eased staff stress and resulted in staff acceptance of peer review principles. Participation in the development of the program, selection of tools, and administrative support of recommendations have also helped to integrate peer review as an accepted component of quality assurance and as a routine staff activity.

Client Satisfaction

Another approach used in the VNA of Omaha quality assurance program is assessment of client satisfaction. Data for assessing client satisfaction are obtained through telephone interviews and written questionnaires. Such data may include information relative to the content of the care, attitudes about the care and care providers, and perceptions of the situation in which the care was provided. Benefits to an agency and its clients realized by client satisfaction surveys have been elaborated by McNeese (1988). They include (1) promotion of use of the research process in evaluating the quality and appropriateness of services, (2) provision of a scientific basis for evaluating and modifying health care delivery systems or models, and (3) identification and integration of individual client and family concerns into quality assurance activities. Client satisfaction surveys are usually designed to protect respondents' identities. This method increases accuracy and completeness of information but does not allow followup to specific comments.

Data for measurement of client satisfaction at the VNA of Omaha are obtained from two sources. One-third of the clients discharged in the previous month are randomly selected to receive a mailed questionnaire. Responses are compiled, and they constitute the first data source. The second source is documentation of verbal or written statements from someone outside the agency expressing satisfaction or dissatisfaction with a personal interaction or service. Written or verbal complaints and compliments are documented on a form that includes a description of the statement and followup action taken. Our standard is that 90% of all responses to the questionnaire and verbal or written comments must indicate that care was satisfactory. Results of both the client satisfaction survey and the complaints and compliments statements are shared with staff.

Supervisory Shared Visits

Supervisory shared visits have two purposes: evaluation of a staff person's performance and documentation of data for quality assurance purposes. At the VNA of Omaha, an immediate supervisor accompanies each staff person on a home visit at least three times per year. Prior to the visit, the supervisor and staff member meet to discuss the purpose of the home visit and to orient the supervisor to the client and family. During the actual home visit, the supervisor observes the staff member and subsequently completes a Supervisory Home Visit Tool. This checklist provides consistency in the way supervisors carry out and document supervisory shared home visits, and it affords tabulation of data for both evaluation and quality assurance purposes. Following the home visit, the supervisor discusses the visit with the staff member. The goals of the conference are to provide feedback for work performed and to develop plans with the staff member to enhance performance. Aggregate data from the supervisory shared home visits are evaluated triannually. The standard for shared supervisory visits is that 90% of all items assessed indicate appropriate care delivery. Items that fail to meet the standard are discussed by the quality assurance committee and a plan for corrective action is developed. The action may include review with staff, an inservice session, or an alteration of the record format. Bridget Young and Carolyn Jorgensen describe the tool that they designed to incorporate the Omaha System Intervention Scheme (Fig. 14–1).

The Visiting Nurse Association of the Midlands
Supervisory Shared Home Visit Tool

Employee Name: _____   Date of Visit: _____

Client Name: _____

		Yes	No	N/A
I.	Format of Home Visit			

A. Greeted client/family appropriately
B. Stated purpose of home visit
C. Carried out home visit in organized, logical manner
D. Informed client about each activity and received his/her consent
E. Stated purpose for next home visit
F. Remained flexible during visit adapting to the client/family needs
G. Comments _____

_____

		Yes	No	N/A
II.	Safety Factors			

A. Handwashing done according to policy
B. VNA bag is properly cared for and protected
C. Supplies and equipment maintained in the home and stored/utilized in appropriate manner
D. Comments _____

_____

		Yes	No	N/A
III.	Health Teaching, Guidance, and Counseling/ Surveillance			

A. Used vocabulary appropriate for client's level of understanding
B. Gave simple, brief explanations
C. Instruction followed logical sequence
D. Steps taken to ensure client's success
E. Plan for teaching allows adequate time for learning to take place
F. Care to be taught was demonstrated
G. Return demonstration planned or carried out
H. Comments _____

_____

A

FIGURE 14–1 ■ (*A and B*) The Supervisory Shared Home Visit Tool is completed after the supervisor observes a staff person's performance during a home visit.

```
IV.  Treatments and Procedures/Surveillance          Yes    No    N/A

     A.  Principles of asepsis and infection control
         applied
     B.  Each medical order was carried out as described  ___   ___   ___
     C.  Observations/assessments made in accordance
         with diagnosis and client need                   ___   ___   ___
     D.  Reported pertinent findings which needed
         immediate report to MD                           ___   ___   ___
     E.  Urged client to seek medical care if indicated   ___   ___   ___
     F.  Assessed for effectiveness and/or side effects
         of medications                                   ___   ___   ___
     G.  Demonstrated sufficient technical skills          ___   ___   ___
     H.  Comments _____


V.   Case Management/Surveillance                    Yes    No    N/A

     A.  All appropriate agency services utilized
     B.  Evidence of supervision of HHA activities         ___   ___   ___
     C.  Community resources utilized                      ___   ___   ___
     D.  Involved client/family in care                    ___   ___   ___
     E.  Evidence of evaluation of total plan of care
         with appropriate revisions, if indicated          ___   ___   ___
     F.  Discharge planning evident                        ___   ___   ___
     G.  Comments _____



Supervisor Signature/Date: _____

Employee Comments: _____

_____

_____

Employee Signature/Date: _____
```

B

FIGURE 14–1 (Continued)

THE SUPERVISORY SHARED HOME VISIT TOOL*

by BRIDGET YOUNG, RN, BSN, Client Service Manager, Visiting Nurse Association of Omaha, Omaha, NE; and CAROLYN JORGENSEN, RN, BSN, Intake Supervisor, Visiting Nurse Association of Omaha, Omaha, NE

The Supervisory Shared Home Visit tool was designed to evaluate elements of the home visit, safety factors, and staff interventions. It was not intended for use in evaluating the documentation of the visit by the staff person. The tool itself contains five sections: I. Format of Home Visit; II. Safety Factors; III. Health Teaching, Guidance, and Counseling/Surveillance; IV. Treatments and Procedures/Surveillance;

and V. Case Management/Surveillance. Each item can be marked yes, no, or not applicable (N/A). There is room for comments under each section as well as a space for a supervisor's signature and date, employee comments, and an employee signature and date.

Format of Home Visit (Section I) involves the way in which staff members conduct home visits and present themselves to clients. The perception of the agency staff by clients is vital to an agency's community image. It is also imperative to a useful, productive home visit that it be carried out with client and family participation. Planning the subsequent home visit with the client provides for continuity of care and can help bridge the gap that often occurs between visits.

*The following contribution is taken from Jorgensen, C., and Young, B. (1989, May/June). The supervisory shared home visit tool. *Home Healthcare Nurse, 7*:33–36. Reprinted by permission of Appleton & Lange, Inc.

Safety Factors (Section II) focus on eliminating potential risks to clients and staff. Handwashing, care of the nursing bag, and care of clients' supplies and equipment can be readily observed and documented. All agencies operate under policies and procedures that address these issues, and the items in this tool should be interpreted according to those policies and procedures.

The final three sections of the tool are organized according to the broad Intervention Scheme categories of the Omaha System. Any home visit includes at least one intervention activity, and the staff document their activities according to the Scheme. The Intervention Scheme of the Omaha System identifies four areas of nursing activities: (1) health teaching, guidance, and counseling; (2) treatments and procedures; (3) case management; (4) surveillance.

Health Teaching, Guidance, and Counseling (Section III) are defined as those activities that range from giving information, anticipating client problems, encouraging client action and responsibility for self-care and coping, to assisting with decision-making and problem-solving. The overlapping actions occur on a continuum, with the variations based on the client's self-direction capabilities. This intervention category was designed to evaluate a nurse's abilities to use effectively the principles of adult learning. To be an effective health teacher, a health professional must be aware that learning is dependent upon the readiness, emotional state, abilities, and potential of the learner. Another important concept to evaluate is the staff's awareness that adults, for the most part, like teaching that is brief, relevant, and has immediate application.

Treatments and Procedures (Section IV) are defined as the technical activities directed toward preventing signs and symptoms, identifying risk factors and early signs and symptoms, and decreasing or alleviating signs and symptoms. Considering the diversity of clients served, this intervention category is intended to allow for the various tasks undertaken during a home visit. It is expected that by meeting the criteria of the intervention category, safe practice can be evaluated.

Case Management (Section V) is defined as activities of coordination, advocacy, and referral. These activities involve facilitating service delivery on behalf of a client, communicating with health and human service providers, promoting assertive client communication, and guiding a client toward use of appropriate community resources. To evaluate a staff member's attention to the needs of an individual client and family besides those presented by an obvious physical diagnosis, the supervisor needs to consider a staff member's ability to provide total case management, including appropriate use of community resources. Effective case management also indicates periodic evaluation of the total plan of care. This may be evident during the course of the home visit or during a pre-visit and post-visit conference between supervisor and staff member when plans for the visit and outcome of the visit are discussed.

Surveillance is defined as those activities of detection, measurement, critical analysis, or monitoring that indicate client status in relation to a given condition or phenomenon. The Omaha System delineates surveillance as one of the four broad interventions. Skilled assessments and surveillance are integral to the other three interventions; for example, when teaching, there must be surveillance of the learner's responses. To avoid redundancy, therefore, surveillance was incorporated into Sections III, IV, and V.

Staff Development

Staff development is a method of providing continual opportunities for professional growth of knowledge applicable to community health care. With the increase of health care technology comes clients with complex care needs, and the role of staff development and clinical specialists in community health agencies is critical. The purpose of the staff development program at the VNA of Omaha is to ensure a high level of quality care to clients by providing educational and practice opportunities for practitioners and professional growth through support of workshop attendance. The agency provides a predetermined number of hours of inservice education for its employees and monetary support for attendance at workshops and other educational opportunities offered by external resources. Topics for agency inservice programs are developed in response to staff interest, external requirements, and areas of deficiency identified through quality assurance activities. The standard for staff development is that 100% of staff must participate in a predetermined number of hours of inservice annually.

Quality Assurance Studies

Quality assurance studies can be designed to focus on an identified problem affecting the agency as a whole or a department or program of the agency. The VNA of Omaha hospice program staff selected the client problem Pain as the focus of a quality assurance study. This problem was chosen because control of untoward signs and symptoms is a major goal of the hospice program, and the majority of hospice clients experience some degree of pain. The method of the study is a retrospective chart audit conducted quarterly. Data are gathered in relation to five indicators that determine the process or outcome of care. The indicators are:

1. The admission assessment includes pain location, severity, and methods of control

2. The interdisciplinary care plan addresses pain control
3. Reassessment occurs regularly
4. The care plan is adjusted as necessary
5. The client reports pain at or below 4 on a pain intensity index, with 0 being no pain and 10 being intense pain

The clinical record serves as the source of data for the study. The data base is reviewed for admission assessment data, the problem ratings and plan of care are examined in relation to problem 24. Pain, and the visit reports are reviewed for evidence of interventions directed at control of pain.

The data are compiled by client and by aggregate. The standard of acceptability for aggregate data is 90%. Results of the study are reviewed by the hospice team, with particular attention given to indicators with results below 90%. Remedial actions have included inservice education programs and alteration in forms and policies regarding documentation of pain.

SUMMARY

Community health nurses throughout history have been concerned about the quality of their services. This concern has been intensified in recent years by a rise in the acuity level of client illness, negative publicity related to community health care, and increasingly restrictive regulations. Federal officials have begun to focus on quality of health care. Current federal initiatives, directed at collection of outcome data and evaluation of care effectiveness, were described by Lang and Marek.

The Omaha System serves as a guide to practice and recording and, as such, can form the basis for a quality assurance program within a community health agency. As a practice framework, the Omaha System is useful in articulating agency standards. As a method of documentation, the System provides clear, concise language that is easily understood by reviewers.

The Omaha System is integrated throughout the quality assurance program at the VNA of Omaha. Further, the components of the Omaha system have served as the basis for tools designed to facilitate several quality assurance processes. Two such tools were described by Scoates and Jorgensen and Young.

REFERENCES

American Bar Association (1986). The black box of home care quality. Report presented to Chairman of the House Select Committee on Aging. Washington, DC, US Government Printing Office.

American Medical Peer Review Association (1989, September). Charting the course of medical effectiveness and outcome assessment. In *Charting the Course for Peer Review.* Proceedings of the 1989 Session and House of Delegates Meeting.

American Nurses' Association (1976). *Quality Assurance Workbook.* Kansas City, MO.

American Nurses' Association (1986). *Standards of Home Health Nursing Practice.* Kansas City, MO.

Barlow, A. (1989, March). A home care quality assurance program. *Caring,* 8:56–59.

Buck, J. (1988, May/June). Measuring the success of home health care. *Home Healthcare Nurse,* 6:17–23.

Congressional Record—House. (1989, November 21). H-9354.

Donabedian, A. (1966, July). Evaluating the quality of medical care. *Milbank Memorial Fund Q.,* 44(2):166–206.

Halamandaris, V. (1988, October). Quality home care: Bridge to the future. *Caring,* 7:5–8.

Jackson, S. (1989, June). Peer review—Why and how to do it. In Glover, S. (Ed.), *Performance Evaluations,* Vol. 1, No. 2 (pp. 60–86). Baltimore, Williams & Wilkins.

Jorgensen, C., & Young, B. (1989, May/June). The supervisory shared home visit tool. *Home Healthcare Nurse,* 7:33–36.

Kane, R., & Kane, R. (1988, Spring). Long-term care: Variations on a quality assurance theme. *Inquiry,* 25:132–146.

Lang, N. (1988, July/August). Non-hospital, non-physician review. *Ampra Rev.,* 5:1–2.

Lieske, A. (1985). Standards: The basis of a quality assurance program. In Meisenheimer, C. (Ed.), *Quality Assurance: A Complete Guide to Effective Programs* (pp. 45–72). Rockville, MD, Aspen.

Lohn, K. (Ed.) (1990). *Medicare: A Strategy for Quality Assurance,* Vol. I. Washington, DC, National Academy Press.

McNeese, B. (1988, May/June). Patient satisfaction: How is it being addressed? *Home Healthcare Nurse,* 6:13–15.

Sovie, M. (1987, January/February). Exceptional executive leadership shapes nursing's future. *Nurs. Econom.,* 5:13–20.

Wagner, D. (1988). *Managing for Quality in Home Health Care.* Rockville, MD, Aspen.

Walton, M. (1975). Quality assurance in health care. In *Quality Assurance: Models for Nursing Education* (pp. 27–32). New York, National League for Nursing.

Wandelt, M. & Phaneuf, M. (1972, August). Three instruments for measuring the quality of nursing care. *Hosp. Topics,* 50:20–23, 29.

BIBLIOGRAPHY

American Nurses' Association (1983). *Standards of School Nursing Practice.* Kansas City, MO.

American Nurses' Association (1986). *Standards of Community Health Nursing Practice.* Kansas City, MO.

Bull, M. (1985). Quality assurance: Its origins, transformations, and prospects. In Meisenheimer, C. (Ed.), *Quality Assurance: A Complete Guide to Effective Programs* (pp. 1–16). Rockville, MD, Aspen.

Federal Register (1989, August 14). *Medicare Program: Home Health Agency Conditions of Participation—Reduction in Record Keeping Requirements,* Vol. 54, No. 155. Washington, DC, US Government Printing Office.

Haley, R. (1986). *Managing Hospital Infection Control for Cost-effectiveness.* Chicago, American Hospital Publishing.

Johnson, N. (1988). Accountability and quality assurance. In Caliandro, G., & Judkins, B. (Eds.), *Primary Nursing Practice* (pp. 47–63). Glenview, IL, Scott, Foresman/Little, Brown.

Kalisch, P., & Kalisch, B. (1986). *The Advance of American Nursing* (2nd ed.). Boston, Little, Brown.

King, P. (1990, February 19). The city and patient. *Newsweek,* 58.

Kornblatt, E., Fisher, M., & MacMillan, D. (1985, October). Impact of DRGs on home health nursing. *Qual. Rev. Bull.,* 11:290–294.

Lang, N. (1979, Spring). Evaluating health and nursing care. *Qual. Assur. Update,* 3:1–5.

Marriner, A. (1979, December). The research process in quality assurance. *Am. J. Nurs.,* 79:2158–2161.

Martin, K., & Scheet, N. (1988, May/June). The Omaha system: Providing a framework for assuring quality of home care. *Home Healthcare Nurse,* 6:24–28.

Meisenheimer, C. (1989). *Quality Assurance for Home Health Care.* Rockville, MD, Aspen.

Mitchell, M. (1988, October). The community health accreditation program. *Caring, 7:*20–24.

Moore, R. (1979). A comprehensive look at quality assurance. In *Pathways to Quality Care* (pp. 7–16). New York, National League for Nursing.

Patterson, C. (1990, May/June). Quality assurance, control, and monitoring. *Comput. Nurs., 8:*105–110.

Rinke, L., & Wilson, A. (Eds.) (1987). *Outcome Measures in Home Care: Vol. II, Service.* New York, National League for Nursing.

Stanhope, M., & Lancaster, J. (1988). *Community Health Nursing: Process and Practice for Promoting Health.* St. Louis, C. V. Mosby.

Tinkham, C., Voorhies, E., & McCarthy, N. (1984). *Community Health Nursing: Evolution and Process in the Family and Community* (3rd ed.). New York, Appleton-Century-Crofts.

Wilson, A. (1988, November/December). Measurable patient outcomes: Putting theory into practice. *Home Healthcare Nurse, 6:*15–18.

Wold, S. (Ed.) (1990). *Community Health Nursing: Issues and Topics.* Norwalk, CT, Appleton & Lange.

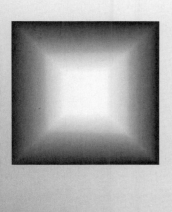

SECTION IV

LOOKING AHEAD

CHAPTER FIFTEEN

*I*t is clear that the health care industry has experienced cataclysmic changes over the past five years. The rapid pace of change no doubt will continue throughout the decade of the nineties and into the 21st century. Patient care has been, and will continue to be, altered by the introduction of advanced and complex diagnostic and treatment modalities. The financing of care also is likely to continue to change as the nation struggles to control escalating health care costs. . . . The pace and scope of change in the health care field pose a significant challenge to all health care professionals and to nurses in particular. (Secretary's Commission on Nursing, 1988, p. 57)

The future of society, health care, and community health nursing is unknown. Past experiences and current trends do provide clues, however, about the future. Clues can be used to help predict larger trends that may be examined and quantified by individuals or groups.

Evidence of the serious, complex issues that will confront future generations, including community health nurses, exists today. To address these issues, community health nurses and their agencies will need many tools like the Problem Classification Scheme, the Problem Rating Scale for Outcomes, and the Intervention Scheme. Emerging issues will not only affect discrete populations but also the entire world population. Changes in world economics and politics and terrorism are critical international concerns. In addition, environmental health, informatics, social issues, health care delivery, and population trends are of special concern to nurses.

INTERNATIONAL HEALTH ISSUES

Environmental health issues including pollution are receiving increasing attention internationally. Will scientific advances employing hazardous materials further reduce the quality of the air, water, and soil throughout the world? Based on research, scientists have predicted serious consequences to all plant and animal life. The general public is beginning to respond to the warnings.

The development of informatics is another important health-related issue. Computers and integrated management information systems already are important, and they will become essential for obtaining accurate, complete, and timely data in the future. Will nurses advocate more effectively for their profession and the consumer as computer technology is developed and installed? If implemented correctly, automation will support and facilitate nursing judgement, not replace it.

Social issues are on the list of growing concerns. Drug and alcohol abuse, violence, suicide, and acquired immune deficiency syndrome (AIDS) are consuming vast quantities of professional energy and public funds. The family unit is changing with an increase in single person and single parent families. Human rights issues, including those specific to women, remain unresolved. Personal and public opinions about women and careers have important implications for the profession of nursing. Will international attitudes change so that more people receive equitable health care, housing, education, jobs, and salaries? Because most social issues are related to cultural, religious, and gender values, intervention and resolution at national and international levels are especially difficult.

Concerns ranging from accessible health care to quality of life increasingly will become international issues. Will enough food, space, money, and health care services be available to support the world population in the future? How will individuals, families, communities, and the world population exert the effort to promote health? At the beginning of the twentieth century, Arnold Toynbee wrote that the health of the whole human race was a practical objective, referring to health as a positive state that emphasizes a preventive rather than a curative orientation. In 1980, members of the World Health Organization established a similar international goal. To reach the goal of health for all by the year 2000, a plan was designed that focused on

Community Health Nursing and the Omaha System

The Future

health promotion and disease prevention by involving health services, health manpower, and higher education. Through case examples, Benner and Wrubel (1989) have clearly described the personal investment required to change less healthy into more healthy living patterns. For any of the predictions about health promotion and improved quality of life to become reality, it will be necessary for consumers to personally and collectively advocate for health.

The dramatic aging trend occurring in the US population only increases the professional, health delivery, ethical, and financial issues related to quality of life. The aging trend is due to scientific discoveries that have saved and extended lives. Although the growth rates of most age subcategories have stabilized or decreased, that of older persons, especially the 85-year and older group, is spiraling. As a result, the incidence of chronic illnesses is increasing. Prevention and cure are relatively unknown for many of these chronic conditions. The rise in the frail elderly population rate will produce extensive long-term care implications for all nurses, including community health nurses. Simultaneously with the aging trend, a world population explosion is occurring as noted below:

6000 BC	5 million people
1 AD	250 million people
1650	500 million people
At present	5.3 billion people
Predicted in 2050	15 billion people

When considered together, the aging trend and population increase will produce serious consequences. As noted previously, those issues relate to the adequacy of food, space, money, and health care services.

FUTURE EFFECTS ON NURSING

Nurses can expect to face new and difficult challenges even if professional and public support increases. Although the total number of employed nurses has grown steadily, experts predict the need for nurses to continue or escalate. Nursing began as an avocation, and became a vocation, then an occupation. It expanded in horizontal and vertical directions until it became a highly complex art and science as well as an evolving profession. During the centuries, nurses have acted as a conscience for the health care system and in that role have enjoyed extensive public support. Nurses also have experienced limited independence in professional decisions and practice, however; in this regard, they have been subject to a negative image with little public or professional support. Resolution of nursing's critical issues is not imminent. Both professional and ethical issues, including the parameters and definitions of the profession as well as licensure and allocation of scarce resources, will continue to be debated. Idealism, humanitarianism, and effective leadership have enabled nursing to survive. These same elements will be required for nursing to remain viable and for nurses to create a positive and preferred future.

Many individuals and groups have questioned the relationship between global issues, public priorities, and the role of the total health care industry. Some experts suggest that a health care crisis already exists. Given the fragmentation within the health care industry, is the nonsystem capable of assuming a positive, aggressive role or only a reactive, responding role? Political activism and collaboration among and within health care disciplines will be necessary for the industry to have a positive impact. Because political influence is directly related to collective strength as evidenced by membership and money, nurses have an obligation to increase their involvement and visibility in professional, interdisciplinary, and related organizations. That involvement must include activities such as policy formulation at the local, state, and national levels.

Increased nursing involvement in serious international issues suggests the need for improved knowledge, competency, and unity. Recent literature documents the trend for more nurses to be baccalaureate, master's, and doctoral program graduates. Nursing education, in conjunction with inservice or continuing education offerings, must prepare nurses to meet the challenges of rapid change in society and in the health care system.

As nursing practice continues to become even more specialized, nurses need to unite as a profession, increasing cooperation and coordination of goals (Donahue, 1985). This does not mean that nurses will reach consensus on all education, practice, and social issues or that they will develop universally accepted systems (Curtin, 1989). The diversity and plurality noted throughout nursing history have been phenomenal sources of strength to the profession and will continue into the future. As noted by Hinshaw (1989), "Diversity is the spice of nursing" (p. 4). Nursing is powerful because of, not in spite of, diversity.

USE OF THE OMAHA SYSTEM

Community health nursing's demand for innovative practice, documentation, and management methods will escalate in relation to changes in nursing and society. Tools that provide structure for the community health setting are urgently needed. As described in this book, the three components of the Omaha System offer important benefits to nurses at staff, supervisory, and administrative levels. A large number of individual practitioners and groups use all or part of the Omaha System. The Problem Classification Scheme, the Problem Rating Scale for Outcomes, and the Intervention Scheme are available in the public domain and have been disseminated through numerous publications and presentations. Therefore, the number of users who have been identified is an underestimate of total users.

Data about Omaha System users have been collected since 1978 through telephone and written correspondence and in conjunction with workshops, speeches, and consultation. Beginning in 1982, surveys were developed to collect more complete and systematic data. The compilation of survey data since that time identified 226 users. For analysis, a user was defined as an agency, a school or college of nursing, or another location or institution regardless of the number of nurses and members of other disciplines that had implemented the Omaha System at any given site. The number of employees per user ranged from one to 600 people. The users were located in 42 states, three Canadian provinces, and in the United Kingdom, Denmark, and the Netherlands.

A revised version of the survey was mailed late in 1989. One hundred forms were returned by persons indicating that they currently used the Omaha System. Within community health agencies, the System was used as a practice guide and documentation framework by nurses and members of other disciplines and as an integral portion of management information systems. Review of data indicated that widespread implementation was occurring in seven states through formal networks. Questionnaire information documented implementation of the Omaha System in multiple settings, a finding that was consistent with analysis of previously identified users. Settings included (1) home health and public health agencies that provide home visit, clinic, group, and school services, (2) ambulatory care, residential, and homeless centers; (3) correctional institutions; (4) migrant worker programs; (5) community-wide programs; and (5) nursing education programs. Nurses, physical therapists, occupational therapists, physicians, nutritionists, social workers, and speech pathologists had implemented the Omaha System.

The 100 respondents were grouped according to those who were employed by (1) local, county, and state community health agencies (72); (2) schools and colleges of nursing (18); and (3) other locations and institutions (10). The community health agencies were subdivided into those that offered both home health and preventive nursing services (22 agencies), preventive services (27 agencies), and home health services (23 agencies). Nursing faculty who responded to the survey had introduced the Omaha System to students at both undergraduate and graduate levels. The majority of the 10 nurse respondents employed at other locations were consultants. Some consultants practiced independently, and others were responsible for a large group of county and local agencies. A nurse employed in an acute care setting and a nurse employed at a residential facility were among the 10 respondents. The total number of nurses and their 100 user agencies, schools and colleges of nursing, and other institutions are depicted in Table 15–1.

OMAHA SYSTEM BENEFITS

Various chapters of this book have included descriptions of the current and future benefits of the three components of the Omaha System. Benefits have been noted for nurses, other health care providers, administrators, clients, third-party payors, and the public. Primary and secondary benefits attributed to the three components are listed below. The Omaha System:

- Allows integration of practice and documentation
- Provides a system of effective feedback loops
- Facilitates precise, comprehensive, standard, professionally acceptable documentation
- Assists staff to focus and direct their energy
- Clarifies linkages between the nursing process and the practice setting

TABLE 15–1 ■ Omaha System Users*

CATEGORY	DESCRIPTION	NUMBER OF NURSES EMPLOYED
Community health nursing agencies N = 72	22 agencies providing home health and preventive services 27 agencies providing preventive services 23 agencies providing home health services	766 1,930 1,038
Total		$\overline{3,734}$
Schools/colleges of nursing N = 18	Undergraduate and graduate faculty	Ranged from one to 8 faculty members per school
Other locations/institutions N = 10	Majority were consultants 1 = acute care setting 1 = residential facility	Ranged from independent to responsible for large number of nurses

*Analysis of 100 individuals/groups identified from 1989 surveys, almost one-half of the total 220 users who have been identified since 1982.

- Offers a holistic model for a client record
- Supplies a framework for sorting essential data
- Provides nomenclature that community health personnel can use to communicate with each other and the general public
- Offers a method to increase the visibility of community health practice
- Expedites organizing and entering client data into a manual or computerized management information system
- Facilitates organization and tracking of client care data
- Provides a sound, client/provider-oriented data base for management decisions
- Offers flexibility for changes in size of agency programs and personnel
- Expedites accurate agency billing
- Facilitates reporting to external regulators and third-party reimbursement sources to enhance fiscal solvency
- Fosters the movement of nursing information into national financial and quality data bases

Practice, Documentation, and Data Management

The Problem Classification Scheme is a taxonomy of nursing diagnoses valuable to community-based nurses, supervisors, administrators, and other providers. The Scheme provides a comprehensive framework and consistent language for collecting, sorting, classifying, documenting, and analyzing data about client concerns. Such data delineate and clarify areas of client need and nursing focus, providing the driving force for organizing the entire documentation system.

The Intervention Scheme is a taxonomy of community health nursing actions or activities. It is intended to offer a system of clues and cues for staff members as they provide and document services. The Scheme generates standard data for supervisors to track and evaluate care. The Scheme also provides a tool for administrators to examine and count client services in a new manner. With increasing frequency, administrators need this type of tool for management information systems. They also need improved service activity data to fulfill the new requirements of third-party payors, accreditation personnel, and external reviewers.

The Problem Rating Scale for Outcomes is a tool designed to measure client progress in relation to specific problems. As such, it is an evaluation method for objective and consistent application by more than one staff member for a given individual client or family. The Scale is used at admission to capture a baseline of client data. It is then used again at intervals throughout the period of service and at dismissal. The comparison of change in ratings provides data to the staff nurse, supervisor, and administrator for evaluating the effectiveness of care.

The Problem Classification Scheme, the Intervention Scheme, and the Problem Rating Scale for Outcomes were designed to be implemented individually or as a unit. When the three components of the Omaha System are used simultaneously, they offer a unique tool applicable to practice, documentation, and clinical data management. As depicted throughout this book, the Omaha System is adaptable to a wide range of orientation and inservice programs, documentation forms, and review and audit procedures. These methods are required by various students, staff, administrators, and agencies. Similarly, the System generates data amenable to either simple or complex analysis.

The three components of the Omaha System provide

a framework for generating uniform and comprehensive data for service and administration. The unit of analysis for Problem Classification Scheme data may be one or many clients. When aggregate data are analyzed, the unit of analysis may be all clients in the caseload of (1) one nurse, (2) a team of staff members, (3) a specific program, (4) the staff assigned to one supervisor, (5) the staff and supervisors within one geographic portion of the agency, or (6) all care delivery staff. Data can be collected and examined at admission, throughout the period of service, and at dismissal. Data from clients' problems, types of services provided, client change/evaluation, program planning, costing, staffing configurations, and quality assurance/staff and agency evaluation can be analyzed both quantitatively and qualitatively. These data may be used within one agency or between agencies. The Omaha System is capable of generating consistent data for comparison and contrast within one program, one community health site, or among multiple sites regardless of geographic location. For analysis to be meaningful, however, the integrity of each component and of the entire Omaha System must be maintained. Reliability and validity have been established for the Problem Classification Scheme, the Problem Rating Scale for Outcomes, and the Intervention Scheme, as described in Chapter 4. If modifications extend beyond those suggested in Chapters 5, 6, and 7, the controls on reliability and validity as well as comparisons of interagency data are not possible.

COMPARISON WITH OTHER TOOLS

Similarities

The Omaha System is *similar* in purpose and focus to other existing practice, documentation, and management tools that give credence to nursing as a profession. Most of the tools have been designed for three reasons. First, developers identified a critical lack of systematic decision-making or clinical judgement tools pertinent to groups of nurses, clients, or settings. Second, developers recognized that "the degree to which the professional society can control and improve nursing practice depends on the ability of the profession to name its phenomena of concern" (Lang, Galliher, & Hirsch, 1989, p. 70). Third, developers had a commitment to excellence in nursing now and in the future.

The Problem Classification Scheme exhibits characteristics similar to those of other nursing diagnosis models. Initial work on most nursing diagnosis models began in the 1970s and was intended to clarify the focus of nursing. Most models are compatible with the nursing process. Some similarity in nomenclature exists among the models.

The development of the Intervention Scheme parallels investigations conducted by others. Recent interest in nursing interventions developed in response to two major forces. First, as members of an emerging profession, nurses are increasingly delineating their practice and recognizing their accountability for that practice. This force is gaining momentum as nurses become more interested in entering the reimbursement system (McCloskey, 1989). Second, the demands from auditors and third-party payors to specify the impact of professional services have escalated. According to Lant (1988), "the inability to define, compare, and contrast the cost of nursing services frequently is cited as a distinct concern in managing the cost of health care" (p. 325).

The development of the Problem Rating Scale for Outcomes is related to a growing interest in measuring effectiveness of care provided. Issues related to professional accountability have stimulated interest in the development of nurse-sensitive outcome measures. External pressure from third-party payors and consumers has contributed to the interest. Client outcomes are being investigated and described by various individuals and groups.

Differences

The Omaha System, when considered in its entirety, is *different* from other nursing tools. Differences involve structure, adaptability, and orientation. In contrast to those models just delineated, the Omaha System was designed to incorporate nursing diagnoses, nursing interventions, and client outcomes into a unified, comprehensive system. When the three components of the Omaha System are used together, they provide a model or conceptual framework for nursing practice as well as data management. The Omaha System is a model for designing forms or software needed to support practice and manual or automated management information systems. It was designed to be compatible with evolving computer technology and reimbursement systems. The advantages of a computerized system relate to the capability of rapidly generating and manipulating individual client/health care provider data as well as diverse aggregate clinical and financial data. Because of the simplicity and flexibility of the Omaha System, the forms or software can be very basic or complicated.

The cost of implementing the Omaha System varies in direct proportion to the complexity of the forms and software. For example, if the entire Omaha System is used to develop a simple, integrated paper record, the cost is equal to or less than other paper records. If the Omaha System is used as the basis for programming personal computer or mainframe software in order to produce extensive outputs, the cost increases substantially. Other costs associated with implementing the Omaha System involve ensuring that the staff continue to use it correctly through orientation and inservice programs. These costs vary with the skill and motivation of agency personnel and with the complexity of agency systems. Although expense is inevitable when implementing the Omaha System, savings result from use of standard language.

The Omaha System differs from existing tools in that it was developed as a research-based model specifically for a community health setting. Because of the trend for the practice of nursing to move from the traditional acute care setting into the community, the value of the Omaha System is likely to increase with time. More nurses and members of other disciplines will be practicing within the community health setting and documenting their services. The increase in numbers of practitioners as well as in the number and size of community health agencies will cause data management and costing requirements to escalate.

Concerned, committed nurses throughout the country are developing innovative practice models designed to address a variety of health issues. As delineated in this book, many nurses are incorporating the Omaha System into their practice and documentation. Sally Lundeen, Nancy Kreuser, and Barbara Friedbacher describe a practice model developed by nursing faculty at the University of Wisconsin-Milwaukee. Their Nursing Center, located in a low-income inner city area, functions collaboratively with a wide variety of human service programs.

OMAHA SYSTEM APPLICATIONS FOR THE FUTURE

by SALLY LUNDEEN, RN, PhD, Nursing Center Director, University of Wisconsin–Milwaukee Nursing Center, Milwaukee, WI;

NANCY KREUSER, RN, MS, Nursing Center Program Manager, University of Wisconsin–Milwaukee Nursing Center, Milwaukee, WI; and

BARBARA FRIEDBACHER, RN, MS, Nursing Center Program Manager, University of Wisconsin–Milwaukee Nursing Center, Milwaukee, WI

The problems facing individuals and families in today's society are staggering. The nation's embarrassing infant mortality and adolescent pregnancy rates and the phenomenal rise in sexually transmitted diseases, substance abuse, child abuse, and child neglect cannot be separated from issues related to poverty, unemployment, inadequate educational systems, homelessness, and racism. The human and monetary costs associated with these problems are of increasing concern to community residents and health and human service providers as well as to local, state, and national policymakers. The solutions require complex assessment and intervention strategies. Furthermore, the evaluation of the impact of particular intervention models is no longer a luxury but rather a necessity as increased accountability in relation to quality and cost-effectiveness is being demanded.

Comprehensive, community-based, coordinated care models may be the best strategies to help families and communities gain control over these interrelated areas of concern. These models use an interdisciplinary team to integrate health, social, education, recreation, employment training, and support services. Community nursing centers offer an opportunity to experiment with comprehensive coordinated models. These centers provide direct client access to professional nurses who serve as care providers as well as coordinators of health care and health-related services. Such innovative delivery models will require powerful, flexible data management tools in order to fully document and evaluate their impact on the targeted population. Furthermore, aggregate data can provide information that will serve to direct policy decisions.

One collaborative, comprehensive, community-based, coordinated care model has been developed by the University of Wisconsin-Milwaukee Nursing Center in conjunction with the Silver Spring Neighborhood Center. Services offered at the Center include day care, meals for elders and low-income children, an alternative middle school program, tutoring and mentoring, job training, recreation for youth and young adults, a graduate equivalency degree (GED) program, and an emergency food pantry. The Nursing Center was implemented in 1986. Staffing is provided by a team of six master's-prepared nurse clinicians who, with the support of nursing faculty, graduate and undergraduate students, and outreach staff, provide services for more than 50 hours per week.

Nursing services include health assessments, risk appraisals and screening, counseling, support groups, wellness programs, health education sessions, home visiting, and health consultations for clients of all ages. In addition, nurse clinicians serve as case managers and coordinators of care across these health-related programs. Approximately 700 direct client encounters are recorded each month.

The Omaha System was selected for this demonstration project after careful consideration. The requirements of a data system included flexibility, power, and applicability across a broad spectrum of issues within a community context. In addition, the tools had to deal simultaneously with assessment, intervention, and outcome analysis. The ability to computerize the data was mandatory due to the strong research components of the project. The Omaha System has provided the means to capture a broad data set; it can generate meaningful information and reports to define client needs, nursing interventions, and outcomes for this low-income, urban population.

Expanded applications of the Omaha System are currently being developed. These applications have important implications for the future use of the System on a nationwide basis. The first application involves implementation across all on-site programs. The staff at the neighborhood house includes nurse practitioners, community health nurses, outreach workers, family advocates, social workers, teachers, day care workers, recreation workers, and a variety of support personnel. Multidisciplinary use of the Omaha System provides a common language for individual client and family assessment as well as for development and implementation of comprehensive, interdisciplinary plans. Consistent documentation of client problems, interventions, and outcomes allows staff to assess program effectiveness.

The second application entails use of the Problem Classification Scheme as a comprehensive intake tool. The domains and categories of the Scheme provide a framework for nurses and non-nurses to comprehensively and systematically review potential problems with individuals and families. In the case of disadvantaged individuals and families, this sort of review is critical to the development of an intervention plan that deals with client strengths as well as problems. Such an assessment guide can provide the structure necessary to complete a comprehensive assessment without distraction of immediate or crisis-related client problems. In addition, a self-assessment tool based on Problem Classification Scheme categories is being considered. Although some modification of the Scheme may be necessary, there are several advantages. Clients who engage in a collaborative process of defining their own needs are much more likely to continue participation in a collaborative problem-solving process with providers. It is critical to optimal client outcomes that the accuracy of staff perceptions of needs and appropriate interventions be measured, at least in part, against the perceptions of the clients themselves. Further research projects could be developed to compare assessments made by clients and staff or by clients and staff of various disciplines.

The third application involves modification of the Omaha System for use with small groups. Many of the interventions directed at clients in community settings, particularly in the areas of prevention and health promotion, are tested in group settings. In a comprehensive practice model, these interventions are part of a program of services provided to clients individually and in groups. Descriptions of problems and interventions provided in group settings are important to the documentation of what nurses and other health-related professionals actually do with clients.

One of the strengths of the Omaha System is its ready conversion to a computerized format. Additional modifica-

tion will be needed to allow linkage of group and individual data in the computerized data base. This linkage will facilitate analysis of all services provided to clients, regardless of the modality. Further, such a linkage will allow providers to better assess the impact of various combinations of interventions with various client populations.

The final application involves use of the Omaha System as a tool for analysis of aggregate client and provider data. Such data analysis is critical for health policy research. Current US health care delivery mechanisms are not effective or efficient in meeting the needs of much of our population. This is true for persons of all ages, ethnic groups, and socioeconomic levels. It is particularly true for those disadvantaged by poverty, lack of education, and lack of employment. We must develop alternative delivery systems that better reach, assess, and intervene with those populations at greatest risk. We must be able to describe the nature of the problems of various populations, that which we do to intervene in those problems, that which works and does not work, and how much specific interventions cost. Such data must be collected by clinicians having the best understanding of and the most consistent access to those populations. Data must be analyzed and disseminated in language that can be easily understood by policy developers and policymakers at local, state, and national levels.

The Omaha System offers a mechanism for aggregation and interpretation of client data routinely collected by clinicians. Software programs can be developed to allow data analysis by various sociodemographic, problem, and intervention groupings. The outcome ratings that are an integral part of the system allow continuous monitoring of the progress of individuals and aggregates. The terminology is understandable to analysts not directly providing health care, making interpretation of the data fairly straightforward and providing a wealth of continuous data for health policy research.

The future of the Omaha System will be determined by the extent to which it is useful to health care practitioners, policymakers, and others in health-related fields. The strength of any classification system lies in its applicability and adaptability. The Omaha System is applicable in a variety of settings and with a variety of disciplines. It is useful as a client assessment tool and a means of generating meaningful data for the health policy arena.

RESEARCH

Further refinement of the Omaha System will result from ongoing research. VNA of Omaha staff began conducting federally funded research as early as 1975. Due to the uniqueness of any research that is proposed and directed by a service setting staff, agency personnel have been widely recognized for their efforts. Even in the 1990s, few nurse clinicians have significant roles in research (Sneed, 1990).

The VNA of Omaha agency staff, management, and board are committed to continuing Omaha System re-

search, improving the client record, and integrating client data with other management data. The agency's fourth research project is funded by the National Center for Nursing Research, the National Institutes of Health. The purpose of the 1989 to 1991 prospective study is to examine the applicability of the entire Omaha System by examining reliability, efficiency, and utility. Discriminate analysis will be used to investigate trends among nursing diagnoses/problems, nursing interventions, and client outcomes among and between sites. Principles of triangulation are being used to guide the 18-month data collection process. Data will be obtained from 4,000 client records, quarterly time studies, shared home visits, staff discussions, and a provider acceptability questionnaire. The results of the study will provide the basis for revising the Omaha System as needed and for future studies involving reimbursement and staffing.

Omaha Project Participants

Home health nursing staff from the VNA of Omaha and three other agencies are essential members of the research team. The other participating agencies are Beatrice (NE) Community Hospital Home Health Care, Visiting Nurse Association of Trenton (NJ), and Polk County (WI) Public Health Nursing Service.

These diverse agencies exhibit several characteristics comparable to diverse home health agencies throughout the US. The characteristics involve (1) agency organization (voluntary, official, and hospital-based), (2) agency location (three distant states), (3) agency size and budget (annual client visits range from 6,000 to 90,000), (4) agency programs (varied), (5) client demographics (across age, economic, cultural, and ethnic groups), (6) nature of staff (employ diverse staff in addition to community health nurses), and (7) previous experience with the Omaha System.

VNA of Omaha staff have used the Problem Classification Scheme since 1976 and all three components of the Omaha System since their completion at the conclusion of the 1986 research project. Polk County nurses began using the Problem Classification Scheme in 1981 and the other two components in 1988. Trenton staff, who began using the Problem Classification Scheme in 1983, were introduced to the Problem Rating Scale for Outcomes and the Intervention Scheme as part of the orientation to the research grant at the onset of data collection in 1990. The community health nurses at Beatrice used a narrative client record until November, 1989, when project orientation was given. At that time, they were introduced to all three components of the Omaha System and a completely revised record.

Other Researchers

Omaha System research is increasing in quantity, quality, and diversity. It is an integrated and essential part of the activities of individuals, groups, and sites described in the previous chapters and in numerous publications listed in the Omaha System Bibliography (Appendix). Doctoral and master's program students are selecting the Omaha System for investigation and are contributing to the knowledge base. Burns and Thompson (1984) used the Problem Classification Scheme to develop a nursing diagnosis classification system specifically for pediatric nurse practitioners. Peters (1988) used the Problem Classification Scheme

to develop a Community Health Intensity Rating Scale for describing nursing care requirements and measuring resource consumption. Like Peters, Hays (1990) investigated nursing care requirements and resource consumption. The nursing diagnoses of the Problem Classification Scheme explained 27% of the variation in the sample of 237 clients. In addition, use of the three modifiers was important in explaining variance. Aden and Warren (1991) examined the use of nursing diagnoses and the Problem Classification Scheme by school health nurses.

SUMMARY

The momentum in nursing and medicine that began during the prehistoric era has continued to accelerate during the twentieth century. These explosive, continuing changes are closely linked to industrialization, science, and technology. Advances in government systems, transportation, and communication have changed daily life. Although prominent nurses of earlier centuries communicated with each other and with leaders in related fields, they experienced many serious obstacles. Collectively, developments have made communication nearly instantaneous and isolation nearly impossible. Except in underdeveloped countries, radical technologic changes have occurred nationally as well as internationally. The Omaha System, as described throughout this book, is an example of a tool that facilitates communication and builds on current technology.

Just as community health nurses were challenged in the past, so will future community health nurses be challenged. Successes of the past are not enough to guarantee successes in the future. Florence Nightingale issued a lofty challenge for 1860, which is applicable for the twenty-first century, when she declared that "no system can endure that does not march" (Nightingale, 1860, p. 448). How far can community health nursing "march" amidst the changes of the future? As far as the passions and systems of the collective body of pragmatists and dreamers, optimists and pessimists, leaders and followers, risk takers and security seekers are willing to go. As far as the wisdom and competence of innovative, pioneering staff nurses, supervisors, directors, researchers, writers, educators, and students have the courage and strength to take the specialty.

REFERENCES

Aden, C., & Warren, J. (1991). A validation study of NANDA's taxonomy I. In Carroll-Johnson, R. (Ed.), *Classification of Nursing Diagnosis: Proceedings of Ninth National Conference.* Philadelphia, J. B. Lippincott.

Benner, P., & Wrubel, J. (1989). *The Primacy of Caring.* Menlo Park, CA, Addison-Wesley.

Burns, C., & Thompson, M. (1984, November/December). Developing a nursing diagnosis classification system for PNPs. *Pediatr. Nurs., 10*:411–414.

Curtin, L. (1989, September). Conflictus avoidus: The humming birds of prey. *Nurs. Manag.*, 20:7–8.

Donahue, M. (1985). *Nursing the Finest Art: An Illustrated History.* St. Louis, C. V. Mosby.

Hays, B. (1990). *Relationships Among Nursing Care Requirements, Selected Patient Factors, Selected Nurse Factors, and Nursing Resource Consumption in Home Health Care.* Unpublished doctoral dissertation, Case Western Reserve University, Cleveland, OH.

Hinshaw, A. (1989). Keynote address: Nursing diagnosis: Forging the link between theory and practice. In Carroll-Johnson, R. (Ed.), *Classification of Nursing Diagnoses: Proceedings of the Eighth Conference* (pp. 3–10). Philadelphia, J. B. Lippincott.

Lang, N., Galliher, J., & Hirsch, I. (1989). Challenge to the profession. In *Classification Systems for Describing Nursing Practice* (pp. 70–73). Kansas City, MO, American Nurses' Association.

Lant, T. (1988). Use of the nursing minimum data set to determine nursing care cost. In Werley, H., Lang N. (Eds.), *Identification of the Nursing Minimum Data Set* (pp. 325–333). New York, Springer.

McCloskey, J. (1989, January). Implications of costing out nursing services for reimbursement. *Nurs. Manag.*, 20:44–49.

Nightingale, F. (1860). *Notes on Nursing.* New York, D. Appleton & Company.

Peters, D. (1988, July/August). Development of a community health intensity rating scale. *Nurs. Res.*, 37:202–207.

Secretary's Commission on Nursing (1988, December). *Secretary's Commission on Nursing: Final Report*, Vol. I. Washington, DC, DHHS.

Sneed, N. (1990, January/February). Curiosity and the year to discover. *Nurs. Outlook*, 38:36–39.

BIBLIOGRAPHY

Abdellah, F. (1957, June). Methods of identifying covert aspects of nursing problems. *Nurs. Res.*, 6:4–23.

Abt Associates (1984). *Home Health Services: An Industry in Transition—Home Health Agency Prospective Payment Demonstration.* Cambridge, MA.

Ahmadi, K. (1990). The American health-care "system": A structural nightmare. In Wold, S. (Ed.), *Community Health Nursing: Issues and Topics* (pp. 57–79). Norwalk, CT, Appleton & Lange.

American Nurses' Association (1980). *Nursing: A Social Policy Statement.* Kansas City, MO.

Aydelotte, M. (1987, May/June). Nursing's preferred future. *Nurs. Outlook*, 35:114–120.

Barnard, K. (1984a, March/April). Commonly understood outcomes. *Matern. Child Nurs.*, 9:99.

Barnard, K. (1984b). *Newborn Nursing Models: Final Report of Project.* Supported by grant No. R01 NJ-00719, Division of Nursing, Bureau of Health Manpower, Health Resources Administration (HRSA), DHHS. Seattle, WA, University of Washington.

Bayer, R., Callahan, D., Caplan, A., et al. (1988, May). Toward justice in health care. *Am. J. Public Health*, 78:583–588.

Benner, P. (1984). *From Novice to Expert.* Menlo Park, CA, Addison-Wesley.

Boesch, D. (Ed.) (1990, January). CHAP develops consumer-oriented outcome standards. *Hosp. Home Health*, 7:1.

Brett, J. (1989). Outcome indicators of quality care. In Henry, B. Arndt, C., DiVincenti, M., et al. (Eds.), *Dimensions of Nursing Administration: Theory, Research, Education, and Practice* (pp. 353–369). Boston, Blackwell.

Brooten, D. Kumar, S., Brown, L., et al. (1986, October 9). A randomized clinical trial of early hospital discharge and home follow-up of very-low-birth-weight infants. *New Engl. J. Med., 315:* 934–939.

Bulechek, G., & McCloskey, J. (1985). *Nursing Interventions: Treatments for Nursing Diagnoses.* Philadelphia, W. B. Saunders.

Caliandro, G., & Judkins, B. (Eds.) (1988). *Primary Nursing Practice.* Glenview, IL, Scott, Foresman.

Campbell, C. (1984). *Nursing Diagnosis and Intervention in Nursing Practice* (2nd ed.). New York, John Wiley & Sons.

Carper, B. (1978, October). Fundamental patterns of knowing in nursing. *Adv. Nurs. Sci.*, 1:13–23.

Carroll-Johnson, R. (Ed.) (1989). *Classification of Nursing Diagnoses: Proceedings of the Eighth Conference.* Philadelphia, J. B. Lippincott.

Caserta, J. (1987, September/October). People, not paper. *Home Healthcare Nurse*, 5:1.

Chaska, N. (Ed.) (1978). *The Nursing Profession: Views Through the Mist.* New York, McGraw-Hill.

Curtin, L. (1986, June). Nursing in the year 2000: Learning from the future. *Nurs. Manag.*, 17:7–8.

Curtin, L. (1987, March). The "employment" of autonomy. *Nurs. Manag.*, 18:9–12.

Daubert, E. (1977, March). A system to evaluate home health care services. *Nurs. Outlook*, 25:168–171.

Diers, D. (1986, June). To profess—To be a professional. *J. Nurs. Admin.*, 16:25–30.

Diers, D. (1988, Fall). On money . . . *Image*, 20:122.

Donabedian, A. (1976). Some basic issues in evaluating the quality of health care. *Issues and Evaluation Research* (pp. 3–28). Kansas City, MO, American Nurses' Association.

Edwards, L., & Dees, R. (1990). Environmental health: The effects of life-style on the world around us. In Wold, S. (Ed.), *Community Health Nursing: Issues and Topics* (pp. 231–265). Norwalk, CT, Appleton & Lange.

Fagin, C. (1989, January/February). Why the quick fix won't fix today's nursing shortage. *Nurs. Econom.*, 7:36–60.

Felton, G. (1987, May/June). Obstacles to nursing's preferred future. *Nurs. Outlook*, 35:126–128.

Goertzen, I. (1987, May/June). Making nursing's vision a reality. *Nurs. Outlook*, 35:121–123.

Gordon, M. (1987). *Nursing Diagnosis: Process and Application* (2nd ed.). New York, McGraw-Hill.

Griffith, E. (1986, August). The home health agency: Past, present, and future. *Caring*, 5:12–15.

Hanlon, J., & Pickett, G. (1984). *Public Health Administration and Practice.* St. Louis, Times Mirror/Mosby.

Henderson, V. (1990, April). Excellence in nursing. *Am. J. Nurs.*, 90:76–77.

Holleran, C. (1988, March/April). Nursing beyond national boundaries: The 21st century. *Nurs. Outlook*, 36:72–75.

Horn, B., & Swain, M. (1977). *Development of Criterion Measures of Nursing Care*, Vol. I. Ann Arbor, MI, University of Michigan.

Hoskins, L., McFarlane, E., Rubenfeld, M., et al. (1986, April). Nursing diagnosis in the chronically ill: Methodology for clinical validation. *Adv. Nurs. Sci.*, 8:80–89.

Jenny, J. (1989). Classification of nursing diagnosis: A self-care approach. In Carroll-Johnson, R. (Ed.), *Classification of Nursing Diagnoses: Proceedings of the Eighth Conference* (pp. 152–157). Philadelphia, J. B. Lippincott.

Joel, L. (1984, January/February). DRGs and RIMs: Implications. *Nurs. Outlook*, 32:42–49.

Johnson, M. (1990). Growing old in America: Health care for the elderly. In Wold, S. (Ed.), *Community Health Nursing: Issues and Topics* (pp. 357–377). Norwalk, CT, Appleton & Lange.

Jones, K. (1990, May). Nurses day is time for change. *Am. Nurse*, 22:5.

Jones, P. (1988, May). Nursing shortage: A caring shortage. *Caring*, 7:15–18.

Kalisch, P., & Kalisch, B. (1986). *The Advance of American Nursing* (2nd ed.). Boston, Little, Brown.

Kelly, L. (1988, May/June). Calculated risk: Big payoff. *Nurs. Outlook*, 36:125.

Kelly, L. (1990, January/February). Nursing's velvet revolution. *Nurs. Outlook*, 38:15.

Lancaster, J. (1986, March). 1986 and beyond: Nursing's future. *J. Nurs. Admin.*, 16:31–37.

Laxton, C. (Ed.) (1988, February). Prospective payment. *Caring*, 7(2):2–3.

Lohn, K. (Ed.) (1990). *Medicare: A Strategy for Quality Assurance*, (Vol. I). Washington, DC, National Academy Press.

Lunney, M. (1990, January–March). Accuracy of nursing diagnoses: Concept development. *Nurs. Diagnosis*, 1:12–17.

Maraldo, P., & Solomon, S. (1987, Summer). Nursing's window of opportunity. *Image*, 19:83–86.

Marek, K. (1989). Classification of outcome measures in nursing care. In *Classification Systems for Describing Nursing Practice* (pp. 37–42). Kansas City, MO, American Nurses' Association.

Martin, K. (1988, June). Research in home care. *Nurs. Clin. North Am., 23*:373–385.

Martin, K., Scheet, N., Crews, C., et al. (1986). *Client Management Information System for Community Health Nursing Agencies: An Implementation Manual.* Rockville, MD, Division of Nursing, US DHHS, Public Health Service (PHS), HRSA.

Mayers, M. (1983). *A Systematic Approach to the Nursing Care Plan* (3rd ed.). Norwalk, CT, Appleton-Century-Crofts.

McCloskey, J., & Grace, H. (Eds.) (1990). *Current Issues in Nursing* (3rd ed.). St. Louis, C. V. Mosby.

Rahman, F. (1990, April 9). A doctor's remedy. *Newsweek*, 10

Rinke, L. (Ed.) (1987). *Outcome Measures in Home Care: Volume I, Research.* New York, National League for Nursing.

Rinke, L., & Wilson, A. (Eds.) (1987). *Outcome Measures in Home Care: Volume II, Service.* New York, National League for Nursing.

Romano, C., McCormick, K., & McNeely, L. (1982, January). Nursing documentation: A model for a computerized data base. *Adv. Nurs. Sci., 4*:43–56.

Secretary's Commission on Nursing (1988, December). *Secretary's Commission on Nursing: Support Studies and Background Information*, Vol. II. Washington, DC, DHHS.

Shamansky, S. (1987, December). Who is listening to the future? *Public Health Nurs. 4*:201.

Sienkiewicz, J. (1984, November/December). Patient classification in community health nursing. *Nurs. Outlook, 32*:319–321.

Simmons, D. (1980). *A Classification Scheme for Client Problems in Community Health Nursing*, No. HRA 80–16. Hyattsville, MD, DHHS, Bureau of Health Professions, Division of Nursing.

Snyder, M. (1985). *Independent Nursing Interventions.* New York, John Wiley & Sons.

Sovie, M. (1990, January/February). Redesigning our future: Whose responsibility is it? *Nurs. Econom., 8*:21–26.

Stevenson, J., & Tripp-Reimer, T. (Eds.) (1990). *Knowledge About Care and Caring: State of the Art and Future Developments.* Kansas City, MO, American Academy of Nursing.

Stewart, M., Innes, J., Searl, S., et al. (Eds.) (1985). *Community Health Nursing in Canada.* Toronto, Ontario, Gage.

Strickland, O., & Waltz, C. (Eds.) (1988). *Measurement of Nursing Outcomes, Vol. 2, Measuring Nursing Performance: Practice, Education, and Research.* New York, Springer.

Tanner, C. (1988). Curriculum revolution: The practice mandate. In *Curriculum Revolution: Mandate for Change* (pp. 201–216). New York, National League for Nursing.

Tinkham, C., Voorhies, E., & McCarthy, N. (1984). *Community Health Nursing: Evolution and Process in Family and Community* (3rd ed.). Norwalk, CT, Appleton-Century-Crofts.

Visiting Nurse & Home Care (1987). Self-management outcome criteria (SMOC) record form. In Rinke, L., & Wilson, A. (Eds.), *Outcome Measures in Home Care, Vol. II, Service* (pp. 255–260). New York, National League for Nursing.

Waltz, C., & Strickland, O. (Eds.) (1988). *Measurement of Nursing Outcomes, Vol. 1, Measuring Client Outcomes.* New York, Springer.

Waltz, C., Strickland, O., & Lenz, E. (1984). *Measurement in Nursing Research.* Philadelphia, F. A. Davis.

Weidmann, J., & North, H. (1987, December). Implementing the Omaha classification system in a public health agency. *Nurs. Clin. North Am., 22*:971–979.

Werley, H. & Lang, N. (Eds.) (1988). *Identification of the Nursing Minimum Data Set.* New York, Springer.

Will, G. (1988, May 23). The dignity of nursing. *Newsweek*, 80.

APPENDIX

INTRODUCTION

The appendix is divided into eight sections. The first six sections conform to portions of the community health clinical record:

■ **Referral Forms**
Form 1: Home Health Referral
Form 2: Public Health Referral

■ **Client Data/Face Sheets**
Form 3: Patient Information Record Worksheet
Form 4: Patient Information Record

■ **Data Base Forms**
Form 5: Data Base/Problem List Worksheet
Form 6: Data Base (Household)
Form 7: Data Base (Adult)
Form 8: Data Base (Child)
Form 9: Data Base Update
Form 10: Data Base Update

■ **Problems/Ratings/Plans Forms**
Form 11: Client Care Plan/Problem Rating Worksheet
Form 12: Problems/Ratings/Plans Data Input Form
Form 13: Problem List
Form 14: Problem Ratings/Plans
Form 15: Nursing Care Plan
Form 16: Problem Rating Scale for Outcomes

■ **Visit Reports**
Form 17: Skilled Visit Report
Form 18: Long Term Care Visit Report
Form 19: Family Visit Report
Form 20: Public Health Nurse Record of Service

■ **Discharge Summaries**
Form 21: Discharge Summary
Form 22: Dismissal/Transfer Summary

The final two sections contain records for use in school health and nurse-managed clinic programs:

■ **Student Health Record**
Form 23: Student Health Record

■ **Health Maintenance Center Record**
Form 24: Data Base
Form 25: Problems/Plans/Ratings/Progress

The forms in the appendix are intended as examples of ways in which staff at the VNA of Omaha and other agencies have incorporated the nursing diagnoses, interventions, and outcome ratings of the Omaha System into clinical records. An introductory portion of each section contains instructions for the forms and identifies the agency that provided each form. Each form was developed for a specific program and group of staff. Therefore, the style of the form and the amount of detail included in the instructions vary accordingly. Refer to Chapters 9 through 13 for record forms that include sample client data.

The forms may be copied as they appear in the appendix or may serve as a starting point as agency staff develop forms to meet their own unique needs.

REFERRAL FORMS

Referral forms provide a way to gather and disseminate client data at the time of intake. Information on these forms includes: (1) source of referral, (2) demographic information, (3) recent hospitalization or other illness data, (4) medical diagnoses, (5) medical orders, and (6) household and account numbers.

The referral form is completed by an intake nurse or hospital coordinator. The form provides a legal document for the record and includes verification of physician's verbal orders.

Two similar, yet different, referral forms are used at the VNA of Omaha:

Form 1: Home Health Referral (p. 339) used for home health and long-term care client referrals; includes medical orders and other information required by Medicare regulations.
Form 2: Public Health Referral (p. 340) used for antepartal, postpartal, and other preventive client referrals; includes sections to identify multiple family members as well as specific mother-infant data.

CLIENT DATA/FACE SHEETS

A Client Data/Face Sheet is used to document demographic data relative to the family as a unit and to the individual family members. Data on this form include: (1) information regarding other providers of health-related services, (2) billing information, and (3) admission status of each individual family member.

Instructions are provided for two VNA of Omaha forms as follows:

Form 3: Patient Information Record Worksheet (p. 341) completed by the staff member conducting the admission visit; serves as a data entry document for creation of the computer-generated Patient Information Record.

Form 4: Patient Information Record (p. 342) generated by the computer and filed as the first form in the clinical record. Much of the information is coded for data entry.

Patient Information Record (PIR) (Form 4, p. 342)

Instructions

The PIR is organized into the following areas:

1. Household Information
2. Patient Address/Emergency Information
3. Admission Information
4. Funding/Employment Information
5. Other Agency Workers
6. Physician Orders

Admission PIRs are initiated by the Intake Department. The nurse/therapist making the admission visit completes a PIR Worksheet that contains additional required data. Information from the PIR Worksheet must be entered into the computer prior to entry of the billing line for the admission visit. When the admission PIR is printed, the case manager reviews the form and makes any necessary corrections or additions. NOTE: The order and titles of the following data items conform to the printed PIR form; move across the PIR from left to right when more than one item appears on a line.

HOUSEHOLD INFORMATION

NOTE: This section includes the following demographic information:

(1) Household number (assigned by Intake)
(2) Station (agency office)
(3) Address #1 (primary address)
(4) Phone
(5) Address #2 (secondary or previous address)
(6) Census tract
(7) City/State/Zip
(8) Monthly Income
(9) Directions
(10) Case manager

EMERGENCY INFORMATION

NOTE: This section contains space for four entries. Each entry should include the following information:
(1) Last name
(2) First name
(3) Relation
(4) Address
(5) Phone

ADMISSION INFORMATION

NOTE: Use code numbers rather than labels for religion, referral source, program, race, medical diagnosis, and discharge reason. If, however, the client will receive three or fewer visits, the discharge code #7 (Inappropriate/Admit and Dismiss) will be written on the admission PIR. Refer to the list of codes.

LIST OF CODES

COST CENTERS		TYPES OF SERVICES	
01	SKILLED NURSING	A1	SKILLED NURSING CARE
02	SPEECH PATHOLOGY	A2	HOME HEALTH AIDE
03	PHYSICAL THERAPY	A3	SPEECH PATHOLOGY
04	OCCUPATIONAL THERAPY	A4	PHYSICAL THERAPY
05	HOME HEALTH AIDE	A5	SOCIAL WORK
06	SOCIAL WORKER	A6	OCCUPATIONAL THERAPY
07	PHYSICIAN	A7	PASTORAL CARE
08	PASTORAL CARE	A8	SKILLED NURSING CARE —LTC FLU SHOT
20	NURSING SUPERVISION	D1	SKILLED NURSING CARE —PER VISIT
21	ADMINISTRATION/ SUPPORT	D3	SPEECH PATHOLOGY— PER VISIT
22	SUPPLY CLERK	D4	PHYSICAL THERAPY— PER VISIT
23	ESCORT	D6	OCCUPATIONAL
24	VOLUNTEER		THERAPY—PER VISIT
25	VOLUNTEER COORDINATOR	D8	SHC—PER VISIT—LTC FLU SHOT
30	MANAGEMENT	P2	HHA PRIVATE DUTY (BILL 2ND PS)
40	MANAGEMENT/ SUPPORT		

ACCOUNT NUMBERS		TYPES OF VISITS	
150	DIRECT SALARIES	AI	IV/BLOOD ADMIT VISIT
151	PDO OTHER/VACATION	AP	ADMISSION & POST HOSPITAL
152	PDO EMPLOYEE ILLNESS	AV	ASSESSMENT VISIT (NONBILLABLE)
155	ADMINISTRATIVE LEAVE		
156	OVERTIME PAID	BV	BEREAVEMENT VISIT
158	COMPTIME ACCRUED	ER	ERRAND VISIT
159	COMPTIME TAKEN	EV	EVALUATION VISIT—HHA
160	COMPTIME PAID		
163	PER VISIT/CLINIC TIME	HO	HOSPITAL/OFFICE VISIT

PROGRAMS			
		HV	REVISIT
Home Visits		IH	INTENSIVE HOME CARE-HOSPICE
201	HOME HEALTH CARE		
202	NON-CERTIFIED HOSPICE	IV	IV/BLOOD VISIT
205	CERTIFIED HOSPICE	NE	NOT HOME VISIT
206	HOME HEALTH AIDE	NF	NOT FOUND VISIT
270	LONG TERM CARE—SNC	PD	PRIVATE DUTY
272	LONG TERM CARE—HHA	PO	PHYSICIAN ORDER VISIT—LTC
General & Administration		SI	SPLIT IV/BLOOD VISIT
603	G & A	SV	SHARED VISIT
		SW	SOCIAL WORK VISIT (NONBILLABLE)

ACTIVITIES		FUNDING SOURCES	
01	RECORDING/REPORTING	01	MEDICARE
02	PLANNING/ARRANGING	02	MEDICAID EXCESS
03	DIRECT CLIENT SERVICE	03	MEDICAID
04	SHARED VISIT	04	VETERANS ADMINISTRATION
05	EVALUATION VISIT		
06	BEREAVEMENT VISIT	05	HMO/SHARE
07	NOT HOME VISIT	06	HMO/HEALTH AMERICA
09	ORIENTATION	07	HMO/OTHER
10	TRAVEL	08	INSURANCE/GENERAL
11	SUPPLIES	09	EXCLUSIVE CARE
12	QUALITY ASSURANCE	10	
14	STUDENTS' PROGRAM		
15	PUBLIC INFORMATION		

LIST OF CODES *continued*

16	MEETINGS/ CONFERENCES	11	PRIVATE PAY
17	ROUNDTABLE	12	
18	STAFF COUNCIL/ COMMITTEES	13	NO CHARGE
19	INSERVICE/WORKSHOP	20	
26	COURT/LEGAL ACTIVITIES	24	
30	ERRAND VISIT	27	SPECIAL CONTACTS
31	NOT FOUND VISIT	32	
		40	MEDICARE HOSPICE
		41	INSURANCE HOSPICE

50	SUPERVISION
51	SUPERVISOR VISIT
53	MANAGEMENT
57	GENERAL SUPPORT SERVICES
61	RESEARCH

LOCATIONS

A1	HOME
A2	HOSPITAL
A3	OFFICE
H1	OTHER SETTINGS

TIME CODES

05	0.1	5 MINUTES
10	0.2	10 MINUTES
15	0.2	15 MINUTES
20	0.3	20 MINUTES
25	0.4	25 MINUTES
30	0.5	30 MINUTES
35	0.6	35 MINUTES
40	0.7	40 MINUTES
45	0.7	45 MINUTES
50	0.8	50 MINUTES
55	0.9	55 MINUTES
60	1.0	60 MINUTES

DISCHARGE REASONS

01	PATIENT RECOVERED
02	PATIENT STABILIZED
03	MOVED OUT OF SERVICE AREA
04	DECEASED
05	ADMITTED TO INSTITUTION
06	REFUSED SERVICE
07	INAPPROPRIATE
08	OTHER
11	ADMIT & DISMISS (A&D)
12	
13	UNABLE TO LOCATE
14	MULTIPLE NOT HOMES
15	TRANSFER TO STUDENT PROGRAM

HOUSEHOLD STATUS

HH	HEAD OF HOUSEHOLD
W	WIFE
H	HUSBAND
D	DAUGHTER
S	SON
0	OTHER

MARITAL STATUS

D	DIVORCED
M	MARRIED
P	SEPARATED
S	SINGLE
W	WIDOWED

RACE

01	CAUCASIAN
02	BLACK
03	NATIVE AMERICAN
04	ORIENTAL
05	HISPANIC
06	BIRACIAL
07	OTHER

RELIGION

1	CATHOLIC
2	PROTESTANT
3	JEWISH
4	SEVENTH DAY ADVENTIST
5	JEHOVAH'S WITNESS
6	CHRISTIAN SCIENCE
7	OTHER

(1) Social Security #
(2) Relation to head of household
(3) Birth date
(4) Religion (use code #)
(5) Admit date
(6) Referral source (use code #)
(7) Refer date
(8) Program (use code #)
(9) First contact
(10) Race (use code #)
(11) Care started (use date)
(12) Sex
(13) Plan established (use date)
(14) Marital status
(15) Discharged (use date)
(16) Discharge reason (use code #)
(17) Special instructions
(18) ICDA diagnosis (use code)
(19) Diagnosis information (use diagnostic code # from Worksheet)

NOTE: "Special Instructions" appears under each individual's admission information. Include here information that is important to know prior to any client contact (e.g., "Does not know diagnosis," or "Does not speak English"). Any known allergies should also be listed.

FUNDING/EMPLOYMENT INFORMATION

1. Funding Source
   (1) Funding source (use code #)
   (2) Billing number
   (3) Comment
   (4) Effective date
   NOTE: Under "Comment" there is space for 20 characters. Comments are especially necessary if there is more than one active pay source, for example:

Funding Source:	Comment:
Medicare	"SNC 1 × 1 month B-12"
Private Pay	"Other SNC visits/HHA"
	or
Medicare	"PT/HHA"
Private Pay	"SNC"

   NOTE: Correct use of "effective date" is essential for billing purposes. This date is the date of the first home visit (by any discipline) that is charged to the corresponding funding source. If more than one funding source is being used, each active funding source must have the same effective date regardless if one of those funding sources has been heretofore active. Leave all previous effective dates on the PIR to serve as a record of funding sources.

2. Medicaid excess remaining $_____
   NOTE: If the client is on Medicaid excess, the amount of excess is entered if known.

3. Private Pay Guarantor
   NOTE: If the client's bill is sent to someone other than the client, that person's name/address is entered, if known.
   (1) Last name
   (2) Address 1
   (3) First name
   (4) Address 2
   (5) Phone
   (6) City/State
   (7) Zip

4. Employment
   (1) Employer
   (2) Phone
   (3) Title
   (4) Hours of work

OTHER AGENCIES

(1) Agency name
(2) Contract agency (use worker name)
(3) *Phone* (enter telephone #)
   NOTE: There is space for 10 names. Include additional physicians, social workers, and other emergency numbers. The name of the primary physician will be entered in Physician Information; the pharmacy will be entered from the PIR Worksheet.

PHYSICIAN INFORMATION

(1) Primary physician name
(2) Physician address
(3) Physician telephone number
(4) Dates of current medical orders

DATA BASE FORMS

The data base is a defined, systematic method of observing and collecting family and household data according to four domains of the Problem Classification Scheme. In addition to nursing information, it may include data from the physician, physical therapist, speech pathologist, occupational therapist, and other health professionals.

Instructions are provided for six VNA of Omaha forms as follows:

Form 5: Data Base/Problem List Worksheet (pp. 343–352) used by home health, long-term care, preventive, and student learning center personnel to generate a data base and problem list. If this Worksheet is selected for use by preventive staff, they would *not* use Forms 6, 7, 8, and 9.

Form 6: Data Base (Household) (p. 353) used by preventive program for all clients/families admitted to service.

Form 7: Data Base (Adult) (pp. 354–355) used by preventive personnel as a supplement to the Data Base on all adult clients admitted to service.

Form 8: Data Base (Child) (pp. 356–357) used by preventive personnel as a supplement to the Data Base for all infants and children admitted to service.

Form 9: Data Base Update (p. 358) used by preventive personnel to document new or changed information gathered during the course of service.

Form 10: Data Base Update (p. 359) used by student learning center personnel to document new or changed information.

Data Base/Problem List Worksheet

(Form 5, pp. 343–352)

Instructions

The worksheet is used on admission to generate the Data Base and Problem List. It is intended for use primarily during the home visit. Completion is required following a maximum of *3* home visits or 2 weeks, whichever occurs first. The worksheet *must* be legible, understandable, and contain a reasonable amount of pertinent information. The form may be entered into the client record as a handwritten document *or* used to produce a typed or data entered document.

IDENTIFYING INFORMATION

Date Admitted:	Enter date of first home visit.
Date Completed:	Enter date data base completed.
Nurse Name:	Enter name of primary nurse.
Family Name:	Enter family surname.
Household #:	Enter household number.
Account #:	Enter number(s) and name(s) of other family members whose data appear on worksheet.

PROBLEM SECTION (Left Side)

Circle ONE item per problem as follows:

Adequate:	Data have been assessed and no actual or potential problem evident.
Not Assessed:	Data not gathered yet but will be at a later date.
Not Applicable:	Area not appropriate to individual/family.
Health Promotion:	Data indicate individual or family interest in activities directed toward developing resources that maintain or enhance well-being in the absence of risk factors, signs, or symptoms. Must also circle F (family) or I (individual). If I circled, indicate individual account number on line in far left column to identify which individual owns the problem. The problem will appear on the problem list as a health promotion problem.
Potential:	Data indicate a health pattern, practice, or behavior of an individual or family and/or the presence of

predisposing factors which increase the probability of occurrence of a health problem and may preclude optimal health. Risk factors must be listed; they may be similar but *not* identical to signs/symptoms. Must also circle F (family) or I (individual). If I circled, indicate account number on line in far left column to identify which individual owns the problem. The problem will appear on the problem list as a potential problem. The risk factors will appear on the data base.

Deficit/
Impairment/
Actual:

Data indicate an existing health problem of an individual or family. One or more signs/ symptoms must also be circled. Further data regarding each circled sign/symptom *must* appear in the comment section. Must also circle F (family) or I (individual). If I circled, indicate account number on line in far left column to identify which individual owns the problem. The problem will appear on the problem list as an actual problem with signs/symptom(s). Supporting data regarding each s/s will appear on the data base, not s/s.

*Items: Each of these items must be completed. Blanks for specific data are provided under selected problems and should be completed as appropriate.

01 Income
*Source—Identify as ADC, SSI, WIC, food stamps, med. insurance, Medicare, Medicaid, etc. Amount to be completed as possible.
03 Residence
*Type—Describe as house, apartment, rooming house, public housing, etc., and circle own or rent.

*Environmental Assessment—A *brief* statement of nursing judgment which summarizes the collected data. Statement may be a comparison to typical or normal standards of environmental health (e.g., "Adequate environment," "Dangerous or unhealthy living conditions exist").

06 Communication with Community Resources
*Transportation Resources—Identify the mode as owns car, public, handicapped van, walks, depends on others (who).
07 Social Contact
*Support System—Indicate who comprises the network such as family, friends, neighbors, church affiliation, or groups. Other information as location may be pertinent.
*Psychosocial Assessment—Refer to Environmental Assessment. This statement may summarize strengths *and* deficits regarding problem-solving ability, use of community resources, family role flexibility, functional vs. dysfunctional patterns (e.g., "Supportive family," "Not coping well with loss," "Much tension in household").
*Physiological Assessment—Refer to Environmental Assessment. Summary will focus on physical strengths and pathology (e.g., "Within normal limits", "Open wound on right knee—no other significant findings," "Compromised respiratory status limits physical activity," "Unstable GU and cardiac findings," "Impaired NMS status related to age/arthritis/general weakness").

41 Health Care Supervision
*Routine and Emergency Care Plans—Identify care provider as None, ER, clinics (which), or physician (who).

*Health Related Behaviors Assessment—Refer to Environmental Assessment. Statement will summarize type and intensity of patterns (e.g., "Many positive health behaviors noted," "Need system for taking medications," "Not following diet," "Serious deficiency in nutritional intake").
*Homebound Status—described factors that interfere with the client's ability to leave home (e.g., "Extreme weakness, limited ambulation," "Gait unsteady, poor endurance").

COMMENTS SECTION (Right Side of Form)
Use for additional data or elaboration of signs/ symptoms that are not self-explanatory. *Elaboration should be provided for circled signs and symptoms.*

HEALTH HISTORY
For the Medical History of Client and Family Members on the last page of the Worksheet, use one column per individual with reasonable identification per column. Be selective when gathering and recording information. When two diagnoses appear together (i.e., asthma/allergies) and information applies to only one, circle pertinent one. To give further information about

a diagnosis such as allergies, write "Allergies" in AS-SESSMENT/COMMENTS section and describe briefly.

DATA BASE UPDATE

A data base update should be completed when there are significant changes in data base information (e.g., following hospitalizations, changes in living situation, change in family structure). Data base updates will be dated and entered after the initial data base. Updates need only to address those categories that reflect change.

Data Base

Instructions

There are four data base forms developed for use by public health staff:

DATA BASE (Form 6, p. 353)
Includes data from the Environmental and Psychosocial Domains relative to the family unit. Completed on all families admitted to service.

DATA BASE (ADULT) (Form 7, pp. 354–355)
Includes data from the Psychosocial, Physiological, and Health Related Behaviors Domains relative to adults. Completed on all adults admitted to service.

DATA BASE (CHILD) (Form 8, pp. 356–357)
Includes data from the Psychosocial, Physiological, and Health Related Behaviors Domains relative to infants and children. Completed on all infants and children admitted to service.

DATA BASE UPDATE (Form 9, p. 358)
Includes space for pertinent information relative to each domain. Completed as needed to document new or changed information obtained later during the course of care.

The data base forms should be completed in conjunction with a review of the Problem Classification Scheme. The blanks should be filled in as completely as possible to accurately describe the family/client situation. Problem numbers indicative of those problems that will appear on the Problem List should be circled. Always complete the assessment statement at the end of each domain. The forms should be completed legibly in black ink.

Data Base Update (Form 10, p. 359)

Instructions

Use this form in two ways. First, use it to complete Data Base/Problem List Worksheet when the original worksheet was initiated by another nurse. Second, use

the form for updates (1) when there are significant changes (e.g., following hospitalizations, changes in living situation, change in family structure such as the birth of baby) *or* (2) when the data base has not been updated for 1 year.

To complete the Data Base Update, write date, your initials, and the domain in columns provided. Write phrases or short, precise sentences in data base narrative column. Refer to Data Base/Problem List Worksheet for instructions about narrative comments.

PROBLEMS/RATINGS/PLANS FORMS

The Problem List is an index to the client's health status. It contains health and health-related problems, each modified by Health Promotion, Potential, or Actual. In addition, each problem is modified by Individual or Family. Problems are identified from the Environmental, Psychosocial, Physiological, and Health Related Behaviors domains. There should be at least one problem identified relevant to each discipline that is providing service (e.g., #27 for Physical Therapy). Some problems may be addressed by more than one discipline.

Only those problems (a small, realistic number) that the nurse and family will be currently addressing should have written plans. Each problem-specific plan must include: (1) ratings from the Problem Rating Scale for Outcomes completed at admission, periodic intervals, and dismissal; (2) time frame for rerating; and (3) anticipated interventions based on the Intervention Scheme.

The Problem List, Client Ratings, and Care Plans may be organized as separate forms or combined in a variety of ways. This section includes six sample forms and instructions. Forms 11 to 14 are from the VNA of Omaha; Forms 15 to 16 are from the Polk County (WI) Public Health Nursing Service.

Form 11: Client Care Plan/Problem Rating Worksheet (p. 360) used by the VNA of Omaha home health personnel as a data entry tool for computer-generated problem ratings/care plans. The problem list, a separate form, is generated from the Data Base/Problem List worksheet (see Form 5).

Form 12: Problems/Ratings/Plans Data Input Form (p. 361) used by the VNA of Omaha public health personnel. The form is designed for incorporation into the clinical record or as a data entry tool for computer-generated problems, ratings, and plans forms.

Form 13: Problem List (p. 362) used by the VNA of Omaha student learning center personnel in conjunction with the Data Base/Problem List Worksheet (see Form 5).

Form 14: Problem Ratings/Plans (p. 363) used by the VNA of Omaha student learning center personnel.

Form 15: Nursing Care Plan (pp. 364–365) used by

the Polk County (WI) Public Health Nursing Service staff.

Form 16: Problem Rating Scale for Outcomes (p. 366) used by the Polk County (WI) Public Health Nursing Service staff.

Client Care Plan/Problem Rating Worksheet (Form 11, p. 360)

Instructions

ADMISSION PROBLEM RATINGS AND PLANS

Problems, ratings, and plans are entered on this Worksheet, which is used to produce a computer-generated Problem Ratings/Plans form. All admission, interim, and dismissal ratings are retained as part of the permanent client record. Information is recorded on the Problem Ratings/Plans Worksheet as follows:

(1) Client name
(2) Household number
(3) Date
(4) Problem number (need only to give number).
(5) Problem Rating Scale for Outcomes.
   a. Knowledge rating—K 1, 2, 3, 4, or 5.
   b. Behavior rating—B 1, 2, 3, 4, or 5
   c. Status rating—S 1, 2, 3, 4, or 5.
(6) Enter intervention category number
(7) Enter number(s) for one or more targets.
(8) Enter client-specific narrative.

When using the same plan or parts of a plan for more than one problem:

(1) For the first problem, complete numbers 4 through 8.
(2) For the next problem(s), complete numbers 4 and 5.
(3) State, "see plan, problem _____" or see plan/problem, _____ numbers _____" (if using only part of the plan).

INTERIM RATINGS/PLANS

This information is data entered and completed when significant client change occurs *or* every 60 days in conjunction with recertification of physician orders. The interim ratings/plans are written on a photocopy of the current Ratings/Plans as follows:

(1) Indicate any change in numeric Knowledge, Behavior, and/or Status ratings for each problem.
(2) Indicate any changes in the plans for each problem. If no change is necessary, write "no change."
(3) If the problem is resolved, indicate at the bottom of the plan for that problem.

DISMISSAL RATINGS

This information is required at the time the client record is closed. On a photocopy of the most recent Problem Ratings/Plans sheet, indicate numeric ratings for Knowledge, Behavior, and Status of each problem. Indicate "client dismissed" at the end of each plan.

Problems/Ratings/Plans Data Input Form (Form 12, p. 361)

Instructions

Problems, ratings, and plans are entered on this Worksheet, which is used to produce a computer-generated Problem List and Problem Ratings/Plans form.

1. Complete identifying information as follows:
   (1) Type of ratings (admission, update, discharge)
   (2) Household number
   (3) Household name
   (4) Nurse name

2. For each problem, complete the following:
   (1) Name of individual or family to whom the problem applies
   (2) Problem number from the Problem Classification Scheme
   (3) F (family) or I (individual)—circle one
   (4) HP (health promotion), P (potential), or A (actual)—circle one
   (5) Signs/symptoms: for actual problems, circle all appropriate numbers from the Problem Classification Scheme

3. For each priority problem, complete the following:
   (1) Ratings: circle one number (1–5) for each concept (Knowledge, Behavior, Status)
   (2) Review: circle one number (2, 3, or 4) indicative of the time frame for planned reassessment of the ratings.

4. For each priority problem, complete the following:
   (1) Interventions: circle each intervention that is being planned (I Health Teaching, Guidance and Counseling; II Treatments and Procedures; III Case Management; IV Surveillance)
   (2) Targets: enter checks to indicate the planned targets of each circled intervention.
   (3) Client-specific Comments: enter a brief description specific to the client for each checked target.

Problem List (Form 13, p. 362)

Instructions

The initial problem list is established on the Data Base/Problem List worksheet. Use this form as a summary to recopy all identified Actual, Potential, and/or Health Promotion problems from the worksheet. Use this form for adding, preventing, or resolving problems. Refer to the Problem Classification Scheme for terminology and numbers to complete this form. Sign your name in column provided.

Problem Ratings/Plans (Form 14,

p. 363)

Instructions

Only those most significant or serious priority problems (a small, realistic number) that the nurse and family will be currently addressing should have written plans. Priority problems should be small in number, realistic, and reflect the significant nurse-client interaction documented on the visit report forms.

Use one-half page for each problem addressed. Each problem-specific plan must include:

(1) Current date
(2) Admission, interim, and dismissal ratings using the Problem Rating Scale for Outcomes
(3) Time frame in weeks or months for when reratings are scheduled
(4) Anticipated interventions (a plan) based on the Intervention Scheme

ADMISSION RATINGS/PLANS

Complete as soon after client admission as reasonable.

(1) Write problem and date in appropriate columns for selected, priority problems.
(2) Thoughtfully select and write a number (1–5) in the rating column for K, B, and S (when rating, always complete all three). Refer to the Problem Rating Scale for Outcomes. Write date in weeks or months when rerating is anticipated. Write your name on the line provided.
(3) In the Plan section, record the date of your entry. Write the three parts of the plan: category, target, and client-specific comments. First, use the letters or codes for (1) Health Teaching, Guidance, and Counseling, (2) Treatments and Procedures, (3) Case Management, or (4) Surveillance listed on the Intervention Scheme. The codes are listed on the Skilled Visit Report. Next, use one or more (a small, realistic number) targets, again referring to the words and codes of the Intervention Scheme. Last, generate and write (*briefly*) client-specific comments, the most detailed portion of the plan.

INTERIM RATINGS/PLANS

At the appropriate update time, review ratings and plans.

(1) Write current date, numerical rating codes, date in weeks or months when rerating is anticipated, and your name.
(2) If no change in the plan, write current date, your initials, and "no change". If changing or adding to a plan, use procedure described in Admission Ratings/Plans. If more space is needed for a plan, turn form over and use back of page.

DISMISSAL RATINGS/PLANS

Review ratings and plans.

(1) Write current date, numerical rating codes, and your name.
(2) Write "client dismissed" after last entry on the page.

Polk County (WI) Public Health Nursing Service Nursing Care Plan (Form 15, pp. 364–365)

CREATING A NURSING CARE PLAN

1. The first page of the nursing care plan with heading information will be generated from the Data Face Sheet. Nursing care plans are due within 7 days of start of care.
2. Identify only those problems from the Problem List for which nursing intervention will be done. The nurse may use professional judgment on what problems will be included in the Nursing Care Plan and when. The nurse should be realistic, practical, and have reasonable expectations. Not all problems can be a priority. Plans may be written for other problems later.
3. It is very important that the intervention categories, targets, and client-specific data are consistent between the plan and the Skilled Visit Report (SVR). In most instances, the nurse cannot carry out an intervention on a SVR if it does not appear on the Nursing Care Plan. Also, if interventions are specified on the Nursing Care Plan and never appear on the SVR, negligence of practice may be suspected.
4. For *each problem* currently on the Nursing Care Plan:
   (1) Select an intervention category.
   (2) Select one or more targets for that category. Multiple targets may be combined for one category if they are similar enough to appear to "go together."
   (3) For each *target*, specify client-specific narrative. Client-specific narrative may reference protocols or doctor orders. Client-specific narrative answers the following questions:
      a. What am I doing about teaching/counseling?
      b. What specific action is taken for a treatment/ procedure?
      c. What do I need to do to carry out case management for a particular target?
      d. What areas specifically are under surveillance?

UPDATING

1. The Nursing Care Plan must be reviewed, but not necessarily altered, at least every 2 months.
2. Problems, categories, targets, or interventions may be changed at any time to reflect client needs.

3. When altering an existing nursing plan of action, the first action must be discontinued and restated as an addition (i.e., reducing frequency of treatment).
4. Face sheets will be revised manually.
5. After hospitalization, dictate a new effective date and update the Face Sheet.

ADDITIONS

1. Problems
   (1) Follow procedure for admitting any problem.
   (2) Additional problems will be entered after the last initial problem on Nursing Care Plan.
2. Categories and Targets—May be added at any time.
3. Nursing Plan of Action—Nursing plan of action may be added at any time.

DISCHARGES

1. Problems—On final discharge, problems are to be discontinued by dating each problem on the nursing care plan and dating and signing the update section on the face sheet.
2. Categories—use revision sheet to discontinue.
3. Targets—Use revision sheet to discontinue.
4. Nursing Plan of Action—Use revision sheet to discontinue nursing plan of action or portion of nursing plan of action. An effective date of discharge will appear directly following statement.

Polk County (WI) Public Health Nursing Service Problem Rating Scale For Outcomes (Form 16, p. 366)

COMPONENTS

1. The Problem Rating Scale is part of the Nursing Care Plan and documents outcome of nursing intervention. The Scale provides an evaluation framework for examining problem-specific client ratings at regular or predictable time intervals. The ratings serve two significant purposes. First, the ratings are a guide for the community health nurse or other health care professionals as client care is planned and provided. Second, the ratings reflect client progress throughout the period of agency service.
2. The rating scale is the last page of the Nursing Care Plan and stays in the chart at all times.
3. The rating scale is produced manually by the nurse.
4. The rating scale measures the concepts of Knowledge, Behavior, and Status.
   (1) Knowledge is the ability of the client to remember and interpret information.
   (2) Behavior is the observable responses, actions, or activities of the client fitting the occasion or purpose.
   (3) Status is the condition of the client in relation to objective and subjective defining characteristics.

5. The rating scale is a five-point Likert scale. Likert scales are subjective in nature. There is no right or wrong numerical rating, but rather the judgement of the individual nurse is recorded. A definition of the five-point ranking for each concept is included on the form.

ADMISSION AND CREATION OF NEW PROBLEMS AFTER ADMISSION

1. Every problem on the Nursing Care Plan (not the Problem List) is entered across the top of the form with the problem number and name (may be abbreviated).
2. Choose the rating for Knowledge, Behavior, and Status for each problem using the nurse's individual best judgement.
3. If the rating refers to the caretaker's Knowledge, Behavior, or Status instead of the patient's, use a subscript "C" within the box with the number. It is likely that Knowledge or Behavior will be ranked for the caretaker, while Status will be ranked for the patient. Any box containing a plan number will be that of the patient.
4. Date and sign each rating.
5. The admission rating should be done within the first three visits. When a new problem is identified, rate on the visit the date the problem is identified.

INTERIM RATINGS AND FREQUENCY

1. Any one or more problems may be rated *whenever* there is a significant change. The nurse can change just one mode (K, B, or S) or any combination for any problem(s). All changes must be dated and signed.
2. Mandatory frequency
   (1) Home Care Skilled—on admission, visit closest to every 2 months, and discharge.
   (2) Home Care Personal Care and Long Term Care —on admission, every 6 months, and on discharge.
   (3) Public Health (face-to-face visits only)—on admission, significant change, or new problem; otherwise interim as appropriate, on discharge.
3. Transfer Public Health/Home Care—Rerate all modes and problems on admission to new service.

DISCHARGE

1. On discharge all problems must have a termination rating.
2. When a *problem* is discharged, rate it and note "D/C'd" in square.
3. If a problem discharge and patient total discharge are close in dates, the nurse can rate all at discharge at nurse's discretion.

TECHNICAL PROCEDURES—SPECIAL CONSIDERATION

1. The technical procedure problem is often unique because the nurse is the one doing it and the patient

is never expected to assume the responsibility for the technical procedure. However, the rating should not reflect the Knowledge, Behavior, or Status of the nurse (i.e., catheter care, IV and Hickman procedures, B12 shots, etc.).

2. Knowledge — Rate the Knowledge level of the patient or caretaker regarding why the procedure is being done. You may also need to rate the knowledge about observing the area or technical equipment while the nurse is not in the home. The patient or caretaker should have some level of knowledge about the technical procedure in order to identify problems when the nurse is not present.

3. Behavior — Rate the patient or caretaker's Behavior in terms of dealing with the technical equipment or site appropriately when the nurse is not there. You may also rank follow-through on teaching done regarding the technical procedure, site, or handling of crisis situations.

4. Status — Rate the Status of the patient's response surrounding the reason they are having a technical procedure done. This may duplicate a Status ranking that has been done under a more diagnostic-related problem, but it is helpful to have it here also. For instance, if a patient has a urinary catheter, the Status of the patient may have been ranked under "Genito-Urinary Problem," but may also be rated under "Technical Procedure" if the nurse is actually doing the insertion or care of a catheter.

SIGNIFICANCE OF RATINGS

NOTE: If the ratings do not change, it does not mean that the nurse has failed. Ratings are not meant to be a grade for the nurse. It may simply mean:

1. The nurse has been successful in preventing a regression on the part of the patient or in preventing a crisis.
2. The patient is not amenable to the intervention and the nurse may want to try a different tactic.
3. The patient is not willing to work with the nurse and the patient should now be evaluated for appropriateness of continuing service.
4. A different resource may be needed in order to affect change.
5. The patient has reached a maintenance level that still calls for nursing care.

VISIT REPORTS

The Visit Report forms are probably the most important professional and legal forms in the record. They are critical to the professional care providers and those who review records for quality assurance and reimbursement purposes. Care activities and professional judgement as well as client progress should be distinctly documented on the Visit Report. Documentation on the Visit Report should be in agreement with the most significant information from the data base

and problem list as well as the problem ratings and plans.

This section includes instructions and samples for five visit report forms as follow:

Form 17: Skilled Visit Report (pp. 367–368) used by all professional disciplines at the VNA of Omaha in the home health program.

Form 18: Long Term Care Visit Report (p. 369) used by nursing staff of the LTC program at the VNA of Omaha.

Form 19: Family Visit Report (p. 370) used by nursing staff of the preventive program at VNA of Omaha.

Form 20: Public Health Nurse Record of Service (p. 371) used by nursing staff at the Midland County (MI) Health Department.

Skilled Visit and Long Term Care Visit Reports (Forms 17 and 18, pp. 367–369)

Instructions

A handwritten Visit Report must be completed within 1 working day of the home visit. Black ink should be used. Identifying information:

(1) Household number
(2) Client name: first and last name
(3) Date: month/day/year
(4)* Time: indicate time visit began and circle a.m. or p.m.
(5)* Unscheduled: check if appropriate and provide a brief description of reason for visit.
(6)* Homebound due to: provide a brief description of the client's functional limitations. N/A (not applicable) may be used *only* if the client is not homebound, regardless of funding source.

CLIENT PROBLEMS

Circle the number of the problem being addressed. If the problem is not listed, write the problem number and name on the blanks under the appropriate domain (Environmental, Psychosocial, Physiological, Health Related Behaviors). NOTE: The entire Problem Classification Scheme is printed on the back of the form. Enter any home visit data in appropriate blanks.

SUBJECTIVE/OBJECTIVE

Enter any data collected during the course of the home visit relative to circled problems. If collected data appears elsewhere on the record, reference the form (e.g., "see Data Base").

CAT/TARG/RX*

Enter the Category Number and Target number from the Intervention Scheme (printed on the right

---

*Skilled Visit Report only

margin) for each intervention performed during the home visit. Enter the appropriate Medicare treatment code (printed on the back of the form) for each intervention performed during the home visit.

INTERVENTIONS/COMMENTS
Enter client-specific narrative to further describe each intervention performed during the home visit.

ASSESSMENT
Enter a brief assessment of the client's status in relation to problems addressed during the visit.

PLAN: FREQUENCY AND REASON
Enter short-term plan data (i.e., actions to be taken prior to the next visit, purpose of next visit, frequency of visits).

SIGNATURE
Legal signature. Circle appropriate discipline and enter employee number.

Family Visit Report (Form 19, p. 370)

Instructions
Complete legibly in black ink to document each home visit. Enter household number; name, patient account number, and age of each individual who received service during the visit; and the visit date.

NURSING PROBLEM/ASSESSMENT PARAMETER
Nutrition, Caretaking/Parenting, Growth and Development, and Family Planning represent problems frequently encountered. Data regarding other problems should be entered in the space provided. The problem name and number must be indicated. Enter subjective and objective data as appropriate.

INTERVENTIONS
Enter the category number and target number from the Intervention Scheme (printed on the right border of the form) and narrative client-specific comments for each intervention provided during the home visit.

ASSESSMENT
Enter a brief statement of the nurse's assessment of the client.

PLAN
Enter information relative to the next planned home visit.

SIGNATURE
Enter legal signature and title.

Midland County (MI) Health Department Public Health Nurse Record of Service
(Form 20, p. 371)

Instructions
1. Write client name, family folder number, and narrative page number on lines provided.
2. In DATE column, write date of service being recorded.
3. In SITE column, write abbreviation for the site of the service being recorded. Use Site abbreviations listed under CODES at the top of the page.
4. In PROB. NO. column, write the number(s) of the problems addressed during the service being recorded. Choose problem numbers from those identified on the client's PROBLEM LIST.
5. In CARE PROVIDED column, write abbreviation for the Care Provided/Interventions used by the nurse during the service being recorded. Use abbreviations listed under CODES at the top of the page.
    (1) Whenever "Assessment" is coded, indicate the basis for that assessment after the code by writing the title of the assessment used. Choose from those listed after "**Basis:" at the top of the page.
    (2) Whenever "Teaching" is coded, indicate the reference for that teaching after the code by writing the title of the reference used and the sections from that reference by chapter or topic and page number.
    (3) Whenever "Coordination, Advocacy and Referral" is coded, write the name of the agency or professional involved after the code.
    (4) Whenever "Surveillance" is coded to indicate such procedures as blood pressure readings or weight checks, write the blood pressure reading, weight, etc., after the code.
6. In NARRATIVE column, write contents of the service using SOAP format. At the end of each NARRATIVE entry, sign your name.
7. In REVISIT DATE column, write the date on which the next visit to the client is planned.

DISCHARGE SUMMARIES

The Discharge Summary serves a dual purpose. First, it documents review of the client's condition, services provided, and reason for discharge for the clinical record. Second, it provides a summary and notification of discharge for the physician. Instructions for two forms are provided as follow:

Form 21: Discharge Summary (p. 372) used by the VNA of Omaha home health personnel.
Form 22: Dismissal/Transfer Summary (p. 373) used by students at the VNA of Omaha Student Learning Center.

Discharge Summary (Form 21, p. 372)

Instructions

The staff person dismissing the client initiates a Discharge Summary form. Items that must be completed by the staff person are:

(1) Date
(2) Client name
(3) Service provided by (check services being discontinued)
(4) Type of service provided (check all that apply)
(5) Comments—as needed. If not all disciplines are discontinuing service, indicate that in this blank
(6) Unresolved problems—as needed
(7) Discharged to
(8) Signature (include discipline)

The Discharge Summary form should be clipped to the Clinical Record and submitted for supervisory review. The supervisor will forward the record for clerical processing.

The clerk will:

1. Complete the Discharge Summary form
   (1) Physician name (from orders)
   (2) Client address
   (3) First visit date (from PIR)
   (4) Last visit date (from Progress Notes)
   (5) Primary diagnosis (from medical orders)
2. Make a photocopy of the form to be retained in the clinical record.
3. Complete the PIR

(1) Date of dismissal
(2) Reason for dismissal
4. Mail the completed Discharge Summary to the appropriate physician(s).

Dismissal/Transfer Summary (Form 22, p. 373)

Instructions

This form allows the nurse to synthesize and summarize care provided during the semester. Usually, one page will provide adequate space for the narrative description although a second page may be used. The completed form becomes part of the permanent client record and is sent to the referral source as a method of showing appreciation for the referral and of indicating continuing client progress. It is essential that your handwriting be legible.

The Summary should include the following sections:

(1) Date service began.
(2) Number and types of visits provided.
(3) Individual or family status when care began *and* at present.
(4) Other resources/agencies contacted.
(5) Disposition/Transfer Plan—particularly important since this justifies the termination or continuation of service.

Text continued on page 374

FORM 1

Date: ____ / ____ / ____ H/Hold #: _____ CT: _____

Account #: _____ , _____ , _____

SS #: _____

Payment Discussed? Y ☐ N ☐ Fax Y ☐ N ☐

Medicare #: _____

Source: (Name) _____

Medicaid #: _____

Relationship: _____ Phone: _____

Ins _____ # _____

Previous VNA Record?: N ☐ Y ☐ Date From ____ / ____ / ____ to ____ / ____ / ____

Other # _____

Rejected? ☐ on ____ / ____ / ____

Patient (Last Name First): _____ Birth Date: ____ / ____ / Sex: M ☐ F ☐ Marital Status: S ☐ M ☐ W ☐ D ☐ Sep ☐

Street Address: _____ City: _____ Zip: _____ Phone: _____

Spouse/Parent: _____ Birth Date: ____ / ____ / ____

Emergency Contact: _____ Relationship: _____ Phone: _____

Hospital: _____ from ____ / ____ / ____ to ____ / ____ / ____ SNF: from ____ / ____ / ____ to ____ / ____ /

Physician: _____ Address: _____ Phone: _____

Physician: _____ Address: _____ Phone: _____

Primary Diagnosis: (Dates) _____

Secondary Diagnosis: (Dates) _____

Mental State:

Alert ☐   Depressed ☐

Forgetful ☐   Disoriented ☐

Other _____ Confused ☐

Functional Limits:

Mental ☐   Ambulation ☐
                 Vision ☐
Speech ☐   Respiratory ☐

Other _____ Hearing ☐

Range of Vital Signs and Lab:

BP _____ P _____ R _____

Blood Sug. _____ Wt. _____

Lives Alone ☐ With Other ☐ _____ H & P Req: Y ☐ N ☐ Pharmacy _____

Significant Information: _____

Service: Nursing ☐   Physical Therapy ☐   Speech Therapy ☐   Occupational Therapy ☐   Home Health Aide ☐

Medical Orders/Plan of Treatment: Medical Social Work ☐

_____

_____   Activity Tolerance: _____

_____   Diet: _____

_____   Allergies: _____

_____   Meds/Dosage: _____

_____

_____

_____

_____

_____

_____

Supplies: _____

M.D. Signature _____   R.N. Signature _____

Additional Information on Attached Sheet: Y ☐ N ☐

FORM 2

DATE: _____ H/HOLD #: _____ CT: _____   URGENT VISIT _____ REASON _____

ACCOUNT #: _____   _____

NOTIFIED HEALTH DEPT. _____ STATION: _____

Payment Discussed Y ☐ N ☐   FAX Y ☐ N ☐   S.S.# _____

MEDICAID # _____ VERIFIED Y ☐

SOURCE NAME: _____   INS. _____

RELATIONSHIP: _____ PHONE _____   POLICY # _____

Previous Record N ☐ Y ☐ DATE FROM _____ TO _____   OTHER # _____

REJECTED? ☐ ON _____   IS CLIENT AWARE OF REFERRAL? _____

HEAD OF HOUSEHOLD (Last Name, First) _____   BIRTH DATE _____ SEX M ☐ F ☐   MARITAL STATUS S ☐ M ☐ W ☐ D ☐ SEP ☐

STREET ADDRESS: _____ CITY _____ ZIP _____ PHONE _____

VNA#	NAME	BIRTH DATE	SEX	VISITS	DATE

EMERGENCY CONTACT NAME: _____ RELATIONSHIP: _____ PHONE: _____

REASON FOR REFERRAL: _____

EXPLANATION OF CARE REQUESTED: TREATMENTS, DRESSINGS, INJECTIONS, TEACHING, OBSERVATIONS, EVALUATIONS, OTHER _____

MOTHER	INFANT

MOTHER

DIAGNOSIS: _____

PHYSICIAN: _____

ADDRESS: _____

PHONE: _____

HOSPITAL _____ DATES: _____ TO _____

E.D.C. _____ BREAST FEEDING: _____

DELIVERY DATE: _____ TYPE _____

BONDING: _____

B.P.: _____ MENTAL STATUS _____

MEDICATION & DOSAGE: _____

M.D. SIGNATURE: _____

INFANT

DIAGNOSIS: _____

PHYSICIAN: _____

ADDRESS: _____

PHONE: _____

HOSPITAL _____

BIRTH WEIGHT: _____

APGAR: _____ 1 MIN _____ 5 MIN _____

GESTATION: _____

FORMULA TYPE: _____ AMT. _____

MEDICATIONS & DOSAGE: _____

RETURN APPOINTMENT _____

R.N. SIGNATURE: _____

ADDITIONAL INFORMATION ATTACHED SHEET Y ☐ N ☐

340

FORM 3

PATIENT INFORMATION RECORD WORKSHEET

Name: _____ Birth Date:_____

Social Security Number:_____

Annual Income	**Religion**	**Race**
1. 0–$4,999	1. Catholic	1. Caucasian
2. $5,000–$9,999	2. Protestant	2. Black
3. $10,000–$19,000	3. Jewish	3. Native American
4. $20,000–$49,000	4. Seventh Day Adventist	4. Oriental
5. $50,000–$99,000	5. Jehovah's Witness	5. Hispanic
6. $100,000 or more	6. Christian Scientist	6. Biracial
	7. Other	7. Other

Allergies: _____

_____

Pharmacy: _____ Phone: _____

FOR OFFICE USE ONLY

Account Number _____

DIAGNOSTIC CODES

Admit Date:_____ First Contact: _____

Program: _____

- 010 Neoplasms
- 011 Malignant
- 012 Non-malignant
- 020 Endocrine, Nutrition, Metabolic
- 021 Diabetes
- 030 Diseases of the Blood and Blood-Forming Organs
- 040 Mental Disorders
- 041 Drug Dependency
- 042 Alcohol Abuse
- 043 Mental Retardation
- 050 Diseases of the Nervous System and Sense Organs
- 051 Multiple Sclerosis
- 052 Disorders of the Eye and Ear
- 053 Muscular Dystrophy
- 060 Diseases of Circulatory System
- 061 Cardiac
- 062 Cerebrovascular Disease
- 063 Hypertension
- 070 Diseases of the Digestive System
- 080 Diseases of the Genitourinary System
- 090 Complications of Pregnancy/Childbirth
- 100 Diseases of Skin and Subcutaneous Tissues
- 110 Diseases of Musculoskeletal System
- 111 Arthritis
- 120 Congenital Anomalies
- 130 Injury and Poisoning
- 131 Fractures
- 140 Diseases of Respiratory System
- 850 AIDS/AIDS–Related Complex

OTHER AGENCY WORKERS

Agency	Worker	Phone
_____	_____	_____
_____	_____	_____
_____	_____	_____
_____	_____	_____

FUNDING SOURCE

#	Billing #	Comment	Effective Date
01	_____	_____	_____
02	_____	_____	_____
03	_____	_____	_____
05	_____	_____	_____
08	_____	_____	_____
11	_____	_____	_____

Case Manager: _____

FORM 4

                        PATIENT INFORMATION RECORD   PAGE

Household #:   Station:
Address 1:   Phone:
Address 2:   Census Tract:
City/St/Zip: Monthly Income:
Directions:
Case Manager:

                         ACCOUNTS IN HOUSEHOLD
Patient's Name: Account #: Birth Date: Rel. to HH:

Patient's Name: Account #:

** EMERGENCY INFORMATION   Relation: Address: Phone:

** ADMISSION INFORMATION
   Soc Sec #:   Rel. to HH:
   Birth Date: Religion:
   Admit Date: Referral Code:
   Refer Date: Program:
   1st Contact: Race:
   Care Started: Sex:
   Plan Establ.:   Marital Sts:
   Discharged: Discharge Reason:
   Special Instructions:
   ICDA Diagnosis:

** DIAGNOSIS INFORMATION

** FUNDING SOURCES   Billing #:   Comment: Effect Date.

** EMPLOYER -

** OTHER AGENCIES   Contact: Phone:

                                         Orders Cover
** PHYSICIAN INFORMATION   From Date: To Date:

FORM 5

DATA BASE/PROBLEM LIST WORKSHEET

Instructions: Circle **one** choice (Adequate, Not Assessed, Not Applicable, Health Promotion, Potential **or** Deficit/Impairment/Actual). CIRCLE F (Family) **or** I (Individual) **only** when using Health Promotion, Potential, or Deficit/Impairment/Actual. If Potential is circled, Risk Factors must be listed. If Deficit/Impairment is circled, one or more Signs/Symptoms (S/S) must be circled. If S/S are circled, elaboration must be included in the comments section. Starred (*) items on the worksheet must be completed.

Date Admitted _____
Date Completed _____
Nurse Name_____
Family Name _____
Household # _____
Account #_____
Account # _____
Account # _____

DOMAIN I. ENVIRONMENTAL

01. INCOME:

Adequate   Not Assessed   Not Applicable   Health Promotion
*Source _____

_____ Amount _____

F **Potential**, Risk Factors:_____
I **Deficit**, S/S: 1) low/no income 2) uninsured medical expenses
\# 3) inadequate money management 4) able to buy only
_____ necessities 5) difficulty buying necessities 6) other _____

02. SANITATION:

Adequate   Not Assessed   Not Applicable   Health Promotion
F **Potential**, Risk Factors:_____
I **Deficit**, S/S: 1) soiled living area 2) inadequate food storage/ disposal 3) insects/ rodents 4) foul odor 5) inadequate water supply 6) inadequate sewage disposal 7) inadequate laundry
\# facilities 8) allergens 9) infectious/contaminating agents
_____ 10) other _____

03. RESIDENCE:

Adequate   Not Assessed   Not Applicable   Health Promotion
*Type _____

Own   Rent

F **Potential**, Risk Factors:_____
I **Deficit**, S/S: 1) structurally unsound 2) inadequate heating/ cooling 3)steep stairs 4)inadequate/obstructed exits/entries 5) cluttered living space 6) unsafe storage of dangerous objects/substances 7) unsafe mats/throw rugs 8) inadequate safety devices 9) presence of lead-based paint 10) unsafe
\# gas/electrical appliances 11) inadequate/crowded living space
_____ 12) homeless 13) other _____

04. NEIGHBORHOOD/WORKPLACE SAFETY:

Adequate   Not Assessed   Not Applicable   Health Promotion
F **Potential**, Risk Factors:_____
I **Deficit**, S/S: 1) high crime rate 2) high pollution level
\# 3) uncontrolled animals 4) physical hazards 5) unsafe play
_____ area 6) other _____

05. OTHER: S/S: 1) other

*Environmental Assessment: _____

FORM 5

DOMAIN II. PSYCHOSOCIAL

Household # _____

06. COMMUNICATION WITH COMMUNITY RESOURCES:

Adequate   Not Assessed   Not Applicable   Health Promotion

*Transportation Resources _____

_____

F   **Potential**, Risk Factors: _____

I   **Impairment**, S/S: 1) unfamiliar with options/procedures for obtaining services 2) difficulty understanding roles/regulations of service providers 3) unable to communicate concerns to

service provider 4) dissatisfaction with services 5) language

_____ barrier 6) inadequate/unavailable resources 7) other _____

_____

07. SOCIAL CONTACT:

Adequate   Not Assessed   Not Applicable   Health Promotion

*Support System _____

_____

F   **Potential**, Risk Factors: _____

I   **Impairment**, S/S: 1) limited social contact 2) uses health care

provider for social contact 3) minimal outside stimulation/

_____ leisure time activities 4) other _____

_____

08. ROLE CHANGE:

Adequate   Not Assessed   Not Applicable   Health Promotion

F   **Potential**, Risk Factors:_____

I   **Impairment**, S/S: 1) involuntary reversal of traditional male/ female roles 2) involuntary reversal of dependent/independent

roles 3) assumes new role 4) loses previous role 5) other

_____

_____

09. INTERPERSONAL RELATIONSHIP:

Adequate   Not Assessed   Not Applicable   Health Promotion

F   **Potential**, Risk Factors: _____

I   **Impairment**, S/S: 1) difficulty establishing/maintaining relationships 2) minimal shared activities 3) incongruent values/ goals 4) inadequate interpersonal communication skills

5) prolonged, unrelieved tension 6) inappropriate suspicion/

_____ manipulation/compulsion/aggression 7) other _____

_____

10. SPIRITUAL DISTRESS:

Adequate   Not Assessed   Not Applicable   Health Promotion

F   **Potential**, Risk Factors: _____

I   **Actual**, S/S: 1) expresses spiritual concerns 2) disrupted

spiritual rituals 3) disrupted spiritual trust 4) conflicting

_____ spiritual beliefs and medical regimen 5) other _____

_____

11. GRIEF:

Adequate   Not Assessed   Not Applicable   Health Promotion

F   **Potential**, Risk Factors: _____

I   **Impairment**, S/S: 1) fails to recognize normal grief responses 2) difficulty coping with grief responses 3) difficulty expressing

grief responses 4) conflicting stages of grief process among

_____ family/individual 5) other _____

_____

344

FORM 5

Household # _____

12. **EMOTIONAL STABILITY:**
      Adequate Not Assessed Not Applicable Health Promotion

F **Potential**, Risk Factors: _____

I   **Impairment**, S/S: 1) sadness/hopelessness/worthlessness
2) apprehension/undefined fear 3) loss of interest/involvement
in activities/self-care 4) narrowed perceptual focus 5) scattering
of attention 6) flat affect 7) irritable/agitated 8) purposeless
activity 9) difficulty managing stress 10) somatic complaints/
\#   chronic fatigue 11) expresses wish to die/attempts suicide
——— 12) other _____

13. **HUMAN SEXUALITY:**
      Adequate Not Assessed Not Applicable Health Promotion

F **Potential**, Risk Factors: _____

I   **Impairment**, S/S: 1) difficulty recognizing consequences of
sexual behavior 2) difficulty expressing intimacy 3) sexual
\#   identity confusion 4) sexual value confusion 5) dissatisfied with
——— sexual relationships 6) other_____

14. **CARETAKING/PARENTING:**
      Adequate Not Assessed Not Applicable Health Promotion
      *Primary Caregiver: _____

F **Potential**, Risk Factors: _____

I   **Impairment**, S/S: 1) difficulty providing physical care/safety
2) difficulty providing emotional nurturance 3) difficulty providing
cognitive learning experiences and activities 4) difficulty
providing preventive and therapeutic health care 5) expectations
incongruent with stage of growth and development
\#   6) dissatisfaction/difficulty with responsibilities 7) neglectful
——— 8) abusive 9) other _____

15. **NEGLECTED CHILD/ADULT:**
      Adequate Not Assessed Not Applicable Health Promotion

F **Potential**, Risk Factors: _____

I   **Actual**, S/S: 1) lacks adequate physical care 2) lacks emotional
nurturance/support 3) lacks appropriate stimulation/cognitive
\#   experiences 4) inappropriately left alone 5) lacks necessary
——— supervision 6) inadequate/ delayed medical care 7) other ____

16. **ABUSED CHILD/ADULT:**
      Adequate Not Assessed Not Applicable Health Promotion

F **Potential**, Risk Factors: _____

I   **Actual**, S/S: 1) harsh/excessive discipline 2) welts/bruises/
burns 3) questionable explanation of injury 4) attacked
verbally 5) fearful/hypervigilant behavior 6) violent
\#   environment 7) consistently negative messages 8) assaulted
——— sexually 9) Other _____

FORM 5

17. GROWTH AND DEVELOPMENT OF CHILD/ADULT:
    Adequate   Not Assessed   Not Applicable   Health Promotion
    Height_____ Weight____ Head Circumference_____
    Feeding_____
    Newborn PA_____

F **Potential,** Risk Factors: _____

I   **Impairment,** S/S: 1) abnormal results of development
    screening tests 2) abnormal weight/height/head circumference
    in relation to growth curve/age 3) age inappropriate behavior

4) inadequate achievement/maintenance of developmental
_____tasks 5) other _____

Household # _____

_____

_____

_____

_____

_____

_____

18. OTHER: S/S: 1) Other

*Psychosocial Assessment: _____

_____

DOMAIN III. PHYSIOLOGICAL

19. HEARING:
    Adequate   Not Assessed   Not Applicable   Health Promotion
    Correction _____

F **Potential**, Risk Factors: _____

I   **Impairment,** R _____ L _____ S/S: 1) difficulty hearing normal

speech tones 2) absent/abnormal response to sound
_____ 3) abnormal results of hearing screening test 4) other _____

_____

_____

_____

_____

_____

20. VISION:
    Adequate   Not Assessed   Not Applicable   Health Promotion
    Correction _____

F **Potential**, Risk Factors: _____

I   **Impairment,** R _____ L _____ S/S: 1) difficulty seeing small print/
    calibrations 2) difficulty seeing distant objects 3) difficulty
    seeing close objects 4) absent/abnormal response to visual
    stimuli 5) abnormal results of vision screening test

6) squinting/blinking/tearing/blurring 7) difficulty differentiating
_____ colors 8) other _____

_____

_____

_____

_____

_____

_____

21. SPEECH AND LANGUAGE:
    Adequate   Not Assessed   Not Applicable   Health Promotion

F **Potential**, Risk Factors: _____

I   **Impairment,** S/S: 1) absent/abnormal ability to speak
    2) absent/abnormal ability to understand 3) lacks alternative
    communication skills 4) inappropriate sentence structure

5) limited enunciation/clarity 6) inappropriate word usage
_____ 7) other _____

_____

_____

_____

_____

_____

22. DENTITION:
    Adequate   Not Assessed   Not Applicable   Health Promotion
    Correction _____

F **Potential**, Risk Factors: _____

I   **Impairment,** S/S: 1) abnormalities of teeth 2) sore/swollen/
    bleeding gums 3) ill-fitting dentures 4) malocclusion 5) other

#
_____

_____

_____

_____

_____

346

FORM 5

23. COGNITION:

          Adequate   Not Assessed   Not Applicable   Health Promotion

F   **Potential,** Risk Factors: _____

I   **Impairment,** S/S: 1) diminished judgment 2) disoriented to time/place/person 3) limited recall of recent events 4) limited recall of long past events 5) limited calculating/sequencing skills 6) limited concentration 7) limited reasoning/abstract

thinking ability 8) impulsiveness 9) repetitious language/

_____ behavior 10) other _____

24. PAIN:

          Adequate   Not Assessed   Not Applicable   Health Promotion

F   **Potential,** Risk Factors: _____

I   **Actual,** Description _____

    Relieved by: _____

    S/S: 1) expresses discomfort/pain 2) elevated pulse/respirations/blood pressure 3) compensated movement/

guarding 4) restless behavior 5) facial grimaces 6) pallor/

_____ perspiration 7) other _____

25. CONSCIOUSNESS:

          Adequate   Not Assessed   Not Applicable   Health Promotion

F   **Potential,** Risk Factors: _____

I   **Impairment,** S/S: 1) lethargic 2) stuporous 3) unresponsive 4) comatose 5) other _____

#

_____

26. INTEGUMENT:

          Adequate   Not Assessed   Not Applicable   Health Promotion

F   **Potential,** Risk Factors: _____

I   **Impairment,** S/S: 1) lesion 2) rash 3) excessively dry

4) excessively oily 5) inflammation 6) pruritus 7) drainage

_____ 8) ecchymosis 9) hypertrophy of nails 10) other _____

27. NEURO-MUSCULO-SKELETAL FUNCTION:

          Adequate   Not Assessed   Not Applicable   Health Promotion

Assistive Devices _____

F   **Potential,** Risk Factors: _____

I   **Impairment,** S/S: 1) limited range of motion 2) decreased muscle strength 3) decreased coordination 4) decreased muscle tone 5) increased muscle tone 6) decreased sensation 7) increased sensation 8) decreased balance

9) gait/ambulation disturbance 10) difficulty managing activities

_____ of daily living 11) tremors/seizures 12) other _____

Household # _____

FORM 5

28. RESPIRATION:
　　Adequate　Not Assessed　Not Applicable　Health Promotion
　　Rate _____ Assistive Devices _____

F　　**Potential**, Risk Factors: _____
I　　**Impairment**, S/S: 1) abnormal breathing patterns 2) unable to breathe independently 3) cough 4) unable to cough/expectorate independently 5) cyanosis 6) abnormal sputum
\#　　7) noisy respirations 8) rhinorrhea 9) abnormal breath sounds
_____ 10) other _____

29. CIRCULATION:
　　Adequate　Not Assessed　Not Applicable　Health Promotion
　　Temp _____ Assistive Devices _____

　　BP: sitting R _____ L _____ ; standing R _____ L _____ ;
　　lying R _____ L _____
　　Pulses: apical _____ radial _____ peripheral _____
F　　**Potential**, Risk Factors: _____
I　　**Impairment**, S/S: 1) edema 2) cramping/pain of extremities
　　3) decreased pulses 4) discoloration of skin/cyanosis
　　5) temperature change in affected area 6) varicosities
　　7) syncopal episodes 8) abnormal blood pressure reading
　　9) pulse deficit 10) irregular heart rate 11) excessively rapid
\#　　heart rate 12) excessively slow heart rate 13) anginal pain
_____ 14) abnormal heart sounds 15) other _____

30. DIGESTION-HYDRATION:
　　Adequate　Not Assessed　Not Applicable　Health Promotion
　　Assistive Devices _____

F　　**Potential**, Risk Factors: _____
I　　**Impairment**, S/S: 1) nausea/vomiting 2) difficulty/inability to chew/swallow/digest 3) indigestion/reflux 4) anorexia
　　5) anemia 6) ascites 7) jaundice/liver enlargement
\#　　8) decreased skin turgor 9) cracked lips/dry mouth
_____ 10) electrolyte imbalance 11) other _____

31. BOWEL FUNCTION:
　　Adequate　Not Assessed　Not Applicable　Health Promotion
　　Assistive Devices _____

F　　**Potential**, Risk Factors: _____
I　　**Impairment**, S/S: 1) abnormal frequency/consistency of stool
　　2) painful defecation 3) decreased bowel sounds 4) blood in
　　stools 5) abnormal color 6) cramping/abdominal discomfort
\#　　7) incontinent of stool 8) other _____

Household # _____

348

FORM 5

32. GENITO-URINARY FUNCTION:

      Adequate Not Assessed Not Applicable Health Promotion

Assistive Devices _____

F **Potential**, Risk Factors: _____

I **Impairment**, S/S: 1) incontinent of urine 2) urgency/frequency
    3) burning/painful urination 4) difficulty emptying bladder
    5) abnormal urinary frequency/amount 6) hematuria
    7) abnormal discharge 8) abnormal menstrual pattern

9) abnormal lumps/swelling/tenderness of male/female
_____ reproductive organs 10) dyspareunia 11) other _____

---

33. ANTEPARTUM/POSTPARTUM:

      Adequate Not Assessed Not Applicable Health Promotion

AP: *TPAL _____ EDC _____ Date OB Care _____
    Fetal Act/FHR _____
    L&D Prep _____ Abn Lab _____
    Danger Sig _____ Preterm Labor _____
PP: Del Date _____ Bonding _____
    8-point check _____

F **Potential**, Risk Factors: _____

I **Impairment**, S/S: 1) difficulty coping with pregnancy/body
    changes 2) inappropriate exercise/rest/diet/behaviors

3) discomforts 4) complications 5) fears delivery procedure
_____ 6) difficulty breast-feeding 7) other _____

*TPAL = Term (36–42 wk), Preterm (under 36 wk), Abortions, Living
Children

---

34. OTHER: S/S: 1) other

*Physiological Assessment: _____
_____

DOMAIN IV. HEALTH RELATED BEHAVIORS

35. NUTRITION:

      Adequate Not Assessed Not Applicable Health Promotion

Height _____ Weight _____ Diet _____

F **Potential**, Risk Factors: _____

I **Impairment**, S/S: 1) weighs 10% more than average
    2) weighs 10% less than average 3) lacks established
    standards for daily caloric/fluid intake 4) exceeds established
    standards for daily caloric/fluid intake 5) unbalanced diet
    6) improper feeding schedule for age 7) nonadherence to

prescribed diet 8) unexplained/progressive weight loss
_____ 9) hypoglycemia 10) hyperglycemia 11) other _____

---

36. SLEEP AND REST PATTERNS:

      Adequate Not Assessed Not Applicable Health Promotion

F **Potential**, Risk Factors: _____

I **Impairment**, S/S: 1) sleep/rest pattern disrupts family
    2) frequently wakes during night 3) somnambulism

4) insomnia 5) nightmares 6) insufficient sleep/rest for age/
_____ physical condition 7) other _____

Household # _____

349

FORM 5

37. PHYSICAL ACTIVITY:
    Adequate   Not Assessed   Not Applicable   Health Promotion

F **Potential**, Risk Factors:_____

I **Impairment**, S/S: 1) sedentary life style 2) inadequate/

inconsistent exercise routine 3) inappropriate type/amount of

_____ exercise for age/physical condition 4) other _____

38. PERSONAL HYGIENE:
    Adequate   Not Assessed   Not Applicable   Health Promotion

F **Potential**, Risk Factors:_____

I **Impairment**, S/S: 1) inadequate laundering of clothing

2) inadequate bathing 3) body odor 4) inadequate

shampooing/combing of hair 5) inadequate brushing/flossing/

_____ mouth care 6) other _____

39. SUBSTANCE USE:
    Adequate   Not Assessed   Not Applicable   Health Promotion

F **Potential**, Risk Factors:

I **Impairment**, S/S: 1) abuses over-the-counter/street drugs

2) abuses alcohol 3) smokes 4) difficulty performing normal

_____ routines 5) reflex disturbances 6) behavior change 7) other

40. FAMILY PLANNING
    Adequate   Not Assessed   Not Applicable   Health Promotion

Methods _____

F **Potential**, Risk Factors: _____

I **Impairment**, S/S: 1) inappropriate/insufficient knowledge of

family planning methods 2) inaccurate/inconsistent use of

family planning methods 3) dissatisfied with present family

_____ planning method 4) other _____

41. HEALTH CARE SUPERVISION:
    Adequate   Not Assessed   Not Applicable   Health Promotion

*Routine care plans _____

*Emergency care plans _____

f **Potential**, Risk Factors:_____

I **Impairment**, S/S: 1) fails to obtain routine medical/dental

evaluation 2) fails to seek care for symptoms requiring

medical/dental evaluation 3) fails to return as requested to

physician/dentist 4) inability to coordinate multiple

appointments/regimens 5) inconsistent source of medical/

dental care 6) inadequate prescribed medical/dental regimen

_____ 7) other _____

42. PRESCRIBED MEDICATION REGIMEN:
    Adequate   Not Assessed   Not Applicable   Health Promotion

F **Potential**, Risk Factors: _____

I **Impairment**, S/S: 1) deviates from prescribed dosage/

schedule 2) demonstrates side effects 3) inadequate system

for taking medication 4) improper storage of medication 5)fails

to obtain refills appropriately 6) fails to obtain immunizations

_____ 7) other _____

Household # _____

350

FORM 5

43. TECHNICAL PROCEDURE:

    Adequate   Not Assessed   Not Applicable   Health Promotion

F **Potential**, Risk Factors: _____

I **Impairment**, S/S: 1) unable to demonstrate/relate procedure
accurately 2) does not follow/demonstrate principles of safe/
aseptic techniques 3) procedure requires nursing skill

4) unable/unwilling to perform procedure without assistance

———5) unable/unwilling to operate special equipment 6) other ____

Household # _____

_____

_____

_____

_____

_____

44. OTHER: S/S: 1) Other

***Health Behavior
Assessment:** _____

_____

_____

_____

_____

Significant Planning Factors: _____

_____

_____

_____

*Homebound Status: _____

_____

_____

_____

HEALTH HISTORY
Significant Medical History of Client(s)

Hospitalizations:

_____

_____

_____

_____

Pregnancies:

_____

_____

_____

_____

Surgeries:

_____

_____

_____

_____

Injuries:

_____

_____

_____

_____

FORM 5

MEDICAL HISTORY OF CLIENT AND FAMILY MEMBERS

Complete column(s) below indicating client's name(s) and relationship of other pertinent family members. Focus on specific family history as it contributes to client care.

Diagnosis	Name/Relationship					
Diabetes						
Epilepsy						
Cardiac Disease						
Hypertension						
CVA						
Arthritis/Gout						
Cancer						
Frequent Headaches/Migraines						
Asthma/Allergies						
Respiratory Disease						
SIDS						
GI Problems/Ulcers						
Kidney/Bladder Problems						
Phlebitis/Varicose Veins						
Drug/Alcohol Abuse						
Mental Retardation						
Mental Illness						
Other						

ASSESSMENT/COMMENTS: _____

_____

_____

_____

FORM 6

DATA BASE
Date_____

Review entire *PCS; then check or fill in the blanks as needed to describe the situation and circle problem numbers.

HH Acct.#_____ Client Name_____ Nurse_____

DOMAIN I. ENVIRONMENTAL

01. **INCOME:** Amount from Sources: Employment_____ ADC_____
SSI_____ Other_____ Food Stamps_____ WIC_____
Medicaid_____ Health Insurance_____

02. **SANITATION:** Adequate cleanliness_____ Unsafe storage_____
Insects/Rodents_____

03. **RESIDENCE:** Type_____ Stability of residency_____
Adequate space_____ Utilities_____
Hazards/Child Safety_____ Phone_____ Rent_____

04. **NEIGHBORHOOD/WORKPLACE SAFETY:** Safe_____ Hazards_____

OTHER PROBLEMS/DATA:_____

_____

ASSESSMENT:_____

_____

_____

DOMAIN II. PSYCHOSOCIAL

06. **COMMUNICATION WITH COMMUNITY RESOURCES:** Transportation: Public_____ Walks_____
Owns reliable car_____ Depends on others (specify)_____
Accessible services: Groceries_____ Laundry_____ Pharmacy_____ Medical care_____
Language barrier_____ Literate_____
School yr. completed: K-12_____ College_____ Now attending_____

07. **SOCIAL CONTACT:** Lives with: Parents_____ Spouse/Significant other_____ Siblings_____
Children_____ Others_____ Network/Support System Outside Household: Parents_____
Spouse/Significant other_____ Siblings_____ Children_____ Friends_____ Church_____
Others_____ Frequency/manner of contact_____

08. **ROLE CHANGE:**

09. **INTERPERSONAL RELATIONSHIP:** Basic cooperation_____
Decision making_____ Tension_____
Relationship with husband/father of children_____

11. **GRIEF:**

13. **HUMAN SEXUALITY:** Recognizes consequences of behavior_____
Satisfaction with relationships_____

OTHER PROBLEMS/DATA:_____

_____

ASSESSMENT:_____

_____

SIGNIFICANT PLANNING FACTORS:_____

*PCS = Problem Classification Scheme

FORM 7

DATA BASE (ADULT)   Date_____

Review entire PCS; then check or fill in the blanks as needed to describe the situation and circle problem numbers.

Pt. Acct.#_____ Client Name _____ Nurse_____

DOMAIN II. PSYCHOSOCIAL (con't)

14. **CARETAKING/PARENTING:** Primary Caregiver_____ Other caregivers/helpers_____
    Physical care skills_____ Emotional/Nurturing skills_____
    Bonding_____ Appropriate expectations_____ Discipline_____
    Satisfaction/comfort_____ Other_____

15. **NEGLECTED CHILD/ADULT:**

16. **ABUSED CHILD/ADULT:**

OTHER PROBLEMS/DATA:_____

ASSESSMENT:_____

DOMAIN III. PHYSIOLOGICAL

23. **COGNITION:** Problem solving ability_____ Recall ability_____

28. **RESPIRATION:** Rate/Quality_____

29. **CIRCULATION:** Temp_____ BP_____ Pulse/Quality_____ Edema_____

32. **GENITO-URINARY FUNCTION:** Urination_____ Menstruation_____

33. **ANTEPARTUM/POSTPARTUM:** AP:EDC_____ *TPAL_____
    Date OB Care_____ Fetal Act/FHR_____
    L&D Prep_____ Abn Lab._____
    Danger Sig_____ Preterm Labor_____
    PP:Del. Date_____ Bonding_____
    8 point check_____

OTHER PROBLEMS/DATA:_____
_____

ASSESSMENT:_____
_____

*TPAL = Term(36-42 wk), Preterm(under 36 wk), Abortions, Living Children

DOMAIN IV. HEALTH RELATED BEHAVIORS

35. **NUTRITION:** Ht.____ Wt.____ Diet_____

36. **SLEEP/REST PATTERNS:**

37. **PHYSICAL ACTIVITY:** Usual_____

38. **PERSONAL HYGIENE:**

39. **SUBSTANCE MISUSE:** Cigarettes_____ Alcohol_____ Drugs_____

40. **FAMILY PLANNING:** Method/Follow through_____

41. **HEALTH CARE SUPERVISION:** MD_____
    DDS_____ Emergency_____ Other_____

42. **PRESCRIBED MEDICATION REGIMEN:** Rx/OTC_____

FORM 7

43. **TECHNICAL PROCEDURE:**
OTHER PROBLEMS/DATA: _____

_____

ASSESSMENT: _____

_____

MEDICAL HISTORY: If not client, indicate M = Maternal, P = Paternal, or identify other

Vision_____ Hearing_____ Birth Defects_____ HIV/STDs_____ Diabetes_____

Hypertension_____ Cancer_____ SIDS_____ Frequent Headaches/Migraines_____

Drug/Alcohol Abuse_____ Epilepsy_____ Arthritis/Gout_____ GI Problems/Ulcers_____

CVA_____ Kidney/Bladder Problems_____ Mental Retardation_____ Cardiac Disease_____

Respiratory Disease_____ Asthma/Allergies_____ Phlebitis/Varicose Veins_____

Mental Illness_____

Describe Significant Hospitalizations/Illnesses/Injuries/Accidents:_____

_____

Assessment: _____

_____

*TPAL = Term (36-42 wk), Preterm (under 36 wk), Abortions, Living Children

FORM 8

DATA BASE (CHILD)   Date_____

Review entire PCS; then check or fill in the blanks as needed to describe the situation and circle problem numbers.

Pt. Acct.#_____ Client Name _____ Nurse_____

Birth Order_____ Age_____

DOMAIN II. PSYCHOSOCIAL (con't)

15. NEGLECTED CHILD/ADULT:

16. ABUSED CHILD/ADULT:

17. GROWTH AND DEVELOPMENT OF CHILD/ADULT:Wt._____ Ht._____ HC._____

Newborn PA_____

Appearance/activity/personality_____ School/preschool day care_____

Parent interaction_____ Sibling interaction_____

OTHER PROBLEMS/DATA:_____

ASSESSMENT:_____

DOMAIN III. PHYSIOLOGICAL

19. HEARING:

20. VISION:

21. SPEECH AND LANGUAGE:

22. DENTITION:

23. COGNITION:

26. INTEGUMENT:Mongolian Spots_____

27. NEURO–MUSCULO–SKELETAL FUNCTION:Reflexes_____

28. RESPIRATION:Rate/Quality_____ Apnea Monitor_____

29. CIRCULATION:Temp_____ BP_____ Pulse/A/R/F_____

30. DIGESTION–HYDRATION:Colic_____ Indigestion/Reflux_____

31. BOWEL FUNCTION:No. of stools/day_____ Color_____ Consistency_____

32. GENITO–URINARY FUNCTION:

OTHER PROBLEMS/DATA:_____

_____

ASSESSMENT:_____

DOMAIN IV. HEALTH RELATED BEHAVIORS

35. NUTRITION:Breast_____ Formula/Type/24 hour_____

Solids_____ Eating habits_____

FORM 8

36. **SLEEP/REST PATTERNS:** Hours _____

37. **PHYSICAL ACTIVITY:**

38. **PERSONAL HYGIENE:**

41. **HEALTH CARE SUPERVISION:** MD _____
     DDS _____ Emergency _____ Other _____

42. **PRESCRIBED MEDICATION REGIMEN:** Rx/OTC _____
     OTHER PROBLEMS/DATA: _____
     _____

ASSESSMENT: _____
     _____

MEDICAL HISTORY: If not client, indicate M = Maternal, P = Paternal, or identify other

Vision _____ Hearing _____ Birth Defects _____ HIV/STDs _____ Diabetes _____

Hypertension _____ Cancer _____ SIDS _____ Frequent Headaches/Migraines _____

Drug/Alcohol Abuse _____ Epilepsy _____ Arthritis/Gout _____ GI Problems/Ulcers _____

CVA _____ Kidney/Bladder Problems _____ Mental Retardation _____ Cardiac Disease _____

Respiratory Disease _____ Asthma/Allergies _____ Phlebitis/Varicose Veins _____

Mental Illness _____

Describe Significant Hospitalizations/Illnesses/Injuries/Accidents: _____
_____
_____

Assessment: _____
_____

FORM 9

DATA BASE UPDATE

Date_____

P ACCT #_____   Client Name _____   Nurse_____

<u>DOMAIN I. Environmental</u>

<u>DOMAIN II. Psychosocial</u>

<u>DOMAIN III. Physiological</u>

<u>DOMAIN IV. Health Related Behaviors</u>

FORM 10

$*$ $*$ $*$ D A T A   B A S E   U P D A T E $*$ $*$ $*$

Client Name _____ Account # _____

Date	Initials	Domain	Data Base

FORM 11

CLIENT CARE PLAN/PROBLEM RATING WORKSHEET

NAME: _____ DATE: _____

HH# _____ ACCOUNT #_____ ADMIT DATE: _____

PROBLEM CLASSIFICATION SCHEME

DOMAIN I. ENVIRONMENTAL
01. Income
02. Sanitation
03. Residence
04. Neighborhood/workplace safety
05. Other

DOMAIN II. PSYCHOSOCIAL
06. Communication with community resources
07. Social contact
08. Role change
09. Interpersonal relationship
10. Spiritual distress
11. Grief
12. Emotional stability
13. Human sexuality
14. Caretaking/parenting
15. Neglected child/adult
16. Abused child/adult
17. Growth and development
18. Other

DOMAIN III. PHYSIOLOGICAL
19. Hearing
20. Vision
21. Speech and language
22. Dentition
23. Cognition
24. Pain
25. Consciousness
26. Integument
27. Neuro-musculo-skeletal function
28. Respiration
29. Circulation
30. Digestion-hydration
31. Bowel function
32. Genito-urinary function
33. Antepartum/postpartum
34. Other

DOMAIN IV. HEALTH RELATED BEHAVIORS
35. Nutrition
36. Sleep and rest patterns
37. Physical activity
38. Personal hygiene
39. Substance use
40. Family planning
41. Health care supervision
42. Prescribed medication regimen
43. Technical procedure
44. Other

Problem Rating Scale For Outcome

1	2	3	4	5
Poor	Fair	Average	Good	Excellent

INTERVENTION SCHEME CATEGORIES

I. Health Teaching, Guidance, and Counseling
II. Treatments and Procedures
III. Case Management
IV. Surveillance

TARGETS

01. Anatomy/physiology
02. Behavior modification
03. Bladder care
04. Bonding
05. Bowel care
06. Bronchial hygiene
07. Cardiac care
08. Caretaking/parenting skills
09. Cast care
10. Communication
11. Coping skills
12. Day care/respite
13. Discipline
14. Dressing change/wound care
15. Durable medical equipment
16. Education
17. Employment
18. Environment
19. Exercises
20. Family planning
21. Feeding procedures
22. Finances
23. Food
24. Gait training
25. Growth/development
26. Homemaking
27. Housing
28. Interaction
29. Lab findings
30. Legal system
31. Medical/dental care
32. Medication action/side effects
33. Medication administration
34. Medication setup
35. Mobility/transfers
36. Nursing care, supplementary
37. Nutrition
38. Nutritionist
39. Ostomy care
40. Other community resource
41. Personal care
42. Positioning
43. Rehabilitation
44. Relaxation/breathing techniques
45. Rest/sleep
46. Safety
47. Screening
48. Sickness/injury care
49. Signs/symptoms-mental, emotional
50. Signs/symptoms-physical
51. Skin care
52. Social work/counseling
53. Specimen collection
54. Spiritual care
55. Stimulation/nurturance
56. Stress management
57. Substance use
58. Supplies
59. Support group
60. Support system
61. Transportation
62. Wellness
63. Other (specify)

PROBLEM _____

RATINGS
Knowledge_____ Behavior_____ Status_____

PLANS

Category _____ Target _____ Specifics _____
_____

Category _____ Target _____ Specifics _____
_____

Category _____ Target _____ Specifics _____
_____

Category _____ Target _____ Specifics _____
_____

Category _____ Target _____ Specifics _____
_____

PROBLEM _____

RATINGS
Knowledge_____ Behavior_____ Status_____

PLANS

Category _____ Target _____ Specifics _____
_____

Category _____ Target _____ Specifics _____
_____

Category _____ Target _____ Specifics _____
_____

Category _____ Target _____ Specifics _____
_____

Category _____ Target _____ Specifics _____
_____

CASE MANAGER _____

360

FORM 12

PROBLEMS/RATINGS/PLANS
DATA INPUT FORM

ADMISSION _____
UPDATE _____
DISCHARGE _____

HHACCT #: _____   HOUSEHOLD NAME: _____   NURSE: _____

DATE: _____   PACCT # _____   PACCT # _____

NAME _____   NAME _____

PROBLEM NO: ____ F I   **PROBLEM NO:** ____ F I

	HP	P	A	
SIGNS/SYMPTOMS:	01	05	09	13
	02	06	10	14
	03	07	11	15
	04	08	12	16

RATINGS:
KNOWLEDGE 1 2 3 4 5
BEHAVIOR   1 2 3 4 5
STATUS   1 2 3 4 5

REVIEW: (MONTHS)   1   2   3   4

INTERVENTIONS: I   II   III   IV

	HP	P	A	
	01	05	09	13
	02	06	10	14
	03	07	11	15
	04	08	12	16

1 2 3 4 5
1 2 3 4 5
1 2 3 4 5

1   2   3   4

I   II   III   IV

CLIENT SPECIFIC COMMENTS

CLIENT SPECIFIC COMMENTS

TARGETS:

ANATOMY/PHYSIOLOGY	01
BEHAVIOR MODIFICATION	02
BLADDER CARE	03
BONDING	04
BOWEL CARE	05
BRONCHIAL HYGIENE	06
CARDIAC CARE	07
CARETAKING/PARENTING SKILLS	08
CAST CARE	09
COMMUNICATION	10
COPING SKILLS	11
DAY CARE/RESPITE	12
DISCIPLINE	13
DRESSING CHG/WOUND CARE	14
DURABLE MEDICAL EQUIP	15
EDUCATION	16
EMPLOYMENT	17
ENVIRONMENT	18
EXERCISES	19
FAMILY PLANNING	20
FEEDING PROCEDURES	21
FINANCES	22
FOOD	23
GAIT TRAINING	24
GROWTH/DEVELOPMENT	25
HOMEMAKING	26
HOUSING	27
INTERACTION	28
LAB FINDINGS	29
LEGAL SYSTEM	30
MEDICAL/DENTAL CARE	31
MED ACTN/SIDE EFFECTS	32
MEDICATION ADMIN	33
MEDICATION SETUP	34
MOBILITY/TRANSFERS	35
NURSING CARE, SUPPLEMENTARY	36
NUTRITION	37
NUTRITIONIST	38
OSTOMY CARE	39
OTHER COMMUNITY RESOURCE	40
PERSONAL CARE	41
POSITIONING	42
REHABILITATION	43
RELAXATION/BREATHING TECH	44
REST/SLEEP	45
SAFETY	46
SCREENING	47
SICKNESS/INJURY CARE	48
SIGNS/SYMP-MENTAL/EMOTION	49
SIGNS/SYMP-PHYSICAL	50
SKIN CARE	51
SOCIAL WORK/COUNSELING	52
SPECIMEN COLLECTION	53
SPIRITUAL CARE	54
STIMULATION/NURTURANCE	55
STRESS MANAGEMENT	56
SUBSTANCE USE	57
SUPPLIES	58
SUPPORT GROUP	59
SUPPORT SYSTEM	60
TRANSPORTATION	61
WELLNESS	62
OTHER	63

FORM 13

----

* * * P R O B L E M   L I S T   (Actual, Potential, and Health Promotion) * * *

Client Name _____ Account # _____

Date Identi- fied	Signa- ture	Problem (Name, Number, Modifier, and S/S[1])	Problem Change and Date[2]

----

[1]Copy problem information from Data Base/Problem List Worksheet. Name and number = write those of 40 problems which were identified. Modifier = write A (Actual), P (Potential), or HP (Health Promotion) as was identified for each problem. S/S = one or more must be recorded for an actual problem.

[2]To describe change, use Resolved for actual problems, Prevented for Health Promotion or Potential, or leave blank if record closed and problem still exists.

362

FORM 14

---
* * * P R O B L E M   R A T I N G S / P L A N S * * *

Client Name _____ Account # _____

Problem _____

Date _____	Date _____	Date _____	Date _____	Date _____	Date _____
(Initial	(Interim/	(Interim/	(Interim/	(Interim/	(Interim/
Rating)	Dismissal)	Dismissal)	Dismissal)	Dismissal)	Dismissal)
K _____	K _____	K _____	K _____	K _____	K _____
B _____	B _____	B _____	B _____	B _____	B _____
S _____	S _____	S _____	S _____	S _____	S _____
*_____ wks/	_____ wks/	_____ wks/	_____ wks/	_____ wks/	_____ wks/
months	months	months	months	months	months
Signature	Signature	Signature	Signature	Signature	Signature

Plan & Date:

_____

_____

_____

_____

_____

Problem _____

Date _____	Date _____	Date _____	Date _____	Date _____	Date _____
(Initial	(Interim/	(Interim/	(Interim/	(Interim/	(Interim/
Rating)	Dismissal)	Dismissal)	Dismissal)	Dismissal)	Dismissal)
K _____	K _____	K _____	K _____	K _____	K _____
B _____	B _____	B _____	B _____	B _____	B _____
S _____	S _____	S _____	S _____	S _____	S _____
*_____ wks/	_____ wks/	_____ wks/	_____ wks/	_____ wks/	_____ wks/
months	months	months	months	months	months
Signature	Signature	Signature	Signature	Signature	Signature

Plan & Date:

_____

_____

_____

_____

KBS Numerical rating codes: 1=Poor   2=Fair   3=Average   4=Good   5=Excellent
* Rerate scheduled
Plan: Use format from Intervention Scheme (i.e., 1 category: 1 or more
targets: client specific comments).

FORM 15

NURSING CARE PLAN

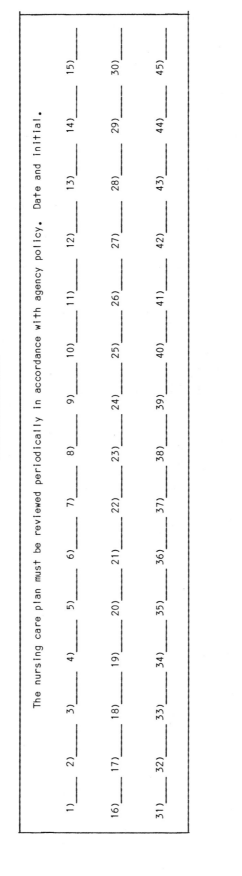

The nursing care plan must be reviewed periodically in accordance with agency policy. Date and initial.

1)_____ 2)_____ 3)_____ 4)_____ 5)_____ 6)_____ 7)_____ 8)_____ 9)_____ 10)_____ 11)_____ 12)_____ 13)_____ 14)_____ 15)_____

16)_____ 17)_____ 18)_____ 19)_____ 20)_____ 21)_____ 22)_____ 23)_____ 24)_____ 25)_____ 26)_____ 27)_____ 28)_____ 29)_____ 30)_____

31)_____ 32)_____ 33)_____ 34)_____ 35)_____ 36)_____ 37)_____ 38)_____ 39)_____ 40)_____ 41)_____ 42)_____ 43)_____ 44)_____ 45)_____

NAME _____ CASE NO. _____ B.D. _____ PHONE _____

ADDRESS _____

CARETAKER _____ RELATIONSHIP _____ PHONE _____ ADDRESS _____

EMERGENCY CARE PLAN:

364

FORM 15

<u>NURSING CARE PLAN</u>

PATIENT NAME:
PATIENT NUMBER:
PAGE:

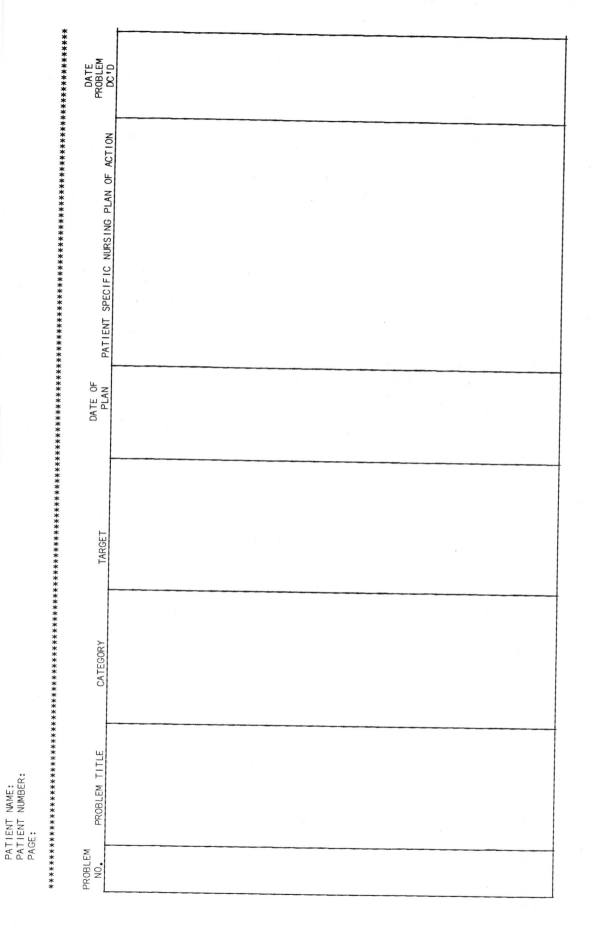

PROBLEM NO.	PROBLEM TITLE	CATEGORY	TARGET	DATE OF PLAN	PATIENT SPECIFIC NURSING PLAN OF ACTION	DATE PROBLEM DC'D

FORM 16

NURSING CARE PLAN
PROBLEM RATING SCALE FOR OUTCOMES

Patient Name _____

Patient Number _____

K = knowledge
B = behavior
S = status
C = caretaker

Problem Number and Name																														Nurse's Signature
Date	K	B	S	K	B	S	K	B	S	K	B	S	K	B	S	K	B	S	K	B	S	K	B	S	K	B	S	K	B	S	

CONCEPT		1	2	3	4	5
KNOWLEDGE:	The ability of the client to remember and interpret information	(no knowledge)	(minimal knowledge)	(basic knowledge)	(adequate knowledge)	(superior knowledge)
BEHAVIOR:	The observable responses, actions, or activities of the client	(never appropriate)	(rarely appropriate)	(inconsistently appropriate)	(usually appropriate)	(consistently appropriate)
STATUS:	The condition of the client in relation to objective and subjective defining characteristics	(extreme signs/symp)	(severe signs/symp)	(moderate signs/symp)	(minimal signs/symp)	(no signs/symp)

FORM 17

SKILLED VISIT REPORT

H.H. # _____ Client Name _____

Homebound Due to _____

Date _____ Time _____ a.m. Unscheduled ( ) Explain _____
p.m.

CLIENT PROBLEMS *(Circle #)*

ENVIRONMENTAL:

PSYCHOSOCIAL:

PHYSIOLOGICAL:
21. Speech and language:
24. Pain:
26. Integument:
   Lesion
   Depth
   Diameter
   Drainage
27. Neuro-musculo-skeletal function:
28. Respiration:
   Rate ___ Resting ___ Activity ___
   Lung Sounds ___
29. Circulation:
   Pulse ___ Apical ___ Radial ___ Pedal ___
   B/P ___ Lying ___ Sitting ___ Standing ___
   Edema ___
   Weight ___ Temp. ___
30. Digestion-hydration:
31. Bowel function:

32. Genito-urinary function:
   Incontinent ( )
   _____ (Other)
HEALTH RELATED BEHAVIORS:
35. Nutrition:
   Intake ___
38. Personal hygiene: HHA SUPERVISORY VISIT
   POC ( ) Appropriate ( ) Inappropriate
41. Health care supervision
   MD Visit Date ___
42. Prescribed med(s): Know   Comply
   Yes/No   Yes/No
   Yes/No   Yes/No
43. Technical procedure:

   _____ (Other)

Assessment _____

Plan: Frequency and Reason _____

Signature _____

SUBJECTIVE/OBJECTIVE

CAT   TARG   RX

INTERVENTIONS/COMMENTS

INTERVENTION SCHEME

CATEGORIES
I. Health Teaching, Guidance, and Counseling
II. Treatments and Procedures
III. Case Management
IV. Surveillance

TARGETS
01. Anatomy/physiology
02. Behavior modification
03. Bladder care
04. Bonding
05. Bowel care
06. Bronchial hygiene
07. Cardiac care
08. Caretaking/parenting skills
09. Cast care
10. Communication
11. Coping skills
12. Daycare/respite
13. Discipline
14. Dressing change/wound care
15. Durable medical equipment
16. Education
17. Employment
18. Environment
19. Exercises
20. Family planning
21. Feeding procedures
22. Finances
23. Food
24. Gait training
25. Growth/development
26. Homemaking
27. Housing
28. Interaction
29. Lab findings
30. Legal system
31. Medical/dental care
32. Medication action/side effects
33. Medication administration
34. Medication set-up
35. Mobility/transfers
36. Nursing care, supplementary
37. Nutrition
38. Nutritionl
39. Ostomy care
40. Other community resource
41. Personal care
42. Positioning
43. Rehabilitation
44. Relaxation/breathing techniques
45. Rest/sleep
46. Safety
47. Screening
48. Sickness/injury care
49. Signs/symptoms-mental/emotional
50. Signs/symptoms-physical
51. Skin care
52. Social work/counseling
53. Specimen collection
54. Spiritual care
55. Stimulation/nurturance
56. Stress management
57. Substance use
58. Supplies
59. Support group
60. Support system
61. Transportation
62. Wellness
63. Other (specify)

RN   LPN   RPT   OTR   SP   MSS   Employee #

FORM 17

PROBLEM CLASSIFICATION SCHEME

DOMAIN I: ENVIRONMENTAL
01. Income
02. Sanitation
03. Residence
04. Neighborhood/workplace safety
05. Other

DOMAIN II: PSYCHOSOCIAL
06. Communication with community resources
07. Social contact
08. Role change
09. Interpersonal relationship
10. Spiritual distress
11. Grief
12. Emotional stability
13. Human sexuality
14. Caretaking/parenting
15. Neglected child/adult
16. Abused child/adult
17. Growth and development
18. Other

DOMAIN III: PHYSIOLOGICAL
19. Hearing
20. Vision
21. Speech and language
22. Dentition
23. Cognition
24. Pain
25. Consciousness
26. Integument
27. Neuro-musculo-skeletal function
28. Respiration
29. Circulation
30. Digestion-hydration
31. Bowel function
32. Genito-urinary function
33. Antepartum/postpartum
34. Other

DOMAIN IV: HEALTH RELATED BEHAVIORS
35. Nutrition
36. Sleep and rest patterns
37. Physical activity
38. Personal hygiene
39. Substance misuse
40. Family planning
41. Health care supervision
42. Prescribed medication regimen
43. Technical procedure
44. Other

TREATMENT CODES FOR PROFESSIONAL SERVICES REQUIRED (MEDICARE)

Code Service

A. Skilled Nursing (SN)
A1. Skilled Observation (Inc. V.S., Response to Med., etc.)
A2. Foley Insertion
A3. Bladder Instillation
A4. Wound Care/Dressing
A5. Decubitus Care - Stage 3, 4, 5,
A6. Venipuncture
A7. Restorative Nursing
A8. Post Cataract Care
A9. Bowel/Bladder Training
A10. Chest Physio (Inc. Postural drainage)
A11. Adm. of Vitamin B/12
A12. Adm. Insulin
A13. Adm. Other IM/Subq.
A14. Adm. IV's/Clysis
A15. Teach Ostomy or Ileo Conduit Care
A16. Teach Nasogastric Feeding

B. Physical Therapy (PT)
B1. Evaluation
B2. Therapeutic
B3. Transfer Training
B4. Home Program
B5. Gait Training
B6. Chest Physiotherapy
B7. Ultra Sound

C. Speech Therapy (ST)
C1. Evaluation
C2. Voice Disorders Treatments
C3. Speech Articulation Disorders Treatments
C4. Dysphagia Treatments
C5. Language Disorders Treatments

D. Occupational Therapy (OT)
D1. Evaluation
D2. Independent Living/Daily Living Skills (ADL Training)
D3. Muscle Re-education
D5. Perceptual Motor Training
D6. Fine Motor Coordination

E. Medical Social Services (MSS)
E1. Assessment of Social and Emotional Factors
E2. Counseling for Long-Range Planning and Decision Making
E3. Community Resource Planning

F. Home Health Aide (AIDE)
F1. Tub/Shower Bath
F2. Partial/Complete Bed Bath
F4. Personal Care
F6. Catheter Care
F8. Assist with Ambulation

Code Service

A.
A17. Reinsertion of Nasogastric Feeding Tube
A18. Teach Gastrostomy Feeding
A19. Teach Parenteral Feeding
A20. Teach Care of Trach.
A21. Adm. Care of Trach.
A22. Teach Inhalation RX
A23. Adm. Inhalation RX
A24. Teach Adm. of Injection
A25. Teach Diabetic Care
A26. Disimpaction/Follow-Up Enema
A27. Other (Specify Under Orders)
A28. Wound Care/Dressing - Closed Incision/Suture Line
A29. Decubitus Care - Stage 1, 2
A30. Teaching Care of Any Indwelling Catheter
A31. Mgt./Eval. Pt Care Plan
A32. Teach/Train (Other)

B8. Electro Therapy
B9. Prosthetic Training
B10. Fabricate Temp. Devices
B11. Muscle Re-ed.
B12. Mgt./Eval. Pt Care Plan
B15. Others (Specify Under Orders)

C6. Aural Rehabilitation
C8. Non-Oral Communication
C9. Other (Specify Under Orders)

D7. Neuro-developmental Treatment
D8. Sensory Treatment
D9. Orthotics/Splinting
D10. Adaptive Equipment (fabrication and training)
D11. Other (Specify Under Orders)

E4. Short Term Therapy
E6. Other (Specify Under Orders)

F10. Exercises
F11. Prepare Meal
F12. Grocery Shop
F13. Wash Clothes
F14. Housekeeping
F15. Other (Specify Under Orders)

FORM 18

LONG TERM CARE VISIT REPORT

Pt. Act.# _____   Client Name _____   Date ____/____/____

CLIENT PROBLEMS	SUBJECTIVE/OBJECTIVE NC = No Change	CAT.	TARG.	INTERVENTIONS/COMMENTS
ENVIRONMENTAL/PSYCHOSOCIAL:				
26. Integument:				
Lesion				
Diameter				
Drainage				
27. Neuro-musculo-skeletal function:				
Ambulation				
28. Respiration:				
Rate Resting Activity				
Lung Sounds				
29. Circulation:				
Pulse Apical Radial Pedal				
B/P Lying Sitting Standing				
Edema				
Weight				
31. Bowel function:				
Continency				
32. Genito-urinary function:				
Continency				
35. Nutrition: Intake				
MOW				
36. Sleep/rest:				
38. Personal hygiene:				
HHA Sup. POC ( )Approp. ( )Inapp.				
Satisfied ____ Unsat. ____				
Needs HHA due to.				
41. Medical/dental supervision:				
MD visit Date ____/____/____				
42. Prescribed med(s): Know Comply				
Yes/No Yes/No				
Yes/No Yes/No				
(Other Problems)				

INTERVENTION SCHEME

CATEGORIES

I. Health Teaching, Guidance, and Counseling
II. Treatments and Procedures
III. Case Management
IV. Surveillance

TARGETS

01. Anatomy/physiology
02. Behavior modification
03. Bladder care
04. Bonding
05. Bowel care
06. Bronchial hygiene
07. Cardiac care
08. Caretaking/parenting skills
09. Cast care
10. Communication
11. Coping skills
12. Day care/respite
13. Discipline
14. Dressing change/wound care
15. Durable medical equipment
16. Education
17. Employment
18. Environment
19. Exercises
20. Family planning
21. Feeding procedures
22. Finances
23. Food
24. Gait training
25. Growth/development
26. Homemaking
27. Housing
28. Interaction
29. Lab findings
30. Legal system
31. Medical/dental care
32. Medication action/side effects
33. Medication administration
34. Medication set-up
35. Mobility/exercise
36. Nursing care, supplementary
37. Nutrition
38. Nutritionist
39. Ostomy care
40. Other community resource
41. Personal care
42. Positioning
43. Rehabilitation
44. Relaxation/breathing techniques
45. Rest/sleep
46. Safety
47. Screening
48. Sickness/injury care
49. Signs/symptoms - mental/emotional
50. Signs/symptoms - physical
51. Skin care
52. Social work/counseling
53. Specimen collection
54. Spiritual care
55. Stimulation/nurturance
56. Stress management
57. Substance use
58. Supplies
59. Support group
60. Support system
61. Transportation
62. Wellness
63. Other (specify)

Assessment: _____

Plan: Frequency and Reason _____

_____ Nurse Signature: _____ Employee #: _____

FORM 19

FAMILY VISIT REPORT

Household Number _____
Client Name _____
Age _____ # _____ Date _____

Nursing Problem/Assessment Parameter	CAT	TAR	INTERVENTIONS
35. NUTRITION			
14. CARETAKING/PARENTING			
17. GROWTH AND DEVELOPMENT			
33. ANTEPARTUM/POSTPARTUM			
40. FAMILY PLANNING			
OTHER PROBLEM			

PLAN: (REVISIT—WHEN, PURPOSE) _____

Nurse's Signature _____

ASSESSMENT:

INTERVENTION SCHEME

CATEGORIES

I Health Teaching, Guidance and Counseling
II Treatments and Procedures
III Case Management
IV Surveillance

TARGETS

01 Anatomy/physiology
02 Behavior modification
03 Bladder care
04 Bonding
05 Bowel care
06 Bronchial hygiene
07 Cardiac care
08 Caretaking/parenting skills
09 Cast care
10 Communication
11 Coping skills
12 Day care/respite
13 Discipline
14 Dressing change/wound care
15 Durable medical equipment
16 Education
17 Employment
18 Environment
19 Exercises
20 Family planning
21 Feeding procedures
22 Finances
23 Food
24 Gait training
25 Growth/development
26 Homemaking
27 Housing
28 Interaction
29 Lab findings
30 Legal system
31 Medical/dental care
32 Medication action/side effects
33 Medication administration
34 Medication set up
35 Mobility/exercise
36 Nursing care, supplementary
37 Nutrition
38 Nutritionist
39 Ostomy care
40 Other community resource
41 Personal care
42 Positioning
43 Rehabilitation
44 Relaxation/breathing techniques
45 Rest/sleep
46 Safety
47 Screening
48 Sickness/injury care
49 Signs/symptoms - mental/emotional
50 Signs/symptoms - physical
51 Skin care
52 Social work/counseling
53 Specimen collection
54 Spiritual care
55 Stimulation/nurturance
56 Stress management
57 Substance use
58 Supplies
59 Support group
60 Support system
61 Transportation
62 Wellness
63 Other (specify)

FORM 20

PUBLIC HEALTH NURSE RECORD OF SERVICE

NAME _____

FF# _____

Page _____

CODES:

Site:

HV = Home
OV = Office
SV = School
TC = Phone
NAH = Not at Home

Care Provided/Interventions:

Assmt = Assessment
HTG&C = Teaching
CAR = Coordination, Advocacy, and Referral
SUV = Surveillance

DATE	SITE	PROB. NO.	CARE PROVIDED	NARRATIVE	REVISIT DATE

FORM 21

DISCHARGE SUMMARY

To: Dr. _____ Date: _____

Re: Client Name _____

Address: _____

1st Visit Date: _____ Last Visit Date: _____

Primary Diagnosis _____

Service provided by:

_____ Nursing   _____ Speech Pathology
_____ Physical Therapy   _____ Medical Social Service
_____ Occupational Therapy   _____ Home Health Aide

Type of Service Provided:

_____ Observation/assessment relative to diagnosis
_____ Technical procedures/direct care
_____ Teaching to implement technical procedures
_____ Teaching health concepts and practices
_____ Assistance in obtaining medical care
_____ Referral to other VNA services
_____ Referral to community resources

Comments: _____

_____

Unresolved Problems: _____

_____

Discharged To:

_____ Self-care [ ] recovered [ ] stable   _____ Hospice
_____ Care of family/friends [ ] recovered [ ] stable   _____ Refused further service
_____ Nursing home   _____ Moved out of service area
                                                     _____ Deceased
_____ Acute hospital   _____ Other: _____
_____ Another home health agency
_____ Long-term care

Thank you for allowing us to be of assistance in caring for your patient. We look forward to working with you in the future.

Sincerely,

FORM 22

```
* * * D I S M I S S A L / T R A N S F E R   S U M M A R Y * * *
```

Client _____ Date _____

Nurse _____ HH # _____

═══

Date service began: _____

Number of visits: _____

Status of client/family when care began and at discharge:

Type of services provided:

Other agencies/resources contacted:

Disposition/Transfer Plan:

STUDENT HEALTH RECORD

The Student Health Record was developed by school nurses at the VNA of Omaha. It is used to organize, document, and communicate health-related information for Kindergarten through Grade 12 pupils. Many of the students are considered well individuals; others have medical and nursing diagnoses that range from mild to severe. Record forms other than Student Health Records are used in conjunction with multiple or profoundly handicapped children. Instructions for recording on the Student Health Record are as follows:

Form 23: Student Health Record (pp. 377–380) is printed on a file folder and consists of:
  (1) Data Base—demographic and immunization data as well as significant health history.
  (2) Screening Results—vision, blood pressure, and hearing data.
  (3) Student Problems and Nursing Interventions—narrative documentation based on the Problem Classification Scheme and the Intervention Scheme.

Student Health Record (Form 23, pp. 377–380)

Instructions

I. Each student has an individual permanent school health record. School health records, although a part of the cumulative folder, are kept in a central separate file for use by the school health assistant, nurse, and teacher. Due to the Family Education and Privacy Act of 1974, parents of students also have access to school records. Student cumulative folders are kept either in each individual teacher's file or in the principal's office. If a student leaves the school, the health card must be refiled into the student's cumulative folder.

II. Recording to be done on the school health record by the School Nurse, School Health Assistants, teachers, or others will include personal data, immunization dates, screening results, referral and follow-up, pertinent health history, emergency and special health information, and physical and dental exam data. (Principal may designate volunteer or school secretary to record routine screening results.)

  A. Personal Data
    Information at the top left on the front of the record may be typed or printed by the secretary, volunteer, or assistant. Address and telephone number should be written in pencil. School name and date student entered should be noted in pencil in the midsection on the front of the record. New or transfer students entering school throughout the school year are issued a health record. (The nurse should remind the school secretary or assistant of the need for health records on new or transfer students.)

  B. Emergency and Special Health Information and Significant Health History
    The school nurse interviews all new students and assesses health information from previous school records as available. Emergency and special health information should be noted on the upper right portion on the front (e.g., "Call Emergency Medical System if seizure activity does not subside in 5 minutes"). Significant health history information should be noted in the section immediately below. All health entries are dated and student's current grade level is specified. The upper left-hand corner circle is filled in with red ink by the nurse if the student is in need of special consideration.

  C. Immunizations
    1. The month and year, and in some instances the day (when the MMR falls in the month of the first birthday), of all immunizations are recorded by the nurse or personnel designated by the principal.
    2. If no immunizations, state why: and if waiver has been signed, state date and reason under "Pertinent Immunization Notes" and insert signed waiver in health record. Record a "W" in pencil in place of the date to identify that an exempt waiver has been signed. Record HIB and chicken pox vaccines if received (not required by law).
    3. Immunization status number (in pencil) at upper right-hand corner indicates level of compliance or non-compliance with State law. The dot is filled in with green ink to identify the child who has been immunized for measles between 12 and 15 months of age. The "OK" is circled if measles was received on or after 15 months of age.

  D. Physical Examinations/Dental Reports
    1. Physical examinations and dental reports are recorded on any student presenting a completed physical and dental exam. This routinely occurs at entrance to school and seventh grade and for transfer from out-of-state students.
      a. Physical examinations—record in midsection on front of record noting data and findings (e.g., 9–20–90, WNL. No restrictions, Dr. Blank). Note additional information on inside portion of record.
      b. Record the year of disease or accident histories under Significant Health History.
    2. Dental—record date and findings of exam in the dental exam area. Additional dental exam dates may be added as needed.
    3. TB Test—note date and results (positive or negative).

  E. Screening
    1. All screening results are recorded under the appropriate grade level in the screening section. Screenings marked #1 should reflect actual findings. Screenings marked #2 should be coded as:

a. "N"—normal.
b. "A"—abnormal.
c. "Ref" if used beside the "A" to indicate referral was made.
d. "FU"—follow-up notes indicated on inside section of record.
e. "UT"—under treatment for condition. Notes on inside section of record.
f. "T"—audiometer threshold results noted inside on bottom right of record.
g. "W" ("Watch")—findings noted on inside of record for future comparison.
h. "D"—diagnosed condition.

2. Vision screening—record results (e.g., (R) 20/20, (L) 20/30, both 20/20) noting with or without correction.

3. Audiometer screening—record as (N) normal or (A) abnormal.
   If screening is failed and threshold results are abnormal, record results on bottom right inside record

	500	1000	2000	3000	4000	6000	8000
DT 1/90 R	10	15	30	35	45	15	15
GR 3 L	10	5	5	10	10	15	15

Referral and follow-up notes are noted above in the Additional Information section.

4. Impedance screening—not routinely performed but may be done in conjunction with hearing assessment. Referral and follow-up notes on inside folder.

5. Blood pressure—record results with referral and follow-up noted on inside folder.

6. Color vision screening—record normal (N) or abnormal (A) results with referral and follow-up noted on inside folder.

7. Scoliosis screening—record normal (N) or abnormal (A) results. "W" (Watch) indicates screening findings noted on inside of folder. "D" designates diagnosis by physician as noted on inside of folder.

8. Stature and weight screening—record findings on back side of record noting date, age, stature in *inches* and weight in *pounds.* Parents' stature may also be noted. Girls' growth is plotted on the left chart marked with physical growth pattern percentiles established from data from the National Center for Health Statistics. Boys' results are plotted on the right chart.
   To graph stature measurements:
   a. Choose appropriate growth chart.
   b. Find the age on the horizontal (bottom) scale.
   c. Follow a vertical line from that point up to the level of the child's stature measurement on the stature (left) scale.
   d. Where the two lines intersect, mark with ink dot.
   To graph weight measurement:
   a. Choose appropriate growth chart.
   b. Find the age on the horizontal (bottom) scale.
   c. Follow a vertical lined from that point up to the level of the child's measurement on the weight (right) scale.
   d. Where the two lines intersect, mark with ink dot.
   When the child is measured again, join the new set of marks to the previous set by straight lines (stature to stature and weight to weight).

   Each chart contains a series of curved lines numbered to show selected percentiles. These refer to the rank of a measure in a group of 100. Thus, when a mark is on the 95th percentile line of weight for age, it means that only five children among 100 of the corresponding age and sex have weights greater than this child's recorded weight.

9. Other assessments/screenings performed but not listed on the folder should be noted on the inside under Additional Information.

F. **Additional Information Regarding Health Problems and Follow-up** (Recorded on inside of folder.)

1. Problem oriented entries will be guided by the Problem Classification Scheme and Intervention Scheme of the Omaha System. The major parts of the System are identified at the bottom left side on the inside of the folder.
   a. Date.
   b. Appropriate nursing problem number (e.g., "#20" coded at beginning of entry). It is not necessary to name the problem.
   c. Subjective/objective information—narrative, descriptors of the problem (e.g., "#20 Failed rescreen using Goodlite (R) 20/40, (L) 20/50, both 20/40").
   d. Intervention category(ies) I, II, III, and/or IV.
   e. Targets appropriate to Intervention (e.g., "III 10, 31 Referral for medical evaluation sent to parents").
   f. Nurse's signature placed directly after recording. No initials.

Example #1: Vision
10/20/89 #20 Failed rescreen using Goodlite (R) 20/40, (L) 20/50, both 20/40. III 10, 31 Referral for medical evaluation sent to parents. Sally Jones, RN

Example #2: Hearing
01/10/89 #19, #24 c/o (L) ear pain past 4 hours, teacher reports frequent infection and slight hearing loss. II 50, 47 Otoscopic exam—(L) TM red. Audio threshold done. III 10, 31 TCM with results of threshold

and otoscopic findings. Referred for medical evaluation. Sally Jones, RN

01/15/89 #19, #24 Dr. Smith saw 1/11/89. DX—Acute Otitis Media with antibiotic treatment. Requests repeat audio in 1 week. Ear pain resolved. IV 47 will repeat audio 1/19/89. Sally Jones, RN

01/19/89 #19 Repeat audio normal. III 10 Results sent home. Sally Jones, RN

Example #3: Injury

09/08/90 #24 States fell on playground and hit forehead on pavement. 2-cm elevation over (R) eye with tenderness. Alert, steady gait, pupils equal and reactive, no loss of consciousness or other injury reported. II 48, 50 Ice applied—30 minutes. Neuro signs checked q 5 min. III 10, 50 Return to class, teacher aware of injury and symptoms to observe. TCM. Notified of injury and head injury form to be sent home with student. Sally Jones, RN

2. Not all recording will reflect the problem-oriented system.
   a. Health and parent updates would be recorded as such (e.g., "9/19/89—Parent update—fracture (L) wrist 6/89"). Sally Jones, RN
   b. Normal rescreening results (e.g., "Vision rescreen with Goodlite (R) 20/20, (L) 20/20, both 20/20"). Sally Jones, RN
3. All completed referrals are recorded. Information from physicians is written in *red* ink.
4. Medications—(when long-term) may be recorded along with a problem-oriented entry or alone as appropriate.

G. Organization

This health record has been designed in folder style to accommodate the insertion of medical reports, previous school health information, physical exam reports, or any additional information the nurse deems important enough to become a part of the health record. These attachments should not be stapled or attached to the record but simply inserted.

Text continued on page 381

FORM 23

STUDENT HEALTH RECORD

Confidential Information
For Use By Professional Personnel

(Red)

Immunization Status No.: _____ ○ OK
(in pencil)   (green) (circle)

EMERGENCY & SPECIAL HEALTH INFORMATION

Name _____ (Last) _____ (First) _____ (M.I.)

Birthdate _____   Sex (M F)   Circle Race (W B Other)

School: _____
1. _____
Parent or Guardian   (pencil)

Address (in pencil) _____   Phone _____
2. _____
                      (pencil)

Physician _____   Phone _____
3. _____
                      (pencil)

Entry Date: _____

SIGNIFICANT HEALTH HISTORY

Allergies: **Other:**

____ Bee Sting   ____ Asthma   ____ Heart Disease
____ Medication   ____ Cancer   ____ Hepatitis
____ Food, Pollens   ____ Chicken Pox   ____ Seizure Disorder
____ Other   ____ Diabetes

Other significant illness, accidents, operations, limitations, medication

_____
_____

IMMUNIZATIONS

If waiver signed state date and reason. Attach to Student Health Card. *

	(Month/Year)
DPT/TD (Diphtheria — Tetanus — Pertussis)	1 __ / 2 __ / 3 __ / 4 __ / 5 __ / 6 __
Polio — Oral trivalent	1 __ / 2 __ / 3 __ / 4 __ / 5 __
	(Month/Date/Year)
Measles (10 day)	1 __ / __ / __
Rubella (3 day)	1 __ / __ / __
Mumps	1 __ / __ / __
M-M-R Combined	1 __ / __ / __
HIB	1 __ / __ / __
Chicken Pox	1 __ / __ / __
Other	1 __ / __ / __

*Pertinent Immunization Notes:
_____
_____

Grade Level	
Kdg.	1 __ / __ / __
7th Grade	1 __ / __ / __
Transfer	1 __ / __ / __
Other	1 __ / __ / __

Physical Examination: (Date and findings — See inside for added notes)

_____
_____

TB Test _____   Dental Exam (Date and findings) _____

SCREENING

		K	1	2	3	4	5	6	7	8	9	10	11	12
Date														
Vision [1]	R	20/	20/	20/	20/	20/	20/	20/	20/	20/	20/	20/	20/	20/
	L	20/	20/	20/	20/	20/	20/	20/	20/	20/	20/	20/	20/	20/
Both Eyes [1]		20/	20/	20/	20/	20/	20/	20/	20/	20/	20/	20/	20/	20/
Vision [1] /c Correction	R	20/	20/	20/	20/	20/	20/	20/	20/	20/	20/	20/	20/	20/
	L	20/	20/	20/	20/	20/	20/	20/	20/	20/	20/	20/	20/	20/
Both Eyes [1] /c Correction		20/	20/	20/	20/	20/	20/	20/	20/	20/	20/	20/	20/	20/
Audiometer [2]	R													
	L													
Impedance [2]	R													
	L													
Blood Pressure [1]														
Color Vision (1st grade)				Scoliosis [2]										

NOTES: [1] Record Findings [2] Code: N-Normal A-Abnormal W-Watch D-Diagnosed Ref-Referred FU-Follow-up (Inside) T-Threshold (Inside) UT-Under Treatment

377

FORM 23

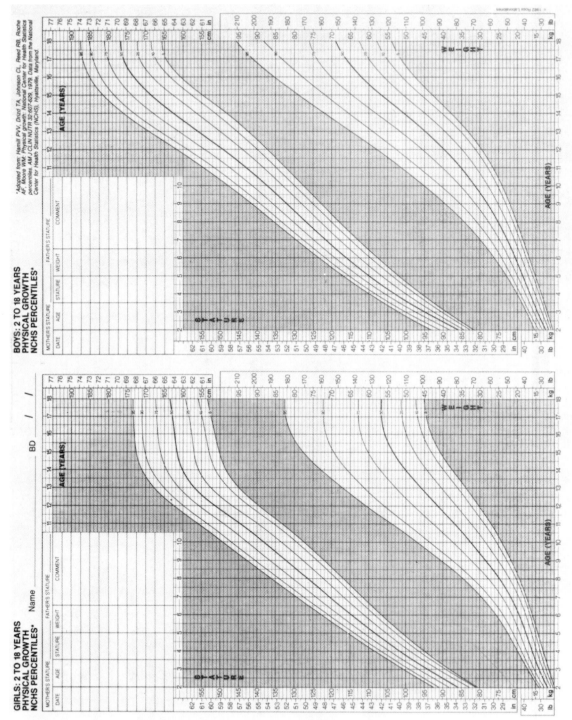

GIRLS: 2 TO 18 YEARS
PHYSICAL GROWTH
NCHS PERCENTILES*

BOYS: 2 TO 18 YEARS
PHYSICAL GROWTH
NCHS PERCENTILES*

*Adapted from: Hamill PVV, Drizd TA, Johnson CL, Reed RB, Roche AF, Moore WM. Physical growth National Center for Health Statistics percentile. AM J CLIN NUTR 32:607-629, 1979. Data from the National Center for Health Statistics (NCHS), Hyattsville, Maryland.

378

FORM 23

Name _____ BD ___ / ___ / ___

ADDITIONAL INFORMATION REGARDING HEALTH PROBLEMS AND FOLLOW-UP
(See problem classification and intervention schemes below. Also audio thresholds.)

DATE		Sign name/title directly after recording. (no initials)

FORM 23

PROBLEM CLASSIFICATION SCHEME

Environmental
- 01 Income
- 02 Sanitation
- 03 Residence
- 04 Neighborhood/workplace safety
- 05 Other

Psychosocial
- 06 Communication with community resources
- 07 Social contact
- 08 Role change
- 09 Interpersonal relationship
- 10 Spiritual distress
- 11 Grief
- 12 Emotional stability
- 13 Human sexuality
- 14 Caretaking/parenting
- 15 Neglected child/adult
- 16 Abused child/adult
- 17 Growth and development
- 18 Other

Physiological
- 19 Hearing
- 20 Vision
- 21 Speech and language
- 22 Dentition
- 23 Cognition
- 24 Pain
- 25 Consciousness
- 26 Integument
- 27 Neuro-musculo-skeletal function
- 28 Respiration
- 29 Circulation
- 30 Digestion-hydration
- 31 Bowel function
- 32 Genito-urinary function
- 33 Antepartum/postpartum
- 34 Other

Health Related Behaviors
- 35 Nutrition
- 36 Sleep and rest patterns
- 37 Physical activity
- 38 Personal hygiene
- 39 Substance misuse
- 40 Family planning
- 41 Medical/dental supervision
- 42 Prescribed medication regimen
- 43 Technical procedure
- 44 Other

INTERVENTION SCHEME

Categories
- I Health Teaching, Guidance, and Counseling
- II Treatments and Procedures
- III Case Management
- IV Surveillance

Targets
- 01 Anatomy/physiology
- 02 Behavior modification
- 03 Bladder care
- 04 Bonding
- 05 Bowel care
- 06 Bronchial hygiene
- 07 Cardiac care
- 08 Caretaking/parenting skills
- 09 Cast care
- 10 Communication
- 11 Coping skills
- 12 Day care/respite
- 13 Discipline
- 14 Dressing change/wound care
- 15 Durable medical equipment
- 16 Education
- 17 Employment
- 18 Environment
- 19 Exercises
- 20 Family planning
- 21 Feeding procedures
- 22 Finances
- 23 Food
- 24 Gait training
- 25 Growth/development
- 26 Homemaking
- 27 Housing
- 28 Interaction
- 29 Lab findings
- 30 Legal system
- 31 Medical/dental care
- 32 Medication action/side effects
- 33 Medication administration
- 34 Medication set-up
- 35 Mobility/exercise
- 36 Nursing care, supplementary
- 37 Nutrition
- 38 Nutritionist
- 39 Ostomy care
- 40 Other community resource
- 41 Personal care
- 42 Positioning
- 43 Rehabilitation
- 44 Relaxation/breathing techniques
- 45 Rest/sleep
- 46 Safety
- 47 Screening
- 48 Sickness/injury care
- 49 Signs/symptoms - mental/emotional
- 50 Signs/symptoms - physical
- 51 Skin care
- 52 Social work/counseling
- 53 Specimen collection
- 54 Spiritual care
- 55 Stimulation/nurturance
- 56 Stress management
- 57 Substance use
- 58 Supplies
- 59 Support group
- 60 Support system
- 61 Transportation
- 62 Wellness
- 63 Other

AUDIOMETER THRESHOLD SCREENINGS
(Frequencies Recorded in Decibel Intensity)

		500	1000	2000	3000	4000	6000	8000
DT	R							
GR	L							
DT	R							
GR	L							
DT	R							
GR	L							
DT	R							
GR	L							
DT	R							
GR	L							
DT	R							
GR	L							
DT	R							
GR	L							
DT	R							
GR	L							
DT	R							
GR	L							
DT	R							
GR	L							

HEALTH MAINTENANCE CENTER RECORD

The Health Maintenance Center Record was developed by clinic nurses at the VNA of Omaha. It is used to organize, document, and communicate health-related information for ambulatory adults. Many of the adults who visit the clinics are considered well individuals; others have acute or chronic illnesses that range from mild to severe. Sample forms and instructions for their use are included as follow:

Form 24: Data Base (pp. 383–384)—physiological, health-related behavior, psychosocial, and environmental data.

Form 25: Problems/Plans/Ratings/Progress (p. 385) —combination of problem-specific flow sheet and narrative data that incorporates the Problem Rating Scale for Outcomes and the Intervention Scheme.

Data Base (Form 24, pp. 383–384)

Instructions

The Data Base is designed to assist the nurse in generating baseline information and the nursing problem list. It is intended to guide the initial appraisal and subsequent interviews and data collection. It is designed to be used on an ongoing basis. It is anticipated that within 3 months of the initial visit, there will be a reasonable amount of data recorded in each category to support a client profile (summary statement). The primary nurse will be responsible for formulating the profile, signing, and dating the initial appraisal.

The summary statement is designed as an assessment statement relative to the client's general health status, specific health problems, functional status, self-care abilities, health-promoting behaviors, and compliance with health care provider recommendations.

DATA BASE UPDATE

Additions may be made to the Data Base at any time, especially when there are significant changes (e.g., following hospitalization, a new diagnosis, change in self-care status). In addition, comprehensive client reappraisal is required at specific intervals. Reappraisal will necessitate that notations of changes in the domains be recorded to the right of the initial notation, creating three vertical columns on the data base form.

ORGANIZATION

1. The domains of the Problem Classification Scheme:
   - III. Physiological
   - IV. Health related behaviors
   - I. Environmental
   - II. Psychosocial

   The ordering of the domains is intended to facilitate recording data collected during the interview and review of systems.

2. A summary statement (client profile): See above
3. Date/Signature/Title:
   - Column 1: Date of initial assessment series (within 3 months of admission date)
   - Column 2: Date of comprehensive reappraisal (at 6 months after admission)
   - Column 3: Date of comprehensive reappraisal (at 1 year after admission)

A new Data Base will be utilized at the second year appraisal and every 3 years thereafter.

Problems/Plans/Ratings/Progress (Form 25, p. 385)

Instructions

PROBLEMS

Client problems are actual or potential health problems which are amenable to solution through nursing. Only those problems which the nurse and client will be addressing are to be listed. Those problems should be listed in priority order relative to frequency of assessment, potential for change, and impact on the plan of care. It is anticipated that, generally speaking, no more than four active nursing problems will be recorded for any one client. The problem list will be initiated on the first visit, updated at 6 months, and at least yearly thereafter. New problems may be added at any time. Likewise, as problems are resolved, it will be so noted on the problem list. Numbers from the Problem Classification Scheme may be used, but are not necessary.

SAMPLE ■ Circ. imp. (29: Circulation: impairment)

PLANS

Each identified nursing problem will have a problem-specific plan. The plan is defined as actions or activities designed by a nurse to establish a course of client care.

SAMPLE ■ Circ. imp.: check edema/time of day/elev. (i.e., problem is circulation. Plan is to check edema, ascertain onset/remission by time of day; encourage to elevate legs)

SAMPLE ■ Tech. pro. deficit: give B_{12} (i.e., this client has a technical procedure deficit: he requires a vitamin B_{12} injection, is unable to do so. Therefore, nurse will administer)

PROBLEM RATING SCALE FOR OUTCOMES

The Problem Rating Scale for Outcomes is a framework for measuring problem-specific client responses to nursing interventions at specified points in time. Problems are rated according to Knowledge, Behavior, and Status at the time the problem is identified, at the 6 month reappraisal, and yearly thereafter. The Rating Scale for any given problem may be updated at any time when the nurse notes a significant change in any of the three categories. Refer to Problem Rating Scale for Outcomes sheet.

PROGRESS NOTES

Each visit must be recorded. The form is designed to accommodate observable measurement parameters (i.e., BP, wt., BSL reading), the problem number, and a brief narrative of findings and interventions.

Interventions are defined as actions or activities implemented by the nurse to address a specific client problem to prevent illness, and to improve, maintain, or restore health. Categories within the Intervention Scheme include Health Teaching, Guidance, and Counseling (HTGC), Treatments and Procedures (T&P), Case Management (CM), and Surveillance (S). Targets in the Scheme are numbered from 1-63. The nurse may choose to use the numbers or abbreviations of the targets in the recording.

CASE EXAMPLE ■ A women has a nursing problem of circulation impairment, evidenced primarily by peripheral edema. The nurse has identified the necessary nursing activities to be monitoring the edema (this, of course, includes measuring, comparing, etc.) and teaching/reinforcing positioning (i.e., elevating legs).

SAMPLE PLAN ■ Circ. imp.: check edema/time of day/elev.

Documenting interventions required giving information, anticipating client problems, encouraging ac-

tion and responsibility for self-care (I), and measurement, critical analysis and monitoring (IV).

SAMPLE

Date	BP	P/R			Prob	Comments
9/01/91	120/80	AP 82 Reg	140	10″	Circ.	I, IV. 40. 1+ pitting bi Elev. qid ———— Sig.

OR

Temporary Problems ■ Problems requiring nursing assessment but predicted to be of short duration will be identified as Temporary Problems. Such problems will not be placed on the Problem List; but will be addressed in the Progress section.

SAMPLE

Date	BP	P/R		Prob	Comments
10/10/91				Temp	Eczematous area on back; itching. Has used Cortaid in past with relief. HTGC regarding spacing application. ———— Sig.

FORM 24

HMC Data Base

Name _____

Admission Date _____

DOMAIN III. PHYSIOLOGICAL

Vision

Hearing

Dentition

Bowel Function

GU Function

Circulation

Respiration

Skin

Neuro-musculo-skeletal

Pain

Cognition

DOMAIN IV.   HEALTH RELATED BEHAVIORS

Smoking   No__ Yes__

Caffeine Drinks No__ Yes__

Alcohol   No__ Yes__

Sleep/Relaxation

Physical Exercise

Nutrition/Hydration

Health Care Supervision

Immunization

BSE/TSE

Mammography

Pap test

Colorectal screening

FORM 24

DOMAIN II.   PSYCHOSOCIAL
Relatives

Social Activities

DOMAIN I.   ENVIRONMENTAL
Bathroom/Bathtub

Steps

Throw rugs

Neighborhood

Summary: Summary: Summary:

_____   _____   _____
Date/Signature/Title   Date/Sig   Date/Sig

FORM 25

PROBLEMS/PLANS/RATINGS/PROGRESS

Name _____

Problem . . . Plan:

Page _____

_____

_____

_____

_____

_____

Date						Date					
Prob						Prob					
Rate	K B S	K B S	K B S	K B S	K B S	Rate	K B S	K B S	K B S	K B S	K B S	K B S

Date						Date					
Prob						Prob					
Rate	K B S	K B S	K B S	K B S	K B S	Rate	K B S	K B S	K B S	K B S	K B S	K B S

Date	BP	P/R			Prob	Comments

OMAHA SYSTEM
BIBLIOGRAPHY

VISITING NURSE ASSOCIATION OF OMAHA PUBLICATIONS

Crews, C., Connolly, K., Whitted, P., et al. (1986, January/February). Computerized central intake: Streamlining community health-care admissions. *Nurs. Economics, 4*:31–36.

Jorgensen, C., & Young, B. (1989, May/June). The supervisory shared home visit tool. *Home Healthcare Nurse, 7*:33–36.

Martin, K. (1981, May). Improving recording and practice: The Omaha project. *Qual. Assur. Update, 8.*

Martin, K. (1982, November/December). A client classification system adaptable for computerization. *Nurs. Outlook, 30*:515–517.

Martin, K. (1982). Community health research in nursing diagnosis: The Omaha study (1980). In Kim, M., & Moritz, D. (Eds.), *Classification of Nursing Diagnoses: Proceedings of the Third and Fourth National Conferences* (pp. 167–175). New York, McGraw–Hill.

Martin, K. (1987). The Omaha system and NANDA: Similar or Different? In McLane, A. (Ed.), *Classification of Nursing Diagnoses: Proceedings of the Seventh Conference* (p. 422). St. Louis: C. V. Mosby.

Martin, K. (1988). Nursing minimum data set requirements for the community setting. In Werley, H., & Lang, N. (Eds.), *Identification of the Nursing Minimum Data Set* (pp. 214–222). New York, Springer.

Martin, K. (1988, June). Research in home care. *Nurs. Clin. of North Am., 23*:373–385.

Martin, K. (1989). Omaha system. In *Classification Systems for Describing Nursing Practice* (pp. 43–47). Kansas City, MO, American Nurses' Association.

Martin, K., Rich, R., & Bargstadt, G. (1979, Spring). Nursing problem classification scheme for community health. *Qual. Assur. Update, 3*:5–6.

Martin, K., Scheet, N., Crews, C., et al. (1986). *Client Management Information System for Community Health Nursing Agencies: An Implementation Manual,* No. HRP-0907023. Rockville, MD: Division of Nursing, US DHHS, PHS, HRSA.

Martin, K., Scheet, N., Crews, C., et al. (1986). *Client Management Information System for Community Health Nursing Agencies: Final Report.* [Unpublished.]

Martin, K., & Scheet, N. (1985). The Omaha system: Implications for costing community health nursing. In Shaffer, F. (Ed.), *Costing Out Nursing: Pricing Our Product* (pp. 197–206). New York, National League for Nursing.

Martin, K., & Scheet, N. (1988, May/June). The Omaha system: Providing a framework for assuring quality of home care. *Home Healthcare Nurse, 6*:24–28.

Martin, K., & Scheet, N. (1989). Nursing diagnosis in home health: The Omaha system. In Martinson, I., & Widmer, (Eds.), *Home Health Care Nursing* (pp. 67–72). Philadelphia, W. B. Saunders.

Matthis, E. (1974). The problem-oriented system in public health nursing. In *The Problem-Oriented System—A Multi-disciplinary Approach* (pp. 48–54). New York, National League for Nursing.

Simmons, D. (1980). *A Classification Scheme for Client Problems in Community Health Nursing.* Hyattsville, MD, US DHHS, BHPr—Division of Nursing.

Simmons, D. (1984). Computer implementation in ambulatory care: A community health model. In *Computer Technology and Nursing* (pp. 19–23). Bethesda, MD, US DHHS.

Simmons, D. (1985). Recent innovations and installations of nursing information systems. In Hannah, K., Guilleman, G., & Conklin, D. (Eds.), *Nursing Uses of Computers and Information Science* (pp. 31–35). New York, North-Holland.

Simmons, D. (1986). Implementation of nursing diagnosis in a community health setting. In Hurley, M. (Ed.), *Classification of Nursing Diagnoses: Proceedings of the Sixth Conference* (pp. 151–158). St. Louis, C. V. Mosby.

Simmons, D., & Hailey, R. (1988). Management information systems. In Benefield, L. (Ed.), *Home Health Care Management* (pp. 39–51). Englewood Cliffs, NJ, Prentice-Hall.

Visiting Nurse Association of Omaha (1976). *Development of a Problem Classification Scheme, a Methodology for its use and a System Designed to Computerize the Scheme for Community Health Nursing Services.* [Unpublished.]

Visiting Nurse Association of Omaha (1980). *Field Testing of a Problem Classification Scheme and Development and Field Testing of Expected Outcome-Outcome Criterion Schemes With a Methodology for Use.* [Unpublished.]

PUBLICATIONS RELATING TO THE OMAHA SYSTEM

Barkauskas, V. Home health care: Responding to need, growth, and cost containment. In Chaska, N. (Ed.), *The Nursing Profession: Turning Points* (pp. 394–404). St. Louis, C. V. Mosby, 1990.

Buck, J. Measuring the success of home health care. *Home Healthcare Nurse, 6*(May–June, 1988):17–23.

Bulau, J. *Home Health Care Quality Assurance Policies and Procedures.* Rockville, MD, Aspen, 1989.

Bulechek, G., & McCloskey, J. Nursing intervention taxonomy development. In McCloskey, J., & Grace, H. (Eds.), *Current Issues in Nursing* (pp. 23–28). St. Louis, C. V. Mosby, 1990.

Burns, C., & Thompson, M. Developing a nursing diagnosis classification system for PNPs. *Pediatric Nursing* (November–December, 1984):411–414.

Burns, C., & Thompson, M. Testing a nursing diagnosis classification system for pediatric nurse practitioners. In McLane, A. (Ed.), *Classification of Nursing Diagnoses: Proceedings of the Seventh Conference* (pp. 405–410). St. Louis, C. V. Mosby, 1987.

Carlson, J., Craft, C., McGuire, A., et al. *Nursing Diagnosis: A Case Study Approach.* Philadelphia, W. B. Saunders, 1991.

Cell, P., Peters, D., & Gordon, J. Implementing a nursing diagnosis system through research: The New Jersey experience. *Home Healthcare Nurse, 2*(January–February, 1984):26–32.

Douglas, D., & Murphy, E. Nursing process, nursing diagnosis, and emerging taxonomies. In McCloskey, J., & Grace, H. (Eds.) *Current Issues in Nursing* (pp. 17–22). St. Louis, C. V. Mosby, 1990.

Feldman, J., & Richard, R. A measure of nursing outcomes for home health care. In Waltz, C., & Strickland, O. (Eds.), *Measurement of Nursing Outcomes* (pp. 475–495). New York, Springer, 1988.

Gilbey, Valerie. The use of a computerized health problem classification system in an adult health assessment clinic. In Coward, I., & Brown, J. (Eds.), *Improving Community Health Through Applied Technology Conference Proceedings* (pp. 65–69). Victoria, BC, Canada, 1990.

Gilbey, Valerie. Screening and counselling clinic evaluation project. *Can. J. Nurs. Res.*, 22(Fall, 1990):23–38.

Grobe, S. *Computer Primer and Resource Guide for Nurses.* Philadelphia, J. B. Lippincott, 1984.

Grobe, S. Nursing intervention lexicon and taxonomy study: Language and classification methods. *Adv. Nurs. Sci.*, 13(December, 1990):22–33.

Helberg, J. Reliability of a problem-classification index for well mothers and children in community health nursing. *Public Health Nurs.*, 5(March, 1988):24–29.

Helberg, J. Reliability of the nursing classification index for home healthcare. *Nurs. Manag.*, 20(March, 1989):48–56.

Jewell, M., & Peters, D. An assessment guide for community health nurses. *Home Healthcare Nurse*, 7(September–October, 1989): 32–36.

Lang, N., & Marek, K. The classification of patient outcomes. *J. Prof. Nurs.*, 6(1990, May/June):158–163.

Marek, K. Classification of outcome measures in nursing care. In *Classification Systems for Describing Nursing Practice* (pp. 37–42). Kansas City, MO, American Nurses' Association, 1988.

McCormick, K. Nursing diagnosis and computers. In Hannah, K., Reimer, M., Mills, W., et al. (Eds.), *Clinical Judgement and Decision Making: The Future with Nursing Diagnosis* (pp. 534–539). New York, John Wiley & Sons, 1987.

Mundt, M. An analysis of nurse recording in family health clinics of a county health department. *J. Community Health Nurs.*, 5(May, 1988):3–10.

Neufeld, A., & Misselbrook, C. Classification and use of nursing diagnosis in community health nursing. In Hannah, K., Reimer, M., Mills, W., et al. *Clinical Judgement and Decision Making: The Future with Nursing Diagnosis* (pp. 349–351). New York, John Wiley & Sons, 1987.

Pasquale, D. A basis for prospective payment for home care. *Image*, 19(Winter, 1987):186–191.

Peters, D. Classifying patients using a nursing diagnosis taxonomy. In Harris, M. (Ed.), *Home Health Administration* (pp. 311–322). Owings Mills, MD, Rynd Communications, 1988.

Peters, D. Development of a community health intensity rating scale. *Nurs. Res.*, 37(July–August, 1988):202–207.

Peters, D. An overview of current research relating to long-term outcomes. *Nurs. Health Care*, 10(March, 1989):133–136.

Schmele, J. Teaching nurses how to improve their documentation. *Home Healthcare Nurse*, 4(July–August, 1986):6–10.

Weidmann, J., & North, H. Implementing the Omaha Classification System in a public health agency. *Nurs. Clin. North Am.*, 22(December, 1987):971–979.

Zielstorff, R., Jette, A., & Barnett, G. Issues in designing an automated record system for clinical care and research. *Adv. Nurs. Sci.*, 13(December, 1990):75–88.

GLOSSARY

GENERAL GLOSSARY

Acute Care. Health services provided for the purpose of addressing actual signs/symptoms of illness.

Advanced Beginner. The second stage in the Dreyfus model of skill acquisition in which the practitioner has enough background experience to recognize recurring meaningful aspects of a situation and can demonstrate marginally acceptable performance (Benner, 1984, p. 291).

Ambulatory Care. Non-emergency health services provided in a clinic or outpatient department.

Autonomous Nursing Functions. Actions that are implemented by nurses as a result of professional knowledge and intuition.

Case Mix. An aggregate of clients grouped by acuity of illness and amount of care required.

Client. An individual, family, group, or community that is the recipient of community health service.

Clinical Judgement. A diagnosis or management plan derived from analytic reasoning and/or intuitive knowledge.

Clinical Record. Legal documents completed by community health agency personnel that may include client identification and demographic data, assessment data, care planning data, reports of services provided, and evidence of client progress; may also include health history, laboratory data, screening reports, and other information pertinent to client care.

Collaborative Nursing Functions. Actions that are implemented by nurses as a result of professional relationships with members of other health, social, and technical groups.

Combined Agency. A community health agency that offers preventive services in homes and clinic settings and home health care to acutely and chronically ill individuals and is supported by public and private money.

Community Health Nursing. A synthesis of nursing and public health practice that is comprehensive and is intended to promote and preserve the health of populations.

Community Health Practitioner. A health professional who provides service in a community setting, such as a nurse, social worker, physical therapist, speech pathologist, occupational therapist, nutritionist, physician, or dentist.

Competent. The third stage in the Dreyfus model of skill acquisition typified by considerable conscious, de-liberate planning, and an increased level of efficiency (Benner, 1984, p. 292).

Data Assessment. Analysis of collected information in relation to environment, psychosocial status, physiologic status, and health-related behaviors.

Data Collection. Systematic gathering of client information in relation to a defined data base through observation and interviews with clients and other health team members.

Data Element. The smallest unit of meaningful information within a computer data bank.

Data Set. A group of data elements.

Defined Data Base. Designated subjective and objective information relative to each family member, the family member, the family as an interacting unit, and the sociocultural and physical environment.

Empirical Data. Actual client data gathered and recorded by practicing community health nurses.

Etiology. Causal factors.

Evaluation. A process designed to ascertain value or amount or to compare accomplishments with some standards.

Evaluation Criteria. Statements describing specific, measurable qualities of a standard.

Expert. The fifth stage in the Dreyfus model of skill acquisition in which the practitioner with an enormous amount of background experience has an intuitive grasp of each situation and accurately identifies the problem without consideration of a large number of alternatives (Benner, 1984, p. 32).

Formative Evaluation. The continuous, ongoing process of measuring client progress toward goals throughout the period of service.

Hardware. Computer equipment including processors, disk drives, tape drives, printers, and terminals.

Home Health Nursing. A subspecialty of community health nursing that focuses, to a large degree, on clients with one or more physiologic problems.

Inductive Reasoning. The process of developing generalizations from specific observations.

Long-term Care. Health care and supportive services for clients in need of help with performance of activities of daily living.

Management Information System. An integrated, systematic data methodology that uses client and general agency data for entry, manipulates or processes data, and produces various client and agency reports.

Module. A portion of a computer system that has freestanding characteristics.

Novice. The first stage in the Dreyfus model of skill acquisition where no background understanding of the situation exists, so that context-free rules and attributes are required for safe entry and performance in the situation (Benner, 1984, p. 296).

Nurse Practitioner. A registered nurse who has completed education such as a master's degree or certificate program and is prepared to provide care to a specific group of clients.

Nursing Diagnosis. A clinical judgement about individual, family, or community responses to actual and potential health problems/life processes which provides the basis for selection of nursing interventions to achieve outcomes for which the nurse is accountable (Carroll-Johnson, 1990, p. 50).

Nursing Process. A logical, dynamic, and problem-solving process by which the community health nurse implements systematic, individualized, and comprehensive care assisting the client to attain the highest possible level of functioning and wellness.

Objective Data. Information and responses to treatment based on observations and measurements by the health care professional.

Official Agency. A community health agency that provides preventive health services in homes and clinics and is supported by tax funds and administered by a governmental subdivision.

Ordinal Scale. A scale on which one instance of the attribute being measured can be judged to be greater than, less than, or the same as another instance of the attribute but which does not have equal intervals between its units of measurement or an absolute zero point.

Outcome Standards. Standards that focus on the results of care in terms of improved health, restored or improved physical and social functioning, and patient satisfaction.

Peer Review. The process by which nurses who provide similar services appraise the quality of nursing care in a given situation relative to established practice standards.

Planning. An analytic process that involves establishing priorities and selecting a course of action from among identified alternatives.

Primary Prevention. Measures designed to promote optimal health and to provide specific protection against illness, injuries, and disabilities for individuals and families.

Process Standards. Standards that focus on the clinical practice activities of health care professionals as well as documentation and other related activities.

Proficient. The fourth stage in the Dreyfus model of skill acquisition in which the practitioner perceives situations as wholes and performance is guided by maxims based upon a deep background understanding (Benner, 1984, p. 297).

Proprietary Agency. A community health agency that provides primarily home health services and is privately owned.

Public Health Nursing. A subspecialty of community health nursing that focuses, to a large degree, on clients who are physically well.

Quality Assurance. Activities to estimate and increase the level of excellence in the alteration of the health status of consumers, attained through review of providers' performance of diagnostic, therapeutic, prognostic, and other health care activities.

Relationship Development. The art of establishing open verbal and nonverbal communication between nurse and client by combining understanding, self-respect, motivation, professionalism, nursing skills, and a genuine concern for others.

Reliability. The degree of consistency with which an instrument measures the attribute it is designed to measure.

Secondary Prevention. Measures designed to reduce the deleterious effects of illness, chiefly by shortening the duration of illness through early identification of the problem and provision of effective health care.

Software. Programs, languages, and/or routines that control the operation of a computer.

Standards. Broad statements of acceptable levels of achievement.

Structure Standards. Standards that focus on resources used to provide care, such as physical facilities, equipment, qualified personnel, and the manner in which these resources are organized.

Subjective Data. Information obtained from the client or another person that reflects the client's viewpoint.

Summative Evaluation. The terminal process of measuring client progress toward goals completed at the end of service.

Taxonomy. The science of classification.

Tertiary Prevention. Measures aimed at reducing residual defects and disabilities following the course of an illness, chiefly by rehabilitating the client to the maximum use of remaining capacities.

Utilization Review. Evaluation directed toward assuring that services provided are needed and that the level of care is both appropriate and cost-effective.

Validity. The degree to which an instrument measures what it is designed to measure.

Voluntary Agency. A community health agency that provides primarily home health services, is privately funded, and is governed by a community-based board of directors.

OMAHA SYSTEM GLOSSARY
General Terms

Clinical Components. The three Schemes that comprise the Omaha System: Problem Classification Scheme, Intervention Scheme, and Problem Rating Scale for Outcomes.

Omaha System. A method of community health nursing practice, documentation, and data management based on a nursing process model and incorporating standardized schemes of nursing diagnoses, interventions, and ratings of client problems.

Problem Classification Scheme Terms

Client Problems. The 40 nursing diagnoses that represent matters of difficulty and concern that historically, presently, or potentially adversely affect any aspect of the client's well-being; accurate identification of client problems enables the professional to focus interventions; used synonymously with nursing diagnosis; the second level of the Problem Classification Scheme.

Deficit/Impairment/Actual. Client status characterized by one or more existing signs/symptoms that may preclude optimal health; a problem modifier that appears at the third level of the Problem Classification Scheme.

Domains. The four general areas that represent community health practice and provide organizational groupings for client problems; the first level of the Problem Classification Scheme.

Environmental Domain. The material resources, physical surroundings, and substances both internal and external to the client, home, neighborhood, and broader community; appears at the first level of the Problem Classification Scheme.

Family. A social unit or related group of individuals who live together and who experience a health-related problem; a problem modifier that appears at the third level of the Problem Classification Scheme.

Health Promotion. Client interest in increasing knowledge, behavior, and health expectations as well as developing resources that maintain or enhance well-being in the absence of risk factors, signs, or symptoms; a problem modifier that appears at the third level of the Problem Classification Scheme.

Health Related Behaviors Domain. Activities that maintain or promote wellness, promote recovery, or maximize rehabilitation potential; appears at the first level of the Problem Classification Scheme.

Individual. A person who lives alone or a single family member who experiences a health-related problem; a problem modifier that appears at the third level of the Problem Classification Scheme.

Modifiers. The two sets of terms used in conjunction with problems allowing the nurse to identify ownership of the problem and degree of severity in relation to client interest, risk factors, and signs/symptoms; appears at the third level of the Problem Classification Scheme.

Physiological Domain. Functional status of processes that maintain life; appears at the first level of the Problem Classification Scheme.

Potential. Client status characterized by the absence of signs/symptoms and the presence of certain health patterns, practices, behaviors, or risk factors that may preclude optimal health; a problem modifier that appears at the third level of the Problem Classification Scheme.

Problem Classification Scheme. A taxonomy of nursing diagnoses; one of the three clinical components of the Omaha System.

Psychosocial Domain. Patterns of behavior, communication, relationships, and development; appears at the first level of the Problem Classification Scheme.

Risk Factors. Environmental, psychosocial, or physiologic events or health-related behaviors that occur in the past, present, or future and increase the client's exposure or vulnerability to the development of an actual problem; the nurse's knowledge base of risk factors is used to identify problems having the modifier Potential.

Signs. The objective evidence of a client's problem observed by a community health nurse or other health care provider; used with the problem modifier Actual; appear at the fourth level of the Problem Classification Scheme.

Symptoms. The subjective evidence of a client's problem reported by the client or by significant others; used with the problem modifier Actual; appear at the fourth level of the Problem Classification Scheme.

Intervention Scheme Terms

Case Management. Nursing activities of coordination, advocacy, and referral that involve facilitating service delivery on behalf of the client, communicating with health and human service providers, promoting assertive client communication, and guiding the client toward use of appropriate community resources; appears at the first level of the Intervention Scheme.

Categories. The four broad areas that provide a structure for describing community health nursing actions or activities; the first level of the Intervention Scheme.

Client-specific Information. The detailed portion of a plan or intervention statement that is generated by the community health nurse or other health care professional; the third level of a plan or intervention statement.

Health Teaching, Guidance, and Counseling. Nursing activities that include giving information, anticipating client problems, encouraging client action and responsibility for self-care and coping, and assisting with decision-making and problem-solving; overlapping concepts that occur on a continuum with the variation due to the client's self-direction capabilities; appears at the first level of the Intervention Scheme.

Intervention. An action or activity implemented to address a specific client problem and to improve, maintain, or restore health or prevent illness; an intervention statement always includes a category and target; it usually includes client-specific information.

Plan. The action(s) or activity(ies) designed to establish a course of client care; this analytic process includes establishing priorities and selecting a course of action from identified alternatives. The plan statement always includes a category and a target(s); it usually includes client-specific information.

Surveillance. Nursing activities of detection, measurement, critical analysis, and monitoring to indicate client status in relation to a given condition or phenomenon; appears at the first level of the Intervention Scheme.

Targets. The 62 objects of nursing actions or activities that serve to further describe interventions; the second level of the Intervention Scheme.

Treatments and Procedures. Technical nursing activities directed toward preventing signs and symptoms, identifying risk factors and early signs and symptoms, and decreasing or alleviating signs and symptoms; appears at the first level of the Intervention Scheme.

Problem Rating Scale for Outcomes Terms

Admission Rating. Problem-specific numeric ratings for the concepts of Knowledge, Behavior, and Status completed at the time of admission to community health service.

Behavior. The observable responses, actions, or activities of the client fitting the occasion or purpose; a concept of the Problem Rating Scale for Outcomes.

Concepts. The three major areas that represent basic community health client issues of knowing, doing, and being; these areas provide a realistic and usable framework for measuring the effectiveness of care provided to a client in relation to a specific problem using the Problem Rating Scale for Outcomes.

Dismissal Rating. Problem-specific numeric ratings for the concepts of Knowledge, Behavior, and Status

completed at the time of client discharge from community health service.

Evaluation. Measurement of client progress by comparing Client Knowledge, Behavior, and Status ratings at admission, regular intervals, and dismissal.

Interim Rating. Problem-specific numeric ratings for the concepts of Knowledge, Behavior, and Status completed at periodic intervals during the course of community health service.

Knowledge. The ability of the client to remember and interpret information; a concept of the Problem Rating Scale for Outcomes.

Problem Rating Scale for Outcomes. A framework for measuring problem-specific knowledge, behavior, and status relative to the client; one of the three clinical components of the Omaha System.

Ratings. The five numeric levels representing continua that depict the most negative to the most positive state of a problem in relation to client Knowledge, Behavior, and Status ratings; a part of the Problem Rating Scale for Outcomes.

Status. The condition of the client in relation to objective and subjective defining characteristics; a concept of the Problem Rating Scale for Outcomes.

REFERENCES

Benner, P. (1984). *From Novice to Expert.* Menlo Park, CA, Addison-Wesley.

Carroll-Johnson, R. (1990, April-June). Editorial: Reflections on the 9th biennial conference. *Nurs. Diagnosis, 1:*49–50.

INDEX

Page numbers in *italics* refer to record forms and illustrations; numbers followed by t indicate tables.

The Visiting Nurse Association of Omaha wants to identify users and to gather current data about users' experiences with the Problem Classification Scheme (PCS), the Intervention Scheme (IS), and the Problem Rating Scale (PRS) for Outcomes. Please remove page or photocopy, complete blanks, and return. Your cooperation is appreciated.

Your Name _____ Title _____

Your Organization _____ Phone (____) _____

Address _____ Zip _____

National Accreditation: NLN _____ JCAHO _____ Other (specify) _____

1. How did you learn about the Omaha System? _____

_____

2. Do you use (1) PCS _____ (2) IS _____ (3) PRS for Outcomes _____

3. For service setting:
   a. Services offered: Home Health _____ Preventive Health _____ Clinics _____
      Inpatient _____ Ambulatory Care _____ Schools _____ Other (specify) _____
   b. Approximate number of staff users: RNs _____ PTs _____
      OTs _____ Speech Ps _____ Soc workers _____ Nutritionists _____
      Other (specify) _____

4. For educational setting:
   a. Nursing education programs offered: AD ___ Dip ___ Bacc ___ Grad ___ Cont Ed ___
   b. Approximate annual number of student users: AD _____ Dip _____
      Bacc _____ Grad _____ Cont Ed _____
      Other (specify) _____

5. From your implementation experiences, can you offer suggestions? Describe any adaptations you have made.

_____

_____

6. Is your agency/institution's client record (1) dictated/typed _____ (2) handwritten _____ (3) computerized _____
   (4) combination (describe) _____

7. If you do not currently use the Omaha System, do you plan to implement the (1) PCS _____
   (2) IS _____ (3) PRS for Outcomes _____

8. May we provide additional materials or information that would be of assistance to you?

_____